Women's Global Health and Human Rights

Edited by

Padmini Murthy, MD, MPH, MS, MPhil, CHES
Assistant Professor, Department of Health Policy and Management
Global Health Program Director
New York Medical School of Public Health, Valhalla, NY
Medical Women's International Association
Representative to the United Nations, New York, NY
American Public Health Association Committee Member on Women's Rights
American Public Health Association International Health Section Counselor
International Health Awareness Network, Program Director

Clyde Lanford Smith, MD, MPH, DTM&H, FACP
Assistant Professor of Clinical Medicine and Clinical Family and Social Medicine
Residency Programs in Primary Care and Social Internal Medicine
Montefiore Medical Center, Albert Einstein College of Medicine
Global Health Advisor, Albert Einstein College of Medicine
Founder, President's Council and Liberation Medicine Counsel
Doctors for Global Health
Global Steering Group, People's Health Movement

JONES AND BARTLETT PUBLISHERS
Sudbury, Massachusetts
BOSTON   TORONTO   LONDON   SINGAPORE

World Headquarters
Jones and Bartlett Publishers
40 Tall Pine Drive
Sudbury, MA 01776
978-443-5000
info@jbpub.com
www.jbpub.com

Jones and Bartlett Publishers Canada
6339 Ormindale Way
Mississauga, Ontario L5V 1J2
Canada

Jones and Bartlett Publishers International
Barb House, Barb Mews
London W6 7PA
United Kingdom

Jones and Bartlett's books and products are available through most bookstores and online booksellers. To contact Jones and Bartlett Publishers directly, call 800-832-0034, fax 978-443-8000, or visit our website www.jbpub.com.

Substantial discounts on bulk quantities of Jones and Bartlett's publications are available to corporations, professional associations, and other qualified organizations. For details and specific discount information, contact the special sales department at Jones and Bartlett via the above contact information or send an email to specialsales@jbpub.com.

This publication is designed to provide accurate and authoritative information in regard to the Subject Matter covered. It is sold with the understanding that the publisher is not engaged in rendering legal, accounting, or other professional service. If legal advice or other expert assistance is required, the service of a competent professional person should be sought.

Production Credits
Publisher: Michael Brown
Production Director: Amy Rose
Associate Editor: Katey Birtcher
Editorial Assistant: Catie Heverling
Senior Production Editor: Tracey Chapman
Production Assistant: Roya Millard
Marketing Manager: Sophie Fleck
Associate Marketing Manager: Jessica Cormier
Manufacturing and Inventory Control Supervisor: Amy Bacus
Composition: Atlis Graphics
Cover Design: Kate Ternullo
Cover Images: Clockwise from top left
    © Alex Staroseltsev/ShutterStock, Inc.,
    © Bnilesh/Dreamstime.com,
    © Delphine Mayeur/Dreamstime.com,
    © Mika Heittola/ShutterStock, Inc.,
    © Muellek/ShutterStock, Inc.
Printing and Binding: Courier Stoughton
Cover Printing: Courier Stoughton

Library of Congress Cataloging-in-Publication Data
Women's global health and human rights / [edited by] Padmini Murthy and Clyde Lanford Smith.
    p. ; cm.
Includes bibliographical references and index.
ISBN 978-0-7637-5631-4 (pbk.)
1. Women--Health and hygiene.   2. Women's rights.   3. World health.   I. Murthy, Padmini. II. Smith, Clyde Lanford.
[DNLM: 1. Women's Health.   2. Women's Rights.   3. World Health.   WA 309.1 W8726 2010]
RA778.W7516 2010
362.1082--dc22

2008050177

6048
Printed in the United States of America
13 12 11 10 09   10 9 8 7 6 5 4 3 2 1

DISCLAIMER
The views expressed by the contributors and the editors are theirs and not necessarily those expressed by institutions or organizations with which they are affiliated.

Dedication

This book is dedicated to the memory of two extraordinary people who have contributed to improving the lives of women by upholding their human rights: my beloved father, M. K. Kashinath and my mentor, Suman Mehta.

This book is also dedicated to my mother, Krishna Kashinath, who taught me to respect my fellow global citizens.

Padmini Murthy

My dedication is to my parents, Celia Renée Lanford Smith and Clyde Copeland Smith, the persons who first and always have oriented me toward health and human rights.

Clyde Lanford Smith

We also dedicate this to the memory of the disappeared, of the survivors, of all women who have suffered just by reason of their gender, and of all women who have fought for the integrity of their and every person's health and human rights.

Padmini Murthy
Clyde Lanford Smith

Acknowledgments

Grateful appreciation to our contributors, authors, and individuals who have helped us at every stage of the book production. We deeply appreciate the support and guidance of our dear friend, Dr. Cathey E. Falvo, who has helped us in more ways than one throughout this journey.

I would also like to express my heartfelt thanks to Dr. Satty Gill Keswani, Dr. Sorosh Roshan, Professor Annette Choolfaian, and Dr. Gopal Sankaran for their continued support and encouragement to me.

Last but not least I would like to express my gratitude to my family: my daughter Aishu, my husband S.M., and my sister Apu, for being there for me.

Padmini Murthy

I acknowledge Zenaida Izquierdo, Union Organizer of 1199/SEIU;. "Nina Silveria," midwife in Naranjeras, Morazan, El Salvador, who showed me the meaning of *alta-alegremia* (high blood-happiness) in promoting women's health and human rights; the volunteers and community partners of Doctors for Global Health; and the South Bronx patients who call me their doctor.

Clyde Lanford Smith

We would also like to acknowledge Patience Ameyaw, Diana Cunningham, Nina M. Luppino, and Shirley Novack for their assistance in the preparation of the manuscript.

We would like to acknowledge the superb guidance and support provided to us by Roya Millard, Sophie Fleck, Katey Birtcher, and Mike Brown of Jones and Bartlett, who helped us realize our dream.

Padmini Murthy
Clyde Lanford Smith

Table of Contents

Foreword

A Prayer for the Girl-Child

When I grow up
Please let me:
Be safe.
Learn to read and write.
Live with my parents
And my brothers and sisters.
Not be sold to work
As an indentured servant
Or a sex slave.
Have enough food
And clean water
To enable me to have
A healthy body and mind.
Keep my sexual organs
Intact and not mutilated.
Allowed to love and marry
The person of my choice.
Enabled to keep
The children that I bear,
And to bear as many as I choose.
When I grow up
May I discover
A world populated
By all who honor
Peace.
And one another.
When I grow up,
May we all be
As one.

Suzanne Stutman, PhD

Dr. Stutman is a Professor of English, American Studies, and Women's Studies at Penn State University and Abington College, as well as a poet and human rights activist.

Preface

Globalization has changed the fabric of society, while the health and human rights of women are remaining stagnant or growing worse in many parts of the world. Some of what the statistics document is so ugly as to seem incompatible with the word *civilization*. Women in this day and age are denied their fundamental right to enjoy a complete state of health as defined by the World Health Organization. Causes include structural violence as well as other disease entities, many of which are dealt with superficially in current public health texts, if they are mentioned at all.

This book is unique in that it addresses the similarities and differences in health and human rights challenges faced by women in different regions of the world. The diversity of backgrounds and geographic locations of the invited authors contributes to the book's richness of content. It is meant to be a text that inspires and educates its readers toward positive action.

The book has been divided into seven sections. The first section gives an introduction to women's global health in a human rights context. The second section addresses the effects of gender-based violence, disasters including war, environmental factors, health policies, and transnational violence on women and the girl-child. The third section discusses the effect economics has on women's human rights. Section four explores the health problems and challenges specific to women within a human rights framework and the global burden they cause. Section five discusses the effects of cultural practices on the health and well-being of women and the girl-child. The sixth section re-views progress made and challenges faced by women and practitioners of public health in reducing gender disparities and human rights violations. The seventh section is the conclusion, which summarizes the long and difficult path women have to travel before they can enjoy a complete state of health within a human rights context.

Women's Global Health and Human Rights was conceived as a tool for all who find the health and human rights of women imperative to their professional and personal lives (including those who are literally not yet able to read it due to issues of literacy and access). We have written toward a readership of global practitioners and students of public health and social justice, including those in the field as well as persons influencing policy nearer the decision makers. However, we hope, and expect, our readers will surprise us with their diversity of action and potential, meaning with the breadth of what and how they are engaging diverse actors toward our one goal of making women's health and human rights a reality recognized and cherished by everyone everywhere.

Because understanding women's global health and human rights is essential to public health best practice, our principal challenge has been to connect author practice experts with others engaged in or learning toward becoming public health practitioners and promoters of social justice.

Our end goal is expressed most eloquently by the poetry of our Foreword: "when I grow up,/ may we all be/ as one."

Padmini Murthy
Clyde Lanford Smith

Contributor List

Kwasi Odoi-Agarko, MD, PhD
Executive Director
Rural Help Integrated
Ghana

Natasha Anandaraja, MD
Assistant Professor
Department of Medical Education
Mt. Sinai School of Medicine
New York, NY

Amy Ansehl, RN, MSN, FNPC
Executive Director
Partnership for a Healthy Population
Assistant Professor and Practicum Coordinator
New York Medical College
School of Public Health
Valhalla, NY

Mary-Wynne Ashford, MD, PhD
Former Co-President
International Physicians for the Prevention of
  Nuclear War
Victoria, BC, Canada

Hala Azzam, PhD, MPH
Assistant Professor & Program Director
UMB Global Health Resource Center
University of Maryland Baltimore (UMB)
Dept of Epidemiology & Preventative Medicine
International Health Division
Baltimore, MD

Joshua Bardfield, MPH
New York, NY

Heidi L. Behforouz, MD
Medical and Executive Director
PACT Project
Assistant Professor
Harvard Medical School
Associate Physician
Brigham and Women's Hospital
Boston, MA

Didi Bertrand Farmer, MA
Director
Community Health Programs, Partners In Health
Inshuti Mu Buzima, Rwanda

Eliot A. Brinton, MD, FAHA
Cardiovascular Genetics
University of Utah School of Medicine
Salt Lake City, UT

Anwarul K. Chowdhury
Ambassador
Former Under-Secretary-General and High
  Representative
United Nations
New York, NY

Jennifer Chung
Project Coordinator/Executive Assistant to
  Director
PACT Project
Boston, MA

Liliana De Lima, MHA
Executive Director
International Association for Hospice and
  Palliative Care
President
Latin American Association for Palliative Care
Houston, TX

Reilly Anne Dempsey, JD, MPH
Researcher and consultant
Sexual and reproductive health and rights
New York, NY

Michelle R. Detwiler, MA
Consultant
Houston, TX

Gayatri Devi, MD
Director
The New York Memory and Healthy Aging
    Services
Attending Physician
Departments of Medicine (Neurology) and
    Psychiatry
Lenox Hill Hospital
Clinical Associate Professor
Departments of Neurology and Psychiatry
New York University School of Medicine
New York, NY

Cathey Eisner Falvo, MD, MPH
Retired Professor of Public Health and Pediatrics
New York Medical College
Valhalla, NY
President
Physicians for Social Responsibility NYC Chapter
New York, NY

Paul E. Farmer, MD, PhD
Presley Professor
Department of Global Health and Social
    Medicine
Harvard Medical School
Associate Chief
Division of Social Medicine and Health
    Inequalities
Brigham and Women's Hospital
Co-founder
Partners In Health
Cambridge, MA

Anne Foster-Rosales, MD, MPH, FACOG
Chief Medical Officer
Planned Parenthood Golden Gate
San Francisco, CA
Assistant Clinical Professor
Department of Obstetrics, Gynecology, and
    Reproductive Sciences
University of California, San Francisco
San Francisco, CA

Jean Fourcroy, MD, MPH, PhD
Staff Urologist
Walter Reed Army Medical Center and the
    Uniformed Services University of Health
    Science
FDA regulatory consultant, urology and
    endocrinology
Past President
American Medical Women's Association
Washington, DC

**Tom Fryers, MB, ChB, DRCOG, DPH, MD,
    PhD, FFPH**
Professor of Public Mental Health
University of Leicester, UK

Anke Hemmerling, MD, MPH
School of Medicine
Department of Obstetrics, Gynecology and
    Reproductive Sciences
University of California at San Francisco
San Francisco, CA

Nils Henning, MD, PhD
Assistant Professor
Community and Preventive Medicine
Pediatric Infectious Diseases at the Mount Sinai
    School of Medicine
New York, NY

Guillermo Hidalgo, MD
Assistant Professor
Pediatrics
University of Illinois
Chicago, IL

Paul N. Hopkins, MD, MSPH
Professor
Internal Medicine, Cardiovascular Genetics
School of Medicine
University of Utah
Salt Lake City, UT

Linda M. Kaljee, PhD
Associate Professor
Pediatric Prevention Research Center
School of Medicine
Wayne State University
Detroit, MI

Marly B. Katz, MPH
Westchester, NY

**Miriam Labbok, MD, MPH, FACPM,
    IBCLC, FABM**
Professor
Practice of Public Health
Director
Center for Infant and Young Child Feeding and
    Care
Department of Maternal and Child Health
School of Public Health
The University of North Carolina at Chapel Hill
Chapel Hill, NC

David Legge, MD
Associate Professor and Director
La Trobe China Health Program
School of Public Health
La Trobe University
Bundoora, Victoria, Australia

Robin C. Leonard, PhD
Associate Professor
Health
College of Health Sciences
West Chester University
West Chester, PA

Eric Li, BA
New York Medical School of Public Health
Valhalla, NY

Purnima Mane, PhD
Deputy Executive Director (Programme)
United Nations Population Fund (UNFPA)
New York, NY

Benjamin Mason Meier, JD, LLM, MPhil
Public Health Law Project Manager
Center for Health Policy
IGERT—International Development and
    Globalization Fellow
Department of Sociomedical Sciences
Columbia University
New York, NY

Caroline Min, MPH
Baltimore, MD

Joia S. Mukherjee, MD, MPH
Medical Director
Partners In Health
Director
Institute for Health and Social Justice
Assistant Professor
Harvard Medical School
Division of Global Health Equity
Brigham and Women's Hospital
Boston, MA

Jaime Mungia, MPH
Jhpiego, an affiliate of Johns Hopkins University
Baltimore, MD

Erica Nakaji, BA
Department of Maternal and Child Health
School of Public Health
The University of North Carolina at Chapel Hill
Chapel Hill, NC

Aishwarya Narasimhadevara
Boston University
Boston, MA

Eleanor Nwadinobi, MBBS
President
Widows Development Organisation
Sub-Saharan Africa Regional Chair
United Nations NGO/DPI
Executive Director
The Tabitha Infirmary Foundation
Nigeria

Ellen C. O'Connell, MPA, MA
Vice President
Administration and Board Relations
International Rescue Committee
New York, NY

Martin Patwell, EdD
Director
Office of Services for Students with Disabilities
West Chester University
West Chester, PA

Roshni D. Persaud, JD, MPH
Staff Attorney
New York City Health and Hospitals
    Corporation's Office of Legal Affairs
New York, NY
Adjunct Assistant Professor
Hofstra University
Hempstead, NY

Michael J. Reilly, MPH, NREMT-PMICP
Assistant Director
Center for Disaster Medicine
Assistant Professor
Public Health Practice
School of Public Health
New York Medical College
Valhalla, NY

Allan Rosenfield, MD, FACOG
Dean Emeritus
Professor, Population and Family Health
DeLamar Professor Emeritus of Public Health
    Practice
Mailman School of Public Health
Professor of Obstetrics and Gynecology
College of Physicians and Surgeons
Columbia University
New York, NY

Fred T. Sai, MB, BS, FRCP, MPH
Advisor to the President of Ghana on
    Reproductive Health
HIV/AIDS Professor, Community Health
Director of Medical Services in Ghana
Nutrition Advisor to the Africa region of FAO
Former President of the International Planned
    Parenthood Federation (IPPF)
Population Advisor to the World Bank
Ghana

Monica Sanchez
Insurer
Campaign Education
Web Director
Campaign for America's Future
Vice President of the Board of Directors
Doctors for Global Health
Previously Deputy Director, Medicare Rights
    Center
New York, NY

Harshadkumar Sanghvi, MD
Vice President & Medical Director
Jhpiego, an affiliate of Johns Hopkins University
Baltimore, MD

Gopal Sankaran, MD, DrPH
Professor
Department of Health
College of Health Sciences
West Chester University
West Chester, PA

Claudio Schuftan, MD
Consultant in public health and nutrition
Ho Chi Minh City, Vietnam
Adjunct Associate Professor
Department of International Health
Tulane School of Public Health
New Orleans, LA

Peter Selwyn, MD, MPH
Professor and Chairman
Department of Family and Social Medicine
Montefiore Medical Center
Albert Einstein College of Medicine
New York, NY

Amartya K. Sen, PhD
Master of Trinity College, Cambridge, UK
Former Professor of Economics at Oxford, UK
Lamont University Professor Emeritus
Harvard University
Cambridge, MA

Donald A. Smith, MD, MPH
Associate Professor
Medicine and Community Medicine
Mount Sinai School of Medicine
New York, NY

Anitha Srinivasan, MD, MPH, FACS
Assistant Professor
New York Medical College
Attending Surgeon
Metropolitan Hospital
New York, NY

Jennifer Staple, BS
Founder, President & CEO
Unite For Sight
Newton, CT

Suzanne Stutman, PhD
Professor
English, American Studies, and Women's Studies
Penn State University & Abington College
Abington, PA

Kimberley Templeton, MD
Associate Professor Orthopedic Surgery
University of Kansas Medical Center
Kansas City, KS

Mitsuru Toda, BA
Cambridge, MA

Ushma D. Upadhyay, PhD, MPH
Consultant
San Francisco, CA

Deborah Viola, PhD
Assistant Professor and Director
Masters in Public Health Program
Department of Health Policy and Management
School of Public Health
New York Medical College
Valhalla, NY

Hema Viswanathan, MA, PGDBA
ICG Consultants
Mumbai, India

Dima Yeshou, MD
Department of Endocrinology
Mt. Sinai School of Medicine
New York, NY

Marie Yezzo, MPH
Westchester Medical Center
Westchester, NY

About the Editors

Padmini (Mini) Murthy is a physician and an activist who did her residency in obstetrics and gynecology. She has practiced medicine in various countries. She has a masters in public health and a masters in management from New York University (NYU). She is also a certified health education specialist. Murthy has been the recipient of several awards and has presented at numerous national and international conferences. She has been the recipient of the Dean's Award for Excellence at NYU School of Education and was named Robert F. Wagner Public Service Scholar at NYU. She is a member of the Phi Theta Lambda Honor Society and was awarded Best Physician Award by the Ministry of Health in Saudi Arabia. Murthy has served as a consultant to the United Nations and serves on the executive board of several national and international health nongovernmental organizations. Currently she is Assistant Professor, Department of Health Policy and Management and Global Health Program Director at New York Medical College School of Public Health. Murthy is the NGO representative of the Medical Women International Association to the United Nations. As program Director of International Health Awareness Network (an international NGO) she has been actively working with other board members to improve the lives of women and children in developing countries. She serves as American Public Health Association Committee Member on Women's Rights and Section Councilor in the International Health Section. Her research interests include women's health with an emphasis on violence against women and HIV/AIDS. Murthy has been a champion of women's rights issues with a focus on gender inequalities in healthcare delivery and policies. Murthy is married to a physician and is the mother of a teenage daughter who is a college sophomore.

Clyde Lanford (Lanny) Smith is a writer and a physician, having majored in English literature and trained in primary care internal medicine, tropical medicine, and preventive medicine. He earned a masters in public health from Harvard School of Public Health and a diploma in tropical medicine and hygiene from the London School of Hygiene and Tropical Medicine. From 1992 to 1998 he lived in El Salvador as Country Director of Médecins du Monde (Physicians of the World) France. Smith is a Fellow of the American College of Physicians and member of the Alpha Omega Alpha Medical Honor Society. He has been the recipient of Davidson College's John Kuykendall Community Service Award for leadership in service to humankind and of the Mid-Career Award in International Health of the American Public Health Association. He serves on the board of the Global Health Education Consortium (GHEC) and on the global Steering Committee of the People's Health Movement (PHM). Founder of Doctors for Global Health (DGH, www.dghonline.org) and its first president from 1995–2000, he continues to serve on its board with the President's Council and as Liberation Medicine Counsel. He is cofounder of the *Journal of Social Medicine* (www.socialmedicine.info) and serves on its editorial board. He is on the editorial board of the journal *Revista De Educação Popular* of the Universidade Federal de Uberlândia, Minas Gerais, Brasil. Currently, he is an Assistant Professor of Clinical Medicine and Clinical Family & Social Medicine in the Residency Programs in Primary Care and Social Internal Medicine, Montefiore Medical Center, Albert Einstein College of Medicine (AECOM) and serves as Global Health Advisor at AECOM. Within Montefiore, he is Director of the Opportunities Pro-Immigrant Elderly and Newcomer and International Travel (OPEN IT) Program, Assistant Director of the Bronx Human Rights Clinic for Survivors of Torture, and cares for patients regularly as a primary care physician in the South Bronx Comprehensive Health Care Center. His research interests include social medicine, liberation medicine, community-oriented primary care, tropical medicine, and health education. Smith has lived in the Bronx since 2000 and works locally and globally to promote liberation medicine, "the conscious, conscientious use of health to promote social justice and human dignity." His upcoming book *Una Sola Vida: Lecciones hasta la Salud y la Justicia Social (One Life Only: Lessons Toward Health and Social Justice)* will be available in July 2009 from Ediciones Corpus Lirio, Rosario, Argentina.

Introduction

This section explores the various challenges women and girls in developing countries face that effect their health and well-being. It is the goal of this section to make the readers aware of the irrevocable link between women's global health and human rights.

Women's empowerment is intertwined with respect for human rights.

—*Mahnaz Afkhami*

Founder and President, Women's Learning Partnership for Rights, Development, and Peace (WLP)

A Portrait of Women's Health in Developing Countries

CHAPTER 1

Global Women's Health and Human Rights

Women in developing countries face a number of challenges to their health and well-being. Some 200 million women in developing countries, or about one in seven women of reproductive age, have an unmet need for effective contraceptives.[1] Over half a million women die each year from complications during pregnancy and childbirth, the vast majority of them in Africa and Asia.[2] This includes nearly 70,000 deaths from unsafe abortion.

More women than ever before are being affected by AIDS. Globally, nearly 16 million women are living with HIV and constitute almost half (48%) of all HIV-positive adults.[3] In sub-Saharan Africa, the impact of HIV on women is especially severe—an estimated 61% of adults living with HIV in sub-Saharan Africa are women. In areas of Asia, Eastern Europe, and Latin America, the number of women infected with HIV is increasing rapidly. With regard to curable sexually transmitted infections (STIs), there are approximately 340 million new cases each year, and the burden of STIs for women is more than five times that of men.[4]

Violence against women and girls is pervasive and is experienced in a wide range of settings, including the home, community, and situations of armed conflict. At least one in three women will be the victim of abuse—physical, sexual, or psychological—at some point in her life. Intimate partner violence is the most common form of violence reported by women, with the lifetime prevalence of physical or sexual partner violence ranging from 15% to 71% across locations. In certain settings, as many as 30% of women report that their first sexual experience was forced, and the younger they were at initiation, the greater the likelihood that it was forced.[5] Women and girls are often subjected to sexual harassment in the workplace and at school. Today, estimates indicate that over a hundred million girls and women live with the scars of female genital mutilation and cutting, mostly in Africa, but also in parts of Asia, the Middle East, and in immigrant communities in Europe, North America, and Australia.[6] In conflict settings, violence against women and girls, particularly sexual violence including rape, is a frequently used weapon of war. The consequences of violence on women's lives are far reaching and

Allan Rosenfield, MD;
Caroline Min, MPH;
Joshua Bardfield, MPH

Allan Rosenfield, MD, is the Dean Emeritus, Mailman School of Public Health, a Professor of Population and Family Health and DeLamar Professor Emeritus of Public Health Practice at the Mailman School of Public Health, as well as a Professor of Obstetrics and Gynecology at the College of Physicians and Surgeons, Columbia University, New York. He is a recipient of the American Public Health Association's Martha May Elliot and Carl Schultz Awards, the New York Academy of Medicine Stephen Smith Award, Planned Parenthood Federation of America Margaret Sanger Award, Doctors of the World Health and Human Rights Leadership Award, American Legacy Foundation Leadership Award for Extraordinary Leadership in Public Health, the International Women's Health Coalition and the United Nations Population Award.

Caroline Min, MPH, of Columbia University.

Joshua Bardfield MPH, of Columbia University.

include the psychological impact of violence, loss of personal freedom, diminished capacity to participate in public life, and a dramatically increased risk of acquiring HIV and other STIs.[7]

Adolescent girls and young women are especially at risk of dying during pregnancy and acquiring HIV or STIs. In many parts of the world, girls are married at a young age, often to older men, and begin childbearing early. This is most common in sub-Saharan Africa and South Asia where more than 30% of girls aged 15 to 19 are married.[8] Girls aged 15 to 19 are twice as likely to die in childbirth as those in their twenties.[9] In sub-Saharan Africa, young women aged 15–24 are between two and six times more likely be HIV-positive than young men.[4]

Fundamentally, these health problems are a reflection of the inequalities of power that exist between women and men in many societies around the world. Women are often marginalized and denied equal opportunities compared to men. They typically do not enjoy the same access to education and economic resources such as income and employment. They may confront legal and customary restrictions on land and property ownership. They are also limited in their ability to participate in government and civil society and are unable to influence national and local decisions that affect their own lives. Within their own households, women often have little power to make decisions with regard to marriage, childbearing, or even their own health care. In short, women are often left with few ways to reduce their vulnerability and protect their own health.

Sexual and reproductive health conditions account for a significant portion of women's disease burden, but women also confront other health challenges, many of which are outlined in this book, including infectious and chronic diseases and mental health conditions. Taken together, statistics on women's health reveal hardship experienced on an immense scale.

Putting Women's Health and Human Rights on the Global Development Agenda

Ensuring women's health and human rights are important priorities for the global health and develop-ment communities, but it has taken decades of work on the part of advocates to make these issues a foremost concern. In the early stages of global public health assistance, mothers and children were identified as vulnerable groups. Indeed, the Universal Declaration of Human Rights, adopted by the United Nations (UN) in 1948, states that "Everyone has the right to a standard of living adequate for the health and well-being of himself and of his family," and "Motherhood and childhood are entitled to special care and assistance."[10] One of the functions of the World Health Organization (WHO), established in 1948, is "to promote maternal and child health and welfare."[11] Maternal and child health, or MCH, became the dominant approach to service delivery in many developing countries.

In reality, conventional MCH programs did little to improve the health of mothers. In the early 1980s, the United Nations Children's Fund (UNICEF), under the leadership of James Grant, launched the most effective worldwide campaign for child survival calling for mass coverage of relatively cheap and easy-to-deliver interventions, such as immunization and oral rehydration therapy. The child survival revolution significantly decreased child mortality rates, although progress began to stall in the mid-1990s prompting renewed calls for action. Unfortunately, as in many areas of maternal and child health, UNICEF's program focused almost entirely on child health, and women's issues were not a key component.

In contrast, the poor state of maternal health in developing countries has gone virtually unnoticed. In part, the lack of data on maternal deaths for a time obscured the scale of the problem. There was also a perception among public health professionals that providing adequate maternity care to women would require high technology at large hospitals, an impossibility in resource-poor settings. Underlying these hesitations was the fact that women simply were not valued as productive members of their communities and as individuals entitled to basic human rights. As Halfdan Mahler, former director-general of WHO, once put it, maternal mortality was "neglected because those who suffer from it are neglected people, with the least power and influence over how national resources shall be spent; they are poor, the rural peasants, and, above all, women."[12]

In 1985, an important article in the *Lancet* voiced the question, "Where is the *M* in *MCH*?"[13]

in order to call attention to the severe neglect of women's health and mortality. The WHO also announced its estimate that half a million women were dying each year from pregnancy-related complications, almost entirely in poor countries, drawing the attention of women's health advocates around the world. Two years later, in part as a result of the *Lancet* article, the World Bank, WHO, and the United Nations Population Fund (UNFPA) convened the Safe Motherhood Conference in Nairobi, Kenya, an event that launched a global campaign to reduce maternal mortality in developing countries. Although the Safe Motherhood Initiative initially pursued strategies that were ineffective at reducing maternal mortality, it has provided much needed advocacy on maternal health, and there is currently greater consensus about what strategies are appropriate.[14]

Maternal health was long a neglected field, but women in poor countries were not left entirely without health services. In the 1950s and 1960s, censuses in developing countries revealed high rates of population growth. Alarm over the possible economic consequences of rapid population growth led many countries to establish national family planning programs, with the support of a number of donor agencies. These programs have played a critical role in the remarkable global decline in fertility that has occurred in the past half century. However, the demographic focus of family planning programs drew some criticism from a number of women's advocate groups, and some countries set inappropriate targets for contraceptive "acceptors" that created potentially coercive situations. Nonetheless, the contraceptive prevalence rate steadily rose worldwide from less than 10% in the 1960s to over 50% in the 1990s, and many women have benefited from the increased availability of contraceptives.

The International Conference on Population and Development (ICPD) held in Cairo in 1994 marked a significant paradigm shift in women's health—a conceptual shift from population to reproductive health. The ICPD was the culmination of efforts on the part of women's advocates to fundamentally alter the rationale of family planning programs from population control to women's health and human rights. Reproductive health was defined broadly to include family planning, prevention of HIV/STIs, maternal health, and sexual health. Also, for the first time, gender equality and women's rights and empowerment were recognized as essential development goals, a theme that was later reiterated at the Fourth World Conference in Beijing in 1995. Unfortunately, donor agencies and developing countries have failed to meet the financial targets they committed to in support of the ICPD Programme of Action.

In 2000, at the United Nations Millennium Summit, 189 nations agreed to a set of eight Millennium Development Goals (MDGs) to be achieved by 2015 that address critical development challenges. Among them are goals to improve maternal health, promote gender equality and empower women, but a goal to ensure reproductive health is noticeably absent from the list. (Several years later, the UN did agree that reproductive health issues should be part of the MDGs). Fortunately, the global health community has acknowledged that greater investments in sexual and reproductive health, as articulated in the ICPD Programme of Action, are essential to achieving the MDGs. While progress varies by region and country, the MDGs hold much promise and have generated an unprecedented level of support from governments and multilateral agencies.

Looking Ahead

Women throughout the world, particularly in Asia and Africa, continue to face enormous obstacles in access to reproductive health services, including contraception, emergency obstetric care, and safe abortion services. The ICPD Programme of Action and Millennium Development Goals are a critical step toward the promise of global improvements in maternal health, though much work remains in order to decrease the worldwide burden of maternal mortality, including a fundamental recognition of the value of maternal health both within the context of MCH and in the broader public health arena. Issues of reproductive health and choice must take center stage within the framework of global health goals as defined in international development programs such as the MDGs, particularly if those objectives are to be achieved.

As demonstrated by over 30 years of research and evidence-based practice, family planning services in poor countries are increasingly delivered by persons other than doctors and nurses, trained in a variety of essential procedures, including prescription and insertion of birth control methods. As evidenced in the 1970s in Thailand, where the training of auxiliary midwives to prescribe oral contraceptives produced a dramatic increase in the number of women using that birth control method, a focus on outreach is an essential factor in successful national policies dedicated to the reduction of unplanned pregnancies and greater reproductive freedom.[15] In terms of maternal health, access to emergency obstetric care and the training of nonphysicians in rural areas is essential, particularly given the absence of obstetricians and very few physicians working in those regions. In Mozambique, for example, the training of nonphysicians to perform emergency obstetrical surgery, including cesarean deliveries, is a major national accomplishment, allowing for many emergency obstetrical procedures, once unimaginable in rural settings, to be successfully conducted in local hospitals.[16]

Conclusion

Today, proven and cost-effective interventions exist to prevent and battle complications from pregnancy and childbirth and save women's lives. The challenge is to guarantee that every woman that needs care gets it. This means international commitment on the part of governments, nongovernmental organizations (NGOs), and civil society institutions—from the community level and beyond—toward capacity building and the development of innovative strategies that address systematic shortages of medical supplies, services, and personnel so common throughout the developing world, particularly in rural areas. Financial targets must be realized, and donor agencies must be committed to undertaking these ambitious tasks.

The HIV/AIDS epidemic continues to represent a serious and rapidly growing crisis, affecting nearly 18 million women worldwide. The global health community must continue to invest in prevention education and treatment interventions (without abstinence-only initiatives and with heavy focus on condom use) in order to stem this vast global dilemma. Prevention measures should include not only education, outreach, and advocacy, but also coordinated policy efforts to guarantee women's rights as equal members of society. These fundamental rights must include access to education, employment, and property ownership. Policies supporting women's empowerment serve to alleviate inequitable gender roles based on antiquated and discriminatory traditions, many of which frequently lead to physical and psychological violence and repression.

Women's rights are also fundamental in the struggle to end the global affliction of violence against women, a universal crisis affecting one in three women and girls throughout the world, and 20% of women in the United States. A commitment to policy reform is needed to protect the rights of women, ensuring equal treatment in society and open access to life-saving reproductive health services.

Numerous international public health challenges persist in the global struggle toward equitable health and rights for women. These are concerns that must be faced unconditionally in order to achieve genuine progress in the fight to save lives. Recognizing that women are vital and equal members of society will not only establish a healthier global norm, but may finally lead to a long-overdue reduction in worldwide maternal morbidity and mortality, decreased rates of HIV/AIDS transmission, and an end to violence against women on a truly global scale.

REFERENCES

1. Abou Zahr C, Wardlaw T. Maternal mortality in 2000: estimates developed by WHO, UNICEF and UNFPA. 2004. http://www.reliefweb.int/library/documents/2003/who-saf-22oct.pdf. Accessed July 29, 2008.

2. Singh S, Darroch JE, Vlassoff M, Nadeau J. Adding it up: the benefits of investing in sexual and reproductive health care. 2003. http://www.guttmacher.org/pubs/addingitup.pdf. Accessed July 29, 2008.

3. UNAIDS. 2007 Report on the Global AIDS Epidemic. http://www.unaids.org/en /KnowledgeCentre/HIVData/EpiUpdate/EpiUpdArchive/2007/default.asp. Accessed July 29, 2008.

4. UNAIDS. 2006 Report on the Global AIDS Epidemic. 2006. http://www.unaids.org/en /KnowledgeCentre/HIVData/GlobalReport/2006/. Accessed July 29, 2008.

5. Garcia-Moreno C, Jansen H, Ellsberg M, Heise L, Watts C. WHO multi-country study on women's health and violence and domestic violence against women: initial results on prevalence, health outcomes and women's responses. 2005. http://www.who.int/gender /violence/who_multicountry_study/summary_report/summary_report_English2.pdf. Accessed July 29, 2008.

6. UNICEF. 2008. http://www.unicef.org/protection/index_genitalmutilation.html. Accessed July 29, 2008.

7. In-depth study on all forms of violence against women. Report of the Secretary-General. 2006. http://www.un.org/womenwatch/daw/vaw/SGstudyvaw.htm. Accessed July 29, 2008.

8. Mathur S, Greene M, Malhotra A. 2003. Too young to wed: the lives, rights, and health of young married girls. http://www.icrw.org/docs/tooyoungtowed_1003.pdf. Accessed July 29, 2008.

9. United Nations Population Fund. 2008. http://www.unfpa.org/adolescents/facts.htm. Accessed July 29, 2008.

10. Universal Declaration of Human Rights, Article 25. 1948. http://www.un.org/Overview /rights.html. Accessed July 29, 2008.

11. Constitution of the World Health Organization, Article 2(l). 1948. http://www.opbw .org/int_inst/health_docs/WHO-CONSTITUTION.pdf. Accessed July 29, 2008.

12. Mahler H. The safe motherhood initiative: a call to action. *Lancet.* 1987;329(8534):668-670.

13. Rosenfield A, Maine D. Maternal mortality–a neglected tragedy. Where is the M in MCH? *Lancet.* 1985;2(8446):83-85.

14. Starrs AM. Safe motherhood initiative: 20 years and counting. *Lancet.* 2006;368(9542): 1130-1132.

15. Rosenfield A, Limcharoen C. Auxiliary midwife prescription of oral contraceptives. *Am J Obstet Gynecol.* 1972;114(7):942-949.

16. Rosenfield A, Min C, Freedman L. Making motherhood safe in developing countries. *N Engl J Med.* 2007;356:1395-1397.

Impact of Gender-Based Violence, Conflict, Discrimination, Terrorism, Environmental Factors, and Transnational Trafficking on Women and Girls

Since the beginning of creation women have been the fabric of human existence. Yet, unfortunately, they have been subjected to discrimination, endured different forms of abuse, and their human rights have been violated, often on a daily basis. Unhappily, prevailing cultural practices and existing or lack of specific governmental policies addressing the needs of women and girls translate into an increased incidence of women's morbidity and mortality worldwide.

This section discusses the profound impact gender-based violence, conflict, discrimination, terrorism, and trafficking have on the lives of women and girls. Women and girls need to be cherished and their human rights recognized—not violated.

Health is a state of complete physical, mental, and social well-being and not merely the absence of disease or infirmity.

—Preamble to the Constitution of the World Health Organization

CHAPTER 2

Violence Against Women and Girls: A Silent Global Pandemic

Historically, women have served as nurturers and caregivers in society. Yet they have been subjected to different forms of abuse, and violence against women and girls is a global pandemic that affects women in all walks of life and in all societies. Women have been abused, tortured, and have their human rights violated daily. Globally women's health issues and human rights have been neglected by various stakeholders, and this has translated into an increased incidence of women's mortality and morbidity. These acts of violence against women and girls are often invisible as they can occur behind closed doors and are often culturally acceptable in many societies.

The direct and indirect impact of violence and gender discrimination against women and girls often cannot be measured; however, the resulting economic burden on the society is enormous. According to studies, between 10% and 69% of women report having been assaulted by an intimate male partner at some time in their lives.[1] A comparison of the prevalence of violence among different countries is alarming. A study conducted by Buvinic, Morrison, and Shifter found that in Latin America the proportion of women who were assaulted by their partners is between 10% and 35%, while in sub-Saharan Africa, it is between 13% and 45%.[1] Furthermore, acts of violence against women are often underreported since many women are afraid, ashamed, or often hold themselves accountable for these acts.

Gender-based violence (GBV) is predominantly a crime against women and represents a violation of women's human rights. The cyclic nature of GBV can be described as "cradle to grave."

The UN Declaration on the Elimination of Violence Against Women, Article 1, defines violence against women as any act of gender-based violence that results in, or is likely to result in, physical, sexual, or psychological harm or suffering to women, including threats of such acts, coercion, or arbitrary deprivation of liberty, whether occurring in public or private life.[2]

Societal acceptance of male superiority, domination, and control of women, and reinforcement of such by the family, schools, policy makers, and

Padmini Murthy MD, MPH, MS, CHES;
Ushma Upadhyay PhD, MPH
Eleanor Nwadinobi, MBBS

Padmini Murthy MD, MPH, MS, CHES, is an Assistant Professor in the Department of Health Policy and Management as well as the Director of the Global Health Program, at New York Medical School of Public Health in Valhalla NY. She is the Medical Women's International Association NGO Representative to the United Nations, New York, Robert F Wagner Public Service Scholar New York University.

Ushma Upadhya PhD, MPH, is a Reproductive Health Consultant in San Francisco, CA.

Eleonar Nwadinobi MBBS, is the Sub-Saharan Africa Regional Chair- United Nations NGO/DPI Nigeria.

religious institutions contribute to the prevalence of gender-based violence worldwide.

Forms of Gender-Based Violence (GBV)

Violence can be classified into four categories:

- Physical violence
- Sexual violence
- Psychological and emotional violence (including coercive tactics)
- Threats of physical or sexual violence

Examples of gender-based violence throughout the life of a woman include:[2, 3]

- Prebirth—Sex-selective abortion.
- Infancy—Female infanticide, physical abuse, neglect, poor nutrition, and lack of immunization and medical care.
- Girlhood—Child marriage, female genital mutilation (FGM), trafficking, child prostitution, sexual abuse, poor nutrition, lack of immunizations and medical care, and minimal or lack of educational opportunities.
- Adolescence—Forced marriages, date rape, FGM, limited or lack of social interaction, acid throwing, dowry deaths, sexual harassment at school and workplace, mass rape during war and civil unrest, lack of safe motherhood facilities, forced prostitution, and trafficking. Other types of violence include economic and social discrimination.
- Young and middle-aged women—Intimate partner abuse, marital rape, dowry abuse, psychological and sexual abuse of women at the workplace, rape, widow abuse, and lack of access to health care including access to safe motherhood facilities.
- Elderly women—Physical and mental abuse of elderly woman and widows including rape and neglect.

Factors that make women more vulnerable to gender discrimination and violence include the following:

- Status (for example, single women, including unmarried women and widows).
- Women with disabilities.
- Physical weakness—Women tend to be physically weaker than men and, as such, are often preyed upon or forced to undergo horrific procedures such as genital mutilation, forced marriage, rape, forced abortion, and sexual enslavement.
- Sociocultural factors such as low economic status due to unemployment or low-paying jobs, as well as lack of basic rights that prohibit women from owning property, making women dependent on men.
- Male-dominated societies—When women and girls are restricted from enjoying the same educational opportunities as their male counterparts, their income-generating capacity and standard of living are adversely affected.
- Sexual coercion and lack of empowerment are important contributors to the increasing incidence of HIV/AIDS among women globally. According to the 2007 UN AIDS report the number of women living with HIV in 2007 is 15.4 million, which is an increase of 1.6 million from 2001.[3] Violence against women, including sexual coercion and unsafe sexual practices, are some of the contributing factors to this growing pandemic.
- Mass and systemic rape as a result of war and civil unrest. In times of war or civil unrest, often women and girls are forcibly recruited into armed groups, which can expose them to sexual violence and discrimination. A report released by the United Nations High Commission for Refugees (UNHCR) in 1995 reported that 250,000–500,000 women were raped in Rwanda during the genocide in 1994.[4]
- Lack of access to health care—Girls and women often do not have access to medical care, including safe motherhood facilities, reproductive health care, and informed consent, which contribute to gender inequality and discrimination. Barriers such as poverty, unequal power relationships between men and women, and lack of education and empowerment prevent millions of women worldwide

from having access to health care and from attaining, enjoying, and maintaining good health.[5,6]

- Prevailing governmental policies that are not conducive to women's health. Contributing factors include the following:
  - Lack of specific gender mainstreaming in healthcare policies targeted to serve the needs of women.
  - Lack of political will and underrepresentation of women in parliaments and policy making.
  - Lack of establishment of legal and constitutional frameworks that support both gender equality and availability of resources directed towards creating a positive effect on women's status and well-being.
  - Absence of a strong women's health and/or human rights movement and a culture of active civil society participation.[7]
- Gender inequality and perceived male superiority and the controlling nature of some men

Special Forms of Violence Against Girls and Women

Violence against women and children is not limited to discrimination, physical abuse, and emotional abuse but can take various other forms as well. The societal practices and prevailing culture in different regions of the world have contributed to the various forms of violence against women.

Harmful Practices Against Girls and Women in Asia, Africa, the Middle East, and the Americas

Violence and Gender Discrimination at Birth, Infancy, and Early Childhood According to a report released by the United Nations Population Fund (UNFPA), there has been a gender imbalance in many regions of Asia as a result of harmful practices against women. In India, according to the data released by UNFPA in 1901, there

were 972 women for every 1000 men, but a hundred years later in 2001, this ratio between women and men dropped dramatically to 933 women for every 1000 men.[5] This decrease has been due to special forms of violence against girls and women such as sex selective abortions, female infanticide, and other harmful practices.

According to a study conducted by UNFPA, the abuse against women, girls, and unborn female fetuses has resulted in a shift in the male-to-female ratio in Asia. In Southeast Asia, the female deficit has increased from 7.6% to 8.5% as a result of such practices.[6] The sex ratio at birth (SRB), which denotes the ratio of boys born per 100 girls, has changed as is evident in the data from five countries in west and east Asia with numbers as high as 108 in India and 120 in China.[6]

Some factors contributing to this imbalance include the following:

- Selective sex abortion of female fetuses.
- Neglect of girls, which results in malnutrition. For example, girls may be breastfed less often and for a shorter period of time, while the male children in the house are given more nutritious food.
- Female infanticide, which is common in isolated and rural parts of south and east Asia. The young female infant may be chocked to death or smothered by her parents or relatives since she is often perceived as a financial burden and is unwelcome. In many cases, female infanticide is falsely reported as a stillbirth.
- Immunization coverage is better for male children, and often the female children receive partial or no immunizations at all.
- Parents tend to seek medical aid for a sick male child, and often a sick female child is neglected and can die since she does not receive the necessary medical attention.

In many parts of Asia in both urban and rural areas, there is immense pressure from society and families to produce sons. Some of the reasons for male preference are lineage continuation, perceived support provided to parents in their old age, and source of income from employment and marriage. This marked male preference has resulted in the discrimination and violation of the human rights of girls, and often girls start their lives at a disadvantage.

Acid Attacks　Another harmful practice against women and girls is acid throwing. In an acid attack, which is one of the most heinous of crimes, acid is thrown, usually by a man, onto the face of a girl or woman with the intent of disfiguring her. The most commonly used acid is sulfuric acid as it is easily available, being found in car batteries. One of the most common reasons for this act is a rejected marriage proposal by the victim. Some of the other reasons for acid attacks are refusal by the wife to have sex with the husband or the perceived lack of adequate dowry.

These horrific attacks lead to severe disfigurement due to second and third degree facial burns and even blindness in some instances. In Bangladesh the number of acid attacks on women and adolescents has been increasing since 2000. The data released by the Dhaka-based Acid Survivors Foundation (ASF) estimates that 150 women were subject to acid throwing in 2006 and 133 women in 2007.[7] Unfortunately, most of these victims do not have access to immediate medical care due to lack of facilities. Naripokkho, a women's advocacy organization formed in 1995, and the ASF, a nongovernmental organization (NGO) founded in 1999, have been actively working with the Bangladeshi government and other international agencies to stop this practice.[7]

Dowry Deaths　A dowry is defined as money or property a bride's family gives a groom and his family at the time of the wedding. Unfortunately the practice of dowry abuse, which is a violation of human rights against women, has been increasing in south Asian countries, especially India. A woman is subjected to ill treatment by her husband and in-laws when the dowry she has brought is considered insufficient. She may be abused verbally, physically, or be subjected to humiliation. In severe cases she may be burned alive. According to a UNIFEM report, more than 12 women die every day as a result of being burned alive by their in-laws or husbands due to dowry disputes. Most of these incidents are reported as accidental burnings or suicides.[8,9]

A study conducted in Chandigarh in northern India, reported that married women made up 78% of total female fatalities and that many of these were the result of dowry disputes.[9] In spite of the Indian government recognizing as a criminal offence dowry acceptance and harassment of women as a result of dowry disputes, only a fraction of the perpetrators of these crimes are brought to justice. Some of the reasons for lack of prosecution include underreporting due to fear of social isolation, lack of sufficient evidence to pursue legal action, and the complacent attitude of law enforcement officials.[9,10]

United Nations agencies such as the UNIFEM, UNFPA, UNICEF, and WHO are partnering with local nongovernmental organizations to address the issue of special forms of violence against women including "bride burning," which can occur as a result of dowry disputes. In 2000, UNICEF launched a global campaign to address issues of violence against women including special forms of violence such as dowry-related harassment and deaths.[10]

Child Marriages and Forced Marriages
The ancient tradition of marrying young girls before they attain puberty is still prevalent in many parts of Asia, Africa, and the Middle East. A recent PBS documentary, *Child Brides,* highlighted the plight of young girls forced into arranged marriages against their will.[11]

In some rural areas in northern India girls as young as 6 are married in spite of the fact that marriages performed before the age of 18 are illegal and are punishable under the Indian penal code.[12] According to a report released in 2006, almost 4 million girls below the age of 18 were married against their will by their families in India.[11]

Rajasthan in India has some of the highest rates of child marriages and, according to a report released by UNICEF in 2001, mass child marriages were solemnized between young boys and girls including some who were two or three years old.[13,14] The report also highlights the practice of child marriages in poor neighborhoods of rural Albania where the culture encourages early marriages for their daughters to young men before they migrated to the city in search of better employment.[13]

In Africa, early marriage is common throughout much of the continent with the highest rates of child marriages occurring in Niger.[11,12] According to the World Health Organization:

The probability that a 15-year-old girl will die from a complication related to pregnancy and childbirth during her lifetime is highest in Africa: 1 in 26. In the developed regions it is 1 in 7300. Of all 171 countries and territories for which estimates were made, Niger had the highest estimated lifetime risk of 1 in 7.[12,1]

Some of the adverse effects and consequences of early marriage include prevalence of low literacy rates for women, lack of empowerment, and reduced access to health care. Additional health risks women face as the result of early marriage and child bearing are increased incidence of pregnancy-induced hypertension, eclampsia, molar pregnancy, and delivery of low birth weight and preterm infants.[14]

The rationale behind forced marriages for young girls is to prevent premarital sex since virginity is prized in many societies. Often young girls are restricted from attending coeducational schools and must adhere to a strict dress code. Often girls are not allowed to have social interactions with their peers.[13] Girls who have been forced to marry early are at a psychosocial disadvantage because of a loss of adolescence, forced sexual relations, and the denial of freedom that restricts their personal development. The impact of this trauma can be subtle, prolonged, and often hard to assess since these girls do not have access to counseling services.[13, 14] Thus the practice of child marriage is a violation of the human rights of girls who are deprived of their dignity and self-respect.

Practice of Sati and Devadasis

Sati and *devadasis* are special forms of cultural violence against women and girls prevalent in the Indian subcontinent. The horrific practice of *sati,* or self-immolation, was prevalent in ancient India where the widow was burned on the funeral pyre along with her dead husband. This practice was outlawed by Indian reformers and the British authorities in 1829, and the Indian penal code deemed it an offense punishable by rigorous imprisonment, heavy fines, and even the death penalty.[15,16]

Devadasi tradition is prevalent in south India where the term *devdasi* is derived from Sanskrit and translates as "servant of god." Devadasis are adolescent girls who are lured into prostitution in the name of religion. UNICEF estimates that there around 300,000 young girls who have become prostitutes in this way.[17] Unfortunately many of these girls are at an increased risk of contracting Sexually Transmitted Infections (STI) due to the practice of unsafe sex and often do not have access to reproductive health services. One of the contributing factors to the rapid spread of HIV/AIDS in rural India is the result of unsafe sexual practices between the young devadasi girls and their clients.[18]

According to the Indian Health Organization, devadasis compose nearly 15% of India's approximately 10 million sex workers. The number of devadasis is highest in the states of Karnataka and Maharashtra, where they constitute 80% of all sex workers. By 1994, it had become clear that adherence to the tradition had exacted a deadly toll: in Pune, a city of 2.5 million people in Maharashtra, already more than half the devadasis had become HIV infected.[18(p1)]

These young girls may suffer from depression, post-traumatic stress syndrome, and injuries as a result of physical violence. They are also at increased risk for indulging in unhealthy behaviors such as smoking, increased alcohol intake, and drug use. It is devastating that many of these young girls have been initiated into the devadasi practice by their family members in the name of culture and tradition.

Sexual Violence

The World Health Organization defines sexual violence as:

> Any sexual act, attempt to obtain a sexual act, unwanted sexual comments or advances, or acts to traffic, or otherwise directed, against a person's sexuality using coercion, by any person regardless of their relationship to the victim, in any setting, including but not limited to home and work.[19(p149)]

The following are forms of sexual violence:[19]

- Marital rape
- Date rape
- Rape by strangers

- Systematic rape during armed conflict
- Sexual harassment, which includes demanding sex in return for favors
- Sexual abuse of physically and mentally disabled people
- Sexual abuse of children
- Denial of the right to use contraception or adopt safe sex practices
- Forced abortion
- Female genital mutilation
- Forced virginity inspections
- Forced prostitution and trafficking of women and children for sexual exploitation
- Forced sexual initiation of young girls

A multicountry study on women's health and domestic violence conducted by the World Health Organization shows that many women worldwide have been the victims of sexual assault by an intimate partner. For example, 22–25% of women surveyed in London, Mexico, Nicaragua, Peru, and Zimbabwe reported that they experienced some form of sexual violence by an intimate partner.[19] A study conducted in South Africa among school children found that 32% disclosed rapes committed on school children were by their teachers.[19]

Forms of Cultural and Gender-Based Violence
Prejudices against women are seen in the language, attitude, and practices of people. Discussed here are a few such prevalent cultural practices which have deleterious effects on the health and well-being of African women.[19-29]

In Zimbabwe there is a custom known as *ngozi* in which a young girl is given as a compensation for the death of a man caused by her family. This custom is a violation of her human rights since on attaining puberty the young girl is forced to have sex with male members of the dead man's family in order to beget a male heir to replace the man who was killed by her family.[19]

Another prevailing custom in some African societies is *chimutsa mapfiwa* or wife inheritance, where according to this custom, when a married woman dies, her sister is expected to take her place and have sexual relations with the dead sister's husband.[19]

In some African cultures, wife beating is considered acceptable by both males and females as a method for disciplining one's wife for reasons such as not preparing food on time or refusing sexual advances. A study, conducted in 2005 on the perceptions of Nigerian women on domestic violence, revealed that a large percentage of Nigerian women support wife beating, as evident from 66.4% and 50.4% of never-married and unmarried women respectively who agreed that a husband is justified for hitting or beating his wife under the conditions examined in the paper. The 2003 NDHS revealed that more than 61% of males also supported wife beating. The high level of support expressed for wife beating by both males and females confirms that violence against women is accepted as a cultural norm among Nigerians.[20]

Levirate This is a practice whereby a widow is passed on to the next surviving male relation against her wish. In cases where a man has died of AIDS or where the actual cause of death was unknown due to poor access to health care, the widow may actually be a danger to her inheritor. The effects are even worse in a polygamous marriage.

Confinement Confinement is a period from 28 days to 3 months when the widow should not be seen anywhere outside the gate of her home. During this time, the widow may not leave the confines of her home to pursue income-generating activities such as going to the market or to seek needed medical attention for herself and her children. Studies have shown that it is usually during this period that widows and their children are most vulnerable to ill health. Unfortunately, there have been instances of widows and their children dying from neglect during this period of mandatory seclusion.

Widow Cleansing Widow cleansing is one of the most heinous forms of cultural violence perpetrated against women. In some communities in Africa and Asia, such cleansing generally involves a widow having sexual relations either with a designated village cleanser or with a relative of her late husband. It has traditionally been seen as a way to break with the past and move forward, as well as an attempt to establish a family's ownership over the late husband's property, including his wife. In cases where a husband died of AIDS, this practice is just as risky for the men who are chosen to cleanse as the women who are cleansed. These harmful cultural practices have contributed to the rapid spread of HIV/AIDS among women in Africa and Asia. This practice also prevents women from inheriting the property that has been their family's main source of support.[20] Widows may also be exposed to physical violence in disputes over inheritance and property rights.

Honor Killings Globally, hundreds or even thousands of young girls and women are murdered each year by their families in the name of family honor. These crimes are committed because these girls are perceived to have brought shame upon or tarnished the reputation of their family, and the killing of the girls will restore the lost honor.

Honor killings are perpetrated for a wide range of offenses. Marital infidelity, premarital sex, flirting, inappropriate attire, or even failing to serve a meal on time can all be perceived as impugning the family honor.[22(p2)]

It is ironic that these acts of horrific violence are not regarded as a crime but are justified in many societies. Unfortunately, it is extremely difficult to get the exact numbers on the phenomenon of honor killing since these murders frequently go unreported or are reported as suicides or accidental deaths.[22]

The United Nations Commission on Human Rights (UNCHR) has reported the occurrence of honor killings in Bangladesh, Great Britain, Brazil, Ecuador, Egypt, India, Israel, Italy, Jordan, Pakistan, Morocco, Sweden, Turkey, and Uganda.[22] A report, released in early 2008 by the Centre for Social Cohesion in the UK, discussed the prevalence of forced marriages and the occurrence of 10–12 cases annually of honor killings among the South Asian immigrant community living in the UK.[23] However, the exact number of deaths attributed to honor killings worldwide is difficult to access because it is difficult to define what constitutes an honor killing. The report further highlights that lack of education and low socioeconomic status are not contributing factors for honor killings that have occurred in the United Kingdom. Families in the developing countries and the Western world are driven by a common force, which is to uphold the honor and tradition of their families. Whenever the women in these families are perceived as "violators," they are then killed to protect the families and restore the lost traditions.

Wife Battering Researcher P.C. Herbert described wife battering as "violent acts—psychological, sexual and/or physical assault—by an assailant against his wife and/or partner made with the intent of controlling the partner by inducing fear and pain."[24(p1)] Wife battering occurs among women of all ages and social strata, and often there is a close association between wife battering and child abuse. This has serious implications on the health of the women and children who are subjected to and witness this act of violence.

Incest Incest describes sexual activity between closely related persons (often within the immediate family). In many cultures, it is considered illegal and socially unacceptable.

Unfortunately, many young girls and adolescents worldwide are coerced into such relationships, which have long-term adverse effects on their health and well-being.

Street Children According to the Human Rights Watch:

> The term *street children* refers to children for whom the street more than their family has become their real home. It includes children who might not necessarily be homeless or without families, but who live in situations where there is no protection, supervision, or direction from responsible adults.[25 (p1)]

Child abuse, children orphaned as a result of wars, civil unrest, AIDS, divorce, lure of city life, peer pressure, and desire for economic advancement are the major causes for children leaving home. Unfortunately, a majority of these children do not have the necessary education or skills to earn a living and end up on the streets. Young girls and adolescents who end up as street children are at risk of being trafficked or lured into prostitution. Street children throughout the world have been ill-treated by the police and are often viewed as a blot on society by governments that do not offer them the protection and nurturing that children are entitled to. In countries where there is civil unrest or ongoing wars, street children face a higher risk of being recruited as gang members, trained as militants, or recruited as child soldiers. A UNICEF report describes the plight of young street children in Latin America, who are often seen roaming the streets begging or committing petty crimes or selling drugs to earn their living. The Colombian term used for runaway or abandoned children or street children who live on their own is *gamine*. These children often live in urban slums and store their belongings in a cardboard box and sleep on plastic sheets.[26] This illustrates the pathetic plight of these children, and the lack of social welfare programs in this region is a significant hindrance to achieve Millennium Development Goals 1, 2, and 4 (Goal 1—Eradicate extreme poverty and hunger; Goal 2—Achieve universal primary education; and Goal 4 Reduce child mortality).[27]

Effects of Violence

The effects of violence on children, adolescents, and women can be devastating to their physical, emotional, and social well-being.[19,20,28,29] Violence has both a direct and indirect consequence on women's health, and it can increase women's risk of future ill health and disability.[23,29] Children who witness violence suffer from anxiety, low self-esteem, and other behavioral problems including depression, physical complaints, and eating disorders.[27] The more severe and prolonged the abuse, the greater the impact on the victims.

Physical Consequences of Violence

The effects of physical trauma can be minor or life threatening and can result in permanent disability or death of the victims. Globally an estimated 40–70% of homicides against women are committed by intimate partners.[27]

Effects of physical abuse include:[19,20]

- Injuries to the abdomen and thorax, which can result in damage to the tissues and vital organs such as the heart, lungs and spleen
- Bruises, welts, contusions, and fractures
- Bleeding or hemorrhage (internal and external)
- 1st-, 2nd-, or 3rd-degree burns
- Chronic pain and chronic fatigue syndromes
- Fibromyalgia

- Functional and organic gastrointestinal disorders, which are common in women who have been in chronic abusive relationships[28]
- Ocular damage, which may result in retinal detachment leading to blindness
- Reduced physical movements and body functions that result in abused women missing more days at work than non-abused women[20]

Furthermore, women who have been subjected to physical trauma often do not have access to medical care since they are not permitted to seek assistance by their abusers and must suffer in silence.

Psychological Trauma

The damage caused by psychological abuse is often invisible but the resulting trauma can be far more devastating than that resulting from physical trauma.

Effects of psychological abuse include the following:[19,20,27,28]

- Depression and anxiety—According to a study conducted in Australia, women who are abused by their partners suffer more from depression and anxiety when compared to women who are in non-abusive relationships.[27]
- Eating and sleep disorders—Abused women and girls tend to overeat and suffer from nightmares and insomnia.
- Feelings of shame and guilt—Abused women and children often blame themselves for the violence to which they are subjected.
- Phobias and panic disorder.
- Physical inactivity.
- Poor self-esteem.
- Post-traumatic stress disorder or PTSD (domestic violence, childhood abuse, and rape are among the most common causes of PTSD among women).
- Psychosomatic disorders.
- Smoking, alcohol, and drug abuse—Women who are in chronic abusive relationships and those who have been sexually abused as chil-

dren are more likely to abuse alcohol and drugs even after other risk factors have been controlled. A 2-year US study found that abused women abused alcohol and drugs as a coping mechanism to deal with the abuse.[29]

- Suicidal behavior and self-harm—Multicountry studies conducted in the United States, Nicaragua, and Sweden have shown that violence against women is closely associated with an increased risk of suicide and self-harm.[20]
- Unsafe sexual behavior.
- A slight increase in the incidence of irritable bowel syndrome (IBS)—Abused women tend to blame themselves for being abused and this can lead to an increase in stress levels which in turn exacerbates the symptoms of IBS.[30]
- Sexual dysfunction—Women who have been sexually abused may develop an aversion to sex.

Other Health Outcomes of Violence Against Girls, Adolescents, and Women

Effects of Violence on Reproductive Health

Violence has been shown to affect a woman's reproductive health in many ways.

Unwanted or Unintended Pregnancies Abused women are at a higher risk for unwanted or unintended pregnancies as these women lack reproductive rights and are often forced to have sex without contraceptive use. Sexual abuse of adolescents can lead to unwanted pregnancies.

Unsafe and Forced Abortions Abused women also have a higher incidence of unsafe and forced abortions. Sexually abused adolescents and women who get pregnant may be forced to abort their pregnancies. They also face a higher risk of unsafe abortions due to lack of access to trained healthcare providers; such abortions can have serious implications, often leading to death and disability. According to a report released by WHO in 2005, of the estimated 46 million induced abor-

tions annually, almost 19 million of them are performed in unsanitary and unsafe conditions by unskilled providers. Such horrific procedures result in the death of almost 68,000 girls and women worldwide. Most of these deaths (almost 99%) occur in developing countries. Unsafe abortions account for 13% of all pregnancy-related deaths that occur each year.[31]

Pregnancy Complications Maternal complications brought on by violence can include preterm labor, vaginal infections, and insufficient maternal weight gain during pregnancy as a result of maternal malnutrition. Trauma during pregnancy can also lead to bleeding and precipitate a condition known as "abruptio placenta," which can increase maternal and fetal mortality. A study conducted in British Columbia, Canada, found that women in abusive relationships were 3.5 times more likely to experience hemorrhage as a result of trauma during pregnancy compared to women who were not abused.[32,33]

Fetal Complications Fetal complications brought on by abuse can include low birth weight. In addition, abuse can increase stress that predisposes the mother to maternal hypertension preeclampsia, preterm labor resulting in an abortion, or small-for-age infants. Fetal injury can also occur resulting in preterm birth and intrauterine fetal death. There have been several studies conducted globally that have focused on the relationship between violence in pregnancy and low birth weight outcomes. One such study conducted in Nicaragua found that after controlling for other factors, violence against pregnant women was associated with almost a three-fold increase in the incidence of low birth weight infants born in that particular health center where the research was conducted.[20]

STIs and HIV Sexual abuse in childhood and adolescence increases the risk of sexually transmitted infections. Sexually abused children and adolescents are also at higher risk for indulging in high-risk sexual practices, which further increases their chances of contracting STIs and HIV.[26]

Research undertaken by UNAIDS, WHO, and UNFPA has established links between violence against women and their risk for contracting HIV infections. The following are a few examples that demonstrate the link between HIV infection and violence:[32]

1. Women who have been raped have their risk increased for acquiring HIV infection as a result of the trauma caused to their genitalia, which results in lacerations.
2. Fear of violence and social stigma prevents women from getting tested for HIV, revealing their HIV status, and availing themselves of treatment.
3. Findings from a study conducted on pregnant women in South Africa who attended a health clinic for their prenatal checkup showed that women who are abused and are subjected to controlling behavior by their partners are 1.5 times more likely to be infected by HIV compared to those who are not in abusive relationships.[20]

Pelvic Inflammatory Disease and Infertility
Complications of repeated STIs give rise to pelvic inflammatory disease and lead to infertility, which in turn can increase the risk for women being abused and becoming social outcasts for not being able to bear children.

Effects of Violence on Society

The effects on society of violence against women and girls are both direct and indirect.[19,28,34] A national survey conducted in Canada on violence against women reported that 30% of abused married women could not carry out their daily activities due to the injuries they sustained. Their children who witnessed such abuse were themselves victims of abuse and performed poorly at school.[28] A study of abused women in Managua, Nicaragua, found that abused women earned 46% less than women who did not suffer abuse, even after controlling for other factors that affect earnings.[20] One of the reasons for this was their frequent absenteeism from work as a result of the physical and mental trauma sustained by them.[34] A survey conducted in Nagpur in India found that 13% of working women missed work due to abuse, and this led to a decrease in their earnings.[19] The above exam-

ples are just one of the effects of violence and the economic impact on global society.

Strategies to Reduce and Prevent Gender-Based Violence

Gender-based violence differs from other forms of interpersonal violence since the patterns of violence against women are different from those experienced by men. Women are more likely to experience violence at the hands of men or members of their family, and often the violence extends over a long period of time. It is important to understand these variations when designing interventions to prevent violence against women. Unfortunately, in spite of more than 20 years of activism in the area of gender-based violence, there have been very few interventions or programs that have been implemented to address this growing pandemic.[19,28,35]

When considering programs to combat this problem, it is critical to include the following components:

■ Empowering women and making them understand that the violence they experience is unacceptable is one of the biggest challenges activists encounter.

■ Educating boys from childhood that violence against women is an offense and a violation of human rights is an important step in designing preventive strategies. It is important to educate communities that women are not chattel or movable property but individuals who need to be valued and not abused.[19]

■ Male involvement and input when implementing programs to prevent violence against women has shown to be effective. A report released the by Pan American Health Organization (PAHO) shows that making men aware that when women are subjected to violence it affects all the members in the family, including themselves, has been instrumental in making some men regard their wives and partners as equals in decision making. This has led to sharing of child-rearing responsibilities and allowing women to make choices regarding their reproductive health and child bearing.[35]

- Treatment programs for abusers are found in the United States, Australia, Canada, and in a few developing countries. These programs discuss gender roles and teach the group members skills to cope with stress and anger management issues. Research has shown that in a few programs implemented in the United States, members refrained from resorting to violence for a period of at least two years.[19]

- Support programs for victims have resulted in the establishment of shelters for battered women. Some of the services provided to these women include legal, emotional, and vocational training. Unfortunately women in developing countries do not have access to such services and suffer in silence.[19,28]

- Attention must be given to legal actions and judicial interventions. Over the past two decades, the issue of violence against women and girls has received worldwide attention. The sustained efforts of United Nations agencies, nongovernmental organizations, foundations, and activists have resulted in criminalizing this act in several countries. In the past decade, 24 countries in Latin America and the Caribbean have passed specific legislation on domestic violence.[19] Another interesting judicial intervention that has been implemented in certain parts of India is the establishment of legal aid cells and family courts (known as *lok adalat*) and women's courts (known as *mahila lok adalat*) by the state government to specifically address the issues related to violence against women and children.[19]

- Alternate sanctions should also be considered. Under this intervention, an abusive male partner may be prohibited from contacting or abusing his partner and may be made to leave home by a civil court. He can also be ordered to pay child support and seek counseling and seek treatment for substance abuse.[19]

- Some all-women police stations have been established in recent years in some countries in Latin America and Asia. These police cells have been staffed with all women police personnel to help encourage more abused

women to come forward and seek assistance. Unfortunately, in some parts of India, women have to travel great distances to avail themselves of the services of such police stations and often do not have the immediate assistance they require.[19]

- Intervention by healthcare providers is also critical. A 2002 WHO report on violence and health stated:

> In recent years attention has turned towards reforming the response of healthcare providers to victims of abuse. Most women come into contact with the health system at some point in their lives—when they seek contraception, for instance, or give birth or seek care for their children. This makes the healthcare setting an important place where women undergoing abuse can be identified, provided with support, and referred if necessary to specialized services. Unfortunately, studies show that in most countries, doctors and nurses rarely enquire of women whether they are being abused, or even check for obvious signs of violence.[19(p131)]

- Community efforts include outreach work and programs where peer educators and volunteers from the local communities are in touch with women and children and make them aware of the services available to them. Lawyers, healthcare providers, social workers, and volunteers who live in the local communities often provide free services and assistance to abused women and children.[19,28]

- In recent years women's organizations, NGOs, and other groups working in partnership with local, state, and national governments have organized campaigns to educate the public and raise awareness of the issues of violence against women and children. Such working partnerships have also resulted in raising funds to help abused women and children. United Nations agencies, such as UNIFEM and the UNFPA have partnered with celebrities to raise public awareness and launch campaigns and fund-raising activities to help these unfortunate women and children.

A multisectorial approach to address the issue of violence against women and girls is being adopted in many countries. Partnering between the health sector, legal and judiciary departments, policy makers, and religious leaders will be effective in reducing or preventing violence. Such cooperation will also be economically and socially beneficial since there is sharing of data and best practices and will result in the development and implantation of more coordinated and strategic approaches to address this problem.[19]

Finally, policy makers, activists, and all the various stakeholders must realize the importance of investing in primary prevention against violence against women and girls. Primary prevention strategies must foster the creation of a global social environment that promotes gender equity and sharing of power between men and women. This is a daunting task, but it is of vital importance that initial acts of violence be prevented rather than trying to clean up and fix the aftermath of such attacks.

Conclusion

Violence against women and girls is an important public health issue that cannot be ignored by the global community. In spite of the recent advances made in the fields of medicine, science, and technology, as citizens of this world we cannot claim to have made progress until this silent pandemic of violence against women and girls ceases locally, nationally, and globally.

DISCUSSION QUESTIONS

1. Discuss the etiology of and contributing factors to gender-based violence.
2. Discuss the role of men in working to reduce culturally acceptable practices of violence against women and girls.
3. How would you work with other members of your community in addressing the issues of gender-based violence in your region?
4. Do you agree with the term *silent global pandemic* that is often used to describe violence against women?
5. What are the profound effects of gender-based violence on the global society?

REFERENCES

1. International Center for Research on Women. Violence against women must stop. 2005. http://www.icrw.org/docs/2005_brief_mdg-violence.pdf. Accessed May 3, 2008.
2. Interactive Population Centre. Violence against girls and women. http://www.unfpa.org/intercenter/violence/intro.htm. Accessed May 3, 2008.
3. United Nations Children's Emergency Fund. Domestic violence against women and girls. June 2000. http://www.unicef-irc.org/publications/pdf/digest6e.pdf. Accessed May 3, 2008.

4. United Nations International Research and Training Institute for the Advancement of Women (INSTRAW). Gender, peace and security. 2000. http://www.un-instraw.org. Accessed May 10, 2008.

5. Bruyn M. Violence, pregnancy, and abortion: issues of women's rights and public health. August 2003. http://www.ipas.org/Publications/asset_upload_file299_2460.pdf. Accessed May 10, 2008.

6. Women's Commission. Masculinities: male roles and male involvement in the promotion of gender equality. September 2005. http://www.womenscommission.org/pdf/masc_res.pdf. Accessed May 3, 2008.

7. Acid Survivors Foundation. Acid attack statistics. http://www.acidsurvivors.org/statistics.html. Accessed May 28, 2008.

8. Fox VC. Historical perspectives on violence against women. November 2002. http://www.bridgew.edu/soas/jiws/fall02/historical_perspectives.pdf. Accessed May 3, 2008.

9. World Health Organization South East Asia Region. Intimate partner violence. http://www.searo.who.int/LinkFiles/Disability_Injury_Prevention_&_Rehabilitation_partner.pdf Accessed June 5, 2008

10. United Nations Trust Fund to Eliminate Violence Against Women. Facts and figures about violence against women. February 2007. http://www.searo.who.int/LinkFilesDisability_Injury_Prevention_&_Rehabilitation_partner.pdf. Accessed June 3, 2008

11. Public Broadcasting Service. Child Brides. 2008. http://www.pbs.org/now/shows/341/transcript.html. Accessed June 10, 2008.

12. World Health Organization South-East Asia Region. Adolescence reproductive health behavior. Indonesia reproductive health profile. 2003. http://www.searo.who.int/LinkFiles/Reproductive_Health_Profile_adolescence.pdf. Accessed June 10, 2008.

13. United Nations Children's Emergency Fund Innocenti Research Centre. Early marriages child spouses. March 2001. http://www.childinfo.org/files/childmarriage_Innocentidigest7.pdf. Accessed May 5, 2008.

14. World Health Organization. Early marriage and childbearing: risks and consequences. http://www.who.int/reproductivehealth/publications/towards_adulthood/7.pdf. Accessed June 3, 2008

15. British Broadcasting Corporation. India wife dies on funeral pyre. 2006. http://news.bbc.co.uk/2/hi/south_asia/5273336.stm. Accessed June 15, 2008.

16. Commission on Sati Prevention Act. http://wcd.nic.in/commissionofsatiprevention.htm. Accessed June 20, 2008.

17. World Health Organization. Adolescent health. 2006. http://www.searo.who.int/LinkFiles/Fact_Sheets_India-AHD-07.pdf. Accessed June 28, 2008.

18. Harvard School of Public Health AIDS Initiative. AIDS in India. http://www.aids.harvard.edu/news_publications/har/fall_1995/fall95-4.html. Accessed June 20, 2008.

19. World Health Organization. World report on violence and health. 2002. http://whqlibdoc.who.int/publications/2002/9241545615_eng.pdf. Accessed May 24, 2008.

20. Ellsberg MC, Heise L. *Researching Violence Against Women. A Practical Guide for Researchers and Activists.* Geneva, Switzerland: World Health Organization, PATH; 2005.

21. The Joint United Nations Programme on HIV/ AIDS. A joint report on women and AIDS confronting the crisis. http://www.unfpa.org/hiv/women/report/chapter7.html. Accessed June 10, 2008.

22. National Geographic News. Thousands of women killed for family "honor". 2002. http://www.unfpa.org/hiv/women/report/chapter7.html. Accessed June 10, 2008.

23. Centre for Social Cohesion, UK. Crimes in the community. Honor based killings in the UK. 2008. http://www.socialcohesion.co.uk/pdf/CrimesOfTheCommunity .pdf. Accessed June 10, 2008.

24. Herbert PC. *Wife Battering*. College of Family Physicians of Canada; 1983:2204-2208.

25. Human Rights Watch. Children's rights: street children. 2006. http://www .hrw.org/children/street.htm. Accessed June 10, 2008.

26. Latin America: street children. http://family.jrank.org/pages/1043/Latin-America-Street-Children.html. Accessed June 20, 2008.

27. United Nations Children's Emergency Fund. Child protection from violence, exploitation and abuse. http://www.unicef.org/protection/index_27374.html. Accessed June 15, 2008.

28. Baccini F, Pallotta N, Calabrese E, Pezzotti P, Corazziari E. Prevalence of sexual and physical abuse and its relationship with symptom manifestations in patients with chronic organic and functional gastrointestinal disorders. *Digestive and Liver Disease,* 2003;35(4):254-261.

29. Population Reports. Ending violence against women. December 1999. http://www.infoforhealth.org/pr/l11/violence.pdf. Accessed May 3, 2008.

30. Center for Advancement of Health. Irritable bowel syndrome linked with emotional abuse. 2000. http://www.cfah.org/hbns/newsrelease/irritablebowel1-31-00.cfm. Accessed June 10, 2008.

31. Population Reference Bureau. Unsafe abortion facts and figures. 2006. http://www.prb.org/pdf05/UnsafeAbortion.pdf. Accessed June 10, 2008.

32. World Health Organization. Violence against women and HIV/AIDS information sheet. http://www.who.int/hac/techguidance/pht/InfosheetVaWandHIV.pdf. Accessed on June 20, 2008.

33. Pan American Health Organization. Maternal death due to domestic violence. July 2005. http://www.paho.org/english/ad/ge/FSmaternaldeath-domviol.pdf. Accessed June 10, 2008

34. World Health Organization. Violence against women. Fact sheet. http://www.who.int/mediacentre/factsheets/fs239/en/. Accessed May 2, 2008.

35. Pan American Health Organization. Reinventing macho: men as partners in reproductive health.1997. http://www.paho.org/English/DPI/Number4_article4 .htm. Accessed June 20, 2008.

CHAPTER **3**

Impact and Effects of Terrorism on Women and Girls

Michael J. Reilly, MPH, NREMT-PMICP

Michael J. Reilly, MPH NREMT-PMICP, is an Assistant Professor of Public Health Practice and the Assistant Director, Center for Disaster Medicine at New York Medical College.

Throughout history women have been involved in and affected by wars, conflict, uprisings, and social and civil unrest. In recent years there has been an increase in the prevalence of these types of incidents occurring across the globe, with more and more women and children being affected by, or participating in, terrorist attacks.

Terrorism has been described as the threat, use, or intended use, of force or violence against persons or property to intimidate or coerce a government, civilian population, or any segment thereof, in furtherance of political or social objectives. Many misconceptions exist about terrorism: where it occurs, who the victims or targets are, and what type of individual a terrorist is. Because it is difficult to predict with certainty the type of person who is likely to be a terrorist, and there is no uniformity among terrorist profiles, terrorists can use this uncertainty to create fear and instill terror in their victims. Although this chapter focuses on the impact of terrorism on women and the girl child, the roles of the women and children as perpetrators of terrorism must also be considered.

Many recent reports have shown that women have been the perpetrators of terrorist acts or are being actively recruited by terrorist organizations in various countries around the world. Examples of female-initiated or involved terrorist attacks have been reported in such countries as India, Iraq, Sri Lanka, Lebanon, Syria, Palestine, Israel, Egypt, Uzbekistan, Turkey, Chechnya, and Jordan. Achieving a better understanding of the behavioral, psychological, and socioeconomic factors influencing women into becoming supporters or perpetrators of terrorist activities can assist us in planning, preparing, and deterring terrorist attacks in our home countries and thereby minimize the morbidity and mortality of these events on our populations.

As victims or targets of terrorist attacks, women have unique vulnerabilities and susceptibilities to injury and illness. Many injuries and illnesses are not gender specific, such as blast trauma and certain exposure-related illnesses from infectious diseases (bioterrorism) or chemical or radiological agents (chemical and radiological terrorism). However, the female is prone to certain additional physical and psychological traumas that occur at higher rates than in men, particularly when discussing the impact of terrorism on the pregnant female.

This chapter analyzes the role of women as victims and targets of terrorism as well as their involvement in planning and carrying out terrorist attacks. The ultimate goal of this chapter is to discuss ways to minimize the physical and psychological impact of terrorism on women and the girl child, and attempt to identify the sociocultural and behavioral risk factors for women who may be recruited into terrorist organizations. The hope is that through prevention and intervention, along with the development and piloting of effective intervention programs targeted at women susceptible to recruitment or coercion by terrorist groups, the extent and impact of terror attacks across the globe will be limited.

Women as Perpetrators of Terrorism

In the past several years more examples of terrorist attacks that have involved the use or support of women as the perpetrators have appeared in the media. Shocking and sensationalized, these examples often leave people wondering why or how women could carry out such acts of violence. Examples of women participating in, supporting, nurturing, or planning terrorism are not new. Throughout history women have been involved in and affected by wars, conflict, uprisings, and social and civil unrest. What would make women so affected that they would carry out such acts, causing injury, death, and devastation to so many? Are acts of terrorism perpetrated by women limited to certain areas of the world, or is this a more pervasive trend that exists in a variety of societies and countries around the globe?

Generally, it has been reported that women are not career terrorists with long histories of terrorist activities, but once recruited they usually play a subordinate or supporting role within the organization. In addition to coordinating and participating in terrorist attacks, there have been several additional areas of involvement of women in support of domestic and international terrorism, as well as specific tactical reasons that terrorist organizations seek out vulnerable women to exploit and recruit into roles within their organizations.

Participation of Women in Terrorism

There is no unified explanation as to why women participate in terrorism, particularly in suicide terrorism. The female suicide terrorist is especially difficult to profile, which makes the detection of a female suicide bomber so difficult. This fact is a main reason terrorist organizations choose to employ female suicide bombers in their ranks, providing them with a significant tactical advantage. However, not all terrorist organizations use women to conduct terrorist attacks. Traditionally, women have served in various types of support capacities within a terrorist organization in both passive and active roles.

Passive support roles may consist of providing nurturing support to husbands who are active members of the organization. Women generally provide a role in supporting the culture of terrorism by bringing up children who share similar acceptable views of the importance of the terrorist organization's role and by raising sons who will be born to fight in the ranks of militancy when they get older. Women may also serve the organization in more active roles such as providing food and clothing to members, conducting surveys of targets to identify areas for future attacks, smuggling weapons or bomb-making materials, transporting messages, providing shelter and hiding to members, or assisting in preparing female suicide bombers for their impending attacks.[1,2]

Motivation of Women Participating in Terrorism

A variety of factors that influence women into participating in terrorist activities have been discussed by various authors and researchers. Some of these arise from involuntary, external factors such as exploitation and humiliation, which will be discussed later. However, many of the voluntary factors that would potentially motivate women into terrorism can be attributed to the following categories: religious motives, political motives, socioeconomic motives, and personal or romantic motives.

Many researchers point to the low social status of women in certain cultures where female-involved terrorism is occurring. The patriarchal nature of some states where women are not given equal rights as men has, in some opinions, caused women to be more willing to rise up to carry out terrorist acts in order to be seen as of equal value as men.[1,3,4] Furthermore, women may see radicalism as an alternative to economic or political insecurity by turning to causes that promise protection, safety and security, and more favorable economic circumstances.[2]

Religious motives include the acknowledgement by religious leaders that women should also rise up to become martyrs because it is permitted under Islam. Men should not be the only ones to conduct suicide attacks, and women should conduct *jihad* even without the permission of their husbands.[4,5] Additionally, "flawed" women, such as those who have had extramarital affairs, may in certain cultures feel that the only way to redeem themselves is through martyrdom. By becoming a *shahid* (one who dies in the name of Allah) they will be permitted to enter Paradise and go on to heaven.[1]

Personal or romantic motives may include the need to cleanse oneself of prior bad deeds. Women in certain cultures feel that if they have not acted in line with what their society dictates is appropriate behavior, then their only recourse is to clear their name and the name of their families by becoming a martyr. Examples of these types of deviations from the norm may include lying to their fathers, husbands, or older brothers about their activities; promiscuity; extramarital affairs, infertility, communication with the "enemy," and so on.[1,4]

Why Women? The Terrorist's Tactical Advantage

There are several reasons why terrorists would choose to use a woman to carry out attacks, including suicide bombings. In many cultures the notion or idea of a woman as a terrorist still remains difficult to understand. Terrorists use this common belief to exploit the vulnerabilities of security forces that may be less likely to identify a woman as a possible terrorist or suicide bomber. Studies have shown that security and military personnel, especially in countries where the modesty or privacy of women is held in high regard, often screen or search women with less scrutiny than men. Additionally, women in certain Muslim countries often wear clothing or traditional garments that would hide or conceal a tactical device unless more thorough secondary screening was performed. Terrorists have also adopted the use of pregnancy prosthetics that enable women to carry explosives inside of a simulated pregnant belly. The ability of a suicide bomber to get close to their intended target before potential detection by security, police, or military forces is a significant tactical advantage to the terrorist. Women have been shown to draw less suspicion, have a greater ability to conceal weapons, and draw more sensational headlines and shock following an attack.

Coercion, Manipulation, and Exploitation of Women into Terrorism

Women may sometimes participate in terrorism not by their own choices but because of external pressure, coercion, manipulation, or exploitation by others. Some terrorist handlers or facilitators (i.e., those individuals who coach or train suicide bombers and plan their attacks) value the use of women as a tactical asset, but they may lack willing participants with the necessary social, religious, or personal motivation to volunteer to carry out attacks. Such terrorist handlers instead may resort to blackmail and other tactics to get a woman to perform terrorists acts against her will. The types of women in Islamic culture who are susceptible to coercion, manipulation, or blackmail by handlers are similar to those who may volunteer for such activities: women who have a "tainted" past; who may have had inappropriate relationships with the opposite sex; who may have been promiscuous, committed adultery, or who have a perceived lower social standing due to various indiscretions in their personal life. Sometimes in certain cultures women who have these kinds of backgrounds are thought to bring dishonor or disrespect to their families, and the male figures in their families may be compelled to perform an honor killing of the woman in order to repair the damage to the family name. Terrorists may be able to exploit the guilt associated with bringing dishonor to the family and convince the young woman that by becoming a *shahid* that she can "right a wrong" or prevent this disgrace from affecting her family. This has even been taken one step further by terrorists who have arranged or set up young women into illicit relationships, gotten them pregnant, or even going so far as to arrange their rapes. The corresponding guilt and associated shame that would be associated in acknowledging this "disgrace" publicly can then be used to manipulate these women into performing suicide attacks in order to negate the inevitable dishonor on their families.[6]

The lengths that terrorists will go to in order to use the tactical advantage associated with female suicide bombers is not limited to simple manipulation or coercion. The presumption of many that a suicide bomber must be young, or physically or mentally strong has been challenged. There is new evidence that terrorist groups may be recruiting or using women who are mentally ill, or have developmental disorders such as mental retardation or Down syndrome to conduct terrorist attacks. The ability to convince an individual who does not have the capacity to comprehend or understand what they are being asked to do, or the horrific consequences of such an act, are seen as an advantage to the terrorist handler. Furthermore, a female suicide bomber who may have the physical signs of a disability may reduce suspicions by police, military, or security forces, giving terrorists an added tactical advantage.

Examples of Terrorist Groups Who Use Women in Terrorist Attacks

As discussed earlier, women have been an integral part of terrorist organizations for decades. Suicide bombers are just one way women are involved in acts of terrorism. Examples of organizations whose membership includes women include those prevalent in Western societies including the United States, such as eco-terrorist organizations, single issue groups, or hate groups. Specific examples include Greenpeace, the Earth Liberation Front (ELF), Animal Liberation Front (ALF), People for the Ethical Treatment of Animals (PETA), the Ku Klux Klan, the Women for Aryan Unity, the Weather Underground, Italy's Red Brigade, and Germany's Red Army Faction.

Examples of countries who have documented incidents involving the use or recruitment of female suicide bombers has risen sharply since the first documented use of a female as a suicide bomber by the Syrian Social Nationalist Party (SSNP) in Lebanon in 1985. The list of counties includes Lebanon, India, Palestine, Chechnya, Iraq, Israel, Turkey, Russia, Sri Lanka, Syria, Uzbekistan, and Egypt.[1-6]

Several international terrorist organizations have been associated with the specific use of women in conducting suicide attacks. Some of the more notable organizations have included such groups as the Chechen Black Widows who have participated in such attacks as the school attack in Beslan, Russia, in September 2004 and the attack and raid on a Moscow theater in October 2002. Others include the Sri Lankan Liberation Tigers of Tamil Eelam (LTTE) or Black Tigers whose membership is approximately one-third women, various groups of Iraqi insurgents, the Palestinian Islamic Jihad (PIJ), and Hamas.

Women as Targets of Terrorism

Women are held in high regard and with high value in many societies and cultures around the globe. Societies that value the woman as the mother and caretaker of her husband and children view her as one who should be protected from harm and cherished as a loving nurturer of her family. When women are victims of terrorist attacks it increases the impact of the event on a society. Not only are individual lives lost in the attack, but when women are killed, children lose their mothers and husbands their wives. As such, societies typically view terrorist incidents involving the death or injury of women as more devastating than attacks when only men or soldiers are targeted.

In over 70% of terrorist attacks, incendiary or explosive devices are used. Physically, women have different vulnerabilities than men that make their chances for suffering morbidity and mortality due to terrorism from improvised explosive devices (IEDs) greater than men. Overall, they have a smaller physical stature with less muscle mass and more adipose than men. They also have a greater percentage of vascular soft tissue on the anterior aspect of their bodies and a pelvic girdle designed for childbearing that is less efficient at dissipating energy than the male.

There are not many examples of terrorist attacks that have only targeted women in the social science literature. However, there are examples of terrorist tactics that exploit the unique vulnerabilities of women and who use specific methods to leverage terror on women to increase the impact of terrorism on society at large.

Rape as a Tactic of Terrorism

Rape has been used by terrorists as a way to inflict genocide on societies and populations. In several examples of ethnic and religious uprisings male militants have raped and impregnated enemy women to "dirty" an ethnic line and incite genocide among the population. The terrorist uses the idea that such "infected" women would need to be murdered by the men in their families in order to purify the society. These tactics are also used to demoralize the men, showing that they are unable to protect their women from harm. This further empowers the enemy or terrorist and causes increased psychological distress on combatants. This has been seen in countries like Rwanda and the former Yugoslavia.[2]

Pregnancy: How Women Are Uniquely Vulnerable to Trauma

Trauma is the most frequent non-obstetric cause of mortality in the pregnant woman. The pregnant female is uniquely vulnerable to morbidity and mortality associated with trauma and in secondary exposure of the fetus to environmental exposure to agents of weapons of mass destruction. There are several specific implications for the pregnant female as a victim of terrorism both for her own well-being and the well-being of her unborn child.

Physical Trauma   Studies have shown that pregnant women injured in terror-related multiple casualty incidents have a high incidence of surgical procedures and the need for cesarean delivery following their injuries. They also suggest that the condition of the fetus in these cases may be poor.[7] Although the amniotic fluid may provide cushioning of the fetus and some protection against blunt trauma, the increase in surgical intervention and

resultant cesarean section may be because the gravid uterus is highly vascular, and blunt and penetrating trauma to the abdomen can result in hypoperfusion (shock) in the mother. This condition can trigger a compensatory mechanism resulting in decreased blood flow to the uterus and an ultimate reduction in fetal heart rate. This leads to fetal distress and a high associated fetal mortality in cases where the gravid female is in shock. Any trauma to the abdomen of the pregnant female could cause a variety of conditions that could jeopardize the life of the mother or the unborn child. Premature labor, rupture of the membranes, spontaneous abortion, uterine rupture, and separation of the placenta from the uterine wall all may cause life-threatening injuries.

Toxic Inhalation Effects   Although the effects of toxic inhalation of hazardous materials or chemical weapons would have immediate and severe health effects on any individual, studies looking at the effects of low-level toxic inhalation of dust and debris following the attacks on September 11, 2001, in the United States, have found that even mild exposures can potentially negatively impact the health of pregnant women and their babies.

Dusts and debris from the collapse of the buildings at the World Trade Center (WTC) site were found to have contained a variety of particulate and hazardous materials. Some of the hazardous chemicals included neurodevelopmental toxicants such as polycyclic aromatic hydrocarbons (PAHs), polychlorinated biphenyls (PCBs), and others. Several studies looked at the effects of the inhalation of these substances on women who worked or lived near the WTC site. Particular attention was given to those women who were pregnant at the time of their exposure to these substances.[8-10]

These studies showed that women who worked or lived close to the WTC site on and around 9/11 had high exposures to particulate matter and correspondingly higher blood levels of PAHs and PAH-DNA adducts than women who lived further away from the site.[8] Upon delivery of their children, women who worked or lived near the World Trade Center site gave birth to infants who were of lower birth weight, shorter length, and smaller head circumference. The mothers also had shorter gestations than women who did not live or work close to the site.[9] Further studies of this exposure have also shown that women pregnant at the time of the 9/11 attacks who were exposed to elevated levels of PAHs and environmental tobacco smoke birthed infants who had reduced cognitive development compared to those who did not have these exposures.[10]

Bioterrorism Considerations Pregnancy causes a variety of endocrine and immunologic responses in the mother. These physiological changes are largely protective of the fetus. The modified immune state of a pregnant woman, however, can cause special considerations for bioterrorism, both in planning and preparedness as well as response. Not only are pregnant women more susceptible to certain infections due to their modified immune status, but certain bioterror agents can be transmitted to the fetus, and some medical treatments for those agents can cause harm.[11-13]

In cases of SARS, viral hemorrhagic fever, and smallpox, pregnant women may have more severe responses than non-pregnant women. In smallpox for instance, maternal mortality may reach 50% where the mortality rates among healthy men and women is around 30%.[11] Also it may be more difficult to diagnose these illnesses in pregnant women than non-pregnant women. Vaccines for illnesses such as smallpox may also be less effective in the pregnant female.[12-13] These and many considerations regarding the prophylaxis, diagnosis, and treatment of women exposed to agents of bioterrorism require clinicians charged with the care of the pregnant female to remain informed regarding the best practices for their care.

Psychosocial Impacts The potential for transgenerational psychological symptomology, as well as "baby booms" following major terrorist events have been discussed by researchers investigating the impact of terrorism on women. There are a variety of psychological and social phenomena that occur in response to a terrorist attack, several involve women and reproductive health that warrant discussion.

Post-traumatic stress disorder (PTSD) as well as other types of acute stress reactions and mood disorders have commonly occurred more frequently in women than in men. It has been suggested that women may be more susceptible to stress, anxiety, and depressive symptoms than men. While these are common and well-described psychological norms, researchers looking into the effects of psychological trauma on women who are pregnant when a traumatic event occurs have described some interesting phenomena.

One investigation evaluated mothers and their 1-year-old children following the 9/11 attacks in the United States. Mothers and their babies were tested for salivary cortisol levels and their samples collected. The cortisol levels were lower in mothers and their babies who developed post-traumatic stress disorder following the 9/11 attacks compared to mothers who did not have PTSD symptoms. Low cortisol levels have been associated with risk for development of PTSD. This may suggest that pregnant women who developed PTSD following 9/11 may have caused a biological vulnerability for the development of acute stress reactions in their infant children.[14]

Two additional studies are relevant. A study in the *Journal of Psychosomatic Research* evaluated the birth weight of infants born to women in the Netherlands who were pregnant during the 9/11 attacks in the United States and compared these birth weights with those one year later. Researchers found that pregnant women exposed to the 9/11 attacks through the media had infants with lower overall birth weights and shorter pregnancies than the birth weights of infants born one year later. This finding suggests that the psychological impact of terrorist attacks, even vicariously, can impact reproductive health.[15] A similar study suggests that mothers pregnant during the 9/11 attacks and having symptoms of post-traumatic stress birthed infants with lower head circumference than mothers without symptoms of post-traumatic stress, suggesting that psychological stress effects neurocognitive development.[16]

Researchers looking at the impact of the Madrid train bombings in March 2004 on pregnant females report that these women experienced an increase in the number of term pregnancies presenting at hospitals with premature rupture of the membranes in the days following the attacks. This was not the result of a physical effect on pregnant women who were victims of the bombings.[17] Although the authors of this study admit that they are uncertain what caused this to occur, some have suggested that this may be due to the effects that psychological stress plays on the pregnant female.

In addition to the direct effect traumatization can have on mothers and infants, psychological stress put on women by society can cause psychological health impacts. Researchers investigated the relationship between Arabic-named women and poor birth outcomes following the 9/11 attacks. They hypothesized that experiences of discrimination increased the risk of preterm birth and low birth weight. They found an elevated relative risk of poor birth outcomes in the population studied compared with the population at large following the 9/11 attacks.[18]

In contrast, terrorism can cause families to change their priorities and encourage closeness and bonding between loved ones. Combined with the social anxiety and fear that is sometimes caused after a terrorist attack, this can cause people to spend more time at home rather than go out to public places or locations that (in the mind of the individual) may seem more susceptible to another terror incident. This need for closeness, combined with spending more time indoors, can also have interesting effects following a terrorist event.

In the United States, following both the bombing of the Oklahoma City federal building in 1995 as well as in the months after the September 11 attacks, researchers described an increase in overall births, increase in pregnancy tests, and an increase in the sale of books for expectant mothers. A "baby boomlet" had been described in both cases and may be related to the desire for individuals to rediscover the importance of family or simply is the result of spending increased amounts of time at home with loved ones.[19-20]

Terrorism and the Girl Child

Children as Perpetrators

Children are in many ways as vulnerable as women to recruitment, exploitation, and manipulation by terrorists and terrorist groups. Female adolescents can be used and exploited sexually in many of the same ways as older females. There have been increased reports, particularly in Iraq, of terror organizations recruiting teenage boys to participate in terror attacks including suicide bombings.

Children serve many of the same tactical advantages to terrorists as women. They can often enter an area under less scrutiny by police, military, or security officials. They are generally psychologically coercible and easy to brainwash or manipulate into performing the acts requested by the handler or facilitators. Children can be threatened with harm to their families or loved ones and coerced into performing requested activities. Many teenage boys develop their first relationships with militants by performing passive support activities such as serving as scouts, messengers, or spies. Additionally, by being of less interest to security personnel, children and teens are often allowed more access to locations of interest to the terrorist cause.

Al-Qaida has reportedly started a terrorist group called the Young People of Paradise that is formed of children in their midteens who are being groomed to become terrorists. Some of the members of this group have been reported to be undergoing training as suicide bombers.

Children as Targets of Terrorism

Children have been among the victims of terrorist attacks in virtually every country affected by terrorism. Some terrorist groups have chosen to target children in their attacks owing to the overwhelmingly emotional and powerful societal response a mass attack on children elicits. The school attack and hostage taking in Beslan, Russia, in September 2004 showed the lengths that terrorist groups will go to instill fear into the heart of society by striking at its most vulnerable population. Terrorism affects children in different ways than it affects adults. Children process and handle terrorist events differently than adults. This section explores the unique impact terrorism has on children and how we can improve resiliency among our most vulnerable population.

There are many unique considerations for terrorism on children. Children are at particular risk for morbidity and mortality secondary to terrorism for a variety of physiological, developmental, and clinical reasons. Children are not just small adults. They interact with their environment in different ways than adults, and as such, are more at risk for exposure to agents of terrorism and have developed fewer defense mechanisms to protect themselves from the aftermath. Below we will discuss how children are different than adults in how weapons of mass destruction (WMD) agents and materials affect their health. Weapons of mass destruction agents and materials consist of chemical agents, biological agents, radiological materials, nuclear weapons, and incendiary or explosive devices.

Similar to an adult, the effects or impact of an improvised explosive device (IED) on children is directly proportional to how close the child is to the bomb when detonation occurs. Injury severity scores (ISS) and mortality rates are generally highest among the persons closer to the explosive device during detonation. The effects on a child would be similar in presentation as an adult in the sense that there would be three levels or classifications of injuries: primary injuries consisting of trauma caused by the blast pressure wave, causing damage to internal hollow organs such as the lungs, GI tract, sinuses, ear drums and internal hollow organs; secondary injuries or trauma caused by blunt or penetrating objects from the fragmentation of debris propelled away from the device; and tertiary injuries resulting from blunt or penetrating trauma occurring from the force of the blast wave propelling a victim into a stationary object. Although the injury profiles are similar to adults based on the proximity to the explosion, children are much more severely affected by traumatic injury and have less ability to physiologically compensate for hypoperfusion or shock than adults. Lack of available specialized pediatric trauma care and resuscitation can increase mortality in the severely injured child.

In chemical, biological, and radiological terrorism, agents and materials are different and each certainly has unique considerations for both adult and child victims. However, all three are dependent on a fundamental law of toxicology in order to cause human health effects: The dose makes the poison. The dose, for most toxic agents or materials, is almost always lower in children than in adults. However, all chemical, biological, and radiological agents and materials are reliant on the principles of exposure and dose/response. A susceptible individual must be exposed to a sufficient quantity of agent over a short enough duration in order to produce a health effect. Because of their unique physical, developmental, physiological, and psychological characteristics, children are af-fected faster and more severely than adults to these agents and materials.[21]

Physically and developmentally, children are smaller than adults. This means that their mobility and motor skills are less adept than older individuals. Where an adult can "run away" from a hazard, children are less able to do so with speed. A child cannot run as fast, as far, or as long as an adult. This can lead to a child remaining in an area with a higher concentration of a toxic agent or materials for a longer period of time, increasing exposure to the poison and increasing their overall dose. Children also, due to their psychosocial and cognitive development, lack the ability to perceive and characterize risk.[21] An adult can rapidly assess a situation, identify a hazardous condition or presence of danger, and then instinctively activate the fight-or-flight response causing the adult to rapidly flee the dangerous situation. A child lacks the ability to characterize danger. To characterize our own risk to a particular circumstance, we must first identify a hazardous or dangerous condition and associate it with our (or another's) vulnerability or susceptibility to that hazard or danger. This allows us to cognitively determine if we or others are at risk or are in jeopardy of imminent physical harm, forming a rudimentary risk estimate. Children do not have this ability owing to immature cognitive or psychosocial development. For example, why would a child put her hand on a hot stove? If she is unable to perceive the heat or stove as a potential danger capable of causing physical harm, she cannot keep herself safe and will burn her hand. Lack of risk perception can cause a child to remain in a dangerous situation or environment for longer than they should be, potentially exposing themselves to danger or harm for a greater period of time. A child's innate curiosity can exacerbate this problem.

Another characteristic of children that makes them more susceptible to chemical and biological terrorism is their small size but large body surface area compared to their mass. As certain chemicals can be absorbed through skin and nonintact or poorly protected skin can absorb infectious agents or materials, a child's skin is particularly vulnerable to chemical and biological agents. Large body surface area can cause children to dissipate or lose body heat more rapidly than adults. This is a consideration whenever a child requires decontamination after exposure to a hazardous substance.

Exposing the child to cold or even cool or tepid water in the ambient environment can cause hypothermia and accelerate the worsening of their clinical condition.[21]

Other physiological characteristics of children that make them more susceptible to WMD agents is their high respiratory rate. A child breathes more times in a minute than an adult. This can cause the child to inhale more of a chemical substance in the same time frame than an adult. Combine this with the fact that children will experience symptoms at lower doses than adults due to their lower body mass, and you will find that children can become incapacitated more quickly and at lower doses than adults. Certain toxic chemicals or terrorist chemical agents such as persistent nerve agents, chlorine, and others, can settle to the ground because of their relatively heavy vapor densities. Vapor clouds that are closer to the ground are likely to be in the breathing zones of children and can affect them more quickly than adults.[21]

Finally, when considering the effects of biological and radiological agents on children, fluid loss and respiratory compromise are of particular concern. Children become dehydrated more readily than adults and lack the fluid reserves that adults have. This means that a child can go into hypovolemic shock more quickly than an adult due to excessive vomiting and/or diarrhea, and are in more need of aggressive fluid resuscitation in a hospital.[21]

Psychosocial Effects of Terrorist Attacks

In addition to the physiological effects of terrorism agents on children, the psychological effects of terrorism can affect children in different ways than adults as well. Several researchers have evaluated the psychological impact of certain terrorist events on children. Two studies evaluated how children psychologically cope with terrorism in relationship to how their parents cope. One set of investigators in the United States after the terror attacks of 9/11, showed that adolescents indirectly exposed to the 9/11 attacks exhibited post-traumatic stress symptoms greater when their parents were unavailable to discuss the attacks with them.[22] In another study that looked at the effect of state terrorism and displacement on Guatemalan refugee children, authors reported that there was a positive association with a child's mental health and the overall health status of their mothers. Researchers found that particularly with the girl child, there was a correlation between depressive symptoms and poor health status in their mothers.[23]

In other studies that looked at the resiliency of adolescents to terrorism we notice some differences between the psychological impact of girls and boys. Earlier we mentioned how women are generally more susceptible than men to post-traumatic stress symptoms and in general, depression and anxiety. A study that evaluated the effects of psychological stress on the survivors of the Beslan, Russia, school attacks showed that among adolescents surveyed by the authors one year after the incident, girls reported significantly more psychological distress than boys.[24] Although this is consistent with the findings from a study in Israel, authors there noted an interesting difference among how boys and girls are affected psychologically. The investigators examined adolescent boys and girls who have exposure to ongoing terrorism. The investigators were able to show that although girls show greater severity of PTSD symptoms, boys with symptoms have more functional impairment in social and family domains.[25] Finally, researchers were able to show that among adolescent girls living in areas prone to acts of terrorism, they had less severe post-traumatic stress symptoms and were more willing to make personal sacrifices for their country than girls who did not live in areas prone to terrorism.[26] This may show an increased resilience or sensitization of adolescent girls in this area to terrorism and allow them to develop coping strategies to overcome the continued psychological stressors.

Conclusion

A greater understanding of the psychosocial, behavioral, and socioeconomic factors that influence women and children to become active supporters, facilitators, and/or perpetrators of terrorist acts is essential to mitigating these incidents and protecting the health and safety of the public. Further research is needed to explore methods to identify women who may be vulnerable to recruitment by terrorist groups. Also needed is programmatic research for the design, development, and piloting of effective intervention programs targeted at populations of women susceptible to recruitment or coercion by terrorist groups in order to limit the extent of these attacks on nations across the globe.

As children are uniquely susceptible to acts of terrorism, more should be done to prepare the adults charged with their safety and security to be able to plan for the children's safety and respond to their needs during a crisis. Training medical professionals, teachers, parents, law enforcement officials, and community leaders how to respond to and protect, as well as how to anticipate and prepare for the needs of, those most susceptible in our population, is essential in minimizing the morbidity and mortality of a terrorist attack involving our children.

DISCUSSION QUESTIONS

1. Discuss reasons that terrorist groups would want to utilize women to conduct terrorist attacks.
2. In what ways are women motivated (internally and externally) to participate in terrorism?
3. Describe the unique physical vulnerabilities women possess that make them more susceptible to morbidity and mortality from terrorist incidents.
4. In what ways have women supported terrorist activities?
5. Discuss how psychosocial factors may contribute to women's vulnerability to terrorism.
6. Describe the physical and psychological characteristics of children that influence how they are affected by terrorism.
7. Describe and suggest strategies that could modify the vulnerabilities associated with women and children being motivated to participate in terrorist activities.
8. In what ways would a woman's role in society affect her vulnerability to terrorism? How could changing societal views modify these vulnerabilities?

REFERENCES

1. Berko A, Erez E. Women in terrorism: a Palestinian feminist revolution or gender oppression. International Institute for Counter-Terrorism. http://www.ict .org.il/apage/printv/9102.php. December 6, 2006. Accessed May 14, 2008.
2. Caiazza A. Why gender matters in understanding September 11: Women, militarism, and violence. IWPR Publication #1908. 2001.
3. Abdullaev N. Unraveling Chechen 'black widows'. *Homeland Defense J.* 2007; 5:18-21.
4. Israeli Ministry of Foreign Affairs. The role of Palestinian women in suicide terrorism. [MFA Archives]. January 30, 2003. http://www.mfa.gov.il/MFA /MFAArchive/2000_2009/2003/1. Accessed April 30, 2008.

5. Davis J. *Women and Terrorism in Radical Islam: Planners, Perpetrators, Patrons?* Halifax, Nova Scotia: Dalhousie University, Center for Foreign Policy Studies; 2006.

6. Israeli Ministry of Foreign Affairs. Blackmailing young women into suicide terrorism. [Government Communiqués]. February 12, 2002. http://www.mfa.gov.il /MFA/Government/Communiques/2003/. Accessed April 30, 2008.

7. Sela HY, Shveiky D, Laufer N, Hersch M, Einav S. Pregnant women injured in terror-related multiple casualty incidents: injuries and outcomes. *J Trauma.* 2008; 64:727-732.

8. Wolff MS, Teitelbaum SL, Lioy PJ, et al. Exposures among pregnant women near the World Trade Center site on 11 September 2001. *Environ Health Perspect.* 2005;113:739-748.

9. Lederman SA, Rauh V, Weiss L, et al. The effects of the World Trade Center event on birth outcomes among term deliveries at three lower Manhattan hospitals. *Environ Health Perspect.* 2004;112:1772-1778.

10. Perera FP, Tang D, Rauh V, et al. Relationship between polycyclic aromatic hydrocarbon-DNA adducts, environmental tobacco smoke, and child development in the World Trade Center cohort. *Environ Health Perspect.* 2007;115:1497-1502.

11. White SR, Henretig FM, Dukes RG. Medical management of vulnerable populations and co-morbid conditions of victims of bioterrorism. *Emerg Med Clin North Am.* 2002;2:365-392.

12. Jamieson DJ, Jernigan DB, Ellis JE, Treadwell TA. Emerging infections and pregnancy: West Nile virus, monkeypox, severe acute respiratory syndrome, and bioterrorism. *Clin Perinatol.* 2005;32:765-776.

13. Suarez VR, Hankins GD. Smallpox and pregnancy: from eradicated disease to bioterrorist threat. *Obstet Gynecol.* 2002;100:87-93.

14. Yehuda R, Engel SM, Brand SR, Seckl J, Marcus SM, Berkowitz GS. Transgenerational effects of posttraumatic stress disorder in babies of mothers exposed to the World Trade Center attacks during pregnancy. *J Clin Endocrinol Metab.* 2005; 90:4115-4118.

15. Smits L, Krabbendam L, de Bie R, Essed G, van Os J. Lower birth weight of Dutch neonates who were in utero at the time of the 9/11 attacks. *J Psychosom Res.* 2006;61:715-717.

16. Engel SM, Berkowitz GS, Wolff MS, Yehuda R. Psychological trauma associated with the World Trade Center attacks and its effect on pregnancy outcome. *Paediatr Perinat Epidemiol.* 2005;19:334-341.

17. Santos-Leal E, Vidart-Aragon JA, Coronado-Martin P, Herraiz-Martinez MA, Odent MR. Premature rupture of membranes and Madrid terrorist attack. *Birth.* 2006;33:341.

18. Lauderdale DS. Birth outcomes for Arabic-named women in California before and after September 11. *Demography.* 2006;43:185-201.

19. Scelfo J. A 9-11 Baby Boomlet. Newsweek [serial online]. 2002;139:42. http://search.ebscohost.com/login.aspx?direct=true&db=mfh&AN=6718464&site=ehost-live. Accessed May 29, 2008.

20. Rodgers JL, St John CA, Coleman R. Did fertility go up after the Oklahoma City bombing? An analysis of births in metropolitan counties in Oklahoma, 1990-1999. *Demography.* 2005;42:675-692.

21. Markenson D, Redlener I. Pediatric preparedness for disasters and terrorism. Paper presented at: National Consensus Conference; March 2007; Watergate Hotel and Conference Center, Washington, DC, 2005.

22. Gil-Rivas V, Silver RC, Holman EA, McIntosh DN, Poulin M. Parental response

and adolescent adjustment to the September 11, 2001 terrorist attacks. *J Trauma Stress.* 2007;20:1063-1068.

23. Miller KE. The effects of state terrorism and exile on indigenous Guatemalan refugee children: a mental health assessment and an analysis of children's narratives. *Child Dev.* 1996;67:89-106.

24. Moscardino U, Scrimin S, Capello F, Altoè G, Axia G. Psychological adjustment of adolescents 18 months after the terrorist attack in Beslan, Russia: a cross-sectional study. *J Clin Psychiatry.* 2008;69:854-859.

25. Pat-Horenczyk R, Abramovitz R, Peled O, Brom D , Daie A, Chemtob CM. Adolescent exposure to recurrent terrorism in Israel: posttraumatic distress and functional impairment. *Am J Orthopsychiatry.* 2007;77:76-85.

26. Laor N, Wolmer L, Alon M, Siev J, Samuel E, Toren P. Risk and protective factors mediating psychological symptoms and ideological commitment of adolescents facing continuous terrorism. *J Nerv Ment Dis.* 2006;194:279-286.

CHAPTER 4

War, Women, and Girls

Mary-Wynne Ashford, MD, PhD

Mary-Wynne Ashford, MD, PhD is the former Co-President of the International Physicians for the Prevention of Nuclear War in Victoria, BC, Canada. She is also a Winner of Gandhi Award from Simon Fraser University, and the Governor General of Canada's Medal.

INTRODUCTION

For centuries women and children, especially girl children, have faced unimaginable violence and deprivation in wartime. Like domestic violence, gender-based violence in war was cloaked in silence. Now the cloak has been lifted and the utter depravity of war exposed. As much as battle is part of the story of war, so is the torture, mutilation, rape, displacement, and enslavement of women and children. Today about 90% of those who die in war are civilians, and the majority are women and children.[2]

The number of wars in the world has been decreasing since the end of the Cold War,[3] and new ways of resolving international conflict are evolving. The challenge of addressing gender-based violence must be discussed in this new context because many social movements are converging to bring human rights and the rights of women and children into discussions of peace and security.

The Centre for Human Security at the University of British Columbia reports that since 1991, the number of major wars and genocides has decreased by 90%, and the number of wars in general has decreased by 40%.[3] Fledgling democracies have appeared in many countries. Sixty dictators have been toppled, with only Romania having significant violence. The Centre concludes that the world appears to be turning away from war, and they attribute this change to the strengthening of international law, the successes of the United Nations, and the growing influence of civil society. Although they do not list the empowerment of women as a factor, the significance of women's actions in conflict resolution and peace building is increasingly recognized through the United Nations system.

Largely as a result of the efforts of the women's human rights movement, Amnesty International and other organizations, gender-based offenses are specifically enumerated in the Rome Statute of the International Criminal Court.[4] The offenses explicitly included within the jurisdiction of the court include rape, sexual slavery, enforced prostitution, forced pregnancy, enforced sterilization, and "other forms of sexual violence."[5]

The world reached a great turning point on October 31, 2000. That was the day the United

I sense that the time has come for the growing and hardy band of women legislators to demand that governments everywhere get their priorities right and recognize that if we want peace and human security in the world, we must replace the culture of war with the culture of peace. I am not saying that a world run by women would necessarily be a completely peaceful world, but my political and diplomatic experience indicates to me that the prospects of achieving a more humane world would improve with more women in the decision-making processes of governments.

Senator Douglas Roche's last speech to the
Canadian Senate, March 30, 2004[1]

Nations Security Council unanimously passed Resolution 1325.[6] It is the first resolution ever passed by the Security Council that specifically addresses the impact of war on women and women's contributions to conflict resolution and sustainable peace. The story of Resolution 1325 is cause for optimism that we are beginning to make progress in the struggle to protect women and girls, and in the larger context, to prevent war itself.

Resolution 1325

Women's organizations have been active observers and participants in UN activities for peace and disarmament for many decades. The NGO Working Group on Women, Peace, and Security formed in May 2000 to call for a Security Council resolution that would increase the participation of women in prevention, resolution, and healing of armed conflict.[7] Although civil society groups cannot make presentations to the Security Council in its chambers, the Council agreed to hear the presentations in a building across the street from UN headquarters. When they returned to their chambers, the Council immediately passed the resolution.

Implementation of the resolution has been very slow, but the synergy between women's organizations and supportive governments—Friends of 1325—is beginning to bear fruit. The long years of struggle to ensure equal rights and opportunities for women and girls seem to be paying off as both international law and public opinion shift toward justice. In the words of the Coalition for Women for a Just Peace, "The age of the generals has ended; the era of women has begun."[8] Women are beginning to share leadership in governance in many countries, and women's values are influencing decision makers even in male-dominated societies.

The doors were open just wide enough for women to squeeze into a Security Council debate. But concerned women and men must act upon the words of Resolution 1325 and use those words and those stacks of papers to jam the doors permanently open and to enter the rooms where peace agreements are negotiated and into the rooms where peacekeeping operations are planned.[9]

The Impact of War on Women and Girl Children

When the Security Council passed Resolution 1325, independent experts began an assessment on the impact of armed conflict on women and women's role in peace building. Their report was released in 2002.

Violence against women in conflict is one of history's great silences. We were completely unprepared for the searing magnitude of what we saw and heard in the conflict and postconflict areas we visited. We knew the data, but knowing all this did not prepare us for the horrors women described: Wombs punctured with guns. Women raped and tortured in front of their husbands and children. Rifles forced into vaginas. Pregnant women beaten to induce miscarriages. Fetuses ripped from wombs. Women kidnapped, blindfolded, and beaten on their way to work or school. We saw the scars, the pain, and the humiliation. We saw the scars of brutality so extreme that survival seemed for some a worse fate than death.[9]

In spite of the horrific violations of human rights described by the independent experts, they also commented that women must not be regarded as helpless victims in wartime. They were awed by the courage and dignity shown by many women who, in the most dangerous circumstances, stood up for justice and human rights. The NGO Working Group on Women, Peace, and Security reports on actions that demonstrate the essential place of women in stopping violence and reconciling enemies.[10]

We organized a silent march to protest the war and the use of rape as a weapon. One thousand women participated—an extraordinary number given Bougainville's small population. We were stopped by the Papua New Guinea Defence Force twice. They wanted to arrest someone and asked, "Who is your leader?" We said, "All of us are leaders. We all own this march." The soldiers couldn't arrest anyone. . . . We walked silently carrying banners we had sewn by hand, with messages of peace . . .

Our sisters in Rabaul were so moved by the story that they organized a boat and sailed through Buka Passage, singing peace songs. There was shooting on both sides of the passage before the women arrived. As they sailed through, the shooting stopped. Their singing stopped the guns. It was the women who risked going out into the jungle to persuade our sons, husbands, and brothers to avert war. It was the women who really made peace, not the menfolk. They were busy killing, destroying, and raping women.

—Helen Hakena, Leitana Nehan
Women's Development Agency,
Bougainville, 2003[11]

War evokes extremes of depraved and brutal behavior both from individuals and groups. In particular, war disinhibits cruel and inhuman actions toward the physically weak and vulnerable: women, children, the disabled, and the elderly. For thousands of years women and girl children have been regarded as part of the booty of war. There is even a proverb, "To the victor go the spoils." Taking women and children as slaves and concubines has been regarded as normal behavior in war. A US Marine Corps drill instructor has been quoted as saying:

"This is the reality of war. We Marines like war. We like killing. We like raping females. This is what we do."[12]

Women and children have no voice in the decisions that lead to armed conflict but must suffer the consequences of being targeted. When we hear horrifying accounts of genocide, rape of women and children, forced pregnancy or abortion, torture, mutilation, and enslavement, we are shocked and sickened, but such atrocities are not new. In fact, war is characterized by behavior so abhorrent that most people have difficulty seeing that it is part of a recurrent pattern. The build up of hostility, spread of hate propaganda, dehumanization of enemy, justification of murder and torture, and violations of the rights of women and children are steps on the path to killing. Preventing war means challenging deeply held beliefs and customs that are supported by the glorification of violence.

War is the extreme expression of a culture of violence that has dominated the world for 5000 years. Changing this culture requires deep social change in attitudes and behaviors steeped in tradition and sometimes in religious practices. The problem we face is not that laws are needed to protect women and children in times of armed conflict, but that the conventions and treaties that exist must be enforced. Many of the legal instruments that protect women and children in times of war and complex emergencies are described in Chapter 5, "Women and Children in War and Complex Emergencies: Human Rights, the Humanitarian Endeavor And Progress Towards Equality."

Precombat

Before combat begins there are gender-specific signs that warn of impending conflict: propaganda emphasizing hypermasculinity, gender-specific unemployment, growth of fundamentalism, increase in households headed by single women, perception of women as property, trafficking of women, prostitution, increased sale of valuables, and increased domestic violence.[13]

Active Combat Period

Bombing civil infrastructure is a strategy of war that is often portrayed by military officials as causing few civilian casualties. In fact, this ruthless strategy amounts to a war on public health.[14] Destroying the electricity grid, sewage treatment plants, water purification, and food distribution systems plunges the society into misery, malnutrition, and disease. Concurrent sanctions prevent the reconstruction of the infrastructure because essential materials and equipment are banned or blockaded.

As able-bodied men leave for battle, women are left to care for the children, the elderly, and infirm. Without income, many must turn to prostitution to provide for their dependents. In a daily struggle for survival women leave the relative security of their homes, risking attack in order to forage for food and fuel for cooking and heating.[15] The lack of essential medicines, vaccines, and safe water leads to respiratory and diarrheal illnesses that claim the lives of countless children.

Displaced Persons and Refugees

Women and children make up 75–80% of the approximately 21 million refugees worldwide.[16] In refugee camps, vulnerable and unprotected, women are often subjected to violence and rape by warlords who control food and protection. Maternal and infant mortality is high in conflict zones and refugee camps. Pregnant women forced to deliver their babies in unsanitary conditions, usually without birth attendants, are at high risk of suffering traumatic birth injuries and death of the infant. The spread of sexually transmitted diseases including HIV/AIDS is increased in conflict zones.

The Joint United Nations Programme on HIV/AIDS (UNAIDS) reports that rates of sexually transmitted infections among military populations in peacetime are generally two to five times higher than in civilian populations. During war, they can be 50 or more times higher.[10]

In countries where genital mutilation is common, rape is particularly devastating because it often involves forced penetration with a sharp object, causing tearing of the vaginal opening.[16] Fistulas often result from this trauma or from injuries during delivery. Women with fistulas are incontinent of urine and/or feces and are usually rejected by their husbands and often excluded from their communities. Repairing fistulas requires lengthy, specialized care that is only available in large medical centers.

Women as Combatants

Although women in some countries may become combatants because they have been abducted, many women in other countries enlist in the military voluntarily. Some have a desire to serve their country; others want to gain an education or trade. Some seek adventure or travel. Armed forces must adapt to the different needs and capabilities of women and to the issues arising when women are added to units that are predominantly male. In recent years, increasing numbers of women in the US armed forces have pressed charges of sexual harassment, rape, and assault against men in their units. Many others do not press charges because they fear they will not be believed, that charges will not be taken seriously, and that they will suffer reprisals for lodging complaints.[12]

Brigadier General Janis Karpinski, the highest-ranking official to lose a job because of the Abu Ghraib prison scandal, testified at the Commission of Inquiry for Crimes Against Humanity Committed by the Bush administration. She reported that a surgeon for the coalition's joint task force said in a briefing that several women in the US armed forces in Iraq died of dehydration in the extreme heat because they stopped drinking fluids in the late afternoon, despite temperatures up to 120° F. The women were afraid that if they needed to use the latrine in the night, they would be assaulted and raped. Karpinski alleged that on the death certificates the cause of death was altered to remove dehydration as a possible factor. These charges have been neither corroborated nor disproven. Kathy Gilber, co-chair of the National Lawyers Guild's Military Task Force, stated that "People who report assaults still face command disbelief, illegal efforts to protect the assaulters, and informal harassment from assaulters, their friends, or the command itself."[18]

Post conflict

At the end of armed conflict, combatants, child soldiers, and camp followers who have, voluntarily or involuntarily, provided services to combatants must be reintegrated into their communities. The tolerance of brutality and killing often continues in the aftermath of combat; many people suffer from post-traumatic stress syndrome; weapons are freely available, but paid work is not. Domestic violence increases even in the countries that have been victorious.[19] Women who have been sexually assaulted may be excluded from their community, and gender-based violence continues with impunity.

Military families are at high risk for spousal abuse even in peacetime. In 2002, there were more than 18,000 incidents of spousal abuse reported to the Family Advocacy Program of the US Department of Defense, 84% of which involved physical abuse.[20] The Pentagon has disclosed that, on average, one child or spouse dies each week at the hands of a relative in the US military.[21]

Resolution 1325 refers specifically to the problems resulting from antipersonnel landmines that remain in the ground long after a ceasefire. International law requires that after the end of armed conflict, the army that laid landmines must remove them or at least provide a map of their location. In practice this requirement is rarely fulfilled. Cluster munitions act as landmines when up to 30% of the hundreds of small bomblets dropped in one large bomb fail to explode and lie on the ground until they are triggered—perhaps by the footfall of a soldier, but more likely by a child or a farm animal. In developing countries women are often the farmers who must return to the fields where landmines have been left.

Women's Role in Conflict Resolution, Reconciliation, and Peace Building

Quietly and not so quietly there is a global movement growing: a movement of local, regional and international civil society alliances which have identified the inclusion of women and gender perspectives in all aspects of peace building as imperative to the maintenance of international peace and security.

—Gina Torry, Coordinator of the
NGO Working Group on Women, Peace,
and Security reporting to the 52nd Session
of the Commission on the Status
of Women, 2008.[22]

Women are underrepresented in national parliaments in almost every country. In a 2004 survey of 130 countries, only 15.4% of the elected seats were held by women. The United Nations Development Program concluded that 30% would be the minimum representation required for women as a group to exert meaningful influence in legislative assemblies. In three post-conflict societies women's representation is greatly improved as a result of including electoral measures as part of peace processes. In Rwanda 48.8% of seats are held by women, in South Africa 32.8%, and in Mozambique 30%.[23]

Women have made significant advances in political leadership in recent years. In December 2005, Ellen Johnson-Sirleaf, a Harvard-educated economist, was elected president of Liberia, and in January 2006, Michelle Bachelet was elected president of Chile.[24] Bachelet is a surgeon, pediatri-

cian, and epidemiologist with training in military strategy. She was previously minister of defense. In that position she promoted reconciliation between the military and victims of the dictatorship. The result was a historic declaration that never again would the military subvert democracy in Chile. Bachelet appointed a cabinet of equal numbers of men and women.

In April, 2008 Prime Minister Jose Luis Rodriguez Zapatero of Spain appointed Carme Chacon as defense minister—a 37-year old woman, then 7-months pregnant. Zapatero chose a cabinet of nine women and eight men, continuing his previous policy of gender parity in the cabinet.[25]

Building participatory democracies in which women have full rights and opportunities to vote and stand for elected office is an important step toward sustainable peace. Recent research comparing the status of women over a 30-year period in countries with or without internal war shows that the more equal the society, the less likely it is to use military force.[26] Researchers inferred the status of women from the length of time women had the vote, the fertility rate, percentage of women in the labor force, and percentage of women in the national legislature. Fertility rate is a variable related to women's status, education, empowerment, and employment. Nations with high fertility rates are nearly twice as likely to experience internal conflict as those with low fertility rates.

In general, where most women participate fully in the work force, the country is far less likely to experience internal war than where women are restricted from working outside the home.

"States (nations) characterized by gender discrimination and structural hierarchy are permeated with norms of violence that make internal conflict more likely."[27] As more women participate in governance, a country is more likely to use nonviolent means to resolve conflict. Five percent fewer women in the national legislature correlated with an almost five times greater likelihood of the use of military force.

After the genocide, women rolled up their sleeves and began making society work again.

—Paul Kagame, President of Rwanda [28]

Because so many men were lost in the Rwandan genocide, women had to step into leadership positions. Aloisea Inyumba, for example, at the age of 26, became minister of gender and social affairs, where she was responsible for creating programs to bury 800,000 dead, to find homes for more than 500,000 orphaned children, and resettle refugees. She also created women's councils that fed into the parliament, resulting in the highest percentage of women legislators in the world.[28]

In Cambodia, Nanda Pok leads an organization to train women to hold political office. More than 5000 women have been trained, including 64% of the women elected to local councils in 2002.[28] In the economic sphere, Cambodian women are now being trained as experts in the removal of land mines because the millions of mines left in Cambodia have made farms unworkable. Women are willing to take on this dangerous work not only because there are few jobs for women, but because the work restores the land to productivity.

In Somalia, women were excluded from peace negotiations because only representatives of the five clans were allowed at the table. The women, who crossed clans, asked that they be recognized as a clan themselves. The group agreed, and the women contributed to the negotiations and were able to secure 12% of the seats in the transitional government.[29]

In his June 19, 2008, remarks to the Security Council meeting on women, peace, and security, Secretary General Ban Ki-Moon said "We must do far more to involve women in conflict prevention, peace negotiations, and recovery after the guns fall silent." He called for member states to come forward with more women candidates. He referred to the all female Indian civil police unit in the United Nations mission in Liberia as a possible model for the central role of women in restoring stability in war-ravaged countries.[30]

Signs of Progress

On June 19, 2008, in a follow up to Resolution 1325, the Security Council unanimously adopted Resolution 1820 demanding the immediate and complete cessation, by all parties, of armed conflict and all acts of sexual violence against civilians.[31] The council expressed its deep concern that, despite repeated condemnation, violence and sexual abuse of women and children trapped in war zones was not only continuing, but, in some cases, had become so widespread and systematic as to "reach appalling levels of brutality."[31]

Resolution 1820 notes that rape and other forms of sexual violence can constitute a war crime, a crime against humanity, or a constitutive act with respect to genocide. This emphasizes the need for the exclusion of sexual violence crimes from amnesty provisions in the context of conflict resolution processes, and calls upon member states to comply with their obligations for prosecuting persons responsible for such acts, to ensure that all victims of sexual violence, particularly women and girls, have equal protection under the law and equal access to justice, and emphasizes the importance of ending impunity for such acts as part of a comprehensive approach to seeking sustainable peace, justice, truth, and national reconciliation.

Conclusion

Social movements for human rights, prevention of war, protection of the environment, and the advancement of women bring the influence of civil society to bear on decision makers in governments, international law, and the economic sector. The convergence of these movements supports the deep cultural change needed for women, peace, and security. While we must not forget the horror of continuing violence and abuse of women and children worldwide, and we must not relax in our efforts toward justice, we can be justified in cautious optimism that real change has begun.

DISCUSSION QUESTIONS

1. If you were appointed as the UN Secretary General's Special Advisor on Women and War, what would be your first priority for action?

2. What do you consider to be the major obstacles delaying the meaningful implementation of SC Resolution 1325?

3. Do you think that increasing the number of women in the world's military forces contributes to the advancement of society? Why or why not?

4. The UN reports that 70% of people working for peace and social justice are women. Why do you think more women than men commit themselves to these issues?

REFERENCES

1. Roche D. Women, peace and security. Canadian voice of women for peace. http://home.ca.inter.net/~vow/senRoche.htm. Accessed July 9, 2008.

2. Garfield RM, Neugut AI. The human consequences of war. In: Levy BS, Sidel VW, eds. *War and Public Health,* New York, NY: Oxford University Press; 1997:27-38.

3. Mack A, Nielsen Z, eds. *Human Security Report: War and Peace in the 21st Century.* Vancouver, BC: Oxford University Press; 2005.

4. Making rights a reality: violence against women in armed conflict. Amnesty International. 2005. http://www.amnesty.org/en/library/asset/ACT77/050/2005/en/dom-ACT770502005en.pdf. Accessed July 9, 2008.

5. Rome Statute of the International Criminal Court, adopted on 17 July 1998, UN Doc. A/CONF:183/9, entered into force on 1 July 2002. http://www.un.org/law/icc/statute/romefra.htm. Accessed July 9, 2008.

6. United Nations Security Council Resolution 1325 on women, peace and security. Peace Women, Women's International League for Peace and Freedom. http://www.peacewomen.org/un/sc/1325.html. Accessed July 9, 2008.

7. No Women, No Peace: The importance of women's participation to achieve peace and security. NGO Working Group on Women, Peace and Security. April, 2004. http://www.peacewomen.org/news/1325News/Issue%2040.pdf. Accessed July 9, 2008.

8. Coalition for Women for a Just Peace. http://www.fire.or.cr/junio01/coalition.htm. Accessed July 9, 2008.

9. Poehlman-Doumbouya S, Hill F. Women and peace in the United Nations. Life and Peace Institute, New Routes. 2001;6(3):28-32. http://www.life-peace.org/sajt/filer/pdf/New_Routes/nr200103.pdf. Accessed July 9, 2008.

10. Rehn E, Sirleaf EJ. *Women, War, Peace: The Independent Experts' Assessment on the Impact of Armed Conflict on Women and Women's Role in Peace-Building.* New York, NY: United Nations Development Fund for Women (UNIFEM); 2002.

11. Hakena H. In: *No Women, No Peace: The Importance of Women's Participation to Achieve Peace and Security.* NGO Working Group on Women, Peace and Security for the UN Secretary-General's High-Level Panel on Threats, Challenges and Change. April 2004. http://www.ipb.org/gender2.html. Accessed July 8, 2008.

12. Allison A. An excellent reason not to join the military. 2006. http://www.wiretapmag.org/stories/35792. Accessed July 9, 2008.

13. McPhedran M, Sherret L, Bond J. R2P, Responsibility to Protect Missing Women—Canada's responsibility to perceive. In: *Fragile, Dangerous and Failed States: Implementing Canada's International Policy Statement.* Presented at: Fragile States Conference; 2005; Victoria, BC, November, 2005.

14. Mann J, Drucker E, Tarantola D, McCabe MP. Bosnia: the war against public health. *Med Global Survival.* 1994;1:130-146.

15. Patrick E. *Beyond Firewood: Fuel Alternatives and Protection Strategies for Displaced Women and Girls.* New York, NY: Women's Commission for Refugee Women and Girls; 2006.

16. Global refugee trends: statistical overview of populations of refugees, asylum-seekers, internally displaced persons, stateless persons, and other persons of concern to the United Nations High Commissioner for Refugees. June 9, 2006. http://www.unhcr.org. Accessed July 9, 2008.

17. Human Rights Watch. *Sexual Violence in the Context of Refugees.* New York, NY: Human Rights Watch; 1993.

18. Cohn M. Military hides cause of women soldiers' deaths. Truth out. 2006. http://www.truthout.org/article/military-hides-cause-women-soldiers-deaths. Accessed July 9, 2008.

19. Meintjes S, Pillay A, Turshen M, eds. *The Aftermath: Women in Post-Conflict Transformation.* New York, NY: Zed Books; 2001.

20. National Coalition Against Domestic Violence. http://www.ncdsv.org/images/DOMESTICVIOLENCEINMILITARY.pdf. Accessed Setember 21, 2008.

21. Schmitt E. Domestic abuse rising in military, Pentagon says. *New York Times.* 1994;A1-A2.

22. Torry G. An effective place at the table: women's equal participation in peace processes and peacebuilding. NGO Working Group on Women, Peace and Security. 52nd Commission on the Status of Women. 2008. http://www.womenpeacesecurity.org/media/pdf-interactive_dialogue_2008.pdf. Accessed July 9, 2008.

23. Women and elections: guide to promoting the participation of women in elections. United Nations. 2005. http://www.un.org/womenwatch/osagi/wps/publication/WomenAndElections.pdf. Accessed July 9, 2008.

24. Rohter L. Woman in the news: a leader making peace with Chile's past. *New York Times.* January 16, 2006.

25. Woolls D. Spain absorbing shock over pregnant defense minister. Associated Press. *International Business Times.* http://www.ibtimes.com/articles/20080416/spain-absorbing-shock-over-new-pregnant-defense-minister.htm. April 16, 2008. Accessed July 9, 2008.

26. Caprioli M. Gendered conflict. *J Peace Res.* 2000;37:51-68.

27. Caprioli M. Primed for violence: the role of gender inequality in predicting internal conflict. *Int Stud Quarterly.* 2005;49(2):161-178.

28. The vital role of women in peace building. The Initiative for Inclusive Security. Hunt Alternatives Fund. http://www.huntalternatives.org/pages/460_the_vital_role_of_women_in_peace_building.cfm. Accessed July 9, 2008.

29. UNIFEM. Calls for stronger international support for women's participation in peace processes. New Release UNIFEM. 2005. http://www.unifem.org/news_events/story_detail.php?StoryID=258. Accessed July 9, 2008.

30. Ban K-M. Secretary-General United Nations. SG/SM/11647 SC/9365 WOM /1685. http://www.un.org/News/Press/docs/2008/sgsm11647.doc.htm. Accessed July 9, 2008.

31. Security Council SC/9364. Security council demands immediate and complete halt to acts of sexual violence against civilians in conflict zones, unanimously adopting resolution 1820. 2008. http://www.un.org/News/Press/docs/2008 /sc9364.doc.htm. Accessed July 9, 2008.

The Rise of Humanitarianism and a Human Rights Culture

Humanitarian aid and human rights have undergone radical changes in the past 150 years since the formation of the first humanitarian aid agencies. The humanitarian endeavor and the modern humanitarian movement came into being primarily in reaction to the horrors of war perpetuated by sovereign nation-states. It was the memoirs of a young Swiss businessman traveling to do business with Napoleon that helped form the first international humanitarian aid organization. Henry Dunant's account of the pain and despair of wounded soldiers left lying in the battlefield, *A Memoir of Solferino,* became the inspiration for the International Committee for the Red Cross and ultimately resulted in the signing of the Geneva Convention of 1864 that provided for care and respect of wounded soldiers, and the neutrality of ambulances, military hospitals, and staff during battle.

But neither Dunant's ideals nor the original Geneva Convention could fully foresee the extent of the suffering of civilians in war zones or crimes against humanity committed by nation-states or individuals. They could not foresee the atrocities of the Holocaust, the genocides in Cambodia, Bosnia, or Rwanda, or the human rights abuses in Afghanistan, East Timor, or Sudan. They did not foresee gender-based violence being used as a weapon of war—rape, sexual slavery, mutilation, trafficking, forced prostitution, and forced marriage or impregnation of women and children in war. The humanitarian enterprise would have to change and develop in order to address these more complicated human situations.[1] The first Geneva Convention provided for medical aid for wounded combatants and the neutrality of medical staff in war. The three later addendums to the convention would extend aid to sailors wounded in naval battle, provide for protection and medical care of prisoners of war, and the protection and medical care for civilians in armed conflict.

As the world reacted to the atrocities of the Holocaust in which the "suffering inflicted by

Women and Children in War and Complex Emergencies: Human Rights, the Humanitarian Endeavor, and Progress Towards Equality

Ellen C. O'Connell, MA, MPA

Ellen C. O'Connell MHA, MA is the current Vice President of Administration and Board Relations of the International Rescue Committee based in New York, NY.

Hitler fell outside of the realm of expression,"[2] it developed international institutions and universal declarations to address unthinkable crimes against humanity. In doing so, the humanitarian enterprise and the humanitarian mandate were expanded. The most important human rights documents were almost all a result of the atrocities committed during World War II. The Universal Declaration of Human Rights, the International Covenant on Civil and Political Rights, and the International Covenant on Economic, Social, and Cultural Rights, were "all direct products of World War II."[3(p44)] "The same can be said about the most important humanitarian treaty, the Geneva Convention of 1949, and the Nuremberg Principles, which were established in war crimes trials of Nazi leaders after World War II."[3(p44)]

Even the word *genocide* did not exist until after World War II. It was not until 1945 that the word *genocide* was coined by Raphael Lemkin. "Lemkin had hunted for a term that would describe assaults on all aspects of nationhood—physical, biological, political, social, cultural, economic, and religious. He wanted to connote not only full-scale extermination but also Hitler's other means of destruction: mass deportation, the lowering of the birthrate by separating men from women, economic exploitation, progressive starvation, and the suppression of the intelligentsia who served as national leaders."[4]

Since the 1990s, humanitarianism has been further transformed by geopolitical realities. These changes have been a result of a variety of factors including external political realities, global technological advances, increased attention to the specific needs of women and children, the change in the nature of war, and the formation of a global conscience and rise of a human rights culture. Since international humanitarian law, which outlines the rules of war, was drafted in the early to mid-1900s, the nature of war has changed dramatically. In the post-Cold War era, women and children are disproportionately affected by war and armed conflict. Today's wars are increasingly waged within the borders of a country rather than between sovereign nation-states, and as a result there has been an increased incorporation of civilians into contemporary conflict. The line between combat zone or militarized space and civilian space is no longer clear.[5(p5)] And civilians, who were more traditionally protected from the frontline of battle, are now the main casualties of war.

"Throughout much of the world, war is increasingly waged on the bodies of unarmed civilians. Where it was once the purview of male soldiers who fought enemy forces on battlefields quite separate from people's homes, contemporary conflict blurs such distinctions, rendering civilian women, men, and children its main casualties."[5(p3)]

As Rehn and Sirleaf point out in a 2002 UNIFEM Independent Experts' Assessment on the Progress of the World's Women: "Over the course of the 20th century, civilian casualties in war climbed dramatically from 5% at the turn of the century, to 15% during World War I, to 65% by the end of World War II, to more than 75% in the wars of the 1990s. The shift was accompanied by a changing demographic landscape of war-torn societies seen in terms of a declining male population, changing household size and composition, and increased migration. Conflict causes an overall increase in female- or child-headed households; women and children are among the majority of the displaced in refugee camps and conflict zones."[6] In addition, "The incorporation of civilians into contemporary conflict has been a highly gendered practice."[5(p5)] As Gyles and Hyndman note in *Sites of Violence: Gender and Conflict Zones,* "The idea that (feminized) civilian and (masculinized) military spaces are distinct and separate no longer holds."[5(p5)] Today's wars are fought in the (feminized) civilian space, and it is largely civilian women and children who bear the burden of war. In contemporary war, "Women, as civilians, are more likely to be killed in war than are soldiers."[7] However, women are not only increasingly the direct casualties of war; they are also more likely, along with children, to be refugees and internally displaced persons. They are also more likely to be victims of sexual and gender-based violence, domestic violence, rape, forced prostitution, forced marriage, forced impregnation, and sexual trafficking.

The vast number of those affected by war and conflict are civilians, and the vast majority of those are women and children. The US Committee for Refugees and Immigrants' World Refugee Survey for 2007 estimates that there were 13,948,800 refugees and asylum seekers in the world as of December 31, 2006.[8] This estimate does not include those individuals who have not crossed an international border and are internally displaced within their country due to war and violence. If you include internally displaced, the total number of refugees/IDPs as of the end of 2006 reaches almost 25 million.[9] Since an estimated 80% of refugees in the world at any given time are women and children, and 50% are women and girls, an understanding of the issues facing this population is critical to understanding the interventions that humanitarian aid can have. In addition, understanding the complexities of humanitarian aid and the development of the modern humanitarian movement can shed light on why the international community has been slow to address the needs of women and children in war and complex humanitarian emergencies and perhaps explain why there is still today a gross inequality in the interventions on behalf of women and children in conflict affected areas.

Issues Facing Women and Children in War and Complex Emergencies

The physical and mental health of women and children is compromised by armed conflict, forced migration, and complex humanitarian emergencies. There is an enormous array of issues facing women and children in conflict zones. Lack of access to education and a stable environment can adversely affect children's development and result in lifelong trauma. Children are deprived of an education and safe places to play and develop. Women and the girl-child are victims of gender-based violence, rape, forced marriage, human trafficking, and other human rights abuses during war and violent conflict. Children under five years of age have the highest mortality rates in conflict affected settings.[10] Adolescent girls are particularly vulnerable to gender-based violence in conflicted affected settings.[11] Violence, specifically against women before, during, and after conflict is enormous.[12] Even basic health care is often lacking for women in conflict situations.[12] Women and adolescent girls may face increased exposure to HIV/AIDS as a result of gender-based violence in conflict-affected areas. The turmoil caused by war and violence often disrupts basic social, education, and health services leaving women and children without adequate access to medical and reproductive health services.[13] Pregnant women and those

with small children are particularly vulnerable during war and conflict because they can not move as quickly as others to escape the enemy.[14(p195)]

Malnutrition, access to health care, reproductive health, menstruation needs, pregnancy and delivery, sexually transmitted diseases, the effects of sexual violence, mental health, and the burden for the care of others, among other things, all pose particular issues for women in wartime. However, one of the most pressing and prevalent issues effecting women and girls in conflict is gender-based violence, particularly rape.

"Rape is not an accident of war, or an incidental adjunct to armed conflict. Its widespread use in times of conflict reflects the unique terror it holds for women, the unique power it gives the rapist over his victim, and the unique contempt it displays for its victims. The use of rape in conflict reflects the inequalities women face in their everyday lives in peacetime."[15]

The phenomenon of gender-based violence during wartime is not new. Well-documented incidents of the systematic abuse of women, children, and civilians and war crimes targeting women and children include the Rape of Nanking (1937–1938) and the My Lai massacre in March 1968 during the Vietnam War.

"After capturing the city of Nanking in December 1937, Japanese forces conducted an orgy of cruelty that became known as the 'Rape of Nanking.' They raped tens of thousands of girls and women between the ages of 9 and 75 and they killed at least 300,000 Chinese in the city. The brutality of the killings exceeded anything ever seen, with huge numbers of victims tortured, beheaded, drowned, or shot at point-blank range. The Japanese then looted and burned the city."[16]

During the 1919 pogroms in Russia, Jewish women were raped by Cossacks. The sexual enslavement and rape of Korean women by the Japanese army and the rape of Bengali women by the Pakistani Army during the 1971 war of succession are well documented.[17] The systematic abuse of women's rights and the targeting of women for abuse has occurred in Bosnia, Sierra Leone, Rwanda, Liberia, Congo, Darfur, and many other war zones.

"Mass rape has been documented in Bosnia, Cambodia, Liberia, Peru, Somalia, and Uganda. In Sierra Leone, 94% of displaced households surveyed reported incidents of sexual assault, including rape, torture, and sexual slavery. At least 250,000—and perhaps as many as 500,000—women were raped during the 1994 genocide in Rwanda. During World War II, 100,000 to 200,000 'comfort women' were captured by the Japanese and subjected to years of brutal exploitation."[14(p44)]

The conflicts in today's world are not immune to such atrocities. A groundbreaking report by Human Rights Watch published in 2002, "The War within the War: Sexual Violence against Women and Girls in Eastern Congo," highlighted the widespread use of sexual violence against women and girls as a weapon of war.

"Within the larger war in the eastern Democratic Republic of Congo (Congo) the warring parties carry out another war: that of sexual violence against women and girls. As military activities increase in one area after another, so do rapes and other crimes against women and girls."[18]

Four years later, in 2006, according to the United Nations, 27,000 sexual assaults were reported in South Kivu Province in Congo. Due to underreporting and the difficulty of getting accurate statistics on sexual assaults, the true number could be significantly higher. As John Holmes, the Under Secretary for Humanitarian Affairs said "The sexual violence in Congo is the worst in the world. . . . The sheer numbers, the wholesale brutality, the culture of impunity—it's appalling."[19] As an Amnesty International report notes: "Widely committed and seldom denounced, rape and sexual assault of women in situations of conflict have been viewed more as the spoils of war than as illegitimate acts that violate humanitarian law. As a consequence, women, whether combatants or civilians, have been targeted for rape while their attackers go without punishment."[20]

Gender-Based Violence as Ethnic Cleansing

In situations of ethnic violence, rape and gender-based violence are often used as a tool for ethnic cleansing. According to a 2002 Save the Children report, "A goal of modern civil wars usually is not so much to eliminate the opponents as to destroy their culture and the very fabric of society."[21] Human Rights Watch reported in its report *Rape as a Weapon of War and a Tool for Political Repression*: "The choice of particular women as targets of rape is almost inevitably determined by their identities, for example, as citizens of a particular country, adherents to a certain faith, or members of an ethnic group, a race, or a class. Thus in Somalia, rapists target women from rival clans, and in the former Yugoslavia, Bosnian women are raped by Serbian men."[20]

An Amnesty International Report on the use of rape as a weapon of war in Darfur cites the testimony of Sudanese women that describes a pattern of: "systematic and unlawful attacks on civilians in north, west, and south Darfur states, by government-sponsored militia mostly referred to as 'janjawid' (armed men on horses) or 'Arab Militia' and by the government army, including thorough bombardment of civilian villages by the Sudanese Air Force. In these attacks, men are killed, women are raped, and villagers are forcibly displaced from their homes, which are burnt; their crops and cattle, their main means of subsistence, are burnt or looted."[22]

The wars of the former Yugoslavia and Rwanda focused international attention on the use of rape as a weapon of war—used to undermine "community bonds, weaken resistance to aggression and, in the former Yugoslavia, to perpetuate ethnic cleansing through impregnation."[23] According to UNICEF's *State of the World's Children 1996*:

"In some raids in Rwanda, virtually every adolescent girl who survived an attack by the militia was subsequently raped. Many of those who became pregnant were ostracized by their families and communities. Some abandoned their babies; others committed suicide."[24]

Wars of nationalism are particularly complicated. Much has been written about the construction of gender and the role that gender plays in the construction of and reproduction of ethnic-national ideologies. Research shows that during times of conflict over national identity, "particularly during national liberation movements and the creation of nation-states" that women frequently become the "iconic representation of cultural and/or ethnic-national identity."[5(p9)]

"It has been argued that ethnic nationalism, as a social phenomenon, engenders a kind of structural violence and gender-specific crimes. While all citizens technically bear the same rights as all others, women are exposed to different forms of sexual and nonsexual violence in the context of their relation to nationalist movements and to their respective nation-states."[5(p13)]

As Giles and Hyndman note:

Gender politics and power relations are at the center of both nationalist and ethnic-nationalist projects. A consideration of the ways in which women are simultaneously incorporated into and oppressed by both kinds of movements, particularly with regard to their reproductive functions, has been a central concern of feminist research on militarized violence.[5(p9)]

The fact that gender-based violence and rape are used as a weapon of war is not a new phenomenon. That gender-based violence is so prevalent in today's world and that a culture of impunity continues to exist in most parts of the world is shocking given the enormous progress that the international community has made in constructing a culture of human rights and a global conscience. Until quite recently, violence against women was thought of as "an insignificant form of collateral damage."[23] How the international community has addressed this issue through resolutions and international law has been slow to progress, however, in the past 20 to 30 years the increased attention to this issue has resulted in a variety of important legislative measures.

The International Community's Response to Violence Against Women

The international community has responded to the fact that civilians have increasingly become the direct target of war with increased legislation to make the specific targeting of civilians during war and conflict a crime. However, it is only fairly recently that it has been recognized that war affects women and children differently than it does men. More recently, there have been legal repercussions for crimes against women committed during war.

While it is true that rape has long been viewed as a crime under international rules of war, it has more traditionally been viewed as a "crime against dignity and honor as opposed to a crime of violence."[25(p65)] The 1949 Geneva Conventions and the 1977 protocols that lay down a foundation for the protection of civilians during war explicitly prohibited rape, enforced prostitution, and indecent assault and called for special protections for women. Yet crimes of rape and gender-based violence were treated separately from other crimes of violence, including murder, torture, and cruel treatment.[25(pp63-79)] As Rhonda Copelon notes in her work *Surfacing Gender: Reconceptualizing Crimes Against Women in Time of War,* that where rape and other sexual assaults are referenced in these documents they are considered to be crimes against personal dignity or crimes against honor. Crimes of violence are treated separately. As Copelon writes:

Where rape is considered a crime against honor, the honor of women is called into question and virginity and chastity is often a precondition. Honor implies the loss of station or respect; it reinforces the social view, internalized by women, that the raped woman is dishonorable. And while the concept of dignity potentially embraces more profound concerns, standing alone it obfuscates the fact that rape is fundamentally violence against women— violence against a woman's body, autonomy, integrity, self-hood, security, and self-esteem, as well as her standing in the community. The failure to recognize rape as violence is critical to the traditional lesser or ambiguous state of rape in humanitarian law.[25(p66)]

Treating the crime of rape as a crime against dignity and honor is radically different than treating rape as a grave crime. As Copelan also notes, "The issue is not whether rape is a war crime, but whether it is a crime of the gravest dimension. Under the Geneva Conventions, the term is 'grave breach.'"[25(p66)] Traditionally, "Where rape has been treated as a grave crime, it is because it violates the honor of man and his exclusive right to sexual possession of his women as property...the media often refer to the mass rape in Bosnia as the rape of 'the enemy's women'—the enemy in this formulation being the male combatant and the seemingly all-male nation, religious, and ethnic group."[25(pp65-66)]

The idea that rape is fundamentally violence against women and that the act of one rape, not only mass or systematic rape, might be punishable and treated as a crime of violence has not been the norm. What has only recently begun to be understood is that rape can be a weapon of war, whether it is genocidal rape, rape of women as permitted or systematized as "booty" of war, or as a method of ethnic cleansing as in Rwanda or Serbia where rape was used to make "Muslin women bear Serbian babies."[25(70)] It is only recently that the crime of rape has been treated as a crime of violence—a grave crime.

Despite the difficulties of clearly categorizing rape, genocidal rape, and other forms of crimes against women, the international community has continued to make progress addressing issues affecting women in war. The UN Convention on the Elimination of All Forms of Discrimination against Women (1979) committed the signatories to condemn violence against women and create protections against violence. The subsequent Declaration on the Elimination of Violence Against Women adopted by the UN General Assembly in 1993, the Global Platform for Action adopted by the Beijing Fourth World Conference for Women in 1995, and the 1998 International Criminal Court adoption of the Rome Statute, which redefines crimes against humanity to "include torture, rape, sexual slavery, enforced prostitution, forced pregnancy, enforced sterilization, and other comparably grave acts of sexual violence that are committed as a part of a systematic attack on civilian populations,"[17] are all examples of the increase in legislation and attention that has been paid to this topic by the international community in the last 30 years. However, as a Human Rights Watch report notes "Not until the international outcry rose in response to reports of mass rape in the former Yugoslavia did the international community confront rape as a war crime and begin to take steps to punish those responsible for such abuse."[20]

The groundbreaking sentences delivered by the International Criminal Tribunals for Rwanda and the former Yugoslavia characterized violence against women, including rape and other forms of gender-based violence, as crimes of genocide and crimes against humanity. The recognition that civilians are more and more the victims of war, in particular women and children, has led to additional resolutions of the United Nations such as Resolution 1325, which calls for recognizing the unique experiences and needs of women and girls in conflict zones. Passed in October 2000 the resolution expresses: "concern that civilians, particularly women and children, account for the vast majority of those adversely affected by armed conflict, including as refugees and internally displaced persons, and increasingly are targeted by combatants and armed elements, and recognizing the consequent impact this has on durable peace and reconciliation" calls for increased attention to this population.[26]

In 2002, the *Impact of Violent Conflict on Women and Girls* was issued by the United Nations and in 2002 Secretary General Kofi Annan noted that "Existing inequalities between women and men, and patterns of discrimination against women and girls, tend to be exacerbated in armed conflict. Women and girls become particularly vulnerable to sexual violence and exploitation. Women and children make up the majority of the world's refugees and internally displaced persons. Even in refugee camps, which are meant to be safe havens, the vulnerability of women and girls may continue, especially if there is a proliferation of small arms. And some women may be forced to follow camps of armed forces, providing domestic services and/or being used as sexual slaves."[27]

The growing international apparatus existing to address human rights abuses and provide relief and protection for populations affected by armed conflict and other violence has begun to effectively describe the needs and mechanisms required to provide the necessary protection of individuals affected by armed conflict. Enormous progress has been made in the last few decades to bring awareness to the issues relevant to women in war and to provide protection to the most vulnerable populations. But the apparatus has not always been as effective in translating the narrative into action.

"Women's Rights Are Human Rights"

Why the inequality in the interventions on behalf of women and children persist in a world that is significantly more attuned to humanitarian need and human rights than it ever was is a dilemma. The process of globalization has given rise to "a language and practice of moral universalism, expressed above all in a shared human rights culture,"[28] but the translation of these ideals into intervention and action has been slower to evolve. It was women's advocacy groups that said "women's rights are human rights" at a 1993 UN Conference on Human Rights in Vienna.[21(p11)] As Anne Firth Murray writes in her book *From Outrage to Courage*, "This is an idea that Eleanor Roosevelt would surely have fully understood, but it is an idea that did not make its way into public consciousness until the 1990s."[21(p11)]

Today's world may appear more violent and chaotic than ever, but progress has been made to provide protection and intervention for vulnerable populations based on humanitarian principles and global concepts of human rights. As Michael Ignatieff writes in *The Warrior's Honor*:

> The world is not becoming more chaotic or violent, although our failure to understand and act makes it seem so. Nor has the world become more callous. Weak as the narrative of compassion and moral commitment may be, it is infinitely stronger than it was only 50 years ago. We are scarcely aware of the extent to which our moral imagination has been transformed since 1945 by the growth of a language and practice of moral universalism, expressed above all in a shared human rights culture.[28]

How this new narrative of compassion and moral commitment plays out in the ordinary lives of individuals affected by armed conflict is more complicated. There are enormous inequalities facing women and children in war and complex emergencies that the humanitarian and international community struggles to address even within the framework of a more global human rights culture. Women's rights organizations, nongovernmental organizations, and feminist research have produced a "dynamic and evolving discourse that frames how international humanitarian institutions and organizations have conceptualized violence against women and girls in conflict-affected settings,"[17] but there are a variety of reasons that the implementation of programs to address these concerns has been slow to evolve. As Jeanne Ward wrote in her 2002 work *"If Not Now, When?: Addressing Gender-Based Violence in Refugee, Internally Displaced, and Post-Conflict Settings"*:

> Until the last 10 years, most gender-based violence committed during periods of armed conflict has been either condoned or ignored. This silence is in significant measure a function of deeply embedded cultural assumptions that acquiesce to the 'inevitability' of violence and exploitation of women and girls.[17]

Issues of cultural sensitivity and the unwillingness of Western organizations to be perceived as imposing their values on other cultures has been an issue in the implementation of gender-based violence programs. As Jeanne Ward goes on to point out:

> Focusing on the contexts in which violence occurs is crucial to reducing violence, but there remains in the international humanitarian aid community a fear of imposing Western standards of social organization and behavior on disparate refugee, internally displaced, and post conflict populations across the world. During research for this report, for example, many international representatives of the humanitarian aid community expressed the opinion that acts of gender-based violence were the preserve of culture and therefore outside of the scope of humanitarian intervention. This perspective may be paternalistic in its failure to acknowledge local communities' desire to improve the rights of its own members, but at the same time its concerns are rooted in a respect for difference that should be a feature of all humanitarian work."[17]

Cultural sensitivity in program implementation is of the utmost importance. However, as the world is compressed by forces of globalization, ignoring the inequalities in the world becomes arguably harder and harder. An understanding of the need to intervene, while respecting differences has begun to emerge. On local and international levels, globalization has begun to transform the interventions made by humanitarian actors and nation-states, including local governments.

The Sanctity of the Nation-State in the Post-Cold War Era

An additional problem translating a global culture of human rights into responsive action has been the perceived sanctity of the nation-state. As W.R. Smyser writes in his book *The Humanitarian Conscience:*

> The world today faces a clash between two irreconcilable principles. The principle, that of the humanitarian conscience, has its origins in the ideals of the Greek, Roman, and Medieval philosophers as well as in the beliefs of the great world religions. The other principle, that of absolute sovereignty, has its origins in the nationalist doctrines laid down by the kings of England, France, and Spain over 500 years ago."[16]

Dunant's ideals and the ideals of the first Geneva Convention were designed for a different world, a world in which the sovereignty of a nation-state was sacrosanct and intervention across national boundaries on a humanitarian basis was unthinkable. Since then, international laws and covenants have changed and so has humanitarian work. It is no longer considered acceptable to be neutral in the face of atrocity. Today, there are institutions such as the United Nations and such documents as the Universal Declaration of Human Rights designed to mitigate human suffering. The idea that the international community would intervene militarily for humanitarian reasons is no longer an impossibility. When NATO began bombing Serbia over the treatment of Albanian Kosovars, President Clinton called the bombing of Serbia, "the first humanitarian war." In a September 1999 address to the General Assembly, Kofi Annan said "State sovereignty, in its most basic sense, is being redefined by the forces of globalization and international cooperation."[1(p100)]

In addition, the idea of human rights, including that "women's rights are human rights" and the formation of a truly global conscience has begun to transform the way that international organizations perceive their mandates and implement their programs and missions. There has been an evolution over the past 20 years reflecting a number of developments including new geopolitical realties in the post-Cold War world, that has fundamen-tally changed the relationship between humanitarian and human rights organizations. Larry Minnear writes about a fundamental change in the mandates of human rights and humanitarian organizations that took place as a result of the end of the Cold War. During the Cold War:

> The humanitarian enterprise viewed its task as delivery of emergency aid to needy populations, a full-time job in its own right in an environment of collapsing states and fight-to-the-death insurgencies. Picking up the cudgels for human rights, agencies feared, might jeopardize hard-won access to those in need, which depended on the cooperation, or at least the acquiescence, of the political authorities. As the 1990s proceeded, however, humanitarian organizations proved less and less able to keep their avowed distance from political issues in general and from human rights matters in particular.[1(p39)]

In the 1990s he argues, NGOs and other international actors became increasingly aware of the political dimensions of their work and began to act not on a purely humanitarian basis providing emergency aid, but in a more assertive manner. "Humanitarian action is now understood in more inclusive terms to encompass both the delivery of relief and other life-saving and life-supporting assistance and the protection of basic human rights."[1(p42)]

This change has not only changed the way the nongovernmental and other humanitarian agencies see their work and how they react to injustices that they see on the ground, it also translates that organizations now feel compelled to speak out against gender-based violence, rape, and other human rights abuses that before were only addressed by human rights organizations.

Globalization and a Global Conscience

Globalization has in many ways compressed the world. The world that we live in today has been transformed by enormous changes in communication, technology, and transportation that have profoundly affected the way that individuals, societies, and nation-states interact with and perceive each other. Global interdependence may not be new, but it is arguable that our world is more interconnected than ever and that it is even more impossible than ever for nation-states to exist in hermetically sealed states.[29] In many ways, the age of the sovereign nation-state is over. As the global economy ignores barriers, so too more and more, does the global conscience. It is progressively less possible for societies and individuals to be isolated from universal concepts of human rights and humanitarianism. As women's rights are more regularly seen as human rights, interventions to stop gender-based violence are becoming more common. Pressure on local governments to react to the prevalence of gender-based violence, rape, and sexual assaults within their countries has also grown:

> In 2006, describing sexual violence as a "new form of criminality" that would "not remain unpunished" the Congolese government modified their laws and penalties. The laws detail three types of sexual violence: 1) indecent assaults on minors committed without violence, 2) indecent assaults on minors committed with violence, and 3) rape. Depending on the age of the victim, sentences range from 6 months to 20 years in prison. If the victim dies from sexual violence, the perpetrator is to serve a life sentence"[30]

Although adjustments have been made to the Congolese penal code, the culture of impunity that exists is unlikely to disappear overnight, and the absence of a strong Congolese state will impede the implantation of these statutes. However, the fact that the Congolese penal code has been modified is a testament to the universality of the human rights culture.

Conclusion

Great progress has been made by what can be thought of as the modern humanitarian movement establishing universal concepts of human rights and political liberties. As Amartya Sen writes in *Development as Freedom:*

> The 20th century has established democratic and participatory governance as the

preeminent model of political organization. Concepts of human rights and political liberty are now very much a part of the prevailing rhetoric. People live much longer, on average, than ever before. Also, the different regions of the globe are now more closely linked than they ever have been. This is not only in the fields of trade, commerce, and communication, but also in terms of more interactive ideas and ideals.[31]

Yet, at the same time, today's world is a world polarized by inequality. Despite unprecedented opulence in many countries in the world, and despite an increasing consciousness of human rights and civil liberties around the world, there remains enormous deprivation, poverty, lack of freedom, access to basic human rights, health care, and education. In complex humanitarian emergencies and war zones, human and civil rights abuses, particularly as they relate to women and children, are still common and prevalent. Adolescent girls and women are increasingly the victims of unthinkable crimes during war. With all of the attention now paid to women's rights by the international community, the idea that women's rights are human rights has begun to get traction, but the realities on the ground do not necessarily reflect the progress made in the rhetoric. With all of the mechanisms put into place by the international community, the provisions made through the array of resolutions and international declarations and agreements, it is shocking that in war zones rape and gender-based violence can be so prevalent and brutal.

Ann Jones, the author of *Kabul in Winter: Life without Peace in Afghanistan,* writes five years after the end of war in western Africa in Liberia:

> Many women were raped so incessantly and so brutally—with sticks, knives, gun barrels, burning coals—that they died. Many others were left with injuries and pain that still linger, long after the war. Many still find it hard to sit down or stand up or walk. Some still spit up blood. Some have lost their eyesight or their memories. Many contracted sexually transmitted diseases or HIV.[32]

How this clear violation of human rights and international law can continue in today's globalized world is unimaginable, and yet it does, not only in Liberia but elsewhere in the world's conflict zones:

> Wars put all human rights at risk by its brutal nature. Humanitarian law applies only to armed conflicts and cannot be suspended during hostilities. People around the world continue to suffer, at least in part, because of the lack of effective enforcement mechanisms for human rights and humanitarian law.[3(p49)]

Given the enormous progress that the international community has made in the past 150 years to address fundamental humanitarian needs, the disproportionate suffering of women and children in conflict-affected areas calls for increased attention and scrutiny. Those who commit war crimes and crimes against humanity, including crimes of violence against women, should be held accountable for their actions. Enormous progress has been made by the international community to construct the apparatus to enforce the law; now increased efforts need to be made to enforce these laws and hold those who break them accountable.

DISCUSSION QUESTIONS

1. What is the role of humanitarian law, human rights law, and international criminal law in the protection of civilians, in particular women and children, in armed conflict?

2. How can law guide the conduct of hostilities and/or mitigate the consequences of the use of armed force?

3. While there has been enormous progress in the development of a universal human rights platform and humanitarian endeavor in the past few decades, what gaps still exist between the three fields of international law that are relevant to today's armed conflict (international humanitarian law, human rights law, and international criminal law)?

REFERENCES

1. Minear, L. *The Humanitarian Enterprise*. Bloomfield, CT: Kumarian Press; 2002:39, 42, 100.
2. Power S. *A Problem from Hell: America and the Age of Genocide*. New York, NY: Basic Books; 2002.
3. Annas G, Geiger H J. War and Human Rights. In: Levy BS, Sidel VW, eds. *War and Public Health*. New York, NY: Oxford University Press; 2008:44, 49.
4. Power S. *A Problem from Hell: America in the Age of Genocide*. New York, NY: Basic Books; 2002:40-41.
5. Gyles W, Hyndman J. Introduction. In: Gyles W, Hyndman J, eds. *Sites of Violence: Gender and Conflict Zones*. Berkeley: University of California Press; 2004:3, 5, 9, 13.
6. Rehn E, Sirleaf E. Women, War, The Independent Experts' Assessment. Peace: Progress of the World's Women 2002. UNIFEM. 2002; Volume 1: Introduction 4.

7. Turpin J. Many Faces: Women Confronting War. In: Lorentzen L, Turpin J, eds. *The Women and War Reader.* New York, NY: New York University Press; 1998:3.

8. US Committee for Refugees. World Refugee Survey, 2007. http://www.refugees.org/article.aspx? id=1942. Accessed April 6, 2008

9. Internal Displacement Monitoring Centre, Norwegian Refugee Council. Internal displacement: global overview of trends in development in 2006. http://www.internal-displacement.org/idmc/website/resources/nsf. Accessed April 8, 2008.

10. Horton R. The coming decade for global action on health. *Lancet.* 2006;367:3-5.

11. Women's Commission for Refugee Women and Children. Fact sheet on adolescent girls affected by violent conflict. New York, NY: Women's Commission for Refugee Women and Children; 2005. http://www.womenscommission.org/pdf/AdolGirls.pdf Accessed on March 21, 2008.

12. Rehn R, Sirleaf EJ. *Women, War, Peace.* New York, NY: UNIFEM Progress of the World's Women; 2002:6.

13. Women's Commission for Refugee Women and Children. Partnering with local organizations to support reproductive health of adolescent refugees: a three year analysis. Reproductive Health Project. New York, NY: Women's Commission for Refugee Women and Children; 2003.

14. Ashford MW. The impact of war on woman. In: Levy BS, Sidel VW, eds. *War and Public Health.* New York, NY: Oxford University Press; 2008:44, 195.

15. Amnesty International. Stop violence against women: rape as a tool of war: a fact sheet. http://www.amnestyusa.org/women/rapeinwartime.html. Accessed March 21, 2008.

16. Smyser WR. *The Humanitarian Conscience: Caring for Others in an Age of Terror.* New York, NY: Palgrave Macmillan; 2003:149.

17. Ward J. If not now, when? Addressing gender-based violence in refugee, internally displaced, and post conflict settings. Women's Commission for Refugee Women and Children, April 2002. http://www.reliefweb.int/rw/rwb.nsf. Accessed March 27, 2008.

18. Human Rights Watch. *The War Within the War: Sexual Violence Against Women and Girls in Eastern Congo.* New York, NY: Human Rights Watch; 2002:Summary:1.

19. Gettleman J. Rape epidemic raises trauma of Congo war. *New York Times* [online]. October 7, 2007. http://www.nytimes.com/2007/10/07/world/africa/07congo.html. Accessed April6, 2008

20. Human Rights Watch. Rape as a weapon of war and a tool of political repression. http://www.hrw.org/about/projects/womrep/General-21.htm. Accessed March 27, 2008.

21. Murray F. *From Outrage to Courage.* Monroe, ME: Common Courage Press; 2008: 11, 134.

22. Amnesty International. Darfur: rape as a weapon of war: sexual violence and its consequences. http://www.amnesty.org/en/library/asset/AFR54/076/2004/en/dom-AFR540762004en.html. Accessed April 8, 2008

23. Watts C, Zimmerman C. Violence against women: global scope and magnitude. *Lancet.* 2002. http://www.thelancet.com/journals/lancet/article/PIIS014067360 2082211/fulltext. Accessed March 21, 2008.

24. UNICEF. The state of the world's children 1996. Sexual violence as a weapon of war. http://www.unicef.org/sowc96pk/sexviol.htm. Accessed March 21, 2008.

25. Copelon R. Surfacing gender: reconceptualizing crimes against women in time of war. In: Lorentzen LA, Turpin J, eds. *The Women and War Reader.* New York, NY: New York University Press; 1998:63-79.

26. Women's International League for Peace and Freedom. United Nations security council resolution 1325 on women, peace and security. http://www.peacewomen .org/un/sc/1325.html. Accessed April 14, 2008.

27. United Nations Information Service (UNIS Vienna). Secretary General's statement to security council on women, peace and security, New York, NY: October 28, 2002. http://www.unis.unvienna.org/unis/pressrels/2002/sgsm8461.html. Accessed April 8, 2008.

28. Ignatieff M. *The Warriors Honor: Ethnic War and the Modern Conscience.* New York, NY: Henry Holt and Co; 1998:8.

29. Ohmae K. *The Next Global Stage: Challenges and Opportunities in Our Borderless World.* Upper Saddle River, NJ: Wharton School Publishing; 2007.

30. Feeley R, Thomas-Jensen C. Getting serious about Women's Commission for Refugee Women and Children. Fact sheet on adolescent girls affected by violent conflict. New York, NY: Women's Commission for Refugee Women and Children ending conflict and sexual violence in Congo. Enough! The project to end genocide and crimes against humanity. http://www/enoughproject.org/reports /congoserious. Accessed March 27, 2008.

31. Sen A. *Development as Freedom.* New York, NY: Knopf; 1999: Preface.

32. Jones AA. War on Women. Los Angeles Times. 2008. http://www.latimes.com /news/opinion/la-op-jones17Feb17,0,7418229.story. Accessed February 21, 2008.

CHAPTER **6**

Human Trafficking: A Modern Plague

Human trafficking is the exploitation of men, women, and children for the financial gain of others and has been delineated as a fundamental human rights violation. Generally, those who are most susceptible to falling prey to this illicit activity are women, children, and adolescents. Victims of human trafficking are typically enticed with false promises of a better life or seized from their homes and forced through various methods to engage in work as prostitutes, domestic servants, sweatshop workers, and agricultural laborers. "Apart from causing grave injury to its victims, human trafficking is a burgeoning industry that undermines government authority, fuels organized crime, and poses a significant threat to global health."[1]

The demands of human trafficking have significantly increased, and this operation is now estimated to be a $32 billion industry worldwide.[2] The United States government estimates that it affects approximately 800,000 people each year; the majority of those affected are women and adolescents from developing countries.[3] Since 2000, after the adoption of the United Nations' Protocol to Prevent, Suppress, and Punish Trafficking in Persons, Especially Women and Children, the efforts to combat human trafficking have improved dramatically. Despite an increased awareness about the devastating effects of this horrific practice among policy makers, government officials, intergovernmental and nongovernmental organizations, and researchers, human trafficking continues to be rampant worldwide. Availability of shelters, rehabilitation, reintegration, and vocational training centers are limited for victims of trafficking, and the consequences to the victim's health have not been fully understood nor appreciated. Moreover, the perpetuators of this practice are seldom brought to justice.

This chapter will highlight the recent trends and practices of human trafficking in the United States and internationally. Moreover, it will discuss some of the health consequences the victims have suffered and the legislative efforts that have been implemented to tackle this insidious problem.

Padmini Murthy, MD, MPH, MS, CHES;
Roshni D. Persaud, JD, MPH;
Mitsuru Toda, BA

Padmini Murthy MD, MPH, MS, CHES, is an Assistant Professor in the Department of Health Policy and Management as well as the Director of the Global Health Program, at New York Medical School of Public Health in Valhalla NY. She is the Medical Women's International Association NGO Representative to the United Nations, New York, Robert F Wagner Public Service Scholar New York University.

Roshni D. Persaud, JD, MPH is Staff Attorney for New York City Health and Hospitals Corporation's Office of Legal Affairs, in New York , NY.

Mitsuru Toda, BA, of Harvard University.

Background

Human trafficking is similar to arms and drug trafficking, and is a heinous crime that poses a major threat to the international community. It presents a special threat to women and adolescents, both girls and boys, especially those who have a low socioeconomic status. Trafficking in persons can be separated into two distinct categories: 1) forced labor, and 2) prostitution, also known as sex trafficking. Both forms of human trafficking have been especially driven by the growing demands for cheap, profitable unskilled labor and for sexual exploitation. The Office of the United Nations High Commissioner for Human Rights recognizes it as "one of the world's fastest growing crimes."[4] The United Nations Population Fund's *State of the World Population 2006* report states that human trafficking is the third most lucrative illicit business in the world after arms and drug trafficking.[5]

The profits associated with this crime have led to the global establishment of this industry. As a logical consequence, vast numbers of victims are systematically deprived of their basic human rights.[3] Human trafficking in a quantifiable number of cases is a gender-based human rights violation against women and children (especially the girl-child). Most importantly, this activity has serious ramifications on the health and well-being of communities worldwide. Human trafficking contributes to the spread of sexually transmitted diseases, including devastating diseases such as HIV/AIDS. Additionally, victims of trafficking are at an increased risk for depression, post-traumatic stress disorders, suicide, and substance abuse.

Definition

Human trafficking is defined by the United Nations Protocol to Prevent, Suppress, and Punish Trafficking in Persons, Especially Women and Children, supplementing the United Nations Conventions Against Transnational Crime (A/RES/55/25) as:

the recruitment, transportation, transfer, harboring or receipt of persons. It involves using threat, force, or other forms of coercion, abduction, fraud, and deception, to control another person for the purpose of exploitation.[6]

At present, this definition is widely used by policy makers, law, and government officials, as well as intergovernmental and nongovernmental organizations.

Often the definition of trafficking in persons is confused with human smuggling. Human smuggling entails moving people across national borders with their complete consent into a country of which the person is not a national or a permanent resident. This is a lucrative operation for the smugglers.[7] Human trafficking involves planned exploitation at the intended destination, and this process is undertaken without valid consent. Although a trafficked person or the guardian of a trafficked child may consent to the movement or to a place of employment promised, their consent is nullified if they end up being exploited at the end of the process.[6] Persons are typically delivered to organizations or individuals who have paid for their delivery and the trafficked persons must, after the delivery, repay their debt to the organizers through prostitution or some form of forced labor.[8,9]

The distinction between the two may be especially difficult when individuals involved are children or when the persons involved are moved across borders to communities where they do not speak the language that the local police or law officials speak.[8,9]

Global View of Causes and Tactics of Human Trafficking

The causes of human trafficking are multifaceted and highly complex. Moreover, the precipitating factors that give rise to the ready availability of victims include those who experience socioeconomic disadvantages, such as economic poverty, lack of education, political instability, public and private corruption, and violence. Also, being a woman, child, or adolescent predisposes one to the risk of becoming a victim of trafficking. Sadly, many individuals who are recruited into these lifestyles are attracted to the perceived higher standards of living elsewhere.[3]

In particular, economic and political instability increase the likelihood that a country or a community will become a source of trafficking. In fact, the United States Department of State noted in its 2002 report that in countries with chronic unemployment, widespread poverty, and a lack of opportunities, traffickers use promises of higher wages and good working conditions in foreign countries to lure people into their networks.[8] Factors such as civil unrest, internal armed conflict, and natural disasters also enhance the risks. These incidents destabilize and displace populations, which in turn, increase their vulnerability to trafficking.[8,10] For example, the United Nations Office on Drugs and Crime reported that traffickers exclusively targeted foreign domestic workers during the armed conflict in Lebanon in mid-2006. Some of the 300,000 domestic workers from Sri Lanka, Ethiopia, and the Philippines were left behind when their employers were evacuated during the unrest. The workers suddenly became vulnerable after abruptly losing their official resident status and livelihoods.[11,12]

The estimated number of persons trafficked globally is often perceived as inaccurate due to the clandestine nature of the operation. The International Labor Organization estimates that globally 2.45 million people are trafficked annually both within and across national borders.[11,12] Among those who are trafficked, approximately 80% are women and 50% are children.[3] The majority of those trafficked end up as commercial sex workers; others are used as domestic workers or agricultural laborers who are abused and have long hours at work under unsuitable conditions; and some of them, especially children, are exploited and made to work as street beggars.

Human trafficking occurs in three different stages: recruitment, transportation, and exploitation. Each stage of the operation is specialized and handled by different criminal groups or individuals. A report by the US Congressional Research Services noted that "Chinese and Vietnamese triads, the Japanese Yakuza, South American drug cartels, the Italian mafia, and the Russian gangs increasingly interact with local networks to provide transportation, safe houses, local contacts, and documentation.[12] These groups create a global network where they recruit and transport victims from one location to another, including across national borders, making detection of such operations extremely difficult.

The recruitment tactics are ruthless and cunning. Traffickers use creative ploys to win the confidence of potential victims by promising a better life through marriage, employment, or educational opportunities.[3] They advertise in local newspapers, mislead parents that their children will be taught a useful skill or trade, or even kidnap or abduct potential victims.[8] For example, cross-border networks engaged in the recruitment of children for purposes of trafficking within Pakistan include "relatives and respected members of the community" who often gain the trust and consent of unsuspecting parents."[9] This is one of the examples that demonstrate the devastating tactics utilized in the recruitment process of human trafficking. In other instances, traffickers use threats, intimidation, and violence to force victims to engage in such exploitations for the trafficker's financial profit.

The original country where the victim comes from is known as the "source country," and the final destination is the "destination country." Victims are generally transported through "transit countries" that the perpetrators perceive as safe routes. The trafficked women and children are usually taken to countries where they do not speak the language, and hence are isolated from the local communities and are at the mercy of their perpetrators. Victims are often despondent because they are in unfamiliar surroundings and do not know how to access assistance from law enforcement or legal bodies, nor do they have the ability to escape from their captors.[8] Sadly, they are often subjected to various forms of psychological and physical abuse, as well as torture.

Poor border monitoring and corruption of immigration officials are documented factors facilitating the transit of victims.[8] Traffickers commonly forge documents including visas or landing permits so victims can traverse national and international borders in order to reach their destination. When reaching a destination country, victims are then made to work as bonded laborers or prostitutes. Debt bondage is the most common and confining mechanism used to exploit these victims who are forced to work under inhumane conditions. Traffickers in many instances add the costs of transportation, fees for procurement or falsifying documents, buying clothes, medicine, and lodging into the victims' so-called debt.[13]

Traffickers charge exorbitant fees for their services, often creating a lifetime of debt bondage for their victims. This is comparable to modern-day slavery from which these victims have no means of escape. The recruiters and traffickers use a variety of tactics to enslave huge numbers of people from the same communities.[12] Women and adolescents become especially vulnerable targets of trafficking, and the low status of women and adolescents are contributors to the swelling trafficking industry.[8] Adolescents are particularly vulnerable since they can be coerced easily and lured by false promises of receiving higher education and gainful employment.

Regional Trends

Presently, the issue of human trafficking affects every region in the world. According to the 2006 report released by the US Department of State Trafficking in Persons report "The United States of America is principally a transit and destination country for trafficking in persons. It is estimated that 14,500 to 17,500 people, primarily women and children, are trafficked to the United States annually."[14] In a report released by the United Nations Office of Drugs and Crime, countries in Asia and central and southeastern Europe are the most frequently mentioned countries of origin where traffickers prey and lure their victims, violating their human rights; this is followed by Latin America, the Caribbean, and Southeast Asia. Central America and western Africa are also reported as bustling transit regions.[9]

Asia and the Pacific

In east Asia and the Pacific, many children who are recruited for work are often lured into prostitution. Popular destinations for sex tourism include Thailand, Cambodia, and the Philippines.[15] Furthermore, in south Asia, trafficking is often related to debt bondage, whereby a child is sold to pay off a debt that is deliberately imposed by the exploiter. Countries such as Myanmar, Vietnam, the Philippines, Thailand, the People's Republic of China, Bangladesh, and Nepal are frequently reported as origin countries.[9] Women and children from these countries are usually trafficked to the United States, India, and Europe.

Africa

In Africa, children make up the largest group of trafficked victims, and almost 40% of them are forced into bonded labor.[9] These children are forced to work long hours in mines or on plantations. Western African countries, such as Cote d'Ivoire and Nigeria, are destinations for victims trafficked from other African countries. African children are also trafficked to the United Kingdom, Italy, France, Belgium, the Netherlands, and some Middle Eastern countries.[12]

Europe

In Europe, children are mainly trafficked from places such as central and eastern Europe, Asia, Africa, and the Americas, reflecting the demand for cheap labor and prostitution in the richer countries of the continent.[5,12,15]

Latin America and the Caribbean

In the Americas and the Caribbean, human trafficking is driven by tourism and concentrated in localities that are major tourist attractions. Individuals who are associated with drug smuggling are getting involved in human trafficking across borders.[15] Victims are commonly taken to countries such as the United States, Spain, Italy, Germany, the United Kingdom, Canada, the Netherlands, and Belgium.[9]

North America

The United States is one of the largest destination countries of victims who have been trafficked. Victims from mostly the Ukraine, Mexico, the Russian Federation, China, Malaysia, and Thailand come to the United States. In addition, women from countries such as Colombia, Georgia, and the Philippines are also trafficked to the United

States.[9] The largest trafficking case ever prosecuted in the United States involved 200 Vietnamese and Chinese nationals, mostly young women, who were brought to American Samoa to work as sewing machine operators in a garment factory. However, these young women were actually lured to work as prostitutes.[2]

Human Trafficking and Its Relevance to Global Health

Findings from a global survey commissioned for the Millennium Summit of the United Nations by former UN Secretary General Kofi Annan, found good health was considered the top desire of men and women around the world.[16] Unfortunately young girls, adolescents, and women who have been trafficked have their dignity and human rights violated and are robbed of their opportunity for good health.

Health is important for socioeconomic stability and productivity. Nevertheless, trafficking has a devastating toll on health. As described previously, the most common form of human trafficking is forced prostitution or sex trafficking. Victims of human trafficking commonly suffer physical and emotional abuse, rape, threats against self and family, document theft, and even death.[3] According to the US State Department report, "A 2006 study found that 76% of 207 trafficked women interviewed were physically assaulted by their trafficker, pimp, madam, brothel, and club owner, clients, or boyfriend."[13] The same study determined that 90% of victims reported being physically forced or intimidated into sex or other sexual acts, and 91% of victims reported being threatened with death, beatings, increased debt, harm to their children and families, or retrafficking.[13]

A survey conducted in 2006 of women trafficked for prostitution into the European Union found that 95% of victims had been violently assaulted and coerced into a sexual act, and more than 60% of victims reported fatigue, neurological symptoms, gastrointestinal problems, back pain, and or gynecological infections.[3]

Violence and abuse are at the core of trafficking for sex labor, and there are many physiological as well as psychological symptoms that victims suffer as a consequence of being exposed to sometimes repeated sex trafficking. Despite the compelling evidence on the physical and psychological health consequences, there is limited evidence about the needs of women who have been trafficked.[17] Furthermore, the documentation or research on the health impacts of victims of trafficking has been limited. Research carried out by the London School of Hygiene and Tropical Medicine on the impact of trafficking on victims' health confirmed that, "Even after a woman is no longer being exploited, many are still confronted with risks associated with detention, deportation, or giving criminal evidence, before they move onto the challenges of the integration or reintegration process.[18]

Unfortunately only a fraction of these victims who are rescued have the opportunity to acquire adequate medical, psychological, and social assistance. While there is a great need for coordinated posttrafficking services, there are relatively few organizations established globally that are able to provide the requisite counseling services, economic and social support, and medical care, including screening services.[13,18]

HIV/AIDS

Prostitution or sex trafficking is recognized as "a major gender-based human rights violation with significant individual and public health consequences and is increasingly discussed as a potential critical mechanism in the spread of HIV across developing nations."[18] The potential health consequences that victims of sex trafficking endure are vast. However, the elevated risk of contracting HIV/AIDS and other sexually transmitted diseases is of paramount concern.

Some of the elements that increase a trafficked woman's risk of contracting HIV/AIDS include the following:

1. Intravenous drug use among young girls in Asia and the former Soviet Union.[19]
2. Younger women are prized by clients for their virginity and also because of the mistaken belief that unprotected sex with a young girl is a cure for HIV/AIDS and sexually transmitted diseases.[3]

3. Compensation received by traffickers from brothel owners is greater than twice that received for older trafficked women.

4. Unfortunately, these young girls and adolescents have limited knowledge about safe sexual practices and disease transmission. Moreover, many may not be empowered to negotiate condom use with their clients.

5. A study conducted in Nepal highlighted the social stigma and discrimination faced by young survivors of trafficking, and in many instances, these young girls were at a very high risk for being retrafficked or for working as prostitutes in the local communities.[18]

Mental Health

Significant psychological consequences are common among prostituted women. These include personality disorders, anxiety, and depression. The psychological symptoms may be the most painful health problems these victims experience.[18] Some of the other symptoms victims experience are post-traumatic stress disorder due to repeated physical and mental abuse, insomnia, nightmares, difficulty concentrating, apathy, and low self-esteem.[15] A study conducted in 2001 by the US Department of State revealed that "86% of women trafficked within their countries and 85% of women trafficked across international borders suffer from depression."[3]

Multiple exposures to trauma through human trafficking can have various long-term effects on a woman's health, especially since human trafficking involves violence. The psychological symptoms experienced by these victims are similar to those seen in survivors of torture and can include increased risk for suicide and cognitive impairment. The resulting cognitive impairment experienced by these victims may impair their ability to actively participate in police inquiries, immigration proceedings, and asylum petitions. Often, these women are unable to make independent decisions about their safety and rehabilitation processes and cannot recall details of the crime or identify their perpetrators.[17,19]

Protection and Reintegration Measures

To comprehensively address the special needs of these victims, services should include strategies for crisis intervention, maintaining confidentiality, providing security, shelter, social support, counseling, and access to healthcare providers who have received formal training in cultural competency.[17,19] It is crucial that policy makers initiate measures to help women manage their individual psychological symptoms. Furthermore, law-making bodies need to create and implement laws and judicial procedures that are sensitive to the changes in trafficked women's physical, emotional, and cognitive abilities.[18]

Cooperation among governments, the United Nations, nongovernmental organizations, healthcare professionals, policy makers, and representatives of the legislature and judiciary will help to provide effective services to assist and rehabilitate the survivors of this appalling crime.

Conventions and Treaties that Address Human Trafficking

In 2000, the United Nations passed the Protocol to Prevent, Suppress, and Punish Trafficking in Persons, Especially Women and Children, Supplementing the United Nations Convention Against Transnational Organized Crime (A/RES/55/25. General Assembly 15 November 2000).[6] This protocol, also known as the Palermo protocol, marked a significant milestone in the field of human trafficking and recognized trafficking as one of the major violations of health and human rights. This protocol requires the ratifying state to criminalize trafficking and also address the issue of victims' rights by providing assistance and protection for victims of trafficking.[9]

The Council of Europe Convention on Action Against Trafficking in Human Beings was endorsed by the Committee of Ministers in 2005. The convention expands the definition of trafficking to explicitly include in-state trafficking and trafficking not necessarily involving organized criminal groups.[20]

Legislative Measures Implemented by the United States and Foreign Countries to Combat Human Trafficking

United States

Congressional findings illustrate that legislation and law enforcement efforts in the United States and abroad were inefficient in deterring human trafficking and prosecuting perpetrators of this modern form of slavery.[19] In effect, there was "a failing to reflect the gravity of the offenses involved," and no body of law existed in the United States that punished the entire gamut of potential offenses involved in the human trafficking scheme.[20] Congressional findings also highlighted that even the most atrocious cases of trafficking were punished under laws that were intended for lesser offenses, so inevitably, traffickers would escape full prosecution.[20]

Victims of Trafficking and Violence Protection Act (TVPA)

As a result, the Victims of Trafficking and Violence Protection Act (TVPA) (which was subsequently reauthorized in 2003 and 2005) was drafted and subsequently signed into law on October 19, 2000.[1] The purpose of TVPA is to set forth a harmonized, "transnational effort to safeguard trafficked individuals, criminalize the conduct of traffickers, and punish sex trafficking as if it were a crime as serious as rape, punishable with a sentence of 20 years to life imprisonment."[21] TVPA defines "severe trafficking" as:

> (A) sex trafficking in which a commercial sex act is induced by force, fraud, or coercion, or in which the person induced to perform such act has not attained 18 years of age; or[20]
>
> (B) the recruitment, harboring, transportation, provision, or obtaining of a person for labor or services, through the use of force, fraud, or coercion for the purpose of subjection to involuntary servitude, peonage, debt bondage, or slavery.[20]

Interestingly, a victim does not have to be physically moved from one location to another in order to fall within the purview of this definition.[21,22]

The statutory framework of the TVPA also provides for the establishment of an interagency task force to monitor and combat trafficking.[20] The agency's responsibilities are inclusive of the following: monitoring the success of the US and foreign countries with regard to trafficking prevention; assisting victims of trafficking; and supporting prosecutorial and enforcement activities against traffickers, "which includes the role of public corruption in facilitating trafficking."[21] Moreover, TVPA requires that annual reports be produced that provide information on human rights practices abroad for countries receiving various types of economic assistance from the United States.[20] This mandate to compile and publish a yearly report to assess the efforts of governments in meeting minimum standards to eliminate trafficking is commonly known as the "Trafficking in Persons Report" and is a comprehensive compilation of information on trafficking in countries worldwide. In an effort to deter trafficking, the act also requires the president to support the creation and implementation of various international initiatives in an effort to increase economic opportunity for those who may become potential victims of trafficking.[20,23,25,26]

TVPA also establishes minimum standards for the elimination of trafficking and enables the US government to provide assistance to foreign countries in meeting these minimum standards.[20,23] Such assistance includes support in the drafting of laws to prohibit and punish acts of trafficking and funding for the investigation and prosecution of traffickers.[25,26] Furthermore, nonhumanitarian sanctions may be imposed against governments failing to meet these minimum standards.[27] The act also creates stern sentencing requirements and a credible threat of prosecution for those responsible for this unconscionable crime.[20] Some may even consider TVPA to be "victim-friendly" legislation because it enables victims who experience a severe form of human trafficking the possibility of permanent residency in the United States and a work permit if they assist in the prosecution of their trafficker.[22] More specifically, the Department of Homeland Security (DHS) provides two types of immigration relief: 1) continued presence (CP) to human trafficking victims who are possible witnesses during investigation or prosecution, and 2) T nonimmigrant status or "T visas," a special, self-petitioned visa category for trafficking victims.[22]

TVPA has been described by some scholars as the "most significant human rights legislation of [the US] Congress."[21] It should be noted, however, that there has been criticism that TVPA has its share of "practical and procedural problems," which persist in thwarting the nation's ability to look after and guard victims of human trafficking.[23] More specifically, critics assert that legislative officials and those in law enforcement seem to have disregarded the primary causes of trafficking, "in favor of conflating trafficking with other issues of political interest."[23] Moreover, critics contend that federal agencies are incorrectly interpreting and applying some of the provisions of the legislation thus rendering it an inefficient tool in combating human trafficking.[23]

Evidence also exists that prosecutors have had limited success in locating and punishing traffickers and aiding trafficking victims.[28,29] For example, the Department of Justice only obtained an annual average of 48 convictions for individuals charged with human trafficking crimes for the fiscal years 2001–2007.[24] Further evidence that lends credence to the position of marginal success of TVPA includes the fact that the Department of Health and Human Services only certified an annual average of 197 trafficking victims to receive federally administered benefits, such as health care, financial assistance, and housing for the fiscal years 2001–2007.[24] Also shocking, is that only 150 T visas were processed in 2003, even though 5000 were available.[24] It is plausible that these low numbers may be attributed to the fact that many victims of trafficking are reluctant to seek governmental assistance or cooperate with the prosecution of their traffickers because there is a deep seeded mistrust of government. Victims may also be fearful that if they seek legal redress or assist in any type of prosecution, the traffickers may retaliate against them or their family members. One needs to be attuned to the fact that there are some countries that have legislation that effectively treat victims of trafficking as criminals.[24,28] In certain circumstances, victims have entered the United States or foreign territories illegally and have used fraudulent documents or other illicit means to gain entry to their destination. As a consequence, a victim's case may very well end up being handled as an immigration matter. This poses

significant cause for concern because a victim of trafficking may encounter the threat of deportation from the locale where he or she resides, and in certain instances, the victim of such trafficking activities could be incarcerated if legislative remedies are not in place to prevent such an occurrence. It is imperative to note, however, that TVPA has resulted in a small, but vital, proliferation in arrest and convictions of traffickers both domestically and in some countries abroad, where financial assistance and guidance from the United States have been used effectively to amend existing trafficking laws or develop new laws imitating the TVPA.[20]

Trafficking Victims Protection Reauthorization Act of 2003 (TVPRA 2003) The Trafficking Victims Protection Reauthorization Act of 2003 was signed into law on December 19, 2003, and reauthorized TVPA.[25] The renewed legislation provided victims of human trafficking a private right of action against their trafficker. Essentially, victims would have the unique ability to initiate a civil action against their trafficker in an appropriate district court of the United States in an effort to recover "damages and reasonable attorney's fees."[25] This civil remedy is described as holding great promise to not only aid in suppressing and preventing human trafficking but to also supply much needed compensation to victims of this horrendous crime.[26] TVPRA 2003 also increases the responsibilities of the United States government by requiring the utilization of media campaigns to fight against sex tourism. Moreover, it requires the submission of an annual report from the US Attorney General to Congress. The aforementioned report is expected to delineate matters related to human trafficking, such as the number of individuals in the United States receiving federal benefits authorized by TVPA and the number of individuals who have been granted "continued presence" in the United States as a result of TVPRA. TVPRA 2003 also refined a number of criminal law provisions.[27]

Trafficking Victims Protection Reauthorization Act of 2005 (TVPRA 2005) The Trafficking Victims Protection Reauthorization Act of 2005 was signed into law on January 10, 2006, and it effectively reauthorized TVPA. Moreover, TVPRA 2005 concomitantly authorized new anti-trafficking resources,[22] while providing the US Attorney General the ability to supply grants to state and local law enforcement agencies in an effort to establish, develop, expand, or strengthen programs related to the prevention of human trafficking.[25] TVRPA 2005 also authorized pilot programs for the establishment of residential rehabilitative facilities for victims of human trafficking, in addition to similar pilot programs specially geared to the needs of juveniles.[24] Moreover, in an effort to combat human trafficking abroad, the act provides for "extraterritorial jurisdiction over trafficking offenses committed abroad by persons employed by or accompanying the federal government."[25]

Prosecutorial Remedies and other Tools to End the Exploitation of Children Today (PROTECT)

The United States strengthened its ability to avert child sex tourism by passing the Prosecutorial Remedies and other Tools to End the Exploitation of Children Today (PROTECT) Act in 2003. The act has "extraterritorial effect" and punishes US citizens engaging in sex with minors in countries abroad where sex tourism might be legal.[28]

Additionally, the act increased penalties to a maximum of 30 years in prison for engaging in child sex tourism.[29] Most importantly, the act states that "no statute of limitations that would otherwise preclude prosecution for an offense involving the sexual or physical abuse or kidnapping of a child under the age of 18 years shall preclude such prosecution during the life of the child."[29] Since the passage of the PROTECT Act, there have been approximately 64 convictions of child sex tourists.[30]

Model State Antitrafficking Criminal Statute

Despite the fact that numerous states have legislation that deal with the crime of trafficking in persons, a press release issued by the White House articulates "There is a need for a comprehensive antitrafficking statute to deter and punish the wide range of coercive tactics used by traffickers."[31]To meet this need, the United States Department of Justice recently drafted the Model State Anti-Trafficking Criminal Statute, which is available for adoption by the various states.[32] Currently, the states of Texas, Washington, Minnesota, Missouri, and Florida reportedly have extensive state trafficking laws.[31]

Measures Implemented by Foreign Countries to Combat Trafficking

Because of obsolete antitrafficking laws, victims of trafficking in countries in Latin America, Africa, Asia, and the Middle East face deportation because their situation is handled as a traditional immigration matter.[22] A limited number of countries, however, have used the United States as a role model and granted T visa type benefits and a stay of deportation for victims of trafficking. For instance, Belgium, Italy, and the Netherlands reportedly offer victims of human trafficking a 3-month temporary stay in order to provide victims with enough time to determine whether they would testify against their traffickers.[22] Generally, the expenses for the victims are covered.

In Croatia, "a victim of trafficking is granted a residence permit for 12 months, which can be renewed.[33] The Croatian criminal code calls for prison sentences for human traffickers of one to 10 years. If a victim is a child, the prison sentence for the offender is a minimum of five years.[33]

The government of China approved the China National Plan of Action on Combating Trafficking in Women and Children (2008–2012) on December 13, 2007.[34] The plan of action was created in an effort to do the following:

> Effectively prevent and severely combat the criminal activities of trafficking in women and children; actively provide assistance and give appropriate aftercare to rescued women and children; earnestly safeguard the legal rights and interests of women and children.[34]

Presently, Greece permits trafficking victims willing to testify against traffickers to remain in the country; however, the prosecutor makes the determination as to whether this protection will be offered.[21] Similarly, Israel currently provides shelter and some cash assistance to individual victims willing to testify against their traffickers.[21]

Role of NGOs and Individuals

Nongovernmental organizations (NGOs) work closely with the United Nations agencies and governments and are at the core of the rehabilitation process for victims of human trafficking. They offer vocational training, job placement assistance, and basic education. They also maintain broad community awareness efforts as well as border surveillance programs to identify and intervene in instances of trafficking.[18]

For example, in Armenia, NGO workers cooperate with the local border control officers in order to identify victims of trafficking who have been deported back to the country. Typically, nongovernmental organization workers receive listings of deported persons in advance to facilitate the identification of probable victims of trafficking. The NGO workers also interview potential victims on their arrival at airports, and they generally offer shelter, health care, and other services.[8] Replication of these practices in various countries would serve as an effective means to identify and rescue potential and actual victims of human trafficking.

Best Practices

The US Department of State's annual *Trafficking in Persons Report* lists several commendable initiatives launched globally by various stakeholders to curb and render assistance to the victims of trafficking.[3]

The first initiative described is that of the local NGO Forum for Street Children in Ethiopia. This NGO, in collaboration with international NGOs and local and regional law enforcement, helped to establish child protection units (CPU) in police stations in Addis Ababa and nine other towns around the nation. Each CPU educates law enforcement officials on the rights of children and provides assistance to child victims of exploitation. Since 2000, this NGO has been successful in reuniting over 1000 trafficked and exploited street children with their families.[3]

The second initiative commended in the report is in Panama. The Ministry of Social Development (MIDES), in cooperation with the International Labor Organization (ILO), initiated "Direct Action," a pilot program aimed at proactively addressing trafficking. In addition to medical and psychological care, participants were provided with formal education and vocational training. To alleviate economic hardship and attempt to eliminate the factor in trafficking vulnerability, MIDES provided support to adolescents and their families in the form of basic equipment for cooking and selling prepared food, as an income-generating opportunity.[3]

In Romania, the National Agency against Trafficking in Persons (ANITP) created a centralized national database for law enforcement personnel to input data on individual trafficking victims. Through the use of the database, ANITP was the first to identify an increase in labor trafficking of Romanians to the Czech Republic, and disseminate the information to law enforcement and policy officials. A national database such as this is an effective tool for targeting trafficking trends, and it serves as a wonderful model for other countries to emulate.[15]

Recommendations

Early identification of trafficked persons is a prerequisite for their recognition as victims, and consequently, their access to assistance and protection.[9] Moreover, the collaboration of all individuals and groups who come into contact with victims of human trafficking, such as border patrol guards, police, immigration officers, prosecutors, judges, health professionals, social workers, housing and agricultural inspectors, and the staff of human rights organizations, is essential and should not be underestimated. A multidisciplinary approach of the aforementioned groups of people would have an immense impact on the well-being of possible and actual victims of human trafficking by ensuring much needed services, counseling, protection, advocacy, preventative health care, and in some circumstances, prevention of recruitment into the dark world of human trafficking.

Furthermore, data gathering and sharing and the creation of a global map or database highlighting the main countries involved in human trafficking may be a useful method to identify countries of origin, transit, and destination. It may further facilitate the identification of organized criminal groups in different countries and the main routes used for trafficking.[8] This information will be extremely helpful in developing strategies and increasing cooperation at a grassroots level among the various stake holders, locally, nationally, and internationally in effectively and efficiently averting this human rights violation.

Examples of such comprehensive databases that can be accessed include the United Nations' Department of Drugs and Crime Office's database, the United States' Trafficked Persons Annual Report, and the International Office of Migration countertrafficking module database.[18]

Based on the legal and judicial systems in various countries, the perpetrators of trafficking can be charged and prosecuted as criminals under various categories. Some of these offenses are kidnapping of minors, forced labor, slavery, unlawful coercion and threats, bribery and corruption, debt bondage, theft, falsifying and destruction of legal documents (passports, visas, legal entry permits), sexual assault, forced abortion, homicide, and rape.[9] The ubiquity and variability of trafficking, however, necessitates a specific and consistent prescription of both international and domestic legislation in order to restrict this slave-like practice.[4] Moreover, this type of legislation needs to be culturally sensitive, and it will need universal adoption, adequate funding, and robust criminal provisions that will be wholly enforced.

Conclusion

Human trafficking is a demoralizing operation that violates the most basic human rights of the girl-child, adolescents, and women whose effects are deleterious. It is an act of gender-based violence that affects the health of an individual victim, but it simultaneously poses a threat to national, regional, and international security. Corruption, border control, political instability, lack of education, greed, hatred, and poverty are some of the primary causes of human trafficking. Effective preventive strategies and rehabilitation of victims spotlights the need for government policies and legislation that will adequately ensure the protection of victims, without jeopardizing their human rights, dignity, and security.[5,8]

Most importantly, empowerment of women and adolescents is crucial in order for them not to become vulnerable recruitment targets or victims of human trafficking.[35] As Amartya Sen states in his book, *Development as Freedom,* women are agents for change and the improvement in the rights and health of women will lead to overall health not just for women but to the community[36] The crux of this statement equally applies in the case of human trafficking where empowerment of women and children, via the promotion of education and economic activities, are key elements to halt the acceleration of this exploitative and devastating practice.[35,36] Such efforts will contribute to the laudable goal of eradication of human trafficking and will contribute to the global success of forthcoming generations.

DISCUSSION QUESTIONS

1. This chapter examined various legislative measures implemented to combat human trafficking. If you were in a position to create model legislation what are some of the crucial elements that you feel should be included. Moreover, if you were required to devise a comprehensive set of laws, how would you go about it?

2. From a policy perspective what type of programs do you think would be effective in preventing human trafficking? Moreover, what type of programs would be useful in helping victims of human trafficking? What are some of the key factors that you feel would address human trafficking that have not been discussed in this chapter?

3. As a public health advocate, if you were given the opportunity to work on matters germane to human trafficking, how do you see yourself contributing to such a discipline given your unique talents and skills?

REFERENCES

1. GAO. *Human Trafficking Monitoring and Evaluation of International Projects Are Limited, But Experts Suggest Improvements*. Washington, DC: GAO; 2007.
2. Besler P. Forced labour and human trafficking: estimating the profits. 2005. http://www.ilo.org/dyn/declaris/DECLARATIONWEB.DOWNLOAD_BLOB?Var_DocumentID=5081. Accessed June 23, 2008.
3. Trafficking in persons report. 2007. http://www.state.gov/documents/organization/82902.pdf. Accessed June 20, 2008.
4. Victims of trafficking and violence protection act of 2000: trafficking in persons report. 2002. http://www.state.gov/documents/organization/10492.pdf. Accessed June 10, 2008.
5. Alcala MJ, et al. State of world population 2006. New York: United Nations Population Fund. 2006. http://www.unfpa.org/swp/2006/pdf/en_sowp06.pdf. Accessed July 8, 2008.
6. Protocol to prevent, suppress and punish trafficking in person, especially women and children, supplementing the United Nations convention against transnational organized crime. 2000. http://untreaty.un.org/English/notpubl/18-12-a.E.doc. Accessed February 20, 2008.
7. Trafficking in persons global patterns. 2006. http://www.unodc.org/pdf/traffickinginpersons_report_2006ver2.pdf. Accessed February 19, 2008.
8. Kangaspunta K. Mapping the inhuman trade: preliminary findings of the database on trafficking in human beings. 2008. http://www.unodc.org/pdf/crime/forum/forum3_note1.pdf.
9. Iselin B, Adams M. Distinguishing between human trafficking and people smuggling. 2003. http://www.unodc.un.or.th/material/document/Distinguishing.pdf. Accessed June 10, 2008.
10. UNODC. http://www.unodc.org/unodc/en/human-trafficking/prevention.html. Accessed February 17, 2008.
11. Besler P, Michaelle DC, Mehran F. ILO minimum estimate of forced labour in the world. 2005. http://www.ilo.org/dyn/declaris/DECLARATIONWEB.DOWNLOAD_BLOB?Var_DocumentID=5073. Accessed February 15, 2008.
12. Slillen J, Beddoe C. Rights here, rights now: Recommendations for protecting trafficked children. 2007. http://www.ecpat.org.uk/downloads/RightsHere_RightsNow.pdf. Accessed March 1, 2008.
13. Forced labour outcomes of irregular migration and human trafficking in Europe. 2003. http://www.belgium.iom.int/STOPConference/Conference%20Papers/06.%20ILO%20-%20Final%20Brussels%20Trafficking%20Paper%20Sept.%202002.pdf. Accessed February 15, 2008.
14. Trafficking in persons report. 2006. Available at http://www.state.gov/g/tip/rls/tiprpt/2006/. Accessed June 25, 2008.
15. Seelke CR, Siskin A. Trafficking in persons: U.S. policy and issues for congress. 2008. http://fas.org/sgp/crs/misc/RL30545.pdf. Accessed May 30, 2008.

16. Sachs J. Macroeconomics and health: investing in health for economic development–report of the commission on macroeconomics and health. 2001. http://www.paho.org/English/HDP/HDD/Sachs.pdf. Accessed June 28, 2008.

17. Zimmerman C, et al. Stolen smiles: the physical and psychological health consequences of women and adolescents trafficked in Europe. 2006. http://www.lshtm.ac.uk/hpu/docs/Stolen%20Smiles%20-%20Trafficking%20and%20Health%20(2006).pdf. Accessed February 1, 2008.

18. Silverman JG, et al. HIV prevalence and predictors of infection in sex-trafficked Nepalese girls and women. 2007;298(5):536-542.

19. Zimmerman C, et al. The health of trafficked women: a survey of women entering posttrafficking service in Europe. 2008;98(1):55-59.

20. Victims of Trafficking and Violence Protection Act of 2000, Pub. L. No. 106-386, 114 Stat. 1464 (codified as amended in scattered sections of U.S.C.).

21. Tiefenbrun S. International justice and shifting paradigms. Updating the domestic and international impact of the U.S. Victims of Trafficking Protection Act of 2000: does law deter crime? *Case West Reserve J Int Law*. 2007;249:280.

22. Department of State. Trafficking persons report. 2007. http://www.state.gov/g/tip/rls/tiprpt/2008/. Accessed July 27, 2008.

23. Haynes DF. (Not) Found chained to a bed in a brothel: conceptual, legal, and procedural failures to fulfill the promise of the Trafficking Victims Protection Act. *Geo Immigr L J* 2007; 337-381

24. Department of Justice. Attorney General's annual report to Congress on U.S. government activities to combat trafficking in persons fiscal year 2006, 2007. http://www.usdoj.gov/ag/annualreports/tr2006/agreporthumantrafficing2006.pdf. Accessed July 23, 2008.

25. Trafficking Victims Protection Reauthorization Act of 2003. 108 P.L. 193; 117 Stat. 2875; (codified in 18 U.S.C.).

26. NAM JS. Note: the case of the missing case: examining the civil right of action for human trafficking victims. *Col L Rev*. 2007;107(7)1655:1703.

27. U.S. Department of Justice. Attorney General's annual report to Congress on U.S. government activities to combat trafficking in persons fiscal year 2007, 2008. http://www.usdoj.gov/ag/annualreports/tr2007/agreporthumantrafficing2007.pdf. Accessed July 23, 2008.

28. Tiefenbrun S. Women, children, and victims of massive crimes: legal developments in Africa: child soldiers, slavery and the trafficking of children. *Fordham Intl L J*. 2008;31(2):415–486.

29. Prosecutorial Remedies and Tools Against the Exploitation of Children Today Act of 2003, Pub. L. 108-21, 117 Stat. 650 (codified as amended in scattered sections of U.S.C.).

30. Office to Monitor and Combat Trafficking in Persons. Fact sheet. US government efforts to fight demand fueling human trafficking. http://www.state.gov/g/tip/rls/fs/08/100208.htm. Accessed July 29, 2008.

31. United States White House Press Release. Human trafficking: a modern form of slavery. http://www.whitehouse.gov/infocus/traffic/. Accessed July 31, 2008.

32. U.S. Department of Justice. Model state anti-trafficking criminal statute. http://www.usdoj.gov/olp/pdf/model_state_regulation.pdf. Accessed July 31, 2008.

33. Forced labor outcomes of irregular migration and human trafficking in Europe. 2003. http://www.belgium.iom.int/STOPConference/Conference%20Papers/06.%20ILO%20-%20Final%20Brussels%20Trafficking%20Paper%20Sept.%202002.pdf. Accessed February 15, 2008.

34. State Council of China. (2008-2012). China National Plan of Action on Combating Trafficking in Women and Children. http://www.humantrafficking.org /uploads/govt_laws/China_National_Plan_of_Action_on_Combating_Trafficking _in_Women_and_Children_December_2007.pdf. Accessed July 31 2008.

35. Moccia P, et al. (2005).UNICEF The state of the world's children 2006, 2005. http://www.unicef.org/sowc06/pdfs/sowc06_fullreport.pdf. Accessed July 31, 2008.

36. Sen AK. *Development as Freedom*. New York, NY: Knopf; 1999:366.

Some violations of women's health and human rights are perpetrated just beyond the mainstream consciousness of public health practitioners. These practices are whispered about, perhaps, and on occasion confronted, but rarely feel their due spotlight of outrage and evidence-based scrutiny. Powerful interests enforce this shadow, including the United States and other governments and the transnational companies they protect. This chapter will explore the current practice and recent history of some of the more egregious of these practices, including the global gag rule, inhumane research practices, targeting women and girl-children for destructive products, torture of women, and forced sterilization. Trafficking of women and girl-children, female genital mutilation, domestic violence, and many other forms of violence against women have their own dedicated chapters within this book.

Many human rights violations against women addressed in this chapter are attributable to United States government policies past and present, often in collusion with other governments and in support of or complicit with transnational companies. While many other governments and supporting entities have a similarly shadowed history and current policy, the leadership of the United States in these issues is of special concern. As a democracy and self-proclaimed champion of human rights, the United States of America should set a global example of what can be done well. Perhaps a light focused upon these dismal practices will help preclude their continuation or their repetition.

The Global Gag Rule

Among the most hypocritical and anti-women's rights of United States foreign policies is the global gag rule, officially termed the Mexico City Policy, which is the practice of withholding US aid from any entity that mentions *abortion* in its literature or performs it in practice (even if such education or practice is financed by funding from other

Shadows on the Sunshine of Women's Global Health and Human Rights: the Global Gag Rule, Tuskegee and HIV Studies, Tobacco Marketing, Torture, and Forced Sterilization

Clyde Lanford Smith MD, MPH, DTM&H, FACP

Clyde Lanford Smith MD, MPH, is Assistant Professor, Residency Programs in Primary Care and Social Internal Medicine, at the Montefiore Medical Center, South Bronx, NY and Doctors for Global Health (DGH) People's Health Movement.

sources). President Bush brought this Reagan-era policy, first begun in 1984, back to practice on January 19, 2001.[1]

So pervasive is the negative mentality concerning abortion engendered by current administration policy that for a brief period beginning around March 30, 2008, the federally funded search site POPLINE, managed by the Johns Hopkins Bloomberg School of Public Health, blocked all searches pertaining to *abortion* from its search engine, concealing with that action approximately 25,000 search results. "We recently made all abortion terms stop words," wrote Debbie Dickson, manager of the Johns Hopkins database. "As a federally funded project, we decided this was best for now." Faced with international scandal, the Johns Hopkins School of Public Health Dean, Dr. Michael J. Klag, sent out a memo on April 4, 2008, stating, "I could not disagree more strongly with this decision, and I have directed that the POPLINE administrators restore *abortion* as a search term immediately. The Johns Hopkins Bloomberg School of Public Health is dedicated to the advancement and dissemination of knowledge and not its restriction."[2]

The global gag rule is the international big brother of US domestic policy under President Reagan. The original gag rule was designed to exclude women in clinics funded by federal government sources from receiving their right to choose elective abortion as established in the 1973 *Roe v. Wade* US Supreme Court decision. Effectively, beginning in 1987, health professionals working in National Health Service clinics (by definition serving the poorest persons in the United States) were prohibited from mentioning abortion as an option during their patient care sessions. If a health professional was caught saying the word *abortion* or implicitly putting that service among the options for a pregnant woman, she or he could be fired.[3]

Several studies have measured the impact, actual and potential, of the global gag rule on women's health. One such study, done in Kenya, concludes: "The loss suffered by NGOs that do not agree to the restrictions imposed by the global gag rule is incalculable. The consequent cutbacks in services and supplies effectively tie the hands of service providers and, by doing so, compromise the health and well-being of millions of women, men, and children. The policy erodes trust between health practitioners and their clients, re-

duces access to HIV/AIDS-prevention measures, and, perhaps most poignantly, renders untold numbers of couples vulnerable to unplanned and unwanted pregnancies, which result in more—not fewer—abortions."[4]

Tuskegee and HIV Studies

Another area of policy and practice affecting women in the US and globally is that of unethical scientific investigation. Here there is the double problem of women not being included in scientific studies (with a potentially deleterious impact of these exclusively male studies on women if the results are then applied to both genders, and the conundrum of how to practice evidence-based medicine in the absence of inclusive investigations), and of studies past and current that do target women but ignore or minimize their human rights. One example of a study that included only men yet affected women directly is the infamous Tuskegee Syphilis Study conducted by the US Public Health Service and Centers for Disease Control and Prevention in Tuskegee, Alabama, from 1932 to 1977, despite the uncovering of the study by the Associated Press in 1972. Briefly, African American males infected with syphilis were told they had "bad blood" (not syphilis) and that they were being treated for this condition. However, even after penicillin, the cure for syphilis, became widely available to the general population in 1947, these men were prohibited from receiving penicillin, all the while receiving regular spinal taps and blood draws to monitor the effect of the disease on their bodies. While all of the 399 subjects of the study were African American males, what many texts and exposés ignore is that these men lived in communities and had wives and children and probably girlfriends.[5]

While Harrison's textbook of medicine records that one third of these men died from the cardiac complications of syphilis,[6] it finds less relevant to comment that 40 wives were infected and eventually given lifelong compensation, and 19 children are known to have been born with congenital syphilis, a condition involving both physical and mental deformities that cannot be compensated for monetarily. Of the men's potential to infect extramarital sexual partners, there is no way to really know if there were any, who they were, and whether any of those who were female were infected and transmitted the agent to their children.[7]

The Tuskegee study at least is a case where an American president (Clinton) has apologized, unlike several of the other shadow practices addressed in this chapter. His apology, an example of what the US government could do for the women torture survivors in Argentina and elsewhere, includes these words:

> The eight men who are survivors of the syphilis study at Tuskegee are a living link to a time not so very long ago that many Americans would prefer not to remember, but we dare not forget. It was a time when our nation failed to live up to its ideals, when our nation broke the trust with our people that is the very foundation of our democracy. It is not only in remembering that shameful past that we can make amends and repair our nation, but it is in remembering that past that we can build a better present and a better future. And without remembering it, we cannot make amends and we cannot go forward. . . . So today America does remember the hundreds of men used in research without their knowledge and consent. We remember them and their family members. Men who were poor and African American, without resources and with few alternatives, they believed they had found hope when they were offered free medical care by the United States Public Health Service. They were betrayed. . . . The people who ran the study at Tuskegee diminished the stature of man by abandoning the most basic ethical precepts. They forgot their pledge to heal and repair. They had the power to heal the survivors and all the others, and they did not. Today, all we can do is apologize."[8]

A more recent study protocol that involved women and echoes Tuskegee was the US Army 2000 study of mother-to-child HIV transmission in Thailand. In this study, exposed by a series of articles in the *Washington Post* called "The Body Hunters," the military insisted on a placebo study arm well after scientific studies had already demonstrated a health advantage to the child. Ad-

ministration of AZT to mothers, followed by administration to newborns, had become the standard of care in the United States.[9] Shortly before, in 1996, a controversy at the *New England Journal of Medicine* had caused a shake-up in the editorial board and throughout the HIV/AIDS community over study protocols that insisted on using placebo arms; their ethical arguments included economic pragmatism and the current (dismal) standard of care in the communities being studied—despite the fact that many of the most evident immediate potential beneficiaries of the studies lived in the industrialized world.[10]

The current controversy of whether to provide HIV-positive mothers with formula is at first blush less black and white than the AZT vs. placebo controlled trials might seem in retrospect. At issue is potentially eliminating the infant's established postpartum breastfeeding risk of HIV infection, 13% per two months exposure in one meta-analysis,[11] but putting the infant at risk for death from diarrhea-related illness, as well as being an option far more expensive for governments and international aid entities. A different study concluded that use of formula instead of breast-feeding by HIV positive mothers seems to have prevented 44% of infant HIV infections,[12] while another analysis gives the rate of transmission of HIV during breast-feeding at 0.7% per month during the first 5 months.[13] Studies evaluating formula vs. breast-feeding continue to be conducted with minimal if any ethical fuss. Consideration that "normal" conditions of the developing world where nearly every child is exposed to feces-containing water leading to nearly universal infection with hepatitis A before adolescence and several episodes of diarrhea is not made. Nor is thought given to creating conditions that include a water-quality intervention such as construction of a clean source of water.[14]

At the heart of the issue there remains the fact that in the industrialized world the standard of care is to provide an alternative to breast milk, resulting in a maternal-to-child postpartum HIV transmission which is nearly zero. Whereas in the non-industrialized world, where most of the children are people of color, some persons, foundations, agencies, and governments insist on a standard of care that involves putting children at significant and well-known risk for HIV infection. Some justify this standard through economic pragmatism, citing the difficulty and expense in providing clean water and effective education to the mothers as well as the expense of formula, and citing studies that show that the children of mothers who have formula but not clean water are at higher risk for dying acutely than are children of breast-feeding mothers. However, it is also important to remember that even if HIV is now a treatable chronic illness for those lucky enough to have access to medicines and who can tolerate them, it remains a deadly illness that itself will need expensive treatment for an infected child's entire life.

Muddying the issue of formula for infants at risk for maternal HIV transmission is the historic memory of the largely successful global fight to take Nestle and other infant-formula companies to task for their unethical and deadly marketing practices to mothers in the nonindustrialized world.[15(p48)]

Tobacco Marketing

Another transnational group that is expert in unethical and deadly marketing to women is the cigarette industry, firmly supported in its murderous growth and actions by the International Monetary Fund as country after country has its state tobacco industry privatized and its citizens exposed to a heightened and effective complexity of advertising that targets women and girl-children to become the newest smokers. "In almost all countries, female deaths due to smoking will more than double over the next 30 years, so that by the year 2020 there will be more than a million deaths of women annually."[15(p49)] As smoking decreases in the West, the tobacco industry is aggressively targeting women and girls with expensive and seductive advertising that blatantly exploits ideas of independence, power, emancipation, and slimness.[16] In Argentina, the targeting of young women, including adolescents, by the cigarette industry has been documented time and again.[17-19]

In Turkey, a case study on the privatization of a state cigarette industry documents the growth of similar targeting as transnational companies take over from privatized national companies. "Gender differences in tobacco use are probably inconsequential in societies where tobacco is grown for home consumption, but become increasingly sub-

stantial as manufactured cigarettes replace local tobacco products."[20]

Within the industrialized world, targeting women and girl-children, especially among people of color, has been documented time and again. "Philip Morris, taking pride in its Marlboro brand, the most popular brand among young women: Marlboro dominates in the 17 and younger age category, capturing over 50% of this market." (1979)

"Statistics show that black people living in a society dominated by whites tend to have a higher smoking rate than their white counterparts. In Canada, only 10% of female university graduates smoke, compared with 40% of unemployed women and 73% of Inuit women. Maori women have the highest rate of lung cancer of any group in the world. In America, rates of lung cancer have increased faster among black women than among white women."[21 (pg25)]

Marketing techniques to encourage women and girl-children to begin and continue smoking are quite extraordinary, and include the following: "brand stretching" or the sales of and promotional efforts for nontobacco products such as clothing that promote tobacco product names and imagery; trade promotions and slotting fees to shape product placement in retail operations; free gifts and prizes in exchange for tobacco purchases; coupons, multipack discounts, and other pricing promotions; venue-based marketing, including formal and informal marketing arrangements in nightclubs; "events marketing" involving creation of particularly youth-oriented events to publicize tobacco products; free cigarette distribution; Internet and online marketing; corporate sponsorship; sophisticated packaging and "youth smoking prevention" campaigns that interfere with genuine tobacco control measures and may actually increase youth smoking rates; database mining and direct-mail promotion—collecting consumer information via web sites, sign-up tables at events, sweepstakes forms, and so on (for direct-mail promotions). The multinational companies have proven particularly expert at making smoking appealing to girls and women.[22]

A 1998 fact sheet from the American Lung Association entitled "Teenage Girls as the Target of the Tobacco Industry" noted:

Cigarette sales and advertising targeting women in the late 1960s and early 1970s coincided with a major increase in the number of teenage girls who began smoking. A 1997 survey by the Centers for Disease Control and Prevention shows that among high school students, 34.7% of girls are current smokers; 15.7% of these girls admitted to smoking frequently."[23]

The sophistication used by the cigarette industry to target women is worthy of exploration in part because the marketing is done with death as an associate-partner. The cognitive dissonance required to be a human part of this profit-making killing machine seems reminiscent of that used by persons working in torture camps or anywhere that promotes death as acceptable collateral damage.

Torture

Promoting death and pain is an essential part of the torturer's job, and when practiced on the body and mind of a woman there is literally fertile ground for terror. Torture is defined by the United Nations 1984 Convention for the Prevention of Torture and Inhumane or Degrading Treatment or Punishment as: "any act by which severe pain or suffering, whether physical or mental, is intentionally inflicted on a person for such purposes as obtaining from him or a third person information or a confession." The convention also states that: "No exceptional circumstances whatsoever, whether a state of war or a threat of war, internal political instability, or any other public emergency, may be invoked as a justification for torture."[24]

Torture is alas another field in which the United States government seems to have decided to become a world leader, recently in the spotlight under the current G. W. Bush administration with its famous Abu-Ghraib torture and subsequent nonapology, and its insistence on promoting water-boarding as an activity that it proudly supports as not being a form of torture. However, the US government has tolerated and encouraged governments that torture and it has taught torture techniques in published manuals within the School of the Americas (now called the Western Hemisphere Institute for Security Corporation) for Latin-American military officers for decades.

These manuals were exposed in 1996, provoking a public apology on the part of the US Department of Defense.[25] Among the many graduates of the School of the Americas were military officers from Argentina, where women suffered famously under the Argentina government during the so-called Dirty War from 1976 to 1983. United States Secretary of State Henry Kissinger was an ardent supporter of this military government, telling Argentina's foreign affairs minister César Augusto Guzzetti in 1976 at a meeting in New York's Waldorf Astoria: "If there are things that have to be done, then you should do them quickly," and under Kissinger's guidance the US government promoted, excused, advised, and financed the Argentina regime's practices.[26] No apology from the US government about its support of what Argentina's women suffered has been forthcoming, a fact that is part of this chapter's motivation. Together with similarly repressive governments in Chile, Paraguay, Uruguay, and for a shorter time Brazil, the US government established Operation Condor with Argentina as a Southern Cone coordinating mechanism in the 1970s, such that what is described in this section about Argentina was done to a greater or lesser extent in all of these countries with the complete knowledge and encouragement of the United States military.[27(p20)]

What was done, specifically, to women in Argentina during this time defies imagination yet has been well documented. A group of survivors and their mothers formed the "Madres de la Plaza de Mayo" (Mothers of the May Plaza) and has made its life goal preserving the memory of those who disappeared and enabling the exposure of the torturers. Women were forced to watch their children and husbands tortured in front of them. "Brutalizing a child in front of his or her mother and torturing a man in front of his wife were favorite ways of trying to make the women talk."[27(p19)]

Entire families were tortured together. As one former death-camp survivor described it: "Of all the dramatic situations I witnessed in clandestine prisons, nothing can compare to those family groups that were tortured, often together, sometimes separately but in view of one another, or in different cells while one was aware of the other being tortured." Another reports: "Five-year-old Josefina Sanchez de Vargas was forced to watch the torture of her father so that he would talk.

When she was returned to her grandparent's home, she took a gun from her grandfather's drawer and shot herself."[27(p21)]

Women were raped and mutilated in front of their children and spouses. Girl-children were raped. One woman gave testimony of her rape at age 12 when the military came to their home to take her father.[27(pp21,22)] One aspect of these women's torture that has not received due attention is the torture of pregnant women. "The treatment and torture of pregnant women in captivity reveals an almost unimaginable level of hatred and cruelty."[27(pp24,25)] Pregnant women in the torture camps were often raped, some daily, and beaten. One documented torture technique was to place an ordinary spoon hooked up to an electric current within the vagina until it touched the fetus, at which point the current (220 volts in Argentina) was applied. Sometimes this and other torture would provoke miscarriage.[28]

Many times pregnant women were held until term, then when they delivered (often by C-section against their will, and always without anesthesia) they were killed. The babies were given to high-ranking military families unable to conceive, or sold on the international market.[29] "At least one military physician—Dr. Norberto Artilio Bianco, who worked in that hospital—is known to have kept two of the children born from women prisoners and registered them as his own. After many years as a fugitive living in Paraguay he was extradited to Argentina in early 1997."[30]

Among the activities of the *Madres de la Plaza de Mayo*, together with Physicians for Human Rights (PHR) has been to use DNA to match these lost children with their estranged birth families. As Dr. Victor Penchaszadeh, a geneticist from Argentina and former board member of PHR, put it: "When grandmothers Chicha Mariani and Estela Barnes de Carlotto asked me in New York in 1982 if it was possible to prove the identity of the children, having only grandparents and other relatives alive, they were making a social claim to the science of genetics. . . . The challenge inherent in that claim resulted . . . in the first identification and restitution of one of the victims: Paula Logares. And this made it possible for human genetics, which for so long served death and backward interests, to serve life."[31]

Forced Sterilization

Preventing the right to have a family, to have children, is one of the oldest forms of violence and abuse against women. But forced sterilization and stealth IUD placement, exemplary as forms of genocide when practiced against people of color and especially indigenous persons, are also a matter of very recent and current practice in many places worldwide. The United States has managed to sterilize its Native American populations quite efficiently, with an estimated 40% of Native American women sterilized in the United States during the 1970s.[32]

In Mexico a ruling found the government guilty of the forced sterilization of indigenous men in the state of Guerrero, their wives having often shared a similar but less overtly traumatic fate.[33(pp79,125-127)] Forced sterilization of indigenous women in the state of Chiapas, Mexico, has also been noted in the recent medical literature.[33(p252)]

In Indonesia, called a "success" in terms of its family planning program, there are reports of IUDs having been placed at gunpoint, notably in populations historically in resistance to the government:

> Coercion of women is still much more common, however. A case study of Kembangwangi subdistrict in west Java reveals the role of the military in threatening villagers. . . . In one safari in 1990 family planning workers accompanied by the police went from house to house and took men and women to a site where IUDs were being inserted. Women who refused had the IUDs inserted at gunpoint."[33(p245)]

Such behavior should not be unexpected given the vision of top policy makers in population control. In an article published in 1979, Bernard Berelson, the late president emeritus of the Population Council, and Jonathon Lieberson argue for the "stepladder" approach to population policy: "Start off with soft measures, such as voluntary family planning services, and proceed if necessary to harsher methods, such as disincentives, sanctions, and even violence." Quoting the aforementioned pair, "Overt violence or other potentially injurious coercion is not to be used before noninjurious [sic] coercion has been exhausted."[33(p255)]

Thus in 1976, India under emergency rule sterilized 6.5 million people, "hundreds, if not thousands, died from infections associated with the operation, and in riots and protests against the program."[33(p248)] The sterilizations in India were done under conditions described as "appalling," and often resulted in the woman not being able to work afterward due to complications. Similar results had been reported in Bangladesh and El Salvador.[33(p228)]

Also in 1976 the US General Accounting Office revealed that the federally funded Indian Health Service had sterilized 3000 Native American women in a 4-year period using consent forms "not in compliance . . . with regulations." Many women of color in New York City during these years received hysterectomies rather than the much less dangerous tubal ligation because the operation was performed in teaching hospitals for the poor.[33(p288)] Dr. R.T. Ravenholt asserted that "The United States was seeking to provide the means by which one quarter of the world's women could be voluntarily sterilized." However, in the case of Puerto Ricans, the United States was even more aggressive, with one study showing that "in the early 1980s half of Puerto Rican women of reproductive age had been sterilized in Hartford, Connecticut."[33(p250)]

The United States Agency for International Development (AID), together with the World Bank, has been one of the principle sources of funding for coercive sterilization globally, despite an injunction in 1982-3; the US Foreign Assistance Act prohibiting US funds "to coerce or provide any financial incentive to any person to undergo sterilization." In 1988 in Bangladesh, for example, AID continued financial incentives, calling them "compensation payments."[33]

One element of perversity for sterilization campaigns is that women of lower economic status are rarely offered options. Thus, even those spared overt coercion often face the dilemma of having child after child without child spacing versus never having another child.[33] Alas, there exists a "phenomenon of sterilization regret . . . A 1987 survey in Mexico found that over 10% of women who had been sterilized would not have the operation again if they had a choice."[33]

Conclusion

The government and transnational policies and practices introduced briefly in this chapter, horrible as they are, are but limited examples to the many similar oppressive policies visited on women globally. What can we as public health students and practitioners, clinicians, and citizens of the world do about the unfair practices and policies identified in this chapter? For one thing we must seek to recognize injustice when we encounter it, and do our best in practice not to participate in doing harm. A litmus test of policy involves the question: "Would I be comfortable having such action done on myself, my family and loved ones, in my community, and in my country? Would it even be legal?" These questions insist that one attempt actions motivated by a rights-based approach, rather than by an economic pseudo-justification that nearly always leaves the practitioner among the patronizing privileged, albeit pragmatically so, in any situation involving oppression and injustice.

Another potential action involves informing ourselves and others about the reality of women's global health and human rights, especially the reality for poor women and women of color. Much of this information will not be presented in the average classroom or on the front page of the daily press, though a careful reading of the latter will often provide a plethora of examples for those who read looking to uncover injustice. Also, do whatever is necessary to hold our professional community as well as our governments, local and national, to task in preventing similar policy, and in addressing current problems. Too many health professionals have participated in all of the above atrocities, including torture, but far more have taken the side of the oppressors by remaining covertly "neutral" when they could have made a difference. Finally, there are many women organized in groups, such as the Mothers of the Plaza de Mayo in Argentina, also in Mexico and Iraq, who have suffered and are survivors but refuse to be victims. Consider seeking, learning with, and joining these groups, accompanying their work with scientific acumen (as Physicians for Human Rights has done globally to restore the children of disappeared women) and sharing with them as a scientist and as a fellow, caring human being.

DISCUSSION QUESTIONS

1. How does the global gag rule affect the ability of health professionals, health centers and nongovernmental health and human rights groups internationally to provide optimal health care for women? What effect might it have on the ability of women internationally to have more control of their own health and lives? What right does the United States of America have to disallow discussion or practice of abortion in groups it helps fund when abortion is by Supreme Court decision a women's right within the United States?

2. Why is there a double-standard in what is considered standard of care for people in the industrialized world vs. people in the nonindustrialized world? How is a rights-based approach to policy different from an approach emphasizing the economically feasible? What are potential ways to guard against future Tuskegee-like investigations involving people of color?

3. How does tobacco marketing target women and the girl-child? Why does the International Monetary Fund promote privatization of the tobacco industry, and what are the potential consequences of that privatization for women? How might marketing employees of transnational tobacco companies justify the deadly consequences of their daily work to their children and grandchildren?

4. How did the United States government facilitate the torture of women in Argentina? Imagine yourself as a member of the Mothers of May group: What steps would you take to try and prevent future happenings of torture in Argentina and around the world? What would you ask of the Argentina and United States governments concerning their conduct during the Dirty War?

5. Why do women of color seem to be the ones disproportionately targeted for sterilization around the world? What role has the United States government played in the global sterilization campaign? How might the Mexican health professionals who placed IUDs in indigenous women without their knowledge justify this professional behavior to their colleagues, community, and patients? What would you do if you found yourself as a health professional expected to participate in coerced sterilization of women or in surreptitious IUD placement and your job depended on your not causing problems?

REFERENCES

1. Access Denied. Global Gag Rule. 2008. http://www.globalgagrule.org/index.htm. Accessed August 2, 2008.
2. CBS News. Web Site restores abortion search term. 2008. http://www.cbsnews .com/stories/2008/04/05/health/main3995656.shtml. Accessed August 2, 2008.
3. Cohen SA. Global gag rule: exporting antiabortion ideology at the expense of American values. 2001;3:3. http://www.guttmacher.org/pubs/tgr/04/3 /gr040301.html. Accessed August 2, 2008.
4. Access Denied. NGO rural and youth outreach programs cutback. 2008. http://www.globalgagrule.org/execsum3.htm. Accessed August 2, 2008.

5. Ross S. Clinton's Tuskegee apology also aims to improve relations with blacks. 2008. http://www.tuskegee.edu/global/Story.asp?s=1211670. Accessed August 2, 2008.

6. Braunwald E, ed. *Harrison's Principles of Internal Medicine.* 15th ed. New York, NY: McGraw-Hill; 2000; 1046.

7. White House Office of the Press Secretary. Remarks by the President in apology for study done in Tuskegee. 1997. http://64.233.169.104/search?q=cache: rOeWZHtCwGIJ:clinton4.nara.gov/textonly/New/Remarks/Fri/19970516898 .html. Accessed August 2, 2008.

8. Hassani B. Trials by fire: the case of unethical clinical trials in the countries of the south. 2005. http://www.utmj.org/issues/82.3/Philosophy_and_Medicine__82-3 -212.pdf. Accessed August 2, 2008.

9. Lurie P, Wolfe SM. Unethical trials of interventions to reduce perinatal transmission of the human immunodeficiency virus in developing countries. *NEJM.* 1997;337:853-856.

10. Timing of breast milk HIV-1 transmission: a meta-analysis. *East Afr Med J.* 2001; 78(2):75-79.

11. Nduati R, John G, Mbori-Ngacha D, et al. Effect of breastfeeding and formula feeding on transmission of HIV-1. *JAMA.* 2000;283:1167-1174.

12. Gottlieb S. News extra: vertical transmission of HIV through breast milk most likely to occur soon after birth. *BMJ.* 1999;319:594. http://www.bmj.com/cgi /content/full/319/7210/594/d. Accessed August 2, 2008.

13. Coovadia HM, Rolins NC, Bland RM, et al. Mother-to-child transmission of HIV-1 infection during exclusive breastfeeding in the first 6 months of life: an intervention cohort study. *Lancet.* 2007;369(9567):1107-1116.

14. Baby milk action. Boycott Nestle. 2008. http://www.babymilkaction.org/pages /boycott.html. Accessed August 2, 2008.

15. MaCay J. FRCP. *JAMWA.* 1996;51:481-482.

16. Braun S, Mejia R, Ling PM, Perez-Stable EJ. Tobacco industry targeting youth in Argentina. *Tob Control.* 2008;(2):111-117.

17. Martinez E, Kaplan CP, Guil V, Gregorich SE, Mejia R, J Pérez-Stable E. Smoking behavior and demographic risk factors in Argentina: a population-based survey. *Prev Control.* 2006;(4):187-197.

18. Morello P, Duggan A, Adger H Jr, Anthony JC, Joffe A. Tobacco use among high school students in Buenos Aires, Argentina. *Am J Public Health.* 2001;91(2): 219-224.

19. Sahin Mutlu F, Ayranci U, Ozdamar K. Cigarette smoking habits among men and women in Turkey: a meta regression analysis. *Iran J Public Health.* 2006;35(2): 7-15. http://journals.tums.ac.ir/upload_files/pdf/2352.pdf. Accessed August 2, 2008.

20. Action on Smoking and Health. Big tobacco and women: what the tobacco industry's confidential documents reveal. http://old.ash.org.uk/html/conduct/html /tobexpld8.html#known. Accessed August 2, 2008.

21. Weissman R, White A. International monetary fund support for tobacco privatization and for tobacco tax and tariff reduction, and the cost to public health: an essential action report. 2002. http://www.essentialaction.org/tobacco. Accessed August 2, 2008.

22. American Lung Association. Teenage girls as the target of the tobacco industry. 1998. http://www.ritobaccocontrolnet.com/teengirl.htm. Accessed August 2, 2008.

23. Britannica. Convention against torture and other cruel, inhuman or degrading treatment or punishment. http://www.britannica.com/EBchecked/topic/930734/Convention-against-Torture-and-Other-Cruel-Inhuman-or-Degrading-Treatment-or-Punishment. Accessed August 2, 2008.

24. Virtual Truth Commission. U.S. Army torture manuals. 1998. http://www.geocities.com/~virtualtruth/manuals.htm. Accessed August 2, 2008.

25. Borger J. Kissinger backed dirty war against left in Argentina transcripts show former secretary of state urged violent crackdown on opposition. 2004. http://www.commondreams.org/headlines04/0828-02.htm. Accessed August 2, 2008.

26. National Security Archive. Operation Condor: cable suggest US role. 2001. http://www.gwu.edu/~nsarchiv/news/20010306/. Accessed August 2, 2008.

27. Arditti R. *Searching for Life: The Grandmothers of the Plaza de Mayo and the Disappeared Children of Argentina.* Berkeley: University of California Press; 1999:19-22, 24, 25.

28. Butler L, Granich R, Barrett K. *The Search for Argentina's Disappeared.* http://www.hrcberkeley.org/dna/argentina011.html. Accessed August 2, 2008.

29. Johansen B. Women and children at risk. 1998. http://www.libertadlatina.org/Sterilization_of_Native_American_Women_09-1998.htm. Accessed August 2, 2008.

30. Intercontinental cry. Mexico compensates indigenous men for forced sterilizations. 2008. http://intercontinentalcry.org/mexico-compensates-indigenous-men-for-forced-sterilizations/. Accessed August 2, 2008.

31. Tlachinollan. Parcial cumplimiento de la Ssa a recomendación de la CNDH, por esterilizados de El Camalot. 2008. http://www.tlachinollan.org/notbp/notbp080731.htm. Accessed August 2, 2008.

32. Kirsch JD, Cedeno MA. Informed consent for family planning for poor women in Chiapas, Mexico. *Lancet.* 1999;354(9176):419-420.

33. Hartmann B. *Reproductive Rights and Wrongs: The Global Politics of Population Control.* Cambridge, MA: South End Press; 1995:79, 125-127, 245, 248, 252, 255.

Laws and policies for human rights evolve, with this evolution drawing on the culmination of several facets of social change: the nature of the driving issues, the rhetoric of proponents and adversaries, the strategic decision making of advocates, and the influence of key stakeholders on all sides of the issues.[2] Yet not all movements for social change reach the level of international law. It is only when there is "a set of political/legal concepts or vocabulary by which scientific insights can be reframed into political claims, and a social movement that can press such claims" that new thinking translates in law, policy, or rights.[3] Characterizing this process in human rights evolution through a "tipping point" model of social change, this chapter explores how the international legal language of reproductive rights became nearly synonymous with women's civil rights, laying out a theoretical human rights framework for the largely programmatic public health chapters that follow. Through this review of international legal norms and the social movements that presaged them, we find that this narrowing of human rights discourse in reproduction is due largely to three elements: political climates at specific moments in history; limitations of available legal frameworks; and strong, vocal, and visible social movements for women's equality. These associated elements have created a paradigm shift, restricting reproductive rights to a negative human rights framework (requiring government to cease interferences) rather than a comprehensive framework complemented by positive human rights (requiring government intervention).

Through the 1979 Convention on the Elimination of All Forms of Discrimination Against Women and subsequently in the 1994 International Conference on Population and Development in Cairo and the 1995 Fourth World Conference on Women in Beijing, many of the advocates for women's equality became the lobbyists, the lawyers, and the leaders in the struggle to define and achieve reproductive rights. Bodily integrity, personal autonomy, and the right to choose became the shared discourse for women across the world in realizing freedom from paternalistic

Going Negative: How Reproductive Rights Discourse Has Been Altered from a Positive to a Negative Rights Framework in Support of "Women's Rights"

Reilly Anne Dempsey, JD, MPH;
Benjamin Mason Meier, JD, LLM, MPhil

Reilly Anne Dempsey, JD, MPH, is a researcher and consultant for sexual and reproductive health and rights, based in New York, NY.

Benjamin Mason Meier, JD, LLM, MPhil, is Project Manager for Public Health Law at the Center for Health Policy, as well as an IGERT-International Development and Globalization Fellow in the Department of Sociomedical Sciences at Columbia University, New York, NY.

It would be a sad irony if our efforts to empower women were to be reduced to a debate on abortion, and if the role and well-being of women were to be reduced, once again, to just one aspect and one moment of their lives and reproductive health, however important it may be.[1]

—Hiroshi Nakajima

regimes. Reproductive rights, rather than goals in and of themselves, were originally framed by women's rights advocates as a means to achieve gender equality. While women's equality would not be whole without reproductive freedom, this predominant demand for a negative rights approach has placed reproductive health outside of the legal obligations of the state.

Yet women's health is different from women's civil rights, requiring more than rights to privacy, nondiscrimination, or participation. Although the right to control one's fertility is a pressing reproductive need,[4] reproductive health also encompasses positive rights—the enabling economic, social, and cultural conditions "in which choices are made" and the infrastructure that allows those choices to come to fruition.[3] Women and men in some cultures are simply not in a position to exercise autonomy or privacy in a way that will lead to sexual and reproductive health. For example, the right to control one's own fertility does not mean much if oral contraceptives are inaccessible or family planning clinics are inadequate, or in a nation in which the health system is crumbling and women's voices are stifled. Thus, "the right to privacy is simply not broad enough to ensure that all women have access to the health services."[3] Where reproductive rights are distilled to a debate on the single issue of abortion (critical as though it may be), myriad other aspects of sexual and reproductive health are left outside of legal discourse.[5]

The current reproductive rights legal framework—formulated as negative rights to protect reproductive decision making—is not independently capable of responding to modern public health challenges. The global capitalist economy has exacerbated disparities in underlying determinants of good health, with neoliberal economic development policies and continued fallout from structural adjustment programs having rendered health care a privilege rather than a basic right. Scholars have only begun to analyze the detrimental long-term effects of the free market economy, which has been shown to affect governmental infrastructures, vulnerable groups, and health outcomes.[6] This global economic shift has harmed, if not decimated, state-sponsored (and therefore universally accessible) health systems, systems which could, if given the infrastructures and resources necessary, address inequities in underlying determinants of

women's health.[7] Without economic and social rights to combat these inequities, specifically rights to health and reproductive health care, rights to privacy and bodily integrity cannot fully succeed in improving lives.[8]

In this chapter, we explore how reproductive rights came to fall under this negative rights framework, examining why this strategy dominated the history of ideas on reproductive health as a human right. In Part II of this chapter, we provide an overview of human rights frameworks and discourses, focusing on the historical split between negative and positive rights and contemporary efforts to reunite these interconnected paradigms. In Part III, we trace the historical events that structured the legal framing of reproductive health, highlighting the political debates, the available legal paths, and the social movements that brought reproductive justice to international policy discussions. Part IV then looks to constructivist international relations frameworks, using a tipping point model of norm evolution, to analyze how and why the changing discourses of reproductive health culminated in a negative rights construction. In Part V, we point out the shortcomings of this enduring negative rights framework and posit that current politics, legal paths, and social movements provide a unique opportunity to develop a complementary positive rights discourse for women's health.

Legal Frameworks

Human rights, though at times purporting to represent natural law, are inextricably rooted in historical context, and as a result of this historical construction, can be seen to evolve in response to social movements.[9] The structure of the UN human rights system, from its origins, was tailored to satisfy political will. Although the 1948 Universal Declaration of Human Rights (UDHR) provided the most comprehensive enumeration of all fundamental rights at the time, when it came time for states to ratify legally enforceable instruments based upon the UDHR, international relations necessitated a split. After all, the post-WWII world itself was divided politically. Western countries were primarily pressing civil and political rights, wary of adopting legally enforceable "welfare" rights. Eastern states, many under communist and socialist rule, were in favor of economic and social rights, but were not willing to adopt legally enforceable civil and political rights. In an effort to salvage the human rights enterprise, state representatives entered into lengthy negotiations and reached what may have been one of the most influential human rights compromises of the century: two separate 1967 treaties—the International Covenant on Civil and Political Rights (ICCPR) and the International Covenant on Economic, Social and Cultural Rights (ICESCR). The world was consequently left with an enduring legacy of bifurcation, reifying the historically constructed political split between civil and political rights and economic, social, and cultural rights.[10]

Though arguably superficial in construct, this divide is critical in application. In its most basic form, civil and political rights, enshrined in the ICCPR, are interpreted as "negative" rights. These rights do not purport to require government intervention.[11] Rather, they ask governments to cease engaging in activities such as torture, interference with voting, or intrusion in citizen's private lives. Economic, social, and cultural rights, enshrined in the ICESCR, are typically framed as "positive" rights. These are rights that call for government intervention such as the right to education, the right to housing, and, most importantly for this chapter, the right to the "highest attainable standard" of health.[12] While almost all scholars now agree that there are negative and positive aspects to each human right (e.g., the meaningful realization of the right to vote encompasses both the state ceasing interference and providing a functioning infrastructure),[13] even a codification of this interrelation among rights in the 1993 Vienna Declaration and Programme of Action has done little to mediate the underlying frameworks constructed during the height of the Cold War.

Continued Western influence has led to a more developed jurisprudence for negative rights, which Western scholars continue to term "first-generation rights."[14] As a result, activists often seek to enforce the more acceptable negative aspects of economic and social rights rather than put forward a direct positive rights argument (e.g., a strategic preference for selective violations of the negative right to life over pervasive violations of the positive right to health).[15] Given this legal landscape, reproductive rights advocates have been more readily able to engage civil and political rights than economic, social, and cultural rights as a means to reach their immediate goals of women's freedom, including reproductive freedom. Donna Sullivan summarizes and justifies this strategy:

> Until the mechanisms for supervising and enforcing implementation of social human rights are strengthened . . . the main aspects of individual and community health, including those related to sexual and reproductive health, are probably better protected indirectly, through enforcement of related classical human rights [negative rights], than by way of reliance on the right to health itself.[16]

But just how and why have negative rights become more readily available for the framing of reproductive rights? In the 1979 Convention on the Elimination of all Forms of Discrimination Against Women (CEDAW), state representatives agreed to root gender equity through civil and political rights. Although there are provisions for economic, social, and cultural rights, CEDAW calls predominantly for equality, freedom, and nondiscrimination—all principles of negative rights.[17] It was under the aegis of this convention, and its codification of negative rights for women's empowerment, that women's rights advocates for reproductive freedom found their legal voice.

In this historical predisposition for negative rights (in reproductive rights and beyond), the right to health under the ICESCR has been comparatively underutilized by states, international organizations, and international treaty implementation bodies.[16] It was not until 2000 that the Committee on Economic, Social and Cultural Rights produced General Comment 14 on the right to the highest attainable standard of health, providing the international human rights community with the clarification necessary to determine the meaning of the right to health and to realize the right through enforcement of state obligations.[18] With this elaboration of positive rights for health, reproductive rights advocates have a unique opportunity to expand their human rights discourse to encompass reproductive health issues.

Evolution of Reproductive Rights

Tracing the historical events and political contexts that led up to the modern day conceptualization of reproductive rights, it becomes clear that international legal norms for health correspond historically with social movements. In this part, we trace these movements, discussing the ways in which they pressed for codification of international legal obligations for reproductive rights.

1950s and 1960s: Population Control

The modern era of human rights began with special concern for issues of reproductive decision making, if not reproduction itself. In the 1948 Universal Declaration of Human Rights, states explicitly linked motherhood with health rights and other social services:

- Everyone has the right to a standard of living adequate for the health and well-being of himself and of his family, including food, clothing, housing, and medical care and necessary social services, and the right to security in the event of unemployment, sickness, disability, widowhood, old age, or other lack of livelihood in circumstances beyond his control.
- Motherhood and childhood are entitled to special care and assistance. All children, whether born in or out of wedlock, shall enjoy the same social protection.[19]

Proceeding from the gender equality mission of the Commission on the Status of Women while ensuring paternalistic chivalry for the "special care" of women, these health concerns would soon become the basis for the ICESCR's Article 12 codification of the right to the "highest attainable standard" of health to include state duties for "provision for the reduction of the stillbirth rate and of infant mortality and for the healthy development of the child."[20]

And yet despite this emphasis on reproductive health, reproduction remained in these early years under the rubric of population control (a sovereign state prerogative) rather than rights (a protected individual entitlement). Demographers in the 1950s and 1960s, drawing on Malthusian fears of overpopulation and holding firm to the theoretical remnants of eugenics, pressed for national policies that would restrain the unchecked growth of the developing world. Despite a consistent emphasis on population control, the tools underlying the debate changed in the 1960s with the advent of medical technologies for hormonal control (most prominently, oral contraceptives) and thereby for population control practiced at the individual level (in opposition to pronatalist developing country policies).[21] Reproductive rights arose in part from the confines of this new population control, with demographers using reproductive technologies to conceive of a "family planning agenda" that would impose Western notions of fertility reduction on developing countries under the rhetorical guise of "reproductive rights."[22] Based on previous United Nations declarations recognizing the importance of slowing reproduction to improve living conditions, this human rights consensus is expressed most expansively in the 1968 International Conference on Human Rights in Tehran, which proclaims the right of "parents...to determine freely and responsibly the number and spacing of their children."[23] This invocation of family planning as an individual human right, making available information along with the benefits of advances in science and technology, would frame women's rights to reproductive health services as extending only as far as access to family planning, a negative framing of reproductive rights that would help structure the debates of the decades to come.[24]

1970s and 1980s: The UN Decade of Women

Despite the emergence of "reproductive rights" as family planning, "reproduction" remained synonymous with "pregnancy," and "pregnancy" remained a site for sexism and paternalism. By the 1970s, the women's rights movement for equality was becoming stronger, more active, and more developed. Starting in 1967 in the United Kingdom, a cascade of domestic abortion court cases and laws flowed across the Western world. In 1969, Canada began to permit abortions under limited circumstances; in *R v. Davidson* in Australia, abortion was made legal to protect the life or physical or mental health of the woman; in 1973, the US Supreme Court heard *Roe v. Wade*, framing US constitutional protections of abortion; and from 1973 to 1980, France, West Germany, New Zealand, Italy, and the Netherlands passed laws legalizing abortion under certain circumstances.[25] At the international level, the United Nations Decade of Women and the women in development (W.I.D.) movement began to chip away at notions that continued to equate women with pregnancy. In 1967, with the support of the Commission on the Status of Women, the UN adopted the Declaration on the Elimination of Discrimination against Women, making this Declaration legally binding in the 1979 CEDAW. Through CEDAW, autonomous control over one's own body was seen as the key to participation and development:

12.1. States Parties shall take all appropriate measures to eliminate discrimination against women in the field of health care in order to ensure, on a basis of equality of men and women, access to health care services, including those related to family planning.

12.2. Notwithstanding the provisions of paragraph I of this article, States Parties shall ensure to women appropriate services in connection with pregnancy, confinement and the postnatal period, granting free services where necessary, as well as adequate nutrition during pregnancy and lactation.[17]

With this language, Article 12.1 couches health in terms of equality and access, not as an explicit social right.[17] Article 12.2, addressing access to services, only applies to pregnancy.[17] Advocates felt that women needed to move toward laws providing for gender equity in all aspects of life. The focus was directed on equality in the public sphere, not the enabling underlying conditions traditionally thought to be in the private sphere or the health rights necessary for reproductive health.[26]

Given this attention to women as rights-holders, the 1985 Third International Conference on Women in Nairobi brought violence against women into global public concern, the first international legal consideration of a women's issue that had previously been relegated to the private sphere.[26] A large NGO forum at Nairobi provided the space for women to explore legal frameworks to combat their unique harms.[26] For example, the final report from Nairobi states: "[t]he continuation of women's stereotyped reproductive and productive roles, justified primarily on physiological, social and, cultural grounds, has subordinated them in the general as well as sectoral spheres of development."[27]

1985–1993: Vienna

With a firm underpinning in international law, the next eight years saw the women's rights movement make significant advances in nations throughout the world.[2] Violence against women, rape, and sexual assault also brought gender inequalities and women's rights to the forefront of international concern. Most rights for women were, at the time, not broadly pursued. Yet the right to be free from violence, internationally well defined, became an important and opportunistic entry point to advocate for rights specific to women. In this context, reproduction and sex were characterized as tools of oppression and the situs of both physical and structural violence against women, restraining women from realizing their civil and political rights to participation and development. Although little is written about this time period, some authors show that this was a time of formulating and debating reproductive justice under this new framework.[28] As international relations changed through the fall of communism and rise of the neoliberal economic model, women's rights advocates were gaining strength and power in domestic circles, networking with one another and preparing to advance their agenda in international law.

The landscape of human rights changed in 1993 in Vienna.[29] As part of a larger recognition that all human rights are interrelated, interdependent, indivisible, and universal (purportedly to reconnect positive and negative rights frameworks), women's rights activists from all over the world came together with governmental and nongovernmental representatives to speak out at the Vienna Convention. Their words were memorialized in the Vienna Declaration and Programme of Action (Vienna Declaration) on the future of human rights in the post-Cold War era.[30] With regard to the rights of women, the Vienna Declaration recognized that:

> The human rights of women and of the girl-child are an inalienable, integral, and indivisible part of universal human rights. The full and equal participation of women in political, civil, economic, social, and cultural life, at the national, regional, and international levels, and the eradication of all forms of discrimination on grounds of sex are priority objectives of the international community.
>
> Gender-based violence and all forms of sexual harassment and exploitation, including those resulting from cultural prejudice and international trafficking, are incompatible with the dignity and worth of the human person, and must be eliminated. This can be achieved by legal measures and through national action and international cooperation in such fields as economic and social development, education, safe maternity and health care, and social support.
>
> The human rights of women should form an integral part of the United Nations human rights activities, including the promotion of all human rights instruments relating to women.[31]

While the Vienna Declaration did not result in the promised denouement in rejoining positive and negative rights for reproduction, the Vienna Declaration was an important landmark for "increasing public visibility for the human rights of women," setting the stage for achievements that would arise soon thereafter.[32]

1994–1995: Cairo and Beijing

Standing on these years of advocacy work, foundation-building activism, and international law culminating in the Vienna Declaration, the 1994 International Conference on Population and Development (ICPD) in Cairo was a strategic opportunity to move away from fertility control. Discourse framed reproduction and sexuality as a combination of both civil and political rights and economic and social rights, advancing these issues in terms of (1) bodily integrity and self-determination, (2) equality, and (3) enabling conditions or social

rights.[29] These concepts were constructed as "prerequisites" for women's full participation in society and development, but not yet as rights unto themselves.[29] Just as paternalistic world leaders had used reproductive rights as a rhetorical guise for population control three decades earlier, now population control provided a rhetorical guise for moving reproductive rights forward.

The Fourth World Conference on Women in Beijing took these hortatory statements even further, endorsing a strong rights-based approach to women's equality and reproductive freedom as well as economic and social rights.[33] Yet even with the guiding principles of Cairo focused on economic and social rights—"[p]opulation-related goals and policies are integral parts of cultural, economic, and social development, the principal aim of which is to improve the quality of life of all people," and "[s]tates should take all appropriate measures to ensure, on a basis of equality of men and women, universal access to health-care services, including those related to reproductive health care, which includes family planning and sexual health"—reproductive rights continued to be aligned with negative civil and political rights.[34] Where political will and global economics did not provide the space or opportunity to meaningfully consider enabling conditions and social rights, reproductive rights continued (and continue today) to be strongly associated with autonomy, self-determination, and equality.

The Framing of Reproductive Rights: Turning a Movement into a Right

Flowing from this historical description of the evolution of international law for reproductive rights, this section examines how these historically constructed developments and political contexts worked in tandem to culminate in the utilization of negative rights to codify reproductive and sexual rights as human rights.

This analysis builds on a rise of constructivism in international relations theory,[35] viewing norms as instrumental in ordering state behavior[36] in the language of human rights jurisprudence and examining the development of each international human right as an iterative process indicative of a global set of norms. Rather than a human right serving as an individual norm, it is possible to consider each human right as a collection of multiple norms, each of which can independently emerge, evolve, and spread over time.[37] International law has become the predominant way of memorializing these global human rights norms,[38] and, as a result, recent constructivist scholarship has looked to the expression of norms in international legal institutions.[36] In this sense, international law reflects a negotiated codification of global norms already in existence and reifies those norms until changed through normative evolution and subsequent legislative amendment.[39]

Applying this framework for norm evolution to explore how reproductive rights became codified as negative rights, this analysis applies a "tipping point" model of global norm development.[40] Here, norms are seen to emerge in a single state among a small group of actors; only once a critical mass of states have adopted the norm does the norm reach a "tipping" point, followed thereafter by broad international acceptance. Under this model, networks of nongovernmental actors ("norm entrepreneurs" in the language of international relations) persuade powerful domestic and international actors ("norm leaders") on the correctness of their social movement,[41] swaying states and international organizations to endorse norms and press them into domestic, regional, and then international treaty law. Reaching the tipping point of states necessary for international codification of this changing norm, norms thereafter gain broad international acceptance through what is now termed a "norm cascade."[40] During this process, individual state and nongovernmental representatives harmonize individual state norms and advance these ideas into international legal discourse.[42] The final stage, norm internalization, "generates a legal rule that will guide future transnational interactions between the parties; future transactions will further internalize those norms; and eventually, repeated participation in the process will help to reconstitute the interests and even the identities of the participants in the process."[43]

In social movements to declare a norm of reproductive freedom and codify that norm as a human right, women's equality activists were "norm entrepreneurs." They were motivated to lobby for reproductive freedom as part of their larger agenda for gender equality. Their organizational platform was CEDAW, focusing on civil rights. As the movement to translate reproductive health into legally enforceable human rights grew, the next class of norm entrepreneurs was dependent on this legal path and existing normative frameworks of women's equality and negative rights. At the ICPD and Fourth World Conference on Women, the normative framing of reproductive justice as a series of negative rights reached its tipping point, where women's rights groups reached the critical mass necessary to secure a place on the international agenda for reproductive freedom.[44] By this moment, the existing structures and legal norms for population and development were in place and provided the path and political support needed to move a negative conception of reproductive rights forward.[1] The norm entrepreneurs, the organizational platforms (development and gender equality conferences), and the dependency on existing normative frameworks acted in concert to dictate this negative rights approach.[45] Despite some activists' longstanding warnings of the shortcomings of this negative rights discourse—explaining that women's reproductive decision making does not exist in a vacuum, but rather is highly dependent on social, political, and economic contexts[5]—reproductive justice as a negative right is currently in the third stage of norm evolution, "norm internalization," as states and other actors have begun to apply the negative rights codification of reproduction to guide policies and programs.

In depicting the normative evolution of reproductive health norms into a negative international human right, Figure 8-1 highlights each international legal document in the process, delineating each legal standard by its pursuance of negative rights discourse (below the line) or positive rights discourse (above the line). Viewing norms for reproductive rights in this way, it is clear that the framing of reproductive health has changed over time, flowing from negative to positive and back again. Yet internalization of reproductive rights as negative rights may be stymied by competing normative frameworks, with a new human rights landscape seen in the emergence of positive rights norms for a robust right to health, indicated by the arrows showing a potential reframing of reproductive health norms in responding more fully to modern reproductive health needs.

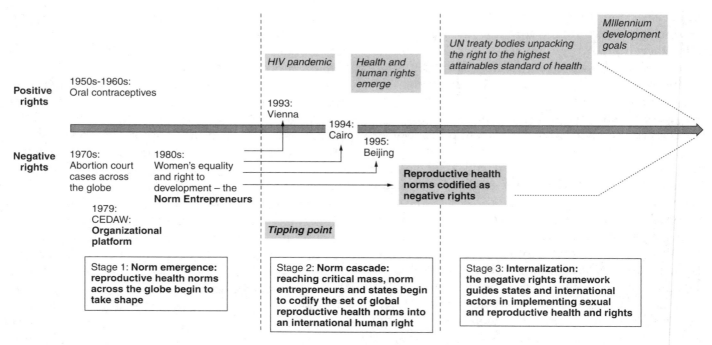

Figure 8-1 Timeline of Human Right's Progress towards the Millennium Goals

Within the normative debate outlined above, although there were likely multiple, overlapping forces acting upon and within the reproductive rights movement, it is clear that the following social movements bear a preponderant role in driving reproductive rights discourse in international law.

First, strange bedfellows—the Vatican and Muslim fundamentalists—found agreement in their strong opposition to reproductive and sexual rights.[32] Throughout the course of modern history, religious groups have been successful in mobilizing to exert influence on global politics.[46] While passing a law against violence or rape was morally acceptable to these groups, progressive ideas such as reproductive freedoms and sexuality rights were not, with implicit and explicit homophobia present at negotiating tables into the early 1990s and beyond.[25] For example, the preamble to the ICPD uses language that carves out exceptions for religious and cultural practices.[34] In opening the door to reproductive and sexual justice, LGBT populations would be authorized to claim rights, thereby weakening the basic tenets of these politically powerful religions. Responding to these pressures, women's groups were constrained to press for reproductive freedoms, not a right to reproductive health.

Second, environmental groups, focused on controlling population growth and fertility, also played a role in shaping the discourse for reproductive rights. Reacting against interest groups pressing for government-sponsored fertility control programs, women's rights activists espoused a "hands off my body" approach to reproductive rights, reinforcing a negative rights framing of reproduction. The emphasis on population control also strongly influenced the burgeoning of the reproductive rights movement in the global south, as northern superpowers began to exert pressure on developing nations to control fertility, evident in some of the language and discourse of Cairo.[46] This struggle also pointed to a negative rights framework to give women rights over their own bodies, if only to stave off "insensitive (if not downright coercive) population control policies."[46]

Finally, the global economy, driven by the effects of the Washington Consensus and international financial institutions' structural adjustment programs, led both developed and developing nations to experience massive cutbacks in social welfare systems, especially health care. In light of this retrenchment in the welfare state under the neo-liberal development model, a reliance on a positive right to health framework in the late 1980s and 1990s would likely have led to few, if any, actual achievements or improvements in reproductive health. Where there lacked the state-level capacity to intervene for sexual and reproductive health through a positive rights framework, there could be few obligations placed on states for conditions largely outside their control.

The legacy of this discourse, a negative framing of reproductive rights, is not sufficient to respond to the changing needs, politics, and economics of today's globalizing world. A negative rights framework obligates states to do little more than cease interfering with the individual right to freely choose the timing and spacing of childbearing and to ensure freedom from sexual violence in the public sphere. (In fact, it has been suggested that states intentionally moved toward a negative rights framework to allow states to provide the bare minimum of health protection and yet still claim that they are fulfilling women's rights.[47]) This framing has not succeeded in achieving bodily integrity and respecting the right to privacy in all parts of the world, nor has it led to equal reproductive justice or sexual and reproductive health in the current neoliberal economy. Women and men will need states to provide a functioning healthcare system and the economic and social conditions that underlie reproductive justice in order to realize sexual and reproductive health.

Moving Forward: Normative Frameworks and Legal Paths

Despite this evolution of reproductive justice as negative rights, reproductive rights are not fixed on this path. Highlighting the ever-present gap between rights and reality, sexual and reproductive health in today's economic and political climate has arguably become even less accessible for many, especially vulnerable populations and communities.[48] With more global attention being paid to social determinants of health and a stronger positive rights framework, the stage is set for shifting reproductive rights away from the negative

rights discourse and framework. While not criticizing the past negative rights discourse of reproductive rights—on the contrary, this was exactly the necessary strategy to translate the social movement for reproductive justice into human rights—it is clear that this framework alone is not appropriate to today's economic, social, and political climate. Given current global health initiatives, the time has come to build on and complement this negative rights jurisprudence by codifying the positive rights inherent in reproductive health.

The Millennium Development Goals

Today's global economy and the international flow of donor funding, both affecting reproductive and sexual health, suggest that a positive rights framework that supports enabling economic and social conditions for sexual and reproductive health is not only desirable but also necessary.[49] International governance has already partially endorsed such a shift with the advancement of the Millennium Development Goals (MDGs).

Though not legally enforceable, the MDGs clarify international consensus on the enabling conditions and social rights necessary for the meaningful and complete realization of reproductive health and rights. In this way, there is a new shared discourse. Creating prescriptions for policies responsive to the needs of the developing world, four of the eight MDGs involve improvements in health—including the reduction of maternal and infant mortality, the prevention of HIV infection, and the eradication of hunger, and one specific to development.[50] For each goal, the United Nations has outlined a number of targets and indicators by which to assess realization of these goals, providing an important roadmap for policies and programs.[51] While these MDGs have been criticized for not taking a legal approach to human rights and for the selection of maternal and infant mortality over health systems more generally,[52] they have become a favored tool in linking reproductive health with development. They may also provide an important link between sexual and reproductive health within a positive rights framework. While the MDGs are a critical step in moving toward a positive rights framework for reproductive rights through the provision of a new shared discourse rooted in development, additional steps will be needed to enforce these rights through international law.

The Right to the Highest Attainable Standard of Health

To codify these positive rights for reproductive health, the human right to health provides a foundation upon which these rights can be built. Ten years ago, the right to health was, to many, an underutilized, underexplored, and unexplained framework for reproductive health.[53] The language of the right itself did not provide specific guidance to states under its funding-dependent framework for achieving "the highest attainable standard of physical and mental health."[20] In the absence of specific public health goals, the ICESCR holds only that states must take affirmative steps necessary for "(a) The provision for the reduction of the stillbirth rate and of infant mortality and for the healthy development of the child; (b) the improvement of all aspects of environmental and industrial hygiene; (c) the prevention, treatment, and control of epidemic, endemic, occupational, and other diseases; (d) the creation of conditions that would assure to all medical service and medical attention in the event of sickness."[20] Although criticized for its ambiguity,[54] the individual right to health has been interpreted to embrace, as part of its minimum core content,[55] basic provisions of emergency health care necessary to save lives, including the treatment of prevalent diseases, the provision of essential drugs, and safeguards against serious environmental health threats.[56]

This ambiguity in human rights for reproductive health was largely washed away beginning at the turn of the century, with UN treaty monitoring bodies clarifying the content of the right to health in CEDAW's General Recommendation 24 on women and health (1999)[57] and the ICESCR's General Comment 14 on the right to health (2000).[18] It is likely that the attention now paid to the right to health has as much to do with the explosion of HIV/AIDS in developing countries as with the inability of neoliberal states to address the fallout from HIV/AIDS in sexual and reproductive health. These general comments provide a foundation to enumerate and clarify state obligations and implement programmatic specification from the expansive language of the right to health.

General Comment 14 provides a useful framework of accessibility, acceptability, availability, and quality ("AAAQ") to evaluate state actions to realize the right to the highest attainable standard of health.[18] To compliment this discourse, General Comment 14 also calls upon states to respect, protect, and fulfill the right, specifically addressing the components of this right necessary for reproductive health by finding that:

> The provision for the reduction of the stillbirth rate and of infant mortality and for the healthy development of the child (Art. 12.2 (a)) may be understood as requiring measures to improve child and maternal health, sexual and reproductive health services, including access to family planning, pre- and post-natal care, emergency obstetric services and access to information, as well as to resources necessary to act on that information).[18]

These specific state obligations, coupled with the AAAQ framework, begin to provide a positive rights framework for reproductive rights in today's globalizing world, where women's equality and freedom necessitate positive rights along with negative rights to attain reproductive health.

New Norm Entrepreneurs: Maternal Mortality as a Human Rights Issue

A newly emerging movement to view maternal mortality as a violation of human rights has galvanized new norm entrepreneurs to advocate for a positive rights agenda in reproductive health.[58] Maternal mortality rates offer a stark example of the impact of changing global economies on reproductive health disparities, highlighting the shortcomings of a negative rights framework.[59] From a public health perspective, maternal mortality cannot be addressed solely through a negative rights discourse; the proven solutions to reducing maternal death and disability are best achieved through a strengthened and functioning health system and a focus on underlying economic and social conditions.[60] The determinants of maternal mortality exist at a systemic level, ranging from a lack of access to contraception to infrastructural deficiencies to an unjust international economic system.[61] While select determinants are captured by the classic negative rights framework, most require something more—a positive rights framework that holds governments accountable for not providing access to acceptable-quality health care and underlying economic and social conditions for reproductive health.[62] Providing an approach that is "sensitive to the historical and political context of the issues, to the dynamics of power, to the impact of language and discourse, and to the agency of multiple actors involved in any given situation,"[60] this systems-based discourse can garner accountability for national improvements in reproductive health. With burgeoning organizational platforms and normative frameworks providing a new path, these new norm entrepreneurs have the language, inspiration, and direction to implement positive rights for reproductive justice.

and dangers, in this case, the threat of backsliding in the progression of reproductive rights. With the resurgence of the Catholic Church and religious fundamentalism in the public sphere, reproductive rights are under attack in a backlash against the successes of previous social movements. In addressing the positive rights inherent in reproduction, advocates must be wary of these forces, which threaten to subordinate the hard-earned freedoms of women. If carefully constructed and negotiated, however, the gains of a positive rights framework, complementing current negative rights frameworks, can overcome these dangers and risks and provide the tools necessary for women and men to achieve the highest attainable standard of reproductive health.

Conclusion and Steps Forward

When laws are opened to rethinking, reframing, and restrategizing, they are also opened to threats

DISCUSSION QUESTIONS

1. What positive and negative aspects of reproductive rights have evolved from moral rights to state accountability under international law?

2. Why have women's rights groups been unable to frame a comprehensive right to women's health?

3. How are reproductive rights enforced? What role do advocacy organizations play in that enforcement process?

REFERENCES

1. United Nations Population Information Network. (1994). *International conference on Population and Development Statement by Dr. Hiroshi Nakajima.* http://www.un.org/popin/icpd/conference/una/940909142950.html. Accessed September 27, 2008.

2. Schuler M. From basic needs to basic rights. In: Schuler M, ed. *From Basic Needs to Basic Rights: Women's Claims to Human Rights*. Washington, DC: Women, Law, and Development; 1995:1-26.

3. Freedman LP. Human rights and the politics of risk and blame: lessons from the reproductive rights movement. *J Am Med Womens Assoc*. 1997;52:165-168.

4. Petchesky R. Cross-country comparisons and political visions. In: Petchesky R, Judd, K, eds. *Negotiating Reproductive Rights: Women's Perspectives Across Countries and Cultures*. London, England: Zed Books; 1998:295-323.

5. Petchesky R. Reproductive freedom: beyond 'a woman's right to choose'. *Signs*. 1980;5:661-668.

6. Globalization Knowledge Network. *Towards Health-Equitable Globalisation: Rights, Regulation, and Redistribution*. Ottawa, Canada: University of Ottawa Institute of Population Health; 2007.

7. Knowledge Network on Health Systems. *Challenging Inequity Through Health Systems*. WHO Commission on the Social Determinants of Health: 2007.

8. The right to the highest attainable standard of physical and mental health. Report of the Special Rapporteur, Paul Hunt. E/CN.4/2004/49: 2004.

9. Otto D. Rethinking the "universality" of human rights law. *Colum Hum Rts L Rev*. 1997;29:10.

10. Donnelly J. *Universal Human Rights in Theory and Practice*. Ithaca, NY: Cornell Univ Press; 2003.

11. Cook R. Human rights and reproductive self-determination. *Am U L Rev*. 1995; 5:975.

12. Steiner H, Alston P. *International Human Rights in Context: Law, Politics, Morals*. Clarendon Press: Oxford; 2000.

13. Landman T. Measuring human rights: Principle, practice, and policy. *Human Rights Q*. 2004;26(4):906-931.

14. Yamin A. Transformative combinations: women's health and human rights. *J Am Med Womens Assoc*. 1997;52:171.

15. Hendricks A. The close connection between classical rights and the right to health, with special reference to the right to sexual and reproductive health. *Med Law*. 1999;18:225-242.

16. Sullivan D. The nature and scope of human rights obligations concerning women's right to health. *Health Hum Rights*. 1995;1:368-398.

17. Convention on the Elimination of All Forms of Discrimination Against Women. New York, NY: United Nations; 1979.

18. Committee on Economic, Social, and Cultural Rights, General Comment 14. The Right to the Highest Attainable Standard of Health. E/C.12/2000/4. New York, NY: United Nations; 2000.

19. Universal Declaration of Human Rights. United Nations General Assembly Resolution 217 A (III). New York, NY: United Nations; 1948.

20. International Covenant on Economic, Social and Cultural Rights. New York, NY: United Nations; 1966.

21. Freedman LP, Isaacs S. Human rights and reproductive choice. *Stud Family Planning*. 1993;24:20-21.

22. Grimes S. From population control to 'reproductive rights': ideological influences in population policy. *Third World Q*. 1998;19:375.

23. United Nations. Final Act of the International Conference on Human Rights. A/Conf.32/41:1968.

24. United Nations. Fertility, Contraception and Population Policies. New York, NY: United Nations; 2003.

25. Rahman A, Katzvie L, Henshaw S. A global review of laws on induced abortion, 1985-1997. *Int Fam Plan Perspect.* 1998;24:56-64.

26. Chesler E. Introduction. In: Chavkin W, Chesler E, eds. *Where Human Rights Begin: Health, Sexuality, and Women in the New Millennium.* New Brunswick, NJ: Rutgers University Press; 2005:1-34.

27. United Nations. *Report of the World Conference to Review and Appraise the Achievements of the United Nations Decade for Women: Equality, Development, and Peace.* Nairobi, Kenya. 1985. Paragraph 93.

28. Hartmann B. *Reproductive Rights and Wrongs: The Global Politics of Population Control & Contraceptive Choice.* New York, NY: Harper & Row; 1987.

29. Copelan R, Petchesky R. Toward an interdependent approach to reproductive and sexual rights as human rights: reflections on the ICPD and beyond. In: Schuler M, ed. *From Basic Needs to Basic Rights: Women's Claims to Human Rights.* Washington, D.C.: Women, Law, and Development International: 1995:343-368.

30. Robinson M. Foreword. In: Chavkin W, Chesler E, eds. *Where Human Rights Begin: Health, Sexuality, and Women in the New Millennium.* New Brunswick, NJ: Rutgers University Press; 2005:ix-xii.

31. Vienna Declaration and Programme of Action, Report of the World Conference on Human Rights. Vienna, Austria: United Nations; 1993.

32. Petchesky R. Introduction. In: Petchesky R, Judd K, eds. *Negotiating Reproductive Rights: Women's Perspectives Across Countries and Cultures.* London, England: Zed Books; 1998:1-30.

33. Beijing Declaration and Platform for Action, adopted September 15, 1995, by the Fourth World Conference on Women: Action for Equality, Development and Peace. In *Women and Human Rights: The Basic Documents.* New York, NY: Center for the Study of Human Rights, Columbia University; 1996.

34. Report of the International Conference on Population and Development. Cairo, Egypt: United Nations; 1994.. United Nations Population Information Network. (1994). *Report of the International Conference on Population and Development.* http://www.un.org/popin/icpd/conference/offeng/poa.html Accessed September 27, 2008.

35. Kratochwill F, Ruggie JG. International organization: a state of the art on an art of the state. *Int Org.* 1986;40:753.

36. Ruggie JG. What makes the world hang together? Neo-utilitarianism and the social constructivist challenge. *Int Org.* 1998;54:855.

37. Sikkink K. Transnational politics, international relations theory, and human rights. *Pol Sci Pol.* 1998;31:516.

38. Finnemore M. Are legal norms distinctive? *Int L Pol.* 2000;32:699.

39. Alston P. Conjuring up new human rights: a proposal for quality control. *Int L.* 1984;78:607.

40. Sunstein C. Social norms and social roles. In: Sunstein C, ed. *Free Markets and Social Justice.* New York, NY: Oxford University Press; 1997.

41. Wiener A. Constructivism: the limits of bridging gaps. *Int Rel Dev.* 2003;6:252.

42. Müller H. International relations as communicative action. In Fierke K, Jorgensen K, eds. *Constructing International Relations: The Next Generation.* New York, NY: M.E. Sharpe; 2001.

43. Koh H. Why do nations obey international law? *Yale L J.* 1997;106:2599.

44. Isaacs S. Incentives, population policy, and reproductive rights: ethical issues. *Stud Fam Plan.* 1995;26:363-367.

45. Mann J, Gruskin S. Women's health and human rights: genesis of Health and Human Rights Movement. *Health Hum Rights.* 1995;1:309-312.

46. Sen G. Southern feminist perspectives on population and reproductive rights: continuing challenges. *Development.* 1999;42(1):25-28.

47. Cardenas S. Norm collision: explaining the effects of international human rights pressure on state behavior. *Int Stud Rev.* 2004;6:213-231.

48. Getgen J. Reproductive injustice: an analysis of Nicaragua's complete abortion ban. *Cornell Int L J.* 2008;41:144-174.

49. Cook R. Women's international human rights law: the way forward. In: Cook R, ed. *The Human Rights of Women: National and International Perspectives.* Philadelphia, PA: University of Penn Press; 1994:3-36.

50. United Nations Millennium Declaration, adopted 8 Sept. 2000, G.A. Res. 55/2, U.N. GAOR, 55th Sess., Supp. No. 49, ¶ 5, U.N. Doc. A/RES/55/2 (2000).

51. Lee K, et al. The challenge to improve global health: financing the millennium development goals. *J Am Med Assoc.* 2004;291:2636.

52. Meier BM, Fox A. Development as health: employing the collective right to development to achieve the goals of the individual right to health. *Hum Rights Q.* 2008;30:259-355.

53. Rahman A, Pine R. An international human right to reproductive health care: toward definition and accountability. *Health Hum Rights.* 1995;1:401-427.

54. Gostin L, Mann J. Toward the development of a human rights impact assessment for the formulation and evaluation of public health policies. *Health Hum Rights.* 1994;1:58-80.

55. Hendriks A. The right to health in national and international jurisprudence. *Euro J Health L.* 1998;5:389.

56. Toebes B. The right to health as a human right. *Int L.* 1999;25:284.

57. Committee on the Elimination of Discrimination against Women. General Recommendation 24; 1999. http://www.un.org/womenwatch/daw/cedaw/recommendations/recomm.htm#recom24. Accessed September 24, 2008.

58. Cook RJ, Dickens BM, Fathalla MF. *Reproductive Health and Human Rights.* Oxford: Oxford University Press; 2003.

59. Rosenfield A, Maine D. Maternal mortality—a neglected tragedy. Where is the M in MCH? *Lancet.* 1985;13:83-85.

60. Freedman LP. Shifting visions: "delegation" policies and the building of a "rights-based" approach to maternal mortality. *J Am Med Womens Assoc.* 2002;54:154-158.

61. Freedman LP. Using human rights in maternal mortality programs: from analysis to strategy. *Int J Gynecol Obstet.* 2001;75:51-60.

62. AbouZahr C. Safe motherhood: a brief history of the global movement. 1947-2002. *Br Med Bull.* 2003;67:13-25.

Women, Economics, and Human Rights

This section explores the historic, economic, and political dimensions of the global health crisis, focusing particularly on the links between the conditions for global health and the prevailing regime of global economic governance. As the benefits of economic growth continue to be highly concentrated and uneven between and within developed and developing countries, policy initiatives must be redefined and health advocacy strengthened to advance the rights of women and improve global health. It is the intent that this section informs and motivates a call to action for those women missing and those women, although accounted for, who struggle daily to endure. Advocacy is nothing new for women.

Her development, her freedom, her independence, must come from and through herself.

—Emma Goldman, Author, Feminist

It is often said that women make up a majority of the world's population. They do not. This mistaken belief is based on generalizing from the contemporary situation in Europe and North America, where the ratio of women to men is typically around 1.05 or 1.06, or higher. In South Asia, West Asia, and China, the ratio of women to men can be as low as 0.94, or even lower, and it varies widely elsewhere in Asia, in Africa, and in Latin America. How can we understand and explain these differences, and react to them?

At birth, boys outnumber girls everywhere in the world, by much the same proportion—there are around 105 or 106 male children for every 100 female children. Just why the biology of reproduction leads to this result remains a subject of debate. But after conception, biology seems on the whole to favor women. Considerable research has shown that if men and women receive similar nutritional and medical attention and general health care, women tend to live noticeably longer than men. Women seem to be, on the whole, more resistant to disease and in general hardier than men, an advantage they enjoy not only after they are 40 years old but also at the beginning of life, especially during the months immediately following birth, and even in the womb. When given the same care as males, females tend to have better survival rates than males.[1]

Women outnumber men substantially in Europe, the United States, and Japan, where, despite the persistence of various types of bias against women (men having distinct advantages in higher education, job specialization, and promotion to senior executive positions, for example), women suffer little discrimination in basic nutrition and health care. The greater number of women in these countries is partly the result of social and environmental differences that increase mortality among men, such as a higher likelihood that men will die from violence, for example, and from diseases related to smoking. But even after these are taken into account, the longer lifetimes enjoyed by women given similar care appear to relate to the biological advantages that women have over men in resisting disease.

CHAPTER 9

More Than 100 Million Women Are Missing*

Amartya Sen

Amartya Sen PhD is a Master of Trinity College, Cambridge, UK, and a former Professor of Economics at Oxford UK. Dr. Sen is also a Lamont University Professor Emeritus at Harvard University in Cambridge MA, and has recieved numerous illustreous awards, including: Nobel laureate Economics, Bharata Ratna, Leontief Prize, International Humanist Award, Eisenhower Medal, for Leadership and Service, and a Lifetime Achievement Award confered by UNESCAP.

* Originally published in *The New York Review of Books*. Volume 37, Number 20 · December 20, 1990. Reprinted with permission from *The New York Review of Books*. Copyright © 1990 NYREV, Inc.

Whether the higher frequency of male births over female births has evolutionary links to this potentially greater survival rate among women is a question of some interest in itself. Women seem to have lower death rates than men at most ages whenever they get roughly similar treatment in matters of life and death.

Status of Women around the World

The fate of women is quite different in most of Asia and North Africa. In these places the failure to give women medical care similar to what men get and to provide them with comparable food and social services results in fewer women surviving than would be the case if they had equal care. In India, for example, except in the period immediately following birth, the death rate is higher for women than for men fairly consistently in all age groups until the late 30s. This relates to higher rates of disease from which women suffer, and ultimately to the relative neglect of females, especially in health care and medical attention.[2] Similar neglect of women vis-à-vis men can be seen also in many other parts of the world. The result is a lower proportion of women than would be the case if they had equal care—in most of Asia and North Africa, and to a lesser extent Latin America.

This pattern is not uniform in all parts of the third world, however. Sub-Saharan Africa, for example, ravaged as it is by extreme poverty, hunger, and famine, has a substantial excess rather than deficit of women, the ratio of women to men being around 1.02. The "third world" in this matter is not a useful category, because it is so diverse. Even within Asia, which has the lowest proportion of women in the world, Southeast Asia and East Asia (apart from China) have a ratio of women to men that is slightly higher than one to one (around 1.01). Indeed, sharp diversities also exist within particular regions—sometimes even within a particular country. For example, the ratio of women to men in the Indian states of Punjab and Haryana, which happen to be among the country's richest, is a remarkably low 0.86, while the state of Kerala in southwestern India has a ratio higher than 1.03, similar to that in Europe, North America, and Japan.

To get an idea of the numbers of people involved in the different ratios of women to men, we can estimate the number of "missing women" in a country, say, China or India, by calculating the number of extra women who would have been in China or India if these countries had the same ratio of women to men as is obtained in areas of the world in which they receive similar care. If we could expect equal populations of the two sexes, the low ratio of 0.94 women to men in South Asia, West Asia, and China would indicate a 6 percent deficit of women; but since, in countries where men and women receive similar care, the ratio is about 1.05, the real shortfall is about 11 percent. In China alone this amounts to 50 million "missing women," taking 1.05 as the benchmark ratio. When that number is added to those in South Asia, West Asia, and North Africa, a great many more than 100 million women are "missing." These numbers tell us, quietly, a terrible story of inequality and neglect leading to the excess mortality of women.

To account for the neglect of women, two simplistic explanations have often been presented or, more often, implicitly assumed. One view emphasizes the cultural contrasts between East and West (or between the Occident and the Orient), claiming that Western civilization is less sexist than Eastern. That women outnumber men in Western countries may appear to lend support to this Kipling-like generalization. (Kipling himself was not, of course, much bothered by concerns about sexism, and even made "the twain" meet in romantically masculine circumstances: "But there is neither East nor West, Border, nor Breed, nor Birth,/When two strong men stand face to face, tho' they come from the ends of the earth!") The other simple argument looks instead at stages of economic development, seeing the unequal nutrition and health care provided for women as a feature of underdevelopment, a characteristic of poor economies awaiting economic advancement.

There may be elements of truth in each of these explanations, but neither is very convincing as a general thesis. To some extent, the two simple explanations, in terms of "economic development" and "East-West" divisions, also tend to undermine each other. A combined cultural and economic analysis would seem to be necessary, and, I will argue, it would have to take note of many other social conditions in addition to the features identified in the simple aggregative theses.

Culture and Women

To take the cultural view first, the East-West explanation is obviously flawed because experiences within the East and West diverge so sharply. Japan, for example, unlike most of Asia, has a ratio of women to men that is not very different from that in Europe or North America. This might suggest, at least superficially, that real income and economic development do more to explain the bias against providing women with the conditions for survival than whether the society is Western or Oriental. In the censuses of 1899 and 1908 Japan had a clear and substantial deficit of women, but by 1940 the numbers of men and women were nearly equal, and in the postwar decades, as Japan became a rich and highly industrialized country, it moved firmly in the direction of a large surplus, rather than a deficit, of women. Some countries in East Asia and Southeast Asia also provide exceptions to the deficit of women; in Thailand and Indonesia, for example, women substantially outnumber men.

In its rudimentary, undiscriminating form, the East-West explanation also fails to take into account other characteristics of these societies. For example, the ratios of women to men in South Asia are among the lowest in the world (around 0.94 in India and Bangladesh, and 0.90 in Pakistan—the lowest ratio for any large country), but that region has been among the pioneers in electing women as top political leaders. Indeed, each of the four large South Asian countries—India, Pakistan, Bangladesh, and Sri Lanka—either has had a woman as the elected head of government (Sri Lanka, India, and Pakistan), or has had women leading the main opposition parties (as in Bangladesh).

Politics and Women

It is, of course, true that these successes in South Asia have been achieved only by upper-class women, and that having a woman head of government has not, by itself, done much for women in general in these countries. However, the point here is only to question the tendency to see the contrast between East and West as simply based on more sexism or less. The large electoral successes of women in achieving high positions in government in South Asia indicate that the analysis has to be more complex.

It is, of course, also true that these women leaders reached their powerful positions with the help of dynastic connections—Indira Gandhi was the daughter of Jawaharlal Nehru, Benazir Bhutto the daughter of Zulfikar Bhutto, and so on. But it would be absurd to overlook—just on that ground—the significance of their rise to power through popular mandate. Dynastic connections are not new in politics and are pervasive features of political succession in many countries. That Indira Gandhi derived her political strength partly from her father's position is not in itself more significant than the fact that Rajiv Gandhi's political credibility derived largely from his mother's political eminence, or the fact (perhaps less well known) that Indira Gandhi's father—the great Jawaharlal Nehru—initially rose to prominence as the son of Motilal Nehru, who had been president of the Congress Party. The dynastic aspects of South Asian politics have certainly helped women to come to power through electoral support, but it is still true that so far as winning elections is concerned, South Asia would seem to be some distance ahead of the United States and most European countries when it comes to discrimination according to gender.

In this context it is useful also to compare the ratios of women in American and Indian legislatures. In the US House of Representatives the proportion of women is 6.4 percent, while in the present and the last lower houses of the Indian Parliament, women's proportions have been respectively 5.3 and 7.9 percent. Only two of the 100 US Senators are women, and this 2 percent ratio contrasts with more than 9 and 10 percent women respectively in the last and present "upper house," Rajya Sabha, in India. (In a different, but not altogether unrelated, sphere, I had a much higher proportion of tenured women colleagues when I was teaching at Delhi University than I now have at Harvard.) The cultural climate in different societies must have a clear relevance to differences between men and women—both in survival and in other ways as well—but it would be hopeless to see the divergences simply as a contrast between the sexist East and the unbiased West.

Economics, Socio-Cultural Factors and Women

How good is the other (i.e., the purely economic) explanation for women's inequality? Certainly all the countries with large deficits of women are more or less poor, if we measure poverty by real incomes, and no sizable country with a high gross national product per head has such a deficit. There are reasons to expect a reduction of differential female mortality with economic progress. For example, the rate of maternal mortality at childbirth can be expected to decrease both with better hospital facilities and the reduction in birth rate that usually accompanies economic development.

However, in this simple form, an economic analysis does not explain very much, since many poor countries do not, in fact, have deficits of women. As was noted earlier, sub-Saharan Africa, poor and underdeveloped as it is, has a substantial excess of women. Southeast and East Asia (but not China) also differ from many other relatively poor countries in this respect, although to a lesser degree. Within India, as was noted earlier, Punjab and Haryana—among the richest and most economically advanced Indian states—have very low ratios of women to men (around 0.86), in contrast to the much poorer state of Kerala, where the ratio is greater than 1.03.

Indeed, economic development is quite often accompanied by a relative worsening in the rate of survival of women (even as life expectancy improves in absolute terms for both men and women). For example, in India the gap between the life expectancy of men and women has narrowed recently, but only after many decades when women's relative position deteriorated. There has been a steady decline in the ratio of women to men in the population, from more than 97 women to 100 men at the turn of the century (in 1901), to 93 women in 1971, and the ratio is only a little higher now. The deterioration in women's position results largely from their unequal sharing in the advantages of medical and social progress. Economic development does not invariably reduce women's disadvantages in mortality.

A significant proportional decline in the population of women occurred in China after the economic and social reforms introduced there in 1979.

The Chinese Statistical Yearbooks show a steady decline in the already very low ratio of women to men in the population, from 94.32 in 1979 to 93.42 in 1985 and 1986. (It has risen since then, to 93.98 in 1989—still lower than what it was in 1979). Life expectancy was significantly higher for females than for males until the economic reforms, but seems to have fallen behind since then.[3] Of course, the years following the reforms were also years of great economic growth and, in many ways, of social progress, yet women's relative prospects for survival deteriorated. These and other cases show that rapid economic development may go hand in hand with worsening relative mortality of women.

Despite their superficial plausibility, neither the alleged contrast between "East" and "West," nor the simple hypothesis of female deprivation as a characteristic of economic "underdevelopment" gives us anything like an adequate understanding of the geography of female deprivation in social well-being and survival. We have to examine the complex ways in which economic, social, and cultural factors can influence the regional differences.

It is certainly true that, for example, the status and power of women in the family differ greatly from one region to another, and there are good reasons to expect that these social features would be related to the economic role and independence of women. For example, employment outside the home and owning assets can both be important for women's economic independence and power; and these factors may have far-reaching effects on the divisions of benefits and chores within the family and can greatly influence what are implicitly accepted as women's "entitlements."

Indeed, men and women have both interests in common and conflicting interests that affect family decisions, and it is possible to see decision making in the family taking the form of the pursuit of cooperation in which solutions for the conflicting aspects of family life are implicitly agreed on. Such "cooperative conflicts" are a general feature of many group relations, and an analysis of cooperative conflicts can provide a useful way of understanding the influences that affect the "deal" that women get in the division of benefits within the family. There are gains to be made by men and women through following implicitly agreed-on patterns of behavior, but there are many possible agreements—some more favorable to one party than others. The choice of one such cooperative arrangement from among the range of possibilities leads to a particular distribution of joint benefits. (Elsewhere, I have tried to analyze the general nature of "cooperative conflicts" and the application of the analysis of such conflicts to family economics.[4])

Conflicts in family life are typically resolved through implicitly agreed-on patterns of behavior that may or may not be particularly egalitarian. The very nature of family living—sharing a home and experiences—requires that the elements of conflict must not be explicitly emphasized (giving persistent attention to conflicts will usually be seen as aberrant behavior), and sometimes the deprived woman would not even have a clear idea of the extent of her relative deprivation. Similarly, the perception of who is doing "productive" work, who is "contributing" how much to the family's prosperity, can be very influential, even though the underlying principles regarding how "contributions" or "productivity" are to be assessed may rarely be discussed explicitly. These issues of social perception are, I believe, of pervasive importance in gender inequality, even in the richer countries, but they can have a particularly powerful influence in sustaining female deprivation in many of the poorer countries.[5]

The division of a family's joint benefits is likely to be less unfavorable to women if (1) they can earn an outside income; (2) their work is recognized as productive (this is easier to achieve with work done outside the home); (3) they own some economic resources and have some rights to fall back on; and (4) there is a clear-headed understanding of the ways in which women are deprived and a recognition of the possibilities of changing this situation. This last category can be much influenced by education for women and by participatory political action.

Considerable empirical evidence, mostly studies of particular localities, suggests that what is usually defined as "gainful" employment (i.e., working outside the home for a wage, or in such "productive" occupations as farming), as opposed to unpaid and unhonored housework—no matter how demanding—can substantially enhance the deal that women get.[6] Indeed, "gainful" employment of women can make the solution of "cooperative conflicts" less unfavorable to women in many ways. First, outside employment for wages can provide women with an income to which they have easier access, and it can also serve as a means of making a living on which women can rely, making them less vulnerable. Second, the social respect that is associated with being a "bread winner" (and a "productive" contributor to the family's joint prosperity) can improve women's status and standing in the family, and may influence the prevailing cultural traditions regarding who gets what in the division of joint benefits. Third, when outside employment takes the form of jobs with some security and legal protection, the corresponding rights that women get can make their economic position much less vulnerable and precarious. Fourth, working outside the home also provides experience of the outside world, and this can be socially important in improving women's position within the family. In this respect, outside work may be "educational" as well.

These factors may not only improve the "deal" women get in the family, they can also counter the relative neglect of girls as they grow up. Boys are preferred in many countries because they are expected to provide more economic security for their parents in old age; but the force of this bias can be weakened if women as well as men can regularly work at paid jobs. Moreover, if the status of women does in general rise and women's contributions become more recognized, female children may receive more attention. Similarly, the exposure of women to the world through work outside the home can weaken, through its educational effect, the hold of traditional beliefs and behavior.

In comparing different regions of Asia and Africa, if we try to relate the relative survival prospects of women to the "gainful employment" of both sexes—i.e., work outside the home, possibly for a wage—we do find a strong association. If the different regions of Asia and Africa (with the exception of China) are ranked according to the proportion of women in so-called gainful employment relative to the proportion of men in such employment, we get the following ranking, in descending order: [7]

1. Sub-Saharan Africa
2. Southeast and Eastern Asia
3. Western Asia
4. Southern Asia
5. Northern Africa

Ranking the ratios of life expectancy of females to those of males produces a remarkably similar ordering:

1. Sub-Saharan Africa
2. Southeast and Eastern Asia
3. Western Asia
4. Northern Africa
5. Southern Asia

That the two rankings are much the same, except for a switch between the two lowest-ranking regions (lowest in terms of both indicators), suggests a link between employment and survival prospects. In addition to the overall correspondence between the two rankings, the particular contrasts between sub-Saharan Africa and North Africa, and that between Southern (and Western) Asia and Southeast (and Eastern) Asia are suggestive distinctions within Africa and Asia respectively, linking women's gainful employment and survival prospects.

It is, of course, possible that what we are seeing here is not a demonstration that gainful employment causes better survival prospects but the influence of some other factor correlated with each. In fact, on the basis of such broad relations, it is very hard to draw any firm conclusion; but evidence of similar relations can be found also in other comparisons.[8] For example, Punjab, the richest Indian state, has the lowest ratio of women to men (0.86) in India; it also has the lowest ratio of women in "gainful" employment compared to men. The influence of outside employment on women's well-being has also been documented in a number of studies of specific communities in different parts of the world.[9]

Women in China

The case of China deserves particular attention. It is a country with a traditional bias against women, but after the revolution the Chinese leaders did pay considerable attention to reducing inequality between men and women.[10] This was helped both by a general expansion of basic health and medical services accessible to all and by the increase in women's gainful employment, along with greater social recognition of the importance of women in the economy and the society.

There has been a remarkable general expansion of longevity, and despite the temporary setback during the terrible famines of 1958–1961 (following the disastrous failure of the so-called Great Leap Forward), the Chinese life expectancy at birth increased from the low 40s around 1950 to the high 60s by the time the economic reforms were introduced in 1979. The sharp reduction in general mortality (including female mortality) is all the more remarkable in view of the fact that it took place despite deep economic problems in the form of widespread industrial inefficiency, a rather stagnant agriculture, and relatively little increase in output per head. Female death rates declined sharply—both as a part of a general mortality reduction and also relatively, vis-à-vis male mortality. Women's life expectancy at birth overtook that of men—itself much enhanced—and was significantly ahead at the time the economic and social reforms were introduced in 1979.

Those reforms immediately increased the rate of economic growth and broke the agricultural stagnation. The official figures suggest a doubling of agricultural output between 1979 and 1986—a remarkable achievement even if some elements of exaggeration are eliminated from these figures. But at the same time, the official figures also record an increase in the general mortality rates after the reforms, with a consistently higher death rate than what China had achieved by 1979. There also seems to be a worsening of the relative survival of women, including a decline, discussed earlier, of the ratio of women to men in the population, which went down from 94.3 in 1979 to 93.4 in 1985 and 1986. There are problems in interpreting the available data and difficulties in arriving at firm conclusions, but the view that women's life expectancy has again become lower than that of men has gained support. For example, the World Bank's most recent World Development Report suggests a life expectancy of 69 years for men and 66 years for women (even though the confounded nature of the subject is well reflected by the fact that the same report also suggests an average life expectancy of 70 years for men and women put together).[11]

Why have women's survival prospects in China deteriorated, especially in relative terms, since 1979? Several experts have noted that recently Chinese leaders have tended, on the whole, to reduce the emphasis on equality for women; it is no longer much discussed, and indeed, as the sociologist Margery Wolf puts it, it is a case of a "revolution postponed."[12] But this fact, while important, does not explain why the relative survival prospects of women would have so deteriorated during the early years of the reforms, just at the time when there was a rapid expansion of overall economic prosperity.

The compulsory measures to control the size of families, which were introduced in 1979, may have been an important factor. In some parts of the country the authorities insisted on the "one-child family." This restriction, given the strong preference for boys in China, led to a neglect of girls that was often severe. Some evidence exists of female infanticide. In the early years after the reforms, infant mortality for girls appeared to increase considerably. Some estimates had suggested that the rate of female infant mortality rose from 37.7 per thousand in 1978 to 67.2 per thousand in 1984.[13] Even if this seems exaggerated in the light of later data, the survival prospects of female children clearly have been unfavorably affected by restrictions on the size of the family. Later legal concessions (including the permission to have a second child if the first one is a girl) reflect some official recognition of these problems.

A second factor relevant to the survival problems of Chinese women is the general crisis in health services since the economic reforms. As the agricultural production brigades and collectives, which had traditionally provided much of the funding for China's extensive rural health programs were dismantled, they were replaced by the so-called "responsibility system," in which agriculture was centered in the family. Agricultural production improved, but cutbacks in communal facilities placed severe financial restrictions on China's extensive rural medical services. Communal agriculture may not have done much for agricultural production as such, but it had been a main source of support for China's innovative and extensive rural medical services. So far as gender is concerned, the effects of the reduced scope of these services are officially neutral, but in view of the pro-male bias in Chinese rural society, the cutback in medical services would have had a particularly severe impact on women and female children. (It is also the pro-male bias in the general culture that made the one-child policy, which too is neutral in form, unfavorable to female children in terms of its actual impact.)

Third, the "responsibility system" arguably has reduced women's involvement in recognized gainful employment in agriculture. In the new system's more traditional arrangement of work responsibilities, women's work in the household economy may again suffer from the lack of recognition that typically affects household work throughout the world.[14] The impact of this change on the status of women within the household may be negative, for the reasons previously described. Expanded employment opportunities for women outside agriculture in some regions may at least partially balance this effect. But the weakening of social security arrangements since the reforms would also have made old age more precarious, and since such insecurity is one of the persistent motives for families' preferring boys over girls, this change too can be contributing to the worsening of care for female children.[15]

Status of Women in East and West

Analyses based on simple conflicts between East and West or on "under-development" clearly do not take us very far. The variables that appear important—for example, female employment or female literacy—combine both economic and cultural effects. To ascribe importance to the influence of gainful employment on women's prospects for survival may superficially look like another attempt at a simple economic explanation, but it would be a mistake to see it this way. The deeper question is why such outside employment is more prevalent in, say, sub-Saharan Africa than in North Africa, or in Southeast and Eastern Asia than in Western and Southern Asia. Here the cultural, including religious, backgrounds of the respective regions are surely important. Economic causes for women's deprivation have to be integrated with other—social and cultural—factors to give depth to the explanation.

Of course, gainful employment is not the only factor affecting women's chances of survival. Women's education and their economic rights—

including property rights—may be crucial variables as well.[16] Consider the state of Kerala in India, which I mentioned earlier. It does not have a deficit of women—its ratio of women to men of more than 1.03 is closer to that of Europe (1.05) than those of China, West Asia, and India as a whole (0.94). The life expectancy of women at birth in Kerala, which had already reached 68 years by the time of the last census in 1981 (and is estimated to be 72 years now), is considerably higher than men's 64 years at that time (and 67 now). While women are generally able to find "gainful employment" in Kerala—certainly much more so than in Punjab—the state is not exceptional in this regard. What is exceptional is Kerala's remarkably high literacy rate; not only is it much higher than elsewhere in India, it is also substantially higher than in China, especially for women.

Kerala's experience of state-funded expansion of basic education, which has been consolidated by left-wing state governments in recent decades, began, in fact, nearly two centuries ago, led by the rulers of the kingdoms of Travancore and Cochin. (These two native states were not part of British India; they were joined together with a small part of the old Madras presidency to form the new state of Kerala after independence.) Indeed, as early as 1817, Rani Gouri Parvathi Bai, the young queen of Travancore, issued clear instructions for public support of education:

The state should defray the entire cost of education of its people in order that there might be no backwardness in the spread of enlightenment among them, that by diffusion of education they might be better subjects and public servants and that the reputation of the state might be advanced thereby.[17]

Moreover, in parts of Kerala, property is usually inherited through the family's female line. These factors, as well as the generally high level of communal medicine, help to explain why women in Kerala do not suffer disadvantages in obtaining the means for survival. While it would be difficult to "split up" the respective contributions made by each of these different influences, it would be a mistake not to include all these factors among the potentially interesting variables that deserve examination.

Conclusion

In view of the enormity of the problems of women's survival in large parts of Asia and Africa, it is surprising that these disadvantages have received such inadequate attention. The numbers of "missing women" in relation to the numbers that could be expected if men and women received similar care in health, medicine, and nutrition, are remarkably large. A great many more than a hundred million women are simply not there because women are neglected compared with men. If this situation is to be corrected by political action and public policy, the reasons why there are so many "missing" women must first be better understood. We confront here what is clearly one of the more momentous, and neglected, problems facing the world today.

REFERENCES

1. An assessment of the available evidence can be found in Ingrid Waldron's "The Role of Genetic and Biological Factors in Sex Differences in Mortality," in A.D. Lopez and L.T. Ruzicka, eds., Sex Differences in Mortality (Canberra: Department of Demography, Australian National University, 1983). On the pervasive cultural influences on mortality and the difficulties in forming a biological view of survival advantages, see Sheila Ryan Johansson, "Mortality, Welfare and Gender: Continuity and Change in Explanations for Male/Female Mortality Differences over Three Centuries," in Continuity and Change, forthcoming.

2. These and related data are presented and assessed in my joint paper with Jocelyn Kynch, "Indian Women: Wellbeing and Survival," Cambridge Journal of Economics, Vol. 7 (1983), and in my Commodities and Capabilities (Amsterdam: North-Holland, 1985), Appendix B. See also Lincoln Chen et al., "Sex Bias in the Family Allocation of Food and Health Care in Rural Bangladesh," in Population and Development Review, Vol. 7 (1981); Barbara Miller, The Endangered Sex: Neglect of Female Children in Rural North India (Cornell University Press, 1981); Pranab Bardhan, Land, Labor, and Rural Poverty (Columbia University Press, 1984); Devaki Jain and Nirmala Banerji, eds., Tyranny of the Household (New Delhi: Vikas, 1985); Barbara Harriss and Elizabeth Watson, "The Sex Ratio in South Asia," in J.H. Momsen and J.G. Townsend, eds., Geography of Gender in the Third World (State University of New York Press, 1987); Monica Das Gupta, "Selective Discrimination against Female Children in Rural Punjab, India," in Population and Development Review, Vol. 13 (1987).

3. See the World Bank's World Development Report 1990 (Oxford University Press, 1990), Table 32. See also Judith Banister, China's Changing Population (Stanford University Press, 1987), Chapter 4, though the change in life expectancy may not have been as large as these early estimates had suggested, as Banister herself has later noted.

4. "Gender and Cooperative Conflicts," Working Paper of the World Institute of Development Economics Research (1986), in Irene Tinker, ed., Persistent Inequalities: Women and World Development (Oxford University Press, 1990). In the same volume see also the papers of Ester Boserup, Hanna Papanek, and Irene Tinker on closely related subjects.

5. The recent literature on the modeling of family relations as "bargaining problems," despite being usefully suggestive and insightful, has suffered a little from giving an inadequate role to the importance of perceptions (as opposed to objectively identified interests) of the parties involved. On the relevance of perception, including perceptual distortions (a variant of what Marx had called "false perception"), in family relations, see my "Gender and Cooperative Conflicts." See also my Resources, Values and Development (Harvard University Press, 1984), Chapters 15 and 16; Gail Wilson, Money in the Family (Avebury/Gower, 1987).

6. See the case studies and the literature cited in my "Gender and Cooperative Conflicts." A pioneering study of some of these issues was provided by Ester Boserup, Women's Role in Economic Development (St. Martin's, 1970). See also Bina Agarwal, "Social Security and the Family," in E. Ahmad, et al., Social Security in Developing Countries, Oxford University Press. 1991.

7. Details can be found in my "Gender and Cooperative Conflicts."

8. For example, see Pranab Bardhan, Land, Labor, and Rural Poverty on different states in India and the literature cited there.

9. See the literature cited in my "Gender and Cooperative Conflicts."

10. See Elisabeth Croll, Chinese Women Since Mao (M.E. Sharpe, 1984).

11. See World Development Report 1990, Tables 1 and 32. See also Banister, China's Changing Population, Chapter 4, and Athar Hussain and Nicholas Stern, On the recent increase in death rate in China, China Paper #8 (London: STICERD /London School of Economics, 1990).

12. See Margery Wolf, Revolution Postponed: Women in Contemporary China (Stanford University Press, 1984).

13. See Banister, China's Changing Population, Table 4.12.

14. On this and related matters, see Nahid Aslanbeigui and Gale Summerfield, "The Impact of the Responsibility System on Women in Rural China: A Theoretical

Application of Sen's Theory of Entitlement," in World Development, Vol. 17 (1989).

15. These and other aspects of the problem are discussed more extensively in my joint book with Jean Drèze, Hunger and Public Action (Oxford University Press, 1989).

16. For interesting investigations of the role of education, broadly defined, in influencing women's well-being in Bangladesh and India, see Martha Chen, A Quiet Revolution: Women in Transition in Rural Bangladesh (Schenkman Books, 1983); and Alaka Basu, Culture, the Status of Women and Demographic Behavior (New Delhi: National Council of Applied Economic Research, 1988).

17. Kerala has also had considerable missionary activity in schooling (a fifth of the population is, in fact, Christian), has had international trading and political contacts (both with east and west Asia) for a very long time, and it was from Kerala that the great Hindu philosopher and educator Sankaracarya, who lived during AD 788–820, had launched his big movement of setting up centers of study and worship across India.

Letters
October 24, 1991: Barbara H. Chasin, The Kerala Difference

Missing women*

Social inequality outweighs women's survival advantage in Asia and north Africa

In Europe and North America women tend to outnumber men. For example, in the United Kingdom, France, and the United States the ratio of women to men exceeds 1·05. In many Third World countries, however, especially in Asia and north Africa, the female:male ratio may be as low as 0·95 (Egypt), 0·94 (Bangladesh, China, and west Asia), 0·93 (India), or even 0·90 (Pakistan). These differences are relevant to an assessment of female inequality across the world. [1-6]

Everywhere about 5% more boys than girls are born. But women are hardier than men and, given similar care, survive better at all ages -including in utero.[7] There are other causes for this preponderance of women-for example, some remaining impact of the deaths of men in the last world war and more cigarette smoking and violent deaths among men. But even taking these into account, women would still outnumber men if given similar care.[7]

Social factors must therefore explain the low female:male ratios in Asian and north African countries. These countries would have millions more women if they showed the female:male ratios of Europe and the United States.[4] Calculated on this basis, China is missing more than 50 million women.

Using European or American ratios may not, however, be appropriate. Because of lower female mortality in Europe and America the female:male ratio rises gradually with age. A lower ratio would therefore be expected in Asia and north Africa partly because of a lower life expectancy and higher fertility rate. There are several ways of adjusting for this. One is to adopt the female:male ratios of sub-Saharan Africa, where there is little female disadvantage in terms of relative mortality but where life expectancy is no higher and fertility rates no lower than those in Asia and north Africa.

* BMJ 1992;304:587-8
Reprinted with permission from BMJ

Using the sub-Saharan ratio of 1 022 yields an estimate of 44 million missing women in China, 37 million in India, and a total of more than 100 million worldwide.[5]

Using population models based on Western demographic experience it is possible to estimate roughly how many women there would be without any female disadvantage in survival, given the actual life expectancy and the fertility rates in these countries. Coale estimates 29 million missing women in China, 23 million in India, and an overall total of 60 million for selected countries.[6] Though lower, these numbers are still enormous.

Why is overall mortality for females higher than that for males in these countries? Consider India, where age specific mortality for females consistently exceeds that for males until the fourth decade. Although the excess mortality at childbearing age may be partly due to maternal mortality, obviously no such explanation is possible for female disadvantage in survival in infancy and childhood. Despite occasional distressing accounts of female infanticide, this could not explain the extra mortality or its age distribution. The comparative neglect of female health and nutrition, especially-but not exclusively-during childhood, would seem the prime suspect. Considerable direct evidence exists of neglect of female children in terms of health care, admission to hospitals, and even feeding.[8,9]

Even though the position in India has been more extensively studied than that in other countries, similar evidence of relative neglect of the health and nutrition of female children may be found in other countries in Asia and north Africa. In China some evidence suggests that the extent of neglect may have increased sharply in recent years, particularly since compulsory restrictions on the size of families were introduced in some parts of the country in the late 1970s. There are also some new, ominous signs in China, such as a substantial increase in the reported ratio of male to female births –quite out of line with the rest of the world. It could quite possibly indicate "hiding" of newborn female children (to avoid the rigours of compulsory restriction on the size of the family), but it could, no less plausibly, reflect a higher female infant mortality-whether or not induced (with new births and new deaths both going unreported).

What causes the relative neglect of females, and how can it be changed? Possible influences include traditional cultures and values. But some economic links have also emerged, and some connections between economic status and social standing have been identified. For example, the ability to earn an outside income through paid employment seems to enhance the social standing of a woman (which is the case in sub-Saharan Africa). This makes her contribution to the prosperity of the family more visible. Also, being less dependent on others, she has more voice. The higher status of women also affects ideas on the female child's "due." Secondly, education, especially female literacy, may make a substantial difference. Thirdly, women's economic rights (for example, land ownership and inheritance) may be important.[10,11] Public policy can influence all of these.

The Indian state of Kerala provides an illuminating exception to the prevailing experience. It has the most developed school education system in India, which dates from the early nineteenth century, with strongly supportive state policies in the "native kingdoms" of Travancore and Cochin.[5] Adult literacy rate is now over 90%. Property inheritance passes through the female line for an influential part of the community (the Nairs). Many women participate in "gainful" economic activities. Kerala also has an extensive health care system, which has been built up through public policy. Even though Kerala is one of the poorer Indian states, life expectancy at birth there now exceeds 73 years for women and 67 years for men.

The female:male ratio of the Kerala population is now around 1-04 -similar to that in Europe and America (and most unlike that in the rest of India, Bangladesh, Pakistan, China, west Asia, and north Africa). It seems that the "missing women" may be rescuable, after all, by public policy.

Amartya Sen
Lamont University Professor,
Harvard University,
Cambridge, Massachusetts 02138,
USA

REFERENCES

1. Sen AK. Resources, values and development. Oxford: Blackwell, 1984:346-85.
2. Kynch J. How many women are enough? Sex ratios and the right to life. In: Gauhar A, ed. Third world affairs 1985. London: Third World Foundation, 1985:156-72.
3. Harriss B, Watson E. The sex ratio in south Asia. In: Momson JH, Townsend J, eds. Geography of gender in the Third World. London: Butler and Tanner, 1987:85-115.
4. Sen AK. Women's survival as a development problem. Bulletin ofthe American Academy of Arts and Sciences 1989;43:14-29.
5. Dreze J, Sen AK. Hunger and public action. Oxford:Clarendon Press, 1989:50-9, 221-5.
6. Coale AJ. Excess female mortality and the balance of the sexes in the population: an estimate of the number of "missing females." Population and Development Review 1991;17:517-23.
7. Waldron I. The role of genetic and biological factors in sex differences in mortality. In: Lopez AD, Ruzicka LT, eds. Sex differences in mortality. Canberra: Department of Demography, Australian National University, 1983.
8. Chen L, Huq E, D'Souza S. Sex bias in the family allocation of food and health care in rural Bangladesh. Population and DevelopmentReview 1981;7:55-70.
9. Sen AK. Commodities and capabilities. Amsterdam: North-Holland, 1985:81-104.
10. Boserup E. Women's role in economic development. London: Allen and Unwin, 1970:15-154.
11. Sen AK. Gender and cooperative conflict. In: Tinker I, ed. Persistent inequalities. New York: Oxford University Press, 1990:123-49.

Missing women—revisited*

Reduction in female mortality has been counterbalanced by sex selective abortions

The concept of "missing women," which was presented in an editorial I wrote in this journal 11 years ago, refers to the terrible deficit of women in substantial parts of Asia and north Africa, which arises from sex bias in relative care.[1] The numbers are very large indeed. For example, using as the standard for comparison the female:male ratio of 1.022 observed in sub-Saharan Africa (since women in that region receive less biased treatment), I found the number of missing women in China to be 44m, in India 37m, and so on, with a total that easily exceeded 100m worldwide, a decade or so ago. Others used different methods and got somewhat different numbers—but all very large (for example, Stephan Klasen's sophisticated demographic model yielded 89m for the countries in question).[2]

How have things moved more recently? At one level they have not changed much. The ratio of women to men in the total population, while changing slowly (getting a little worse in China and a little better in India, Bangladesh, Pakistan, and west Asia), has not altered radically in any of these countries. Even though the total numbers of missing women have continued to grow (Klasen's 89m is now 93m for the same countries and 101m for the world as a whole[3]), this has resulted mainly from the absolute growth in population.[4]

But another more important and radical change has occurred over the past decade.[5][6] There have been two opposite movements: female disadvantage in mortality has typically been reduced substantially, but this has been counterbalanced by a new female disadvantage—that in natality—through sex specific

* BMJ 2003;327:1297-8

abortions aimed against the female fetus. The availability of modern techniques to determine the sex of the fetus has made such sex selective abortion possible and easy, and it is being widely used in many societies. Compared with the normal ratio of about 95 girls being born per 100 boys (which is what we observe in Europe and North America), Singapore and Taiwan have 92, South Korea 88, and China a mere 86 girls born per 100 boys. Given the incompleteness of birth registration in India that ratio is difficult to calculate, but going by the closely related ratio of girls to boys among young children (below 6) we find that the female:male ratio has fallen from 94.5 girls per 100 boys in the census of 1991 (almost in line with the ratio in Europe and North America) to 92.7 girls per 100 boys in the census of 2001.

The drop may not look particularly high (especially in comparison with China or Korea), but further grounds for concern exist. Firstly, these could be "early days," and it is possible that, as sex determination of the fetus becomes more standard, the Indian ratio will continue to fall. This is quite possible despite the fact that the Indian parliament has outlawed sex determination of the fetus (except when it is medically required) precisely to prevent its abuse for sex selective abortion. Secondly, variations within India are gigantic, and the all India average hides the fact that in several states—in the north and west of India—the female:male ratio for children is very much lower than the Indian average and lower even than the Chinese and Korean numbers.

Most interestingly, a remarkable division seems to run right across India, splitting the country into two nearly contiguous halves.[6][7] Using the European female: male ratios of children (the German figure of 94.8 girls per 100 boys was used as the dividing line), all the states in the north and the west have ratios that are very substantially below the benchmark figure, led by Punjab, Haryana, Delhi, and Gujarat (between 79.3 and 87.8 girls per 100 boys). On the other side of the divide, the states in the east and the south of India tend to have female:male ratios that equal or exceed the benchmark line of 94.8, with Kerala, Andhra Pradesh, West Bengal, and Assam leading the pack with 96.3 to 96.6 girls per 100 boys. The solitary exception in this half is Tamil Nadu, with a figure just below 94, but that too is close to the European dividing line of 94.8 and well above the numbers for every northern and western state.

The higher incidence of sex-specific abortions in the north and the west cannot be explained by the availability of medical resources (Kerala or West Bengal do not have fewer of these than Bihar or Madhya Pradesh). The difference does not lie in religious background either, since Hindus and Muslims are divided across the country, and the behaviour of both groups conforms to the local pattern of the region. Nor can it be explained by the income level (since the list of deficit states includes the richest, such as Punjab and Haryana, as well as the poorest, like Madhya Pradesh and Uttar Pradesh). Nor can it be explained by variations in economic growth (it includes fast growing Gujarat as well as stagnating Bihar). Even female education, which is so effective in cutting down sex bias in mortality does not seem to have a similar effect in reducing sex bias in natality (as is readily seen from the deficit in high education Himachal Pradesh or Maharashtra or Gujarat, not to mention China, South Korea, Singapore, or Taiwan).

The remarkable division of India (splitting the country into two disparate halves) is particularly puzzling. Are there differences in traditional cultural values that are hidden away? Is there any cultural or deep political significance in the fact that religion based parties have been able to make much bigger inroads precisely in the north and the west and not in the east and the south? A simple but imperfect indication of this can be seen in the fact that in the last general elections (held in 1999), 169 of the 197 parliamentary members of the Hindu right wing parties were elected precisely from northern and western states? Or is all this purely coincidental, especially since the rise of religion centred politics and the emergence of female feticide are both quite new in the parts of India where they have suddenly become common. We do not know the answer to any of these questions, nor to a great many others that can be sensibly asked. Sex bias in natality calls for intensive research today in the same way that sex bias in mortality—the earlier source of "missing women"—did more than a decade ago when I was privileged to write in these pages.

Amartya Sen, *master of Trinity College*
Master's Lodge, Trinity College, Cambridge CB2 1TQ
Competing interests: None declared.

REFERENCES

1. Sen AK. Missing women. BMJ 1992;304: 586-7.
2. Klasen S. Missing women reconsidered. World Dev 1994,22: 1061-71.
3. Klasen S, Wink C. Missing women: revisiting the debate. Feminist Econ 2003;9: 263-300.
4. Klasen S, Wink C. A turning-point in gender bias in mortality? An update on the number of missing women. Population and Development Review 2002;28: 285-312.
5. Sen AK. Many faces of gender inequality. New Republic 2001;(17 September): 35-40.
6. Sen AK. Many faces of gender inequality. Frontline 2001; 19 November;18:4-14. www.hinduonnet.com/fline/fl1822/18220040.htm (accessed 15 Sep 2003).
7. Dreze J, Sen AK. India: development and participation. Delhi: Oxford University Press, 2002: 257-62.

CHAPTER 10

Globalization, Development, and Health: A Political Economic Perspective on the Global Struggle for Health

Fourteen thousand women die every day giving birth. Their deaths, largely from bleeding or sepsis, are almost all preventable. Overwhelmingly they come from poor families and live in low and middle-income countries. Their deaths provide a measure of the tragedy of the global health crisis, but the crisis could be equally measured in terms of farmers' suicides, occupational injury, violence, or deaths through lack of access to health care. The broad dimensions of the global health crisis have been well documented in recent World Health Reports. The purpose of this chapter is to briefly explore the economic and political dimensions of this crisis, focusing, in particular, on the links between the conditions for global health and the prevailing regime of global economic governance ("globalization").

Our focus is on the economic dimensions of globalization and their implications for health. Health systems and pathways to better health are shaped, in large degree, by the economic environment and the social structures and political forces that govern the economy.

Our focus on global economics and health should not discount the other dimensions of crisis reflected by our colleagues in other chapters of this text, such as environmental destabilization, the crisis of inequality, despair, violence, and militarism. Absolutely, "economic causes for women's deprivation have to be integrated with other social and cultural factors to give depth to the explanation."[1]

The preventable deaths of 14,000 young women every day reflect the way the global economy works. We argue in this chapter that the global economy is in crisis and that the contemporary consequences of this crisis are born largely by the peoples in developing countries. We argue that the economic policies implemented to protect the rich world from the crisis exacerbate the existing healthcare crisis for low-income countries.

There are three main parts to this chapter:

1. First we focus on economic history. We review the development of the global economy since the end of the Second World War, highlighting the high growth rates of the long

David Legge, MD; Deborah Viola, PhD

David Legge, MD, BS, BMedSc Melb, FRACP is Associate Professor and Director of the La Trobe China Health Program at the School of Public Health, La Trobe University, Bundoora, Victoria, Australia.

Deborah Viola, PhD is Assistant Professor and Director of the Masters in Public Health Program at the Department of Health Policy and Management, School of Public Health, New York Medical College, Valhalla, NY.

boom (1945–1975) and the slowing pace of growth since then.

2.   In the second part of the chapter we examine the political structures that support and maintain prevailing global economic relationships. Understanding globalization as a regime of global governance provides a useful framework for analyzing both how an unfair and unsustainable global economy is maintained, and for thinking about political strategies through which the global economy might be reformed.

3.   Lastly, we review a number of key episodes over the last 60 years that highlight the links between globalization and health. We show how the changing policies for managing the global economy have shaped the policies and discourses of health development.

We close by presenting some broad conclusions about the relations between globalization and health and a role for advocacy that is becoming increasingly more critical. If in fact women's health is to be improved by political action and public policy, we have no choice but to return to the links between global economic crisis and its various manifestations. These include, first, seeing how the local struggles for health are framed by the wider economic and political environments and factoring the big picture into our local strategies. Second is the importance of building solidarity, shared analyses, and vision across geography, class, and culture. Third is identifying the new forms of struggle that are called for by the contemporary structures of globalizing economic governance. With our improved understanding, another world is possible.

Globalization and Economic Crisis: A Historical Perspective

The decades since the end of the Second World War fall into three periods:

■   The "long boom" and the dominance of Keynesianism (1945–1975)

■   The emergence of stagflation and the rise of monetarism (1975–1985)

■   The looming threat of structural overproduction and the rise of neo-liberalism (1975 onwards)

Any such periodization involves oversimplification. The progressive improvement in living standards associated with the long boom continued (for many) into the 1980s and 1990s and the threat of structural overproduction commenced well before the mid-1970s. However, these three periods provide a framework for tracing the main dynamics operating at the global level over the last 60 years and are briefly summarized. (For further reading about the contemporary global economy, see references 2–5).

The Long Boom (1945–1975)

The 30 years from 1945 to 1975 were characterized by high annual growth rates and relatively short recessions.[5] Two major factors contributed to this. On the demand side was the huge need for reconstruction after the war and the pent-up consumer demand after so much hardship. On the supply side was the huge industrial capacity that had been built up during the war, much of which could be converted to producing for the civilian market.

In addition to these postwar factors, the development of the internal combustion engine, associated with cheap oil, contributed greatly to increasing productivity in many different sectors of production.

This economic regime has been described as Fordism, a regime of mass production, mass employment, and mass consumption. Metaphorically this refers to Ford employees being paid enough in wages to actually buy a Ford motor car. The significance of the metaphor as a descriptor of a broader economic configuration is the concept of workers as consumers and the significance of mass employment and high wages sustaining mass markets.

While the dynamics of the long boom were primarily rooted in the industrialised world there was some "trickle down" to the developing countries. Increasing production in the rich world raised the demand for agricultural products and minerals from developing countries. Newly independent developing countries commenced the process of industrialization using various forms of protection to allow local manufacturers to produce goods for the local market (substituting for imports and therefore described as the "import substitution" approach to economic development). A small number of these countries were able to complete this process and achieve strong industrial economies, notably the "Asian tigers." (The circumstances of the Cold War created particular conditions that facilitated the industrialization of Korea, Taiwan, and the postwar rebuilding of Japan.)

Stagflation and the Rise of Monetarism (1975–1985)

The long boom was replaced during the 1970s by stagflation, a combination of prolonged recession associated with rising inflation. The economic slowdown of the late 1970s reflected a combination of a cyclical slowdown (the cyclical overproduction of the normal business cycle) and the emergence of structural overproduction (defined as global productive capacity exceeding effective demand).

Thus, economic policy makers faced two problems: economic slowdown and inflation. The economic slowdown of the late 1970s suggested the need to stoke the economy (which might have suggested low interest rates), but the need to control inflation suggested the need for high interest rates. The "fight inflation first" slogan prevailed, and the policy makers implemented high interest rate policies that gradually led to the control of inflation but which deeply exacerbated the recession.

The Debt Trap: Set (in 1973) and Sprung (in 1981) Following the first OPEC (Organization of Petroleum Exporting Countries) oil price rise in 1973, the oil producers were flush with cash; more cash than they could spend or invest, so much of it was deposited in commercial banks. The banks sent salesmen around the world lending money at low and even negative interest rates. Interest rates are "negative" when they are lower than the prevailing rate of inflation; effectively paying people to borrow. Much of this lending was to private corporations, particularly in South America, but generally with government guarantees, which meant when the debt crisis was sprung the governments were held accountable for repaying and

servicing these debts. In Africa, most of the lending was directly to governments. Some of the borrowing during this period was well directed, but much of it went to projects that were corrupt or aggrandizing. Much of it was also directed to support the sales of corporations from the developed world. One notorious example was the borrowing by a friend of Ferdinand Marcos in the Philippines to construct a nuclear power station (on a tectonic fault). The power station has never produced any power, but the people of the Philippines continued to service the debt until very recently.

In the early 1980s, under the "fight inflation first" policy, interest rates escalated (to a peak of 17% in the United States in 1981) imposing repayment and servicing burdens that many poor countries could not carry; particularly, in the context of economic recession. We return to the debt trap later in this chapter.

Structural Overproduction (1975 to the Present)

The third phase, from around 1975 to the present, we characterize as "the looming threat of post-Fordist crisis." With increasing productivity, fewer and fewer workers are needed to produce goods for the global market. With the greater use of low-wage production platforms and low-paid casual employment in the rich world, discretionary spending of those who are employed is more and more constrained. The crisis that threatens is a crisis of structural overproduction; *overproduction* meaning that productive capacity exceeds effective demand; *structural* because it reflects the structural changes to patterns of global production and consumption; *post-Fordist* because it represents a delinking of high wage mass employment in mass production from mass consumption.

The global economy is too complex to be summarized simply in terms of one dominant dynamic, in this case the looming threat of post-Fordist crisis. Against this negative dynamic of crisis we can also discern the continuing influence of the (Fordist) dynamic that underscores the long boom: underemployed labor plus capital and technology producing new goods and services for new markets that are themselves motivated by the wages and business expenditure of the new production.

The emergence of China as the global factory since the 1980s epitomizes the continuing significance of the Fordist dynamic. China's explosive growth has involved underemployed labor coming together with capital and technology to produce goods and services that those employees can now buy with their wages, which therefore stokes further consumption continuing the process of capital accumulation. China's economic growth and its industrialization may stand as a metaphor for the continuing significance of the Fordist dynamic in India, Brazil, and other regions.

Nevertheless, despite China and India, the threat of productive capacity outpacing effective demand and precipitating economic crisis remains real with increasing numbers of people excluded from employment because of productivity growth and excluded from consumption because they are unemployed or underemployed.

The threat of crisis is made more urgent by compensatory policies adopted by corporations and governments that tend to exacerbate the threat of overproduction and make the crisis more likely. In the corporate world the threat of crisis is manifest in terms of reduced sales and reduced profitability. The common compensatory strategies include the following:

- Mergers and acquisitions (maintaining market share but further reducing productive employment)

- Increasing market power (e.g., gaining monopoly control over supply or through intellectual property strategies) supporting the successful corporation but exacerbating underconsumption through increasing prices

- Cutting wages (maintaining sales through cheaper prices but further reducing wage-based consumption)

- Replacing labor with technology (further reducing the flow of wages into consumption)

- Transferring production to low-wage platforms (maintaining sales through cheaper prices but further reducing the flow of wages into consumption)

- Expanding the boundaries of the market place (commodifying family, community, and government functions previously conducted outside the marketplace)

- Keeping prices low by transferring the costs of production to the environment (through unregulated pollution) and to the workforce (through lack of occupational safety or financial compensation for occupational injury and disease)

The threat of structural overproduction is understood in the policy world in terms of falling growth rates, which elicit a range of policy responses many of which also further exacerbate the risk of crisis (or impose greater burdens on those already suffering their effects). These policy responses may in fact be similar to those used within the corporate arena, but may also include the following:

- Cutting taxes (reducing the corporate and executive tax burden to compete for new investment in the global market place but also reducing the financial capacity of government to ameliorate the impact of crisis)

- Outsourcing and privatizing government functions (providing new investment and market opportunities for underemployed capital but also transferring the costs of government services from tax payer to user)

- Forcing repayment of debt from developing countries (supporting the profitability of the banks and maintaining living standards in the developed nations and propping up the value of developed or western country currencies thereby keeping the prices of imported goods in the developed nations low)

- Forcing developing countries to open their markets to manufacturers from developed countries

Some of these corporate and policy responses might tend to restore the conditions for sustainable growth. However, most of them further reduce demand through reduced employment and reduced wages. Many of these responses also have adverse consequences in relation to the environment (illustrated by the reluctance to reduce greenhouse gas emissions), in relation to family and community life (the commodification of family and community functions), and the decay of social infrastructure.

Rise of Neoliberalism (1980 to 2000)

Despite some developing countries having achieved economic growth over the last 30 years, for many countries the conditions for health development for the poorer sections of the population have been sacrificed in order to maintain living standards in the West.

This is not the story told in the mainstream financial press or by the politicians meeting each year at the World Economic Forum in Davos, Switzerland. *They* speak of the importance of free trade, reduced taxes, free markets, and small government. This story about the superiority of markets and the dangers of government is commonly described as the new liberalism or neoliberalism.

The term *neoliberalism* is a reference to the rise of economic liberalism during the early development of capitalism in Europe. Liberalism here meant freedom of commerce, in particular the lifting of royal monopolies sanctioned by the king in return for a share of the rent. The new liberalism borrows from this history but in very different conditions.

The underlying logic of the new liberalism is about the greater efficiency of free markets compared with planned and administered program delivery. In many respects the new liberalism was an ideological campaign about the general superiority of markets over governments; it argued for small government, deregulation, reduced reliance on planning, and for program design to follow market principles. It is noteworthy in relation to health development that the commitment to the free market did not extend to intellectual property where monopoly power has been progressively shored up. (See **"Globalization and Health"** in this chapter for examples, specifically the subsections on "Access to Expensive Drugs" and "Agriculture.")

Globalization as Governance

Our purpose in this chapter is to understand how global health conditions are shaped. Our focus so far has been on economic relationships including the flow of goods and services around the world and the corresponding (reverse) flow of money. We have explored briefly some of the system relationships between these flows that we believe can be described in terms of *dynamics*: the dynamic of Fordist stability and the dynamic of post-Fordist instability. An appreciation of these economic dynamics is necessary to understand the ways in which the conditions for global health are determined through the global governance of economic relationships.

The economic "system" we have described is a simplification of a much more complex world. Other conceptual systems applied to the same world will reorganize our experience in different ways, often in ways that will add new insights to our understanding of the problems the global community faces and possible directions which may be taken. A focus on governance, as opposed to the stocks and flows of "the economy," can enhance our understanding of the conditions that shape global health and possible strategies for change. The following are key components:

- Empires, big powers, and nation-states
- Transnational corporations and their peak bodies
- International institutions and conventions
- Nongovernment organizations (local, national, and international)
- Constituencies and movements
- Information (e.g., knowledge, discourses, ideology, and the organizations that support the generation, flow, and engagement of knowledge and discourse)
- Pathways of social change

Our purpose here is not an exhaustive and systematic description of the structures of global governance. Rather we introduce the governance perspective and highlight some of the critical components that are of particular importance to the nexus between globalization and health.

Empires, Big Powers, and Nation-States

Historically, global governance has been the work of empires, in varying degrees of tension with other empires, nation-states, and other political forces. The dominant imperial power in the present era is the United States, and it uses a range of instruments to fulfill its governance responsibilities.

In many respects, however, the global economic regime governs itself, and the role of the governors is merely to adjust the settings from time to time. Markets are self-sustaining mechanisms that, within a particular framework of regulation,[6] reproduce the economic flows and relationships we have discussed above. The rules that characterize this regulatory regime at the global level are formalized and administered by a range of international institutions and conventions that generally mediate the interests of the big powers and big corporations.

The health implications of this "market autonomy within a particular regulatory framework" perspective can be seen in the eclipse of Keynesianism and rise of monetarism in the early 1980s. Keynesianism, with its focus on tax policy and government expenditure, provided space for redistributive policies and public investment in social infrastructure.[7] The rise of monetarism and the neoliberal philosophy of small government weakened the support for such social policies and created the conditions for widening global inequalities with familiar implications for population health.

International Institutions and Conventions

The main groups of institutions that would need to be considered in any account of the global governance of health include:

- United Nations system, especially World Health Organization (WHO), Joint United Nations Program on HIV/AIDS (UNAIDS), and United Nations Children's Fund (UNICEF) on the health side, and United Nations Conference on Trade and Development (UNCTAD) and United Nations Development Programme (UNDP) on the economic side

- Various public–private partnerships in health (e.g., Global Fund to Fight AIDS, Tuberculosis and Malaria [GFATM], Global Alliance for Vaccines and Immunization [GAVI])

- The Bretton Woods institutions (the International Monetary Fund (IMF), World Bank (WB), and WTO)

- The conventions and agreements that set the legal framework internationally (e.g., WTO agreements; various declarations on economic, political, cultural, and social rights; Kyoto Agreement; the International Health Regulations; and Framework Convention on Tobacco Control)

The various public–private partnerships such as the Global Fund to Fight AIDS, Tuberculosis and Malaria (GFATM), and the Global Alliance for Vaccines and Immunization (GAVI), are a relatively late addition to this range of governance institutions. Much of the pressure for the emergence of the global partnerships has been the need to mobilize corporate charity (differential pricing) to alleviate the medications crisis in the developing world and head off the risk of more profound reform to the global intellectual property regime.[8]

These various players do not operate in a vacuum. Beyond the empire, the nation-states, the transnationals, and the international institutions are the more diffused constituencies whom the principal players both lead and follow. We can describe these constituencies in terms of nationalities, ethnicities, classes, castes, and religions although these overlap complexly. When trying to understand the global economy it is useful to think in terms of countries: the countries of the north and the south, or the center and the periphery. However, class alliances (and those of race, language, and religion) cut across national boundaries and are also useful descriptors. Cross-national solidarities are also framed by religion, language, and race. Reich[9] has pointed to the rise of the global middle class with a sense of shared identity and cultural solidarity arising from similar educational experiences and greater international travel (owing to links with government, transnational companies, and universities).

The idea of social movements that cross national boundaries provides further insights into the agency of these more dispersed constituencies. The people's health movement (as an illustration of global social movements generally) is based on a shared consciousness and solidarity arising from a common recognition of, and opposition to, the disease burden arising from globalization.

Information, Knowledge, and Discourses and the Organizations That Support Their Generation, Flow, and Engagement

Any account of governance structures must also include the information dimension (including knowledge, discourse, and ideology,) and the organizational structures that support the generation and dissemination of knowledge and the flow of discourses and the engagement of ideologies. We may characterize the information dimension of global governance in the following terms:

- Information (e.g., population statistics, intelligence, news)
- Knowledge paradigms (e.g., traditional, technicist, interpretive)
- Discourses of health and economics (e.g., neoliberalism, free trade, comprehensive primary health care, cost-effectiveness packages)
- Ideologies (e.g., neoliberalism, liberal democracy, market fundamentalism, religious fundamentalisms, community empowerment)

The organizations that support the generation, flow, and engagement of information, knowledge, discourses, and ideology include the following:

- Academic and other research centers (e.g., London School of Hygiene and Tropical Medicine, the Harvard University School of Public Health, the World Bank)
- Media organizations (e.g., News Corporation, BBC, VOA)
- Discussion platforms (e.g., UN, the Organization for Economic Co-operation and Development [OECD], the World Economic Forum, and the World Social Forum)
- Markets, in particular, the financial markets and the financial media

The idea of an information dimension of global governance (including knowledge, discourse, and ideology) opens up a huge field for description, analysis, and strategy. This is not the place for such a discussion, but we can illustrate the importance of this dimension by simply mentioning two examples:

- The promotion of "cost-effective packages of interventions" as the basis for the World Bank's approach to health sector reform
- Role of progressive Web sites in supporting popular movements around health issues

Since 1993 the World Bank has promoted the principle of cost-effective packages of interventions as the basis for health system planning. In essence this approach assumes a multitiered health system with the middle class relying on insurance and private providers and the minimal packages constituting a safety net for the poor. In promoting this model, a huge infrastructure of data and information has been built up dealing with the burden of disease and cost-effectiveness evaluations of interventions. There is a certain logic to much of this argument, and it has a place in the range of disciplines from which the health planner draws. However, in the context of the broader economic perspective of the World Bank, this body of data, techniques, and ideas has a particular ideological function as well, namely to legitimize an unfair and unstable economic regime; the ideological message is that improved health is possible within this regime.

A counterillustration of the importance of the information dimension of global governance concerns the role of progressive Web sites in supporting popular movements around health issues. This is particularly clear in relation to the various campaigns around the medications crisis: the Treatment Action Campaign in South Africa, the Novartis campaign in India, and the support for the Thai use of compulsory licensing; and in exploring alternatives to the prevailing intellectual property regime.

Pathways of Social Change

An account of global governance that is designed to support the struggle for health needs to go beyond simply describing the structures of global governance. Our main focus in the preceding discussion has been on the policy decisions and structures that maintain the existing regime. We also need a framework for thinking about the pathways through which change occurs and the pressures for change and the ways in which the strategies of the people's health movement might drive change. This is a big field, too big to be properly addressed in this chapter.

However, in the following section we shall review a number of key struggles in health development and seek to draw out of these some principles of activist practice.

Globalization and Health

Our purpose in this chapter is to explore the links between population health and globalization (which we are using to denote the prevailing regime of global economic governance). We began with an overview of the dynamics and transitions of the global economy since the Second World War and proceeded from there to present a framework for analyzing the political regime through which the global economy is governed (and which so powerfully shapes population health).

In this part we give examples of the impact of the economic regime on health development.

Primary Health Care

In many countries under colonial rule, health service development had been largely restricted to the urban centers. This pattern was in many cases continued after decolonization, leaving the rural majority poorly served. However, during the 1960s several countries were experimenting with more comprehensive approaches to health care, moving away from hospital and doctor-based care in the cities to the provision of basic health services in the rural areas. There was also new attention given to appropriate workforce strategies and more focus on community mobilization for prevention. This approach became known as primary health care (PHC) and was formally enshrined in and endorsed by the Alma-Ata Conference and Declaration.[10]

Alma-Ata was a reaction against top-down vertical programs and urban-centered health service development. The declaration called for greater attention to the needs of rural populations and for greater reliance on heath workers with basic training who were accountable to local communities but who were properly supported by clinical and prevention specialists more centrally based.[11]

The Alma-Ata Declaration went well beyond a narrow medical or disease-centered model, recognizing that sustainable economic development was a critical condition for health development in developing countries. Alma-Ata refers explicitly to the 1974 call by the Non-Aligned Movement for a New International Economic Order, a governance regime that might facilitate the sovereign economic development of poor countries. Alma-Ata was driven in large part by the spirit of the Non-

Aligned Movement with support and facilitation from the leaderships of the WHO and UNICEF. By this time Dr. Halfdan Mahler was the Director-General at WHO. Mahler was a committed advocate for the PHC approach although there remained divisions within WHO who were still oriented to the vertical disease focus.[12]

In some ways Alma-Ata was the last hurrah of the hope and confidence of the Non-Aligned Movement. The long boom had petered out, monetarism was on the rise, and the debt trap had been set. Within a few years many developing countries were facing recession and economic restructuring under the control of the IMF. The IMF did not regard health development as particularly important; the debt had to be serviced, and if that meant dismantling health services and terminating food price subsidies then so be it.

PHC Debates and Legitimation Crisis

As early as 1979 there were voices[13] calling for a return to the orthodoxy of narrow vertical programs (now renamed as *selective primary health care*), perhaps recognizing that in the conditions of the time the resources necessary for the implementation of comprehensive PHC were not going to be available. From the point of view of donors (Western governments and philanthropies) the practical challenge was about getting outcomes for the aid dollar. The choices appeared to be either waiting for basic health system infrastructure to be developed or investing in more limited disease-centered and maternal and child health (MCH) programs that at least offered the promise of achievable outcomes. With the rise of AIDS/HIV and the weakening of basic health services associated with structural adjustment, the preference of the donors to return to vertical programs was consolidated. Advocates of vertical programs saw themselves as accepting the *real politic* that comprehensive PHC was not happening; they commonly depicted the advocates of comprehensive PHC as unreal ideologues.

The advocates of comprehensive PHC had two problems with this position.[14] Their first objection was that for many diseases narrow vertical programs simply did not work; smallpox was the exception rather than the paradigm case. Effective prevention and management of such conditions as TB, malaria, and AIDS/HIV require a wide range of

generic programs and services that are either not provided under the vertical programs model or are duplicated specifically for this condition. The second issue motivating the advocates of comprehensive PHC was a concern that fraying livelihoods (e.g., loss of markets and jobs, malnutrition, loss of access to education) and the decay of services under the pressure of economic restructuring (e.g. reduced budgets, user charges) was actually adding to the disease burden of poor people in poor countries, indeed was now one of the most serious threats to health those communities were facing. Particularly for women, the impact on health from job loss and denial of education has been demonstrated to be particularly significant.[15] From this point of view the effect of arguments for selective PHC and vertical programs was to obscure the damage being done by economic restructuring and to project the view that health could be improved despite these influences, thus legitimating an unfair regime.

The human cost of illness is a major motivating factor for health activists; 200,000 women died in childbirth during the writing of this chapter. Primary healthcare practitioners confront the immediate, local, and personal issues that affect their communities, but they can also work with those families and communities to make sense of the upstream factors that reproduce those patterns of pain and to consider ways of more effectively engaging with the structures and forces behind them. In many communities, poverty and lack of healthcare facilities are compounded by gender inequality:

> The prevailing belief in this area [Sub-Saharan Africa] is that the role of a female in society is to marry, have many children, raise the children, and look to her husband for guidance in all matters. Even as we train more clinical officers and try to improve our medical services to women, we must remember that the environment we work in does not allow the women themselves to have a voice in their choices of health care or where and when they will seek medical help.[16]

Access to Expensive Drugs

High prices for life-saving drugs (and denial of access for millions who would benefit from them) is a further illustration of the way neoliberal globalization affects health. High prices for essential medicines are partly a consequence of the global intellectual property regime administered under the WTO. However, this case also shows the role of big power bullying and even how international organizations such as the WHO can be suborned. It also shows how civil society working through south–north partnerships can effect change. The key issue at stake in these struggles has been whether and when generic manufacturers might be authorized to create cheap versions of life-saving drugs.

As early as 1991 the US Trade Representative (USTR) was putting pressure on Thailand because it authorized the manufacture of drugs still under patent in the United States through its government production facilities.[17] Thailand had also modified its patent laws to require advanced notice of new drug approval applications and to make the information provided to the regulators available to generic manufacturers prior to patent expiration in order to accelerate their introduction to the marketplace. The US pharmaceutical lobby maintains a global watch over such threats, and the USTR acts promptly on the urging of big pharmaceutical companies (also a big contributor to politicians' election funds). The USTR threatened Thailand with Super 301, a US trade law which authorizes the US to implement trade sanctions against any country that is found to be harming the interests of US corporations. Similarly Brazil has been subject to threats and pressures by the USTR on behalf of big pharmaceutical companies because of its policies of compulsory licensing and local production of antiretrovirals.

Perhaps the highest profile case was the South African case in 1998 when 38 large pharmaceutical companies took the South African government to court (in South Africa) arguing that the legislative provisions for parallel importation of antiretrovirals (sourcing public purchasing in the cheapest overseas market and bypassing authorized local representatives) contravened South African intellectual property laws. The legal issue was never decided. The case created such an international political storm that in April 2001 the companies withdrew their complaints and agreed to pay the costs of the defendant. The defeat of the drug companies in South Africa involved a massive struggle in South Africa (led by the Treatment Action Campaign) and the organization of a massive global protest (led by Médecins Sans Frontières and resourced by CPTech). The drug companies withdrew because they were bringing into disrepute the intellectual property rights upon which they depend and which are integral to the capitalist system itself. It was a battle about legitimacy, and they lost.

However, even as big pharmaceutical companies were buckling in Johannesburg, the government of Norway was hosting (April 2001) a meeting that included WHO, UNICEF, the World Bank, the global pharmaceutical giants, and a small group of NGOs to discuss strategies to deal with access to expensive drugs by poor countries. The meeting considered all options including compulsory licensing but adopted the more conservative pharma-friendly option of differential pricing. This position was to be expected from the World Bank, but from the WHO it was disappointing—perhaps a warning to those who might have expected more.

The conservatism of this position (differential pricing) was underlined 7 months later when the WTO Ministerial Council meeting in November 2001 in Doha, Qatar adopted the Doha Statement on TRIPS and Public Health. One of the most significant agreements administered through the WTO is the Trade-Related Intellectual Property Rights (TRIPS) agreement, in particular for its implications in relation to pharmaceuticals and specifically, retrovirals for AIDS/HIV.[18] The principle underlying the Doha Statement was that public health should take priority over trade rules. The statement affirmed the legitimacy of compulsory licensing and also addressed the barriers facing small countries unable to use compulsory licensing to meet their own needs because they did not have a domestic generics industry. The Doha meeting commissioned a process to work out the detailed rules and arrangements under which poor countries could use compulsory licensing for domestic or export purposes (to small countries without their own generic industry). In the years that followed the United States mounted a rearguard action to prevent the use of the TRIPS agreement to sanction compulsory licensing in developing countries.

Nevertheless the writing was on the wall with regard to the WTO as a compliant vehicle for US economic policy. The alternative strategy of multiple bilateral and regional free-trade agreements was being implemented at the same time. In October 2002, Bristol Myers Squib was defeated in a long-running case about the Thai government's right to manufacture DDI (an AIDS drug) for local consumption. In the context of the Gore-Bush presidential campaign and under sustained pressure from AIDS activists in the United States, the USTR (under President Clinton) announced in 2000 that the US accept Thailand's right to produce DDI within the terms of its own intellectual property laws. However, in 2003 negotiations commenced between Thailand and the United States towards a US Thai FTA with compulsory licensing, data access, and extended Intellectual property rights (IPRs) on the table.

There is no sign of big pharmaceutical companies withdrawing from this issue. In early 2007, the Swiss giant Novartis commenced proceedings in the India courts seeking to overturn the decision not to grant a patent to imatinib (Glivec) on the grounds that it was not sufficiently innovative in comparison to existing drugs. The criteria for patenting new drugs will remain a tightly contested issue in future years.

Agriculture

While the TRIPS agreement is directly and explicitly relevant to health, the agreement that has the strongest impact on the health of people in developing countries is probably the Agreement on Agriculture (AoA). It allows the United States, Europe, and Japan to protect their domestic markets while forcing agricultural producers in developing countries to open their markets to manufactured and agricultural imports. Structural adjustment packages (SAPs) comprise a set of policies imposed by the International Monetary Fund (IMF) on highly indebted countries seeking to borrow from the IMF as the lender of last resort. SAPs included cuts in public expenditure (on health and food subsidies), devaluation to make exports cheaper (but which made imports more expensive), and a reorientation of agriculture and industry around production for export. The prime purpose of the SAPs was to enable client countries to generate the export earnings needed to repay debts. While they were packaged in the language of economic development, this was not their principal purpose. Indeed, in many ways the SAPs involved a process of deindustrialization and regression with respect to social and economic development. In a relatively small number of countries the SAPs were associated with economic growth and improvements in health and welfare despite widening inequalities. However, in most cases, particularly in Africa, structural adjustments have had a negative impact on health status and on health services.

After several generations of SAPs in which poor countries have been told to switch to producing the same range of agricultural commodities for export, the prices for these products have fallen below cost, leaving the farmers without subsistence and without income. The dumping of subsidized products into the cities of developing countries is a further blow to the farmers in the hinterlands.

While the rhetoric of the WTO is about free trade, it may be more useful to see it as driving towards a somewhat different objective, namely, to ensure that the transnational corporations of the rich world have access to the economies of the developing countries (without any real expectation of exposing the farmers of Europe, Japan, and the United States to international competition).

The pressure on developing countries to provide increased access to agricultural and food imports from the developed countries threatens the livelihood of hundreds of millions of small farmers, unable to compete with protected, subsidized, oil-based industrialized agriculture. Once again, the decreased earnings and employment have also resulted in reduced access to education and healthcare services.

Conclusion

So what conclusions can we draw from this review, and what directions do they suggest? Our purpose in undertaking this review of global health and global economic governance over the last 6 decades was to draw out possible lessons and implications for people's health activists and for health policy and public health practice at the national and global levels. In this final section we discuss these possible lessons and implications.

Health activists need to develop their "global economics literacy" to project clear narratives linking the disease burden carried by their communities with the structures, dynamics, and flows of the current global economic regime and its governance. They also need to be able to read through the half truths of the establishment policy reports.

The impact of TRIPS on access to drugs for AIDS has proved a powerful introduction for many health activists to the workings of the WTO and the role of the WTO in regulating an unfair and unsustainable global trading regime. In terms of sheer burden of disease the Agreement on Agriculture (AoA) is probably the single most health-damaging instrument in the whole complex governance structure. Hundreds of millions of small farmers are being driven off their lands through the swamping of global markets by industrialized agriculture (heavily subsidized in the case of Europe, Japan, and the United States). Only a small proportion of these small farmers will find jobs in the cities. The health consequences associated with this loss of livelihood range from undernutrition to drug use and violence, and from AIDS to TB. It is not wrong to attribute this burden of disease to violence or AIDS, but it does not tell the whole story. Behind violence and AIDS are the stock and flows and dynamics of the global economy that in turn are sustained and reproduced by a governance regime that includes organizations, countries, and transnational corporations. However, even for such powerful forces, their power is not unlimited as demonstrated by the success of the Treatment Action Campaign in South Africa.

The structures of global governance will be determined, in part, through contests over legitimation: how legitimate is the IMF, the WTO, and the USTR in the eyes of various global constituencies. How legitimate is the World Bank in its advocacy for multitiered healthcare systems with minimal safety nets for the poor versus comprehensive PHC and health system capacity building. There are real questions about models for health system development that need to be worked through, but World Bank advocacy for vertical programming and cost-effective interventions are partly about projecting the possibility that health can be improved, for a relatively modest sum, without changing the economic dynamics of alienation and expropriation. How legitimate is this?

Health advocates need new ways of projecting the disease burden of poverty, despair, violence, displacement, and conflict and of the underlying economic relations and structures of economic governance.

Comprehensive PHC, access to essential medicines, and small farmers' livelihoods are important issues in their own right. However, they also provide case material through which to examine in more detail how economic dynamics and governance structures work at the global level. Global health policy advocates need to be able to advance a clear underlying economic analysis that makes sense of these issues.

The story presented in this chapter is not an overriding and eternal truth about the global economy. It is an attempt to make sense of what is in truth impossibly complex. It is a story that knits together some of the salient features of the last 60 years of global capitalism, in particular focusing on the flow of resources and value between rich and poor countries. There is much scope for developing this story, perhaps accommodating more complexity, and for applying it in different ways to different parts of the system.

Another world is possible.

In December 2000 at a venue outside Dakha in Bangladesh, the first International People's Health Assembly (PHA) was held with several thousand delegates representing over 50 countries. Out of the first PHA was formed the People's Health Movement,[20] an international network of grass roots community health activists and policy advocates dedicated to demonstrating that "another world is possible." In July 2005, 1500 delegates participated in the Second People's Health Assembly in Cuenca, Ecuador. The growing strength of the People's Health Movement may be taken as a mark of the growing consciousness of the shared context among health activists world wide and the growing sense of solidarity and common purpose.

We have reviewed the interplay of economics and health at the global level over the past 60 years and drawn some conclusions about strategy for health activists working locally, globally, and at all levels in between. Global health advocates need to keep the need for a fairer regime of global economic governance at the center of activist practice and health policy advocacy. *

> *Rise like lions after slumber*
> *In unvanquishable number!*
> *Shake your chains to earth, like dew*
> *Which in sleep had fallen on you—*
> *Ye are many, they are few!*
> —P. Shelley, 1832[19]

* The authors thank Dr. Peter Arno for his thoughtful and considered review of this chapter.

DISCUSSION QUESTIONS

1. When bilateral or multilateral agreements are developed how should women's global health issues be addressed?

2. How can health activism play a greater role in international trade agreements?

3. What lesson can be learned from how the role of health activists influenced the Doha accord?

4. How can economic growth foster better health outcomes for women and why is this not always the case?

REFERENCES

1. Sen, A. More than 100 Million Women Are Missing. *The New York Review of Books.* Volume 37, Number 20. December 20, 1990.

2. Amin S. *Capitalism in the Age of Globalisation: The Management of Contemporary Society.* London, UK: Zed Books; 1997.

3. Shutt H. *The Trouble with Capitalism: An Enquiry into the Causes of Global Economic Failure.* London, UK: Zed Books; 1998.

4. Went R. *Globalisation: Neoliberal Challenge, Radical Responses.* Drucker P trans., London, UK: Pluto Press with International Institute for Research and Education; 2000.

5. Bello W. The capitalist conjuncture: over-accumulation, financial crises, and the retreat from globalisation. *Third World Quarterly.* 2006;27(8):1345-1367.

6. Jessop B. The regulation approach, governance, and post-Fordism: alternative perspectives on economic and political change? *Econ Soc.* 1995;24(3):307-333.

7. Keynes JM. *The general theory of employment, interest and money.* Amherst, NY: Prometheus Books; 1997.

8. Commission on Intellectual Property Rights Innovation and Public Health. Public Health, Innovation, and Intellectual Property Rights. Geneva, Switzerland: WHO; 2006.

9. Reich RB. *The Work of Nations.* New York, NY: Vintage Books; 1992.

10. World Health Organisation. *Alma-Ata 1978. Primary Health Care.* Geneva, Switzerland: World Health Organisation; 1978.

11. Werner D, Sanders D. *Questioning the Solution: The Politics of Primary Health Care and Child Survival.* Palo Alto, CA: Healthwrights; 1997.

12. Werner D, Sanders D. *Questioning the Solution: The Politics of Primary Health Care and Child Survival.* Palo Alto, CA: Healthwrights; 1997.

13. Walsh JA, Warren KS. Selective primary health care: an interim strategy for disease control in developing countries. *N Engl J Med.* 1979;301:967-974.

14. Werner D. Who killed primary health care? *New Internationalist.* 1995;272:28-30.

15. Sen, A. *More Than 100 Million Women Are Missing. Women's Global Health and Human. Rights.* Boston, MA: Jones and Bartlett; 2009.

16. Makin, S. Saving mothers, one at a time [Opinion]. *New York Times.* http://Kristof .blogs.nytimes.com. Accessed July 23, 2008.

17. Markandya S. Timeline of trade disputes involving Thailand and access to medicines. Consumer Project on Technology, 2001. http://www.cptech.org/ip/health /c/thailand/thailand.html. Accessed April 22, 2008.

18. Khor M. *Rethinking Globalization: Critical Issues and Policy Choices.* London, UK: Zed Books; 2001.

19. Shelley, PB. *The Masque of Anarchy: A Poem.* London, UK: Edward Moxon; 1832.

20. Health for all now! People's Health Movement. http://www.phmovement.org. Accessed April 23, 2008.

Globally, women are often the victims of poor access to health care and discrimination. Often they do not receive assistance and treatment for their ailments and suffer pain and humiliation in silence. This section attempts to discuss the impact various infectious and chronic diseases have on the quality of life for women worldwide.

Health Problems and Challenges Specific to Women, Including Chronic Diseases and Their Global Burden

When will our consciences grow so tender that we will act to prevent human misery rather than avenge it?

—Eleanor Roosevelt, Former First Lady, United States of America

CHAPTER 11

The AIDS Pandemic and Women's Rights

INTRODUCTION

When acquired immune deficiency was first described, case reports of unusual infections and cancers among gay men in New York and San Francisco lead to the predominant view that AIDS was a gay men's disease. One of the first articles suggesting the heterosexual transmission of the disease was published in the prestigious *Journal of the American Medical Association* in 1983 and entitled, "Acquired immunodeficiency . . . in infants born to promiscuous and drug-addicted mothers."[1] It is historically significant that the focus of this article, and indeed the global policy that accompanied it in the subsequent decades, was on the babies as innocent victims of their mothers' bad behavior.[2] Much of discussion, in the ensuing two decades, of providing HIV testing or treatment to women, particularly poor women, in resource poor settings, was based not on a woman's right to receive treatment but rather on a public health approach of preventing the transmission of HIV to their infants. While this public health approach has epidemiological merit in terms of disease prevention for babies; in neglecting women's lives, the strategy of women as drug delivery vessels of HIV drugs promoted a large moral blind spot; one that has not promoted a rights-based approach either in women's access to life-saving treatment or approaches to prevention that take into account the underlying causes of the epidemic. From early in the epidemic, the work of Jonathan Mann and others[3,4] emphasized vulnerability and lack of human rights among those affected by AIDS; yet, much of the coverage of the epidemic in the scientific and lay literature emphasized, then as now, a lack of individual responsibility and the choice of risky behaviors as the engines of the epidemic rather than the risks inherent to the environment of social and economic inequality in which the epidemic thrives.

In the third decade of the AIDS epidemic, there has been a long overdue awareness of women's special vulnerability to the disease. The facts are overwhelming that women *are* being affected by the disease and *do* bear a disproportionate burden of suffering. The situation is indeed dire and growing worse for women. The UNAIDS 2007 AIDS

Joia S. Mukherjee, MD, MPH
Didi Bertrand Farmer, MA
Paul E. Farmer, MD, PhD

Joia S. Mukherjee, MD, MPH is the Medical Director for Partners In Health and the Director for the Institute for Health and Social Justice. Dr. Mukherjee is also an Assistant Professor in the Division of Global Health Equity of Harvard Medical School, and a recipient of Janet Glasgow Memorial Achievement Citation: AMWA.

Didi Bertrand Farmer, MA, is the Director of Community Health Programs for Partners In Health, Inshuti Mu Buzima, Rwanda.

Paul E. Farmer MD, PhD, is the Presley Professor in the Department of Global Health and Social Medicine, at Harvard Medical School. He is also the Associate Chief, Division of Social Medicine and Health Inequalities at Brigham and Women's Hospital and the Co-founder of Partners In Health, Cambridge MA. Dr. Farmer is the recipient of Jimmy and Rosalynn Carter Award for Humanitarian Contributions to the Health of Humankind from the National Foundation for Infectious Diseases, the Salk Institute Medal for Health and Humanity, the Duke University Humanitarian Award, the Margaret Mead Award from the American Anthropological Association, and the American Medical Association's International Physician (Nathan Davis) Award. John D. and Catherine T. MacArthur Foundation "genius award".

Epidemic Update reported that women constitute half of the 30.8 million adults globally who are living with HIV, a proportion that has remained steady for a number of years now. Almost 61 percent of adults living with HIV in the most heavily burdened region, sub-Saharan Africa, are women, and three quarters of people living with HIV in the region who are between 15–24 years old are women. Every region of the world has seen an increase in the number of women living with HIV during the past 2 years.[5]

Women are more susceptible to HIV and constitute a higher proportion of new cases than do men. We know that an HIV-negative woman is at least twice as likely to become infected by an HIV-positive man as an HIV-negative man is likely to become infected by an HIV-positive woman. Girls under the age of 15 are five times more likely to be HIV-positive than boys of their age group. We would make a critical mistake, however, to view this heightened threat to women as solely a matter of biology. While part of the greater transmissibility of HIV from men to women can be explained by basic science, biological vulnerability adds little to our understanding of the disproportionate suffering borne by poor women across the globe at the hands of the AIDS epidemic. When we take a step back from statistics and biology, the bigger picture reveals that AIDS affects women who, struggling under the overarching epidemic of *inequality*, have little control over the factors that put them at risk for this deadly disease. This link between the economic inequality in which women live and their vulnerability to all facets of the pandemic remains unaddressed by the very policies that aim to mitigate the impact of HIV on women.

AIDS as a Window into Structural Violence

The systematic exclusion of a group from the resources needed to develop their full human potential has been called structural violence.[6] The concept of structural violence is useful to understand the barriers that prevent health maintenance and risk mitigation in the HIV epidemic. Access to

treatment is also intertwined with poverty. Active antiretroviral therapy (ART), the three drug "cocktail" that became available in 1995, rapidly returned even the sickest people with AIDS to good health. However, the miracle of ART markedly worsened the inequality of AIDS outcomes between the rich and the poor around the globe. The poor throughout the developing world were systematically excluded from ART; the drugs were said to be too expensive, too complicated, and not sustainable to use in resource-poor settings. The combinations of increased risk for HIV fueled by structural violence and unequal access to treatment led to a global pandemic in which the poor have excess risk of acquiring HIV and, once infected, have less access to lifesaving ART. As a result, the most heavily HIV-burdened countries have become further impoverished due to the epidemic.

Gender inequality continues to affect societies across the globe. Women are less likely to be educated and less likely to find paying work. When working, women earn two-thirds of what men earn. Women also bear the enormous burden of uncompensated work, including caring for children and sick relatives, feeding the family, and managing the home. As a result, women spend twice as much time performing unpaid work than do men.[7] Men are far from immune, however, to the crushing poverty of the developing world. They, too, suffer from desperation, depression, anger, and emasculation, all of which have been linked with resultant so-called social ills such as substance abuse, domestic violence, and other criminal activities.[8] Such social ills are rooted in poverty and inequality. Structural violence, defined as the physical and psychological harm that results from exploitive and unjust social, political, and economic systems, is the dynamic in which the AIDS virus lurks.

Structural Violence Is the Risk

How does structural violence relate to sexually transmitted disease? Sexual violence is a common product of the power structure in which women are trapped in the home, on the street, or during war. Additionally, selling sex as a commodity—whether it is in exchange for money, food, or security—can be a means of survival for the world's poorest women. Neither sexual violence nor commercial sex work are behaviors that one would choose if they had options; rather, these behaviors are imposed upon them by the social structures that continue to oppress poor women.

Rape is a major factor driving the AIDS epidemic. In political conflicts, rape is a common crime and has even been used purposefully as a tool of war. For example, in Rwanda the systemic sexual molestation, rape, and mutilation of women and girls was an integral part of the Hutu plan to annihilate the Tutsi population.[9,10] Similarly, as in all wars, women were forced to exchange sex for food, money or security. As a result, an estimated 70% of the 250,000 women who survived the genocide are now HIV-positive.[11,12] Similarly, studies by the United Nations Children's Fund concluded that over 75% of girls and young women abducted by rebel forces during times of armed conflict in Sierra Leone were sexually abused.[13] In Uganda, the Lord's Resistance Army (LRA) continues to abduct children; in this 15-year conflict, thousands of children have been raped and HIV-infected by the LRA. Ninety percent of northern Uganda's 1.8 million people have been internally displaced and are now crowded into refugee camps. Forty thousand children routinely walk up to several kilometers each night to schools, hospitals, and shelters in the town of Gulu to protect themselves from abduction. Not surprisingly, the HIV prevalence rate in northern Uganda is at least twice that of the rest of the country. In Haiti, since the February 29, 2004, overthrow of the democratically elected president, Jean Bertrand Aristide, human rights violations including rape were documented to increase significantly.[14]

It is not only political violence itself that threatens to spread the virus.[15] While official statistics have not been released, it is now widely recognized that United Nations (UN) peacekeeping forces have contributed to the spread of HIV, through unprotected contact with commercial sex workers, through rape, and through using their position of access to resources to leverage sexual favors. Many UN troops come from countries with high prevalence rates; for example, in 2001 in Sierra Leone, 32% of the 16,630 UN peacekeepers were from countries with prevalence rates greater than 5% and were responsible for an upsurge in HIV prevalence in Sierra Leone.[16] Similarly, UN peacekeepers stationed in Haiti have been implicated in rapes in that country.[17]

Even in times of relative political stability, women in impoverished settings frequently experience violence and sexual harassment as a "normal" component of their workday. One research study of the International Labor Rights Fund in Kenya's coffee, tea, and light manufacturing industries revealed that over 90% of the women interviewed experienced or observed sexual abuse within their workplace; 95% who suffered such abuse feared being fired if they reported the crime; and 70% of the men interviewed believed that the sexual harassment of female workers was "normal and natural behavior."[11,18]

A similar lack of real choice or agency faces women in monogamous relationships who are encouraged to rely on "being faithful" as their means to prevent HIV infection. This strategy, of course, withers against the backdrop of structural violence, as most women are infected as a result of their partners' infidelities, not their own. In fact, in many locations, the main HIV risk factor for a woman is the simple fact of having a stable sexual partner.[19] One study reports that HIV-infection rates were 10% higher for married than for sexually active unmarried girls aged 15–19 years in Kenya and Zambia.[20] A study in rural Uganda found that 88% of HIV-infected women aged 15–19 were married.[21] Because young women in many societies often have significantly older men as their partners, the men are more likely to have had other partners and are therefore more likely to have been exposed to HIV. Additionally, while infidelity is as old as the human species, structural violence often forces men living in poverty to leave their homes to search for work in cities, factories, and mines where there are no provisions for family life. Such necessary migration for meager wages, resulting in long absences from family, sets the stage for multiple sexual partners.

Additionally, condom use is rarely under the control of women. While "success stories" of commercial sex worker labor unions demanding condom use of their clients do exist, few would argue that a society that affords women no option but prostitution should be considered a "success."[22-26] Collective bargaining around the terms of the commercial exchange of sex only highlights the marginalization of women in a society where sex is their only marketable resource. Women in stable relationships may fare even worse than single women in terms of their ability to use condoms for HIV prevention. Many couples decrease condom use because of greater trust, or in an attempt to conceive children, or because the man holds economic sway and refuses to use a condom. Often, if a woman within a stable union demands that her partner use a condom, she is accused of infidelity, physically abused, or even thrown out of the house.[27,28,29]

Global AIDS Prevention: Not as Easy as ABC

Three and a half decades into the AIDS epidemic, prevention programs remain doggedly focused on information, education, and communication about behaviors that put people at risk for HIV, a sexually transmitted disease, ignoring issues of structural violence. AIDS can be prevented, it is reasoned, through behavior change. The answer is often simply stated as prevention and treatment. HIV prevention can be viewed as two interrelated entities: risk avoidance such as abstaining from sex and drug use; and harm reduction that is minimizing risk while conducting behaviors that are associated with HIV risk. This specifically refers to the use of clean injecting needles for drug users and the use of condoms if one is having sex. Prevention is often presented as "lifestyle choices," within the control of the individual. Yet those who live in poverty and lack basic necessities have severely constrained lifestyle choices.

In the last 5 years there has been even a further minimization of prevention strategies into the formulaic *ABCs* (maintaining *A*bstinence, *B*eing faithful to one partner, and using *C*ondoms). This simplistic strategy (the ABCs of HIV prevention) has garnered attention from religious groups and the right wing lead American government responsible for the large majority of AIDS funding. Each of these simple letters entails a choice that many women do not have the power to make. Abstinence relies on the ability to say "no" and have it be heard. Such personal agency is severely constrained by violence of both the structural and physical varieties. Gender inequality through laws or practices from unequal access to education,

housing, paying work, or inheritance continue to place more women than men into destitution. Infidelity more commonly stems from the male partner and is worsened by a shortage of wage-earning jobs available. In such a state, women are more likely to be victimized by rape or forced to use sex as a tradable commodity for survival. Trumpeting calls for abstinence and fidelity without addressing the economic roots of the commoditization of women's bodies is a cynical dismissal of the lives of the most vulnerable in the epidemic. Such an approach fails to take on the fact that violence and brutality, rather than love, trust, or sexual activity, are the forces that most put women at risk for AIDS, death, and unplanned pregnancy.

Even education itself has been associated with risk. In its Fact Sheet on Gender and AIDS, UNAIDS reported:

> Available data show that one in 200 South African women aged 15–49 has been raped by a school teacher before the age of 15. Of the schoolgirls covered by the South African Medical Council survey in 2000, half reported being forced to have sex against their will, one third of them by their teachers. In Zimbabwe, research points to widespread abuse of girls in coeducational schools taking the form of aggressive sexual behavior, intimidation, and physical assault by older boys.[30]

Obviously, these risks do not diminish the critical importance of the education of girls but rather highlight the need for mitigating girls' vulnerability in all sectors through rights-based approaches. Education should focus upon gender equity in access to education, in intramural relationships, and in the pedagogical processes. Lack of access to education presents special vulnerabilities because school is not, in most countries, free nor considered a basic right, families struggle to provide school fees. Such vulnerability is even worse for orphans who are last in the familial line for such resources. For many children, the desire to attend school leads to a Faustian deal of exchanging sex for school fees. Additionally, children's voices are rarely heard in education; creating a culture of silence in the context of HIV can be deadly. Unburdening children from fee-based and patriarchal education structures and replacing them with

The Pandemic Today: A Map of Structural Violence Against Poor Women

Today, many of the world's most populous nations are increasingly affected by AIDS. China has registered more than one million cases of HIV since its first case was diagnosed in 1985 and the scale of the HIV/AIDS problem was publicly acknowledged in 2002. Initial reports focused on infected blood products as the main factor in this country's epidemic, as economic necessity had led to the development of the well-publicized blood trade, where people sold blood for cash income. However, it is now recognized that profound rural poverty in areas bypassed by China's economic boom drove large scale migration for work, causing behavior changes such as increased prostitution and drug use.[31,32,33]

In India, 2.5 million people are infected with HIV. Although the overall prevalence of HIV in the population is still fairly low, the epidemic is clearly generalized beyond typical high-risk groups. Given the weak public health infrastructure, women's low societal status, and the extreme poverty of much of the population, it is unlikely that the rising tide of the epidemic will abate. South Africa currently has the highest number of HIV infections in the world, and while overall prevalence may be leveling off, many areas remain heavily burdened.[34]

In the 1990s, the fastest growing epidemic in the world was in Russia and the other countries of the former Soviet Union. In these countries, the collapse of social safety nets resulted in widespread joblessness and a lack of basic means. Intravenous drug use, commercial sex work, and incarceration skyrocketed, making the countries a fertile ground for HIV transmission.[35,36,37] As the economic situation has improved, the rate of acquisition of HIV has slowed. But the consequences of this period remain among the poor and marginalized. While sex trafficking of women and girls from Eastern to Western Europe along the typical lines of economic inequality has been widely reported, little has been done to provide real economic opportunities for these women in either their home countries or the countries in which they arrive through the sex trade. Harm reduction programs targeted at intravenous drug users are often not accessible to women.[38]

Lastly, there is sub-Saharan Africa. Though most needy in every way with respect to AIDS and the factors that foment its spread, Africans remain last in receiving the benefits of our achievements in the struggle against AIDS. In 2002, over 30 million Africans are living with HIV; fewer than 10% have access to voluntary testing and counseling, and only about 300,000 were on treatment. Large international funding sources—most notable the Global Fund to Fight AIDS, TB and Malaria (GFATM) and the U.S. government's President's Emergency Plan for AIDS Relief (PEPFAR) finally began to address the unmet need for treatment in 2002 and 2003 respectively.[39,40] Yet even with new paradigms in funding of prevention and treatment of AIDS, structural violence continues to fuel the epidemic, the countries of southern Africa in particular, have the highest HIV prevalence in the world. This is hardly surprising, given the legacy of the carefully crafted structural violence of Apartheid. As recounted in Alan Paton's 1948 novel, *Cry, the Beloved Country*, the question of whether African men should be allowed to buy land, build homes, or bring their families to the mining communities in which they work was one of the hotly debated topics of the original Apartheid legislation. Reading this classic novel now gives one a terrible sense of foreboding of the AIDS epidemic that was then still 45 years away. The country of South Africa reports an HIV prevalence of 15.6%. The three countries with the highest prevalence in the world—Botswana, Lesotho, and Swaziland[41]—are intimately tied with South Africa's mining economy. It is only by understanding history and acting to prevent the systemic disregard of social and economic rights throughout the world that the further disastrous consequences of structural violence can be avoided. A critical analysis of the world, evaluated from the point of view of the vulnerable, serves as a basic primer for those who wish to consider structural violence in its rightful context—a vector of the epidemic.

schools to which access is free, equitable, and in which rights are respected structurally and taught pedagogically would serve to decrease risk and empower girls.

Worsening Poverty and Gender

AIDS is making the world's poorest countries poorer, and women bear much of this burden. One only needs to look at the salient economic indicators of family income, food, security, education, and health care to see the impact of AIDS in sub-Saharan Africa. In Zambia, two-thirds of families who lose the head of the household experience an 80% drop in monthly income. In the Ivory Coast, families who lose an adult to HIV experience a 50% decrease in household income. Agricultural productivity in Burkina Faso has fallen by 20% because of AIDS. In Ethiopia, HIV-positive farmers spend between 11.6 and 16.4 hours per week farming compared with 33.6 hours weekly for healthy farmers.[42] In 2007 and 2008 an increased attention to food security was fueled by riots in Haiti and elsewhere.[43] While rising fuel costs and odious trade and aid policies clearly contribute to the critical nature of food insecurity, the reality is much harsher than a short-term crisis. The interrelationship of HIV and food security is bidirectional. AIDS has reduced production, but also hunger and food insecurity is a well-documented risk for infection, particularly among women. A study from Swaziland and Botswana showed that food insufficiency was associated with inconsistent condom use with a nonprimary partner, exchange of sex for food or money, intergenerational sexual relationships, and lack of control in sexual relationships.[44]

As more adults perish, not only is food security compromised but so too is the education of children. The International Labor Organization estimated that in sub-Saharan Africa, 200,000 teachers will die from AIDS by 2010. In Swaziland, school enrollment fell by 36%, mainly because girls left school to care for sick relatives. In addition to women's work contributing to the economic survival of most poor families, women's central role of care provider has expanded to caring for sick relatives and taking in orphans. For many young girls, this means terminating school early, which diminishes their livelihood options and increases vulnerability. Work from Haiti has documented that income inequality within a couple is both a risk factor for forced sex and other HIV risk factors.[45]

Treatment Access and Gender

Today, the biennial International AIDS Conference generates significant animus in the scientific community.[46] Researchers from Europe and North America often choose to avoid the event entirely, as it is a meeting that not only addresses the scientific but also the social aspects of HIV/AIDS. The social voices are loud; they are angry, and they are dissatisfied with the slow progress of the rights-based agenda. Outside the conference center, demonstrators march daily with banners protesting the lack of access to medicine, clean needles, and basic rights associated with both preventing and treating HIV. The protests are directed at the forces that perpetrate injustice and also serve as a way to marshal a global constituency of people who care not only about AIDS but also about poverty, debt, and human rights. Gender and economic disparity continue to play a role not only in risk, as discussed previously in this chapter, but in access to testing, care, and treatment. Several studies have shown that women, particularly rural married women, are less likely to know their HIV status.[47] While women are accessing HIV services, and in some studies more likely to return for their results, fear of domestic violence and stigma continues to constrain women's choices not only for testing but disclosure of their status.[48]

However, perhaps due in some part to the awareness raised by such activism, women do seem to be well represented in HIV treatment cohorts in resource-limited settings.[49] In the large Anti-Retroviral Therapy in Lower Income Countries (ART-LINC) cohort, among 33,164 individuals followed, 19,989 (60.3%) were women. The women in this cohort were, in general, younger than the men and less likely to have advanced HIV infection. Several other groups have documented this trend as well.[50] Equal or even overrepresentation of women in HIV treatment globally is likely caused by several factors. First, women tend to access health services more frequently than do men particularly for prenatal care, family planning, and to accompany their children. This is true in both rich and poor settings. Additionally, with respect to AIDS, the public health focus on prevention of maternal-to-child transmission of HIV predated the scale-up of ART, and many relatively healthy women are diagnosed due to antenatal screening. Yet, even with these relatively positive statistics of treatment access, global scale-up remains slower than needed with HIV testing and treatment available to fewer than 10% of pregnant women in sub-Saharan Africa.

HIV Treatment Scale-Up: Lessons from the Field

In Haiti, where the organization Partners In Health (PIH) and its local partner Zanmi Lasante have worked for over 2 decades, 1994 saw the democratically elected government of President Jean Bertrand Aristide reinstalled after a coup in 1991, with the assistance of the international community. Since that time, Haiti has been one of the few countries to control its AIDS epidemic, even in the face of crushing poverty. Much of this was accomplished through open and extensive prevention programs—targeted towards women, youth, and other vulnerable groups—broadcasted on the radio and in the press. Haiti was also one of the first countries to receive a grant from Global Fund to Fight AIDS, Tuberculosis, and Malaria, in no small part due to its successes in AIDS prevention and high-level political will. Led by the first lady, Mrs. Mildred Aristide, a vocal advocate for the rights of poor women, Haiti's Country Coordinating Mechanism—made up of members of the governmental, educational, religious, commercial, and NGO sectors—served as a model for the world in its ability to coordinate AIDS programs across all sectors so that the new sources of aid would reach the greatest number of people affected by HIV.

Partners In Health has been providing ART to patients with advanced AIDS since 1998 through a program called the HIV Equity Initiative. A decade of experience with a successful community-based tuberculosis program, and the fact that the AIDS and tuberculosis epidemics substantially overlapped, led our Haiti team to decide in 1998 to deliver AIDS care via the same model that we previously used to treat tuberculosis. Community health workers "accompany" their patients through regimens of antiretroviral therapy visiting daily to provide social support, assess secondary effects, and serve as patient advocates at the clinic. Critical to the success of this program is gender equity at its root.[51] The program relies heavily on community health workers, rather than physicians or nurses, to provide the bulk of care—more than half of these are women, and more than half of the patients followed are women, resulting in not only treatment equity but also economic opportunity for the women who bear the enormous burden of this epidemic. Today, the project follows 9000 people living with HIV across two states in Haiti, of whom nearly 3500 are receiving ART. Importantly, with the advent of funding through the Global Fund to Fight AIDS, TB and Malaria, the Partners in Health and Zanmi Lasante team has chosen to work with understaffed and underfunded public clinics as the site for provision of services in the belief that a vital public sector is key to the rights-based framework[52] and that HIV must be delivered within the context of comprehensive primary health care.[53] Rather than drawing resources away from primary health care, using the increased staffing, money for essential drugs (not only ART), training, and infrastructure can have salutary effects on the provision of primary visits, the integration of voluntary testing and counseling with general care, TB case finding, and women's health.

Partners In Health, working together with the Ministry of Health and the Clinton Foundation has replicated this model of using the attention and funding for HIV to integrate HIV services with comprehensive primary care in twelve public facilities in three districts of Rwanda (as of 2008). The key to this program in Rwanda as in Haiti is the employment, training and supervision of community health workers (CHWs) who extend the reach of the clinic in health promotion and disease prevention. CHWs in the (MoH) Minstry of Health /Partners in Health and Inshuti Mu Buzima model not only follow the 2893 people on ARVs (1865 women, 1028 men) (as of 2008) but also deliver more comprehensive primary care, addressing such health and social needs as women, maternal and reproductive health, and family planning, as well as childhood illnesses and socioeconomic needs. At household level, CHWs, informal alliances with household members and informal collaboration with professional healthcare providers are integrated agents of community development and members of larger clinical teams. This alignment between social needs and community and institutional support harnesses partnerships and genuinely engages the community in their own development. This formal endorsement of the community participating in their own development not only allows the community to realize their own agency but simultaneously addresses gender inequality. With over 63% of CHWs being female in one sector in Rwanda, women's societal status is elevated by this important position, women are less financially dependent on their partners as the positions are paid, and through monthly training where their skills are improved and they are able to network with others. In Haiti PIH has seen that the model of HIV and comprehensive primary health care can result in improved health outcomes but has the additional benefit of community development and women's empowerment. This has been successfully replicated in Rwanda since 2005 and is underway in Lesotho, Malawi and Burundi.

Conclusion

The AIDS pandemic, now in its third decade, has taken a major toll on human life and development. No group, however, has born a larger burden than poor women from sub-Saharan Africa. A lack of basic human rights—including the right to education, work, health care, property rights, and gender equity underscore women's vulnerability to infection much more so than individual behavior choice. For prevention programs to be credible they must address women's social and economic rights and provide novel ways to respect, protect, and fulfill these rights. Since governments are the entities held accountable for rights, public-sector approaches provide the best avenue to fulfill a rights-based agenda for HIV prevention and treatment. However, governments of poor countries cannot meet the needs of their population in the pandemic without significant help from the international community. The 2001 call from the United Nation's General Assemble Special Session on AIDS, which created the Global Fund to Fight AIDS, TB and Malaria, was a unique and significant multilateral response in which wealthy nations responded to the needs of not only the poor, but also to the needs of their governments.

The scale-up of antiretroviral therapy has had a surprisingly equitable effect on gender balance given what is known about women's vulnerability. It is likely that young women's utilization of the health services explains most of the trend, but this opportunity should be seized to find more women living with HIV and engage them in work within HIV programs and thus empower other women at the community level. Gender balance in the work force in general and the health work force more specifically could serve to mitigate some of the disproportionate burden that HIV places on women in resource-poor settings.

DISCUSSION QUESTIONS

1. Are there examples of strategies (national and local) that reduce gender disparities in work, school, and homes?
2. How can HIV prevention be made more relevant and within the control of women?
3. How do social and economic rights overlap with women's rights?

4. Is it possible to identify structural interventions (e.g., job creation or changes in the legal system so that widows inherit land) that reduce HIV transmission risks and then to rank them in order of importance and impact?

5. What unexamined models underpin the notion that risk will be reduced, in certain societies, by focusing on the cognitive considerate?

REFERENCES

1. Rubinstein A, Sicklick M, Gupta A, et al. A new syndrome of acquired immunodeficiency with reversed T4/T8 ratios in infants born to promiscuous and drug-addicted mothers. *JAMA.* 1983;249(17):2350-2356.

2. Booth KM. National Mother, Global Whore, and Transnational Femocrats: The Politics of AIDS and the Construction of Women at the World Health Organization. *Feminist Studies.* 1998;24(1):115-139.

3. Mann J, Tarantola D. Responding to HIV/AIDS: A historical perspective. Part I: The roots of vulnerability. *Health Human Rights.* 1998;2(4):5-8.

4. Famer P. On suffering and structural violence: a view from below. *Daedalus.* 1996; 125(1):261-283.

5. Joint United Nations Program on HIV/AIDS, World Health Organization. *AIDS Epidemic Update: December 2007.* Geneva, Switzerland: World Health Organization; 2007.

6. Galtung J. Violence, peace, and peace research. *J Peace Res.* 1969;6(3):167-191.

7. International Labor Organization. *Facts on Women at Work.* Geneva, Switzerland: International Labor Organization; 2004:1. http://www.ilo.org/public/english /bureau/inf/download/women/pdf/factssheet.pdf. Accessed March 20, 2008.

8. Kawachi I, Kennedy BP. Health and social cohesion: why care about income inequality? *Brit Med J.* 1997;314:1037.

9. Donovan P. Rape and HIV/AIDS in Rwanda. *Lancet.* 2002;360(S1):S17-S18.

10. Amnesty International. Rwanda: "Marked for death," rape survivors living with HIV/AIDS in Rwanda. http://www.amnesty.org/en/library/info/AFR47/007 /2004. Accessed March 20, 2008.

11. Human Rights Watch. *Struggling to Survive: Barriers to Justice for Rape Victims in Rwanda.* New York, NY: Human Rights Watch; 2004:7.

12. United Nations Security Council Resolution 1325 on Women, Peace, And Security. http://www.avega.org.rw. Accessed March 20, 2008.

13. Amnesty International. *Sierra Leone. Rape and Other Forms of Sexual Violence Against Girls and Women.* London, UK: Amnesty International; 2000:2.

14. Kolbe AR, Hutson RA. Human rights abuse and other criminal violations in Port-au-Prince, Haiti: a random survey of households. *Lancet.* 2006;368(9538):864-873.

15. Westerhaus MA, Finnegan AC, Zabulon Y, Mukherjee JS. Framing HIV prevention discourse to encompass the complexities of war in northern Uganda. *Am J Public Health.* 2007;97(7):1184-1186.

16. General Accounting Office. UN faces challenges in responding to the impact of HIV/AIDS on peacekeeping operations. Washington, DC: General Accounting Office; 2001:11.

17. UN peacekeepers in Haiti. *Lancet.* 2006;368(9538):816.

18. International Labor Rights Fund. *Violence Against Women in the Workplace in Kenya: Assessment of Workplace Sexual Harassment in the Commercial Agriculture and Textile Manufacturing Sectors in Kenya.* Washington, DC: International Labor Rights Fund; 2002:3.

19. Joint United Nations Program on HIV/AIDS, World Health Organization. *AIDS Epidemic Update: December 2004.* Geneva: World Health Organization; 2004:7-12.

20. Glynn JR, Carael M, Auvert B, et al. Why do young women have a much higher prevalence of HIV than young men? A study in Kisumu, Kenya and Ndola, Zambia. *AIDS.* 2001;(suppl 4):S51-S60.

21. Kelly RJ, Gray RH, Sewankambo NK, et al. Age differences in sexual partners and risk of HIV-1 infection in rural Uganda. *J Acquired Immune Deficiency Syndrome.* 2003;32:446-451.

22. Crossette B. UN fields odd allies as it wages AIDS battle. *New York Times.* December 3,1995:A4.

23. Hanenberg R, Rojanapithayakorn W. Prevention as policy: how Thailand reduced STD and HIV transmission. *Aidscaptions.* 1996;3(1):24-27.

24. Anti-AIDS program to be expanded throughout Cambodia. *AIDS Weekly Plus.* 1999;March:10.

25. Cohen J. Sonagachi sex workers stymie HIV. *Science.* 2004;304(5670):23.

26. Cohen J. Two hard-hit countries offer rare success stories: Thailand and Cambodia. *Science.* 2003;301(5640):1658-1662.

27. Piot, P. HIV/AIDS and violence against women. Presented at: United Nations Commission on the Status of Women, Panel on Women and Health, 43rd Session; March 3, 1999; New York, NY. http://www.thebody.com/content/art690 .html. Accessed March 20, 2008.

28. De Zoysa I, Sweat MD, Denison JA. Faithful but fearful: reducing HIV transmission in stable relationships. *AIDS.* 1996;10(A):S197-S203.

29. Van Der Straten A, King R, Grinstead O, et al. Couple communication, sexual coercion and HIV risk in Kigali, Rwanda. *AIDS.* 1995;(9):935-944.

30. UNAIDS Inter-Agency Task Team on Gender and HIV/AIDS. Resource pack on gender and HIV/AIDS, 2006. Geneva, Switzerland: UNAIDS. http://www.unfpa .org/hiv/docs/rp/factsheets.pdf. Accessed June 20, 2008.

31. World Health Organization. *HIV/AIDS in Asia and the Pacific Region: 2003.* Geneva, Switzerland: World Health Organization; 2003.

32. Thompson D. China's growing AIDS epidemic increasingly affects women. Washington, DC: Population Reference Bureau; 2004. http://www.prb.org/Articles/2004/ChinasGrowingAIDSEpidemicIncreasinglyAffectsWomen.aspx. Accessed March 20, 2008.

33. Volkow P, Del Rio C. Paid donation and plasma trade: unrecognized forces that drive the AIDS epidemic in developing countries. *Inter J STD AIDS.* 2005;16(1):5-8.

34. Joint United Nations Program on HIV/AIDS, World Health Organization. *AIDS Epidemic Update: December 2007.* Geneva, Switzerland: World Health Organization; 2007.

35. Joint United Nations Program on HIV/AIDS, World Health Organization. *AIDS Epidemic Update.* Geneva, Switzerland: World Health Organization; 2003.

36. Drobniewski F, Atun R, Fedorin I, et al. The "bear trap": the colliding epidemics of tuberculosis and HIV in Russia. *Inter J STD AIDS.* 2004;15:641-646.

37. Kelly J, Amirkhanian Y. The newest epidemic: a review of HIV/AIDS in Central and Eastern Europe. *Inter J STD AIDS.* 2003;14(6):361-371.

38. Pinkham S, Malinowska-Sempruch K. Women, harm reduction and HIV. *Reprod Health Matters*. 2008;16(31):168-181.

39. Joint United Nations Program on HIV/AIDS, World Health Organization. *Joint Fact Sheet*. Geneva, Switzerland: World Health Organization; 2005.

40. UNAIDS/WHO/United States Government. Consultative meeting on HIV testing and counseling in the Africa region. November 15-17, 2004. Johannesburg, South Africa. http://data.unaids.org/UNA-docs/consultativemeeting-hivtesting_17nov04_en.pdf. Accessed March 20, 2008.

41. Joint United Nations Program on HIV/AIDS, World Health Organization. *AIDS Epidemic Update: December 2007*. Geneva, Switzerland: World Health Organization; 2007.

42. Food and Agricultural Organization (FAO). *The Impact of HIV/AIDS on Food Security*. Rome, Italy: FAO. http://www.fao.org/docrep/meeting/003/Y0310E.htm. Accessed June 20, 2008.

43. Mukherjee JS, Barry DJ. Feeding Haiti. *Boston Globe*. May 5, 2008. http://www.boston.com/bostonglobe/editorial_opinion/oped/articles/2008/05/05/feeding_haiti/. Accessed June 20, 2008.

44. Weiser SD, Leiter K, Bangsberg DR, et al. Food insufficiency is associated with high risk sexual behavior among women in Botswana and Swaziland. *PLoS Med*. 2007;4(10):e260-e270.

45. Smith Fawzi MC, Lambert W, Singler JM, et al. Factors associated with forced sex among women accessing health services in rural Haiti: implications for the prevention of HIV infection and other sexually transmitted diseases. *Soc Sci Med*. 2005;60(4):679-689.

46. Wells WA. Full of sound and fury, but signifying something: XVI International AIDS Conference. August 13-18, 2006. Toronto, Canada. *J Exp Med*. 2006; 203(11):2394-2403.

47. Wringe A, Isingo R, Urassa M, et al. Uptake of HIV voluntary counseling and testing services in rural Tanzania: implications for effective HIV prevention and equitable access to treatment. 2008. *Trop Med Inter Health*. 2008;13(3):319-327.

48. Weiser SD, Heisler M, Leiter K, et al. Routine HIV testing in Botswana: a population-based study on attitudes, practices, and human rights concerns. *PLoS Med*. 2006;3(7):e261-e270.

49. Braitstein P, Boulle A, Nash D, et al. Antiretroviral therapy in lower income countries (ART-LINC) study group. Gender and the use of antiretroviral treatment in resource-constrained settings: findings from a multicenter collaboration. *J Womens Health*. 2008;17(1):47-55.

50. Muula AS, Ngulube TJ, Siziya S, et al. Gender distribution of adult patients on highly active antiretroviral therapy (HAART) in Southern Africa: a systematic review. *BMC Public Health*. 2007;7:63-71.

51. Mukherjee JS, Eustache E. Community health workers as a cornerstone for integrating HIV and primary healthcare. *AIDS Care*. 2007;19(suppl 1):S73-S82.

52. Mukherjee J. Basing treatment on rights rather than ability to pay: 3 by 5. *Lancet*. 2004;363(9414):1071-1072.

53. Walton DA, Farmer PE, Lambert W, Léandre F, Koenig SP, Mukherjee JS. Integrated HIV prevention and care strengthens primary health care: lessons from rural Haiti. *J Public Health Policy*. 2004;25(2):137-158.

Tuesday Clinic, 10:30 a.m.—Susan

Susan sat down in the chair next to me and started crying. She didn't say anything for a long time, and for a few minutes, I just listened to her hushed sobs with my hand on her knee. "I just can't take it anymore. It's too much." Susan had just come from the vascular surgeon who had told her that her dialysis fistula needed yet another revision. This would be her third surgery in the past 6 months. Her kidneys had failed a few years ago, likely due to the combination of HIV, remote heroin use, and many years of poorly controlled diabetes and hypertension. Susan was only 36 years old. She had already had a stroke, a below-the-knee amputation, and a heart attack. I had planned on talking to her about her latest HIV tests. They showed a declining CD4 count (now 4 cells/microliter) and an HIV viral load of 32,000 copies/ml.* Both of these numbers suggested that she was having trouble taking her antiretroviral therapy (ART), despite a new once-daily regimen that I had prescribed to target her resistant HIV virus. But, I didn't mention the numbers. Clearly, she didn't need to hear this news now. What could I do to stop what I knew was inevitable? I was watching, seemingly helplessly, the imminent untimely death of yet another young black woman in one of the world's most well-resourced countries.

HIV/AIDS Statistics Among U.S. Women

In the United States, particularly in the northeast and in the South, Susan's story is all too familiar.

---

* The CD4 count is a marker of immune system strength. A normal CD4 count is between 600-1500 cells/μl. A CD4 count <200 cells/μl means a patient has AIDS and is at significantly higher risk of opportunistic illness and death. The HIV viral load is a marker of HIV activity in the body: the higher the viral load, the more potential damage to the immune system. ART reduces viral replication, drops the viral load (goal: undetectable), and allows the CD4 count to rebuild.

CHAPTER 12

Poor, Black, and Female: The Growing Face of AIDS in the United States

Heidi Behforouz MD,
Jennifer Chung

Heidi Behforouz, MD, is the Medical and Executive Director of the PACT Project as well as an Assistant Professor in Harvard Medical School and Associate Physician at Brigham and Women's Hospital, Boston, MA.

Jennifer Chung is a Project coordinator for the PACT Project, Boston, MA.

At the beginning of the US HIV epidemic in the early 1980s, women accounted for only 8% of AIDS cases. Today, women comprise almost 30% of the 1.2 million people with HIV/AIDS.[1,2] HIV-positive women in America are predominately poor and nonwhite. Sixty-four percent of women with HIV have annual incomes less than $10,000. Eighty-two percent of women with AIDS in the United States are African-American (66%) or Latina (16%), while only 25% of women in the general population are African-American (12%) or Latina (13%).[1,3] The AIDS case rate among African-American women is 21 times higher than for white women.[1] These poor, minority HIV-positive women are also young: 71% of women with AIDS are between the ages of 25 and 44, with girls aged 13–19 representing 43% of women with AIDS.[4,5]

Overall HIV/AIDS Trends in the United States: Who, How, Where?

Prior to the 1990s, the AIDS epidemic in the United States affected predominantly urban, white, men who had sex with men. Among the small minority of HIV-infected women, most had contracted their disease through injection drug use.[6,7] Over the past two decades, the demographic of those affected by the epidemic has changed; there are approximately 40,000 new cases of HIV infections every year, a number that has not declined in over 10 years, and the disease burden has shifted to disproportionately affect people of color, and has been steadily increasing in women and rural communities.[7(p1075),8-10] The main mode of HIV transmission among men remains sex with men, whereas women are predominantly contracting the disease from heterosexual contact with infected partners. In 2005, 49% of the newly diagnosed HIV/AIDS cases occurred in blacks as opposed to 31% in whites and 18% in Latinos.[1] These statistics show that the populations within which HIV transmission has achieved its highest incidence have experienced shifts across gender, sexual orientation, and racial and ethnic classifications, a phenomenon that requires closer examination and adjustments in the ways we approach treatment and prevention strategies.

Why Are Women, Especially Black Women, Contracting HIV at Higher Rates?

The rate of new infections in the United States has grown faster among women than among men: between 2000 and 2004, women experienced an increase in AIDS cases of 9.9% as compared to an increase of 7.1% in men.[11] Among the factors that heighten a woman's risk of contracting HIV/AIDS is increased biological susceptibility to infection. At a minimum, women are eight times more likely to contract HIV as a result of a single act of inter-

Susan's Story

Susan was born in Roxbury, Massachusetts, a Boston neighborhood with high rates of poverty, substance use, and crime. Four generations ago, her family had moved north from Virginia to make a better life for themselves. They worked in the Longwood Medical Area as hospital housekeepers and kitchen cooks. When Susan was only four, her father was stabbed in an alley behind her house and killed. Her mother, raising four children on her own, worked two jobs to keep the household solvent. She was seldom home. Susan "got in with some bad people" and dropped out of school in the eighth grade. At age 13, she started smoking weed and drinking alcohol and met her 23-year old boyfriend, Anderson. He bought her clothes and CDs and took her dancing. They had unprotected sex. Her mother had told her about condoms, but Anderson did not like using them. When Susan learned that Anderson was secretly hooked on heroin, she ignored it. On her 16th birthday, Anderson gave Susan her first hit of intravenous heroin. It was magical, and shortly thereafter, Susan was using as much as Anderson. She became pregnant, and at 5 months, Anderson started to hit her. Susan stayed with him until finances became tight, and decided to leave. It was around this time that her mother took her to her first prenatal appointment, and she was told she had HIV.

course with an infected man, compared to the likelihood of transmission from woman to man, due to women's anatomically receptive role in heterosexual intercourse. Additionally, the risk of contracting HIV and/or other STDs is increased during menstruation, by use of oral contraceptives, and by having an ectopic cervix.[12] Infection with other STDs can also increase the efficiency of HIV transmission. Women are also more likely to be asymptomatic with STDs, prolonging the period during which they are at higher risk for contracting HIV/AIDS.[12-15]

In addition to the unequal risks of HIV infection that women face from each unprotected sexual encounter, economic, cultural, and social factors may hinder a woman's ability to sufficiently protect herself. Consistent condom use during sexual intercourse is widely accepted as a highly effective practice in reducing HIV transmission. With such high prevalence of HIV in their neighborhoods, why are women not practicing safer sex? The statistics are telling. Women at highest risk for contracting HIV are black, young, and poor, factors that affect a woman's ability to protect herself in multiple ways.

First and foremost, black women in the United States are among the most impoverished individuals in the country. According to the US government census published in 2006, 36.5 million people in the United States were living in poverty (i.e., household income less than $2,614/month for a family of four), with 24.3% of blacks living in poverty as compared to 20.6% of Hispanics, 10.3% of Asians, and 8.2% of non-Hispanic whites. Poverty rates were highest for families headed by single women, especially if they were black or Hispanic. Forty-three percent of black female-headed households (without a husband present) were living in poverty.[16] Almost 70% of black children were born into poor, female-headed households.[17,18]

Poverty is not solely restricted to financial impoverishment but also includes social poverty and marginalization. Black women, dating back to the era of slavery, have had the lowest paying wages for some of society's hardest and most menial work. They live in neighborhoods plagued by poor educational opportunities, joblessness, and drug use. They also live in neighborhoods with a high ratio of women to men, and a significant portion of the men circulate in and out of the prison system where the rate of HIV infection is estimated to be as much as 10 times higher than in the general population. "Black women are no more likely to have unprotected sex, have multiple sexual partners, or use drugs than women of other racial/ethnic groups . . . but they are more likely to have risky sex partners and STDs."[19] In other words, a young black woman in a neighborhood with a high HIV prevalence who has sex with only one man is at much higher risk of getting infected than a young woman who has sex with multiple men in an area with a low prevalence of HIV.

The story of Step County (name fabricated for purposes of anonymity), a county in North Carolina, is a cogent case study demonstrating how the historic factors of low economic opportunity and racial discrimination have created environments that propagate and increase the unequal risk of HIV infection for women of color. Trends in farmland aggregation that took place between 1950 and 1990 disproportionately affected poor black farmers, many of whom lost their land and their livelihoods.[20] The black community was further destabilized by discriminatory practices in federal loan approvals; a 1997 Civil Rights Action Team appointed by the government verified that the US Department of Agriculture withheld aid from black farmers.[21] The depressed economic situation facing the black community resulted in the migration of black men out of Step County as they searched for work elsewhere. Unbalanced male-to-female ratios have been associated with decreased marriage rates, a risk factor for HIV infection,[22] and social-economic networks, defined as "financial support from multiple male or female sex partners as a part of a personal economic strategy" and which include such high-risk behaviors as unprotected sex with several partners.[23] As demonstrated in Step County, when faced with limited opportunity, low-income residents of a community may rely on economic coping strategies that include relationships involving a sexual-economic exchange, government financial assistance, and sales of illegal drugs.[23(p1081)] It is clear that in battling the current HIV epidemic in America, we must confront the ramifications of past mistakes and strive to remedy them.

The black community's history of discrimination and resulting impoverishment may also contribute to current low levels of literacy. A particularly salient factor correlated to the disproportionately rapid spread of HIV within low-income, African-American populations is health literacy, which is defined as "the literacy proficiency needed to properly understand and act on health information."[24] One study investigating the associations between medication adherence of HIV-positive individuals, race, and health literacy demonstrated that health literacy was a significant predictor of nonadherence to medication, whereas race was not. Comparisons of African-American patients to non-African-American patients showed a significantly higher prevalence of marginal or low health literacy skills in the African-American cohort, 52.1% as opposed to 14.3%, suggesting that health literacy may be one of the underlying factors driving the racial disparities in health outcomes among HIV/AIDS patients.[25]

Interventions to Reduce the Spread of HIV Among Vulnerable Women

Effective interventions to reduce the spread of HIV entail a multipronged approach to promote change on an individual level as well as on a structural level, which considers the historical, political, and socioeconomic context within which HIV risk behaviors occur. Current HIV prevention efforts among women focus heavily on increasing women's condom use, as condoms have proven to be a highly effective and relatively low cost means of preventing HIV as well as other STDs. A number of studies testing the efficacy of educational and skill-building interventions targeted at high-risk groups—black and Latino women—reported promising results. Effective interventions were based in social psychological theory and included gender-specific curricula with an emphasis on gender-related influences. These interventions involved peer leaders, culturally competent and sensitive educators, and interactive skill-building exercises.[7(p545),26-28] The various interventions with these characteristics that were successful in significantly changing self-reported high-risk behaviors as well as in reducing the incidence of STDs were tested in a number of different settings and varied in duration from 20 to 250 minutes.

A behavioral change approach, however, concentrates the burden of prevention at the individual level, neglecting to address the potential for enacting effective prevention methods through structural changes. Given the links between poverty, gender inequality and HIV risk, the most effective structural interventions would include equal education and employment opportunities regardless of race or gender, a societal commitment to reducing income inequality, and services and programs to empower women. However, effective structural interventions do not have to be complex. For example, the free distribution of condoms is a straightforward and effective way to reduce high-risk sex. When condoms were made available at no charge at 1000 small businesses across Louisiana, an average of 2000 condoms were dispensed per month at each site, totaling 200,381 condoms per month. When a nominal cost of up to $0.25 was charged for each condom, the number distributed plummeted to 22 per month, per site.[29]

A change in partner notification policy is another example of a structural intervention with a potentially big impact. Through partner notification, the sexual or needle-sharing partners of individuals diagnosed with HIV are identified and alerted to their potential risk. The immediate goal of partner notification is to have all people who have had high-risk contact with an HIV positive person undergo testing and practice safer sex. Partner notification can also aid health professionals in detecting high-risk sexual networks that may be major STD reservoirs.[30-39] Partner notification has not been heretofore adopted due to concerns about loss of patient confidentiality and discrimination as well as placing partners at risk of suicide or domestic violence.[40] However, these fears were more real when the diagnosis of HIV was equal to a death sentence. Today, HIV is a treatable chronic disease. Policy makers are therefore beginning to reexamine the partner notification laws and, it is hoped, will enact a change that will protect more individuals from becoming infected.

Another policy change that would reduce HIV transmission is the lifting of the federal ban on needle exchange. Numerous studies, including four commissioned by the federal government, have shown that needle exchange dramatically reduces HIV transmission rates and does not increase dysfunctional drug use, increase number of drug users, or decrease the age of drug initiates. Despite these data, the federal ban remains.[41-44] Lifting this ban and making clean needles more widely accessible would prevent 10 new cases of HIV disease every day and save the government over hundreds of millions of dollars in avoidable healthcare costs.[45]

Disparate HIV/AIDS Mortality Rates Among Black Women

The disproportionately high rates of HIV/AIDS acquisition in the black population is especially worrisome in light of the fact that blacks have a higher likelihood of dying from the disease once infected. One analysis found that the unequal life expectancy of blacks and whites in the United States is largely attributable to HIV. Although antiretroviral therapy (ART) has been a boon for those who can access and afford treatment and has increased life expectancy to near normal, minority populations have not benefited to the same degree as whites.[46] Once infected with HIV, African-Americans more rapidly develop AIDS and survive for shorter periods of time.[8,47,48] Again, persons dying from HIV increasingly consist of African-Americans (>50%), women, and residents of the South.

Why Does She Die More Often and More Quickly?

As a physician providing care to HIV-positive individuals in inner city Boston, I am faced with troubling questions. How can I help Susan, a poor black woman with AIDS, take her medications? How can I help Elijah, a gay African-American man with HIV disease, stay sober enough to get to his doctor's appointments? How could I have prevented my patient's 14-year old hip-hop loving daughter, from turning seropositive? Although stunning advances have been made in HIV care, we are still faced with the reality that HIV incidence is not going down and that certain populations are experiencing inordinately high AIDS

mortality rates. In Roxbury, Massachusetts, for example, an African-American woman with HIV is 15 times more likely to die from AIDS than a white man in Boston.[49] We can explain these discrepancies in developing nations, but we are pressed to do so in the United States, where access to ART is relatively unlimited.

These questions can only be answered by asking a larger one. Assuming that, in this country, we do have the infrastructural and biomedical capacity to treat patients with HIV disease, what are the barriers to access to health care that preclude desirable outcomes for all? For the purposes of this chapter, I propose a broad definition of access to health care: the culmination of factors needed for a patient to establish and maintain an effective and meaningful relationship with a healthcare provider and achieve the best possible health outcome.

In reviewing the literature on access to health care, it is readily apparent that this is not a simple issue or one that we completely understand. There is a long list of factors that affects access, reviewed in Table 12-1.

It is important to note that patient-related and system-related factors are not truly separable and interact with each other to create diminished access to health care for vulnerable populations. It is not within the scope of this chapter to explore each of these factors in depth. I will choose to focus on the impact of race and ethnicity and depression and stress on differential outcomes, in addition to a brief overview of insurance coverage in the United States.

Insurance

Among the many factors that limit one's ability to have an effective relationship with a healthcare provider is lack of insurance, which has been shown to lead to worse outcomes (in this case, service utilization) among patients with HIV.[50] With at least 70% of HIV-infected individuals relying on public insurance schemes in order to receive care,[51,52] it is necessary to examine what services are actually being provided. The three largest government programs for HIV/AIDS care are Medicaid, Medicare, and Ryan White CARE, all of which limit access to their services through complicated eligibility requirements, spending caps, and waiting lists. For example, Medicare and Medicaid

TABLE 12-1

Factors Affecting Access to Health Care for HIV-Positive Patients	
Patient-Related Factors	**Health Care and Social System-Related Factors**
1. Gender	1. Societal factors:
2. Ethnicity	a. Income inequality
3. Culture	b. Resource inequality
4. Sexual preference	c. Racism, classism, sexism
5. Mental health	d. Stigma against those with HIV/AIDS
6. Household, livelihood, security	and/or substance users
7. Education	2. Healthcare policy:
8. Disease-specific knowledge and health literacy	a. Health insurance
9. Geographic location	b. Drug availability
10. Social support network	3. System infrastructure:
11. Logistics: transportation, childcare	a. Medical resource availability,
12. Substance abuse	responsiveness, and design
13. Domestic or other violence	b. Institutional racism, classism, sexism
14. Internalized stigma	c. Nonmedical resource availability and design
	4. Healthcare professionals:
	a. Physician experience or competence
	b. Physician discrimination

Source: Author created.

require that a person with HIV infection already be disabled before accessing these programs, even at a time when treatments offer the hope of delaying or preventing disability.[53] Though the president's fiscal year 2009 budget requests an increase of 3.6% from 2008 spending levels for domestic HIV/AIDS programs, the finalization of spending levels is still pending, and eligibility criteria will need to be adjusted if low-income HIV-positive patients are to be able to access needed care and medications in a timely manner.[54]

Race and Ethnicity

Numerous studies have been published describing the effect of various factors on healthcare access and healthcare outcomes. One of the factors of greatest concern is differential access to care or treatment based on a person's race or ethnicity. Some authors have posited that the patient's own cultural beliefs about HIV/AIDS and therapeutic preferences may partially account for the disparities. Some studies have suggested that minorities may have a greater mistrust of care providers,[55] a

greater sense of fatalism associated with the disease,[56] and a belief that the HIV epidemic is the white man's attempt to destroy the black race.[47] These perceptions may impact an individual's engagement with health care. These cultural beliefs, though very important in developing culturally relevant care strategies, cannot alone account for the vast racial disparities in access to care. Differences in knowledge of HIV/AIDS may be another significant factor.[57-59] More compelling, perhaps, are data suggesting that minorities are treated differently once engaged in the healthcare system. In recent years, research has revealed that minorities are much less likely than whites to receive many medical services including cardiac catheterization for coronary artery disease,[60-63] treatment for alcoholism,[64] referral to nephrologist for chronic renal failure,[65] renal transplantation,[66] and treatment for prostate, breast,[67] and colorectal cancer.[68]

Healthcare utilization analysis for HIV-infected persons similarly reflects racial disparities in access.[69-72] For example, African-Americans and Latinos are less likely to have a primary care physician and more likely to have preventable emergency room visits. Among a cohort of 571 HIV-infected individuals in Providence, Rhode Island, minorities were admitted 20% more often and had 35% more inpatient days per person-year but only 74% as many HIV clinic visits as white patients.[64] The authors postulated that much of these differences were related to differential access to and utilization of ART. According to multiple studies, minorities are less likely to receive ART or prophylaxis for opportunistic infections such as pneumocystis pneumonia, or PCP.[65,73-77] Whether or not these differential prescribing patterns are due to overt racial discrimination; subtle but unexplored beliefs about a person's ability to adhere to medication regimens based on socioeconomic factors, gender, and education level; poor patient-doctor communication due to the physician's cultural incompetence, or physician burnout is unclear.[78] Studies have documented that physicians have diminished communication with and negative perceptions of patients from lower socioeconomic status or lower educational levels.[66]

Depression

Major depressive disorder is two times more frequent in HIV-positive than HIV-negative adults.[79] Numerous studies have demonstrated an association between depression and higher rates of HIV morbidity and mortality.[80-83] Possible reasons why depression may be related to worse clinical outcomes include delay in ART initiation, prescription of less potent regimens, poor medication adherence, decreased utilization of the healthcare system, high-risk sexual behavior, and substance use.[84] Of all these correlating factors, poor adherence due to depression is commonly viewed as the most powerful. Across adherence studies and in most meta-analyses, depression is the factor that consistently and repeatedly shows a positive association with poor adherence. People with depression usually struggle with hopelessness, memory problems, erratic schedules, and lack

of self-interest; all traits that counteract successful ART adherence. In addition, poor health outcomes may result from lower immune function among depressed individuals. Depression is associated with lower CD4 counts and increased disease progression, independent of adherence.[85-88] Stress appears to have a similar effect on HIV outcomes. A recent study suggested that HIV-positive individuals who had suffered more psychosocial trauma in their lives were almost twice as likely as others to have HIV disease progression.[89] Another study also suggested that those HIV-positive patients with histories of lifetime trauma above the median were three times more likely to die than those with lower trauma scores.[90,91]

These findings may partly explain more rapid disease progression among African-Americans, particularly African-American women, as they contend with higher levels of stress and poorer mental health than their white counterparts.

Susan

During her last trimester, Susan kicked her heroin habit, moved out of her mother's house into a subsidized apartment, and received ART while pregnant with Zachary. He was born without HIV. Although Anderson visited infrequently and gave her money, Susan did not encourage him. She made do with the monthly TANF payment for a few years. She tried to get work, but was not able to afford child care with the salary of a middle school dropout. Her health started to deteriorate, and her diabetes was out of control, even though the doctor and nutritionist advised her to eat better, but prohibitively expensive, food. Life also seemed to get in the way of taking her medications. Zachary was getting into trouble at school, her mother moved to Brockton, and she was having trouble paying her bills. Now that Zachary was in school, Susan decided to take a GED class. At her class, she met Leon, who had just gotten out of jail and was living in a halfway house. After he moved into her apartment, life improved. Leon loved Zachary and Susan and provided day-old breads and pastries from the bakery where he worked and took them to the zoo or the park on his days off. A few months later, however, he was laid off, became depressed and began drinking again. And when he drank, he physically abused Susan. But Susan loved Leon, and did not want to be alone, and so forgave him his behavior. She had just had a stroke and wanted someone around should she become sicker. Leon knew about her diabetes but did not know she had HIV. Having unprotected sex worried Susan, but she was afraid to tell him for fear he would hit her or leave her if he found out.

"Women of lower social class standing are especially at risk for poor mental health outcomes. Having low educational attainment, low personal incomes, and less prestigious occupations is associated with a poor self-concept (self-esteem and self-efficacy). Women with low self-concepts, in turn, report poorer mental health."[92,93] African-American women are also more likely to report discrimination on the basis of their HIV, another factor that negatively contributes to their physical and mental health.[94-96]

In summary, black women are at the intersection of poor mental health, racism, and lifetime stress due to poverty, low self-esteem, internalized stigma, and lack of social mobility, all of which contribute to poorer health outcomes, despite access to and perhaps utilization of available health services and medical technology. Any intervention that aims to improve outcomes among HIV-positive women must acknowledge and address these factors in order to be successful.

Strategies to Equalize HIV/AIDS Health Outcomes

Most HIV health promotion interventions have focused on improving ART adherence. Most are based in cognitive-behavioral theory (CBT) and attempt to change patient behaviors and self-efficacy skills.[97] Although these interventions have demonstrated feasibility and short-term success in improving adherence, they have not yet been tested in large clinical effectiveness trials. Furthermore, they do not address all the factors that influence ART adherence, as described, for example, by Ickovics and Meisler.[98] A recent review of 21 adherence interventions revealed that most interventions increase patient knowledge, reduce patient barriers to compliance, improve self-efficacy, or develop reminder systems, but seldom do they focus on changing factors outside of the individual in a comprehensive or effective manner.[99] There are also concerns that many of the current cognitive-behavioral health promotion interventions that primarily focus on the individual's health risk behaviors do not successfully address the cultural, community, and institutional factors that influence adverse health outcomes.[100] These

other factors may be just as important in effecting long-term well-being. Evidence therefore suggests that interventions should combine strategies that address community and cultural structures with those that address individual change through cognitive-behavioral therapy methodologies. Wilson and Miller also emphasize the importance of creating interventions that address societal and culturally reinforced power dynamics such as illness stigmatization, racism, sexism, and heterosexism, all of which affect a group's ability to access resources or employ healthy behaviors. Few such integrated interventions exist or have been studied in a rigorous manner.[101]

The PACT Project

In response to the earlier stated feelings of hopelessness that I encountered while witnessing the preventable ravages of HIV on poor minority populations within this resource-rich setting, I mobilized a partnership of like-minded individuals to mount a multifaceted and aggressive campaign to address many of the complex social justice and healthcare issues heretofore discussed. The Prevention and Access to Care and Treatment (PACT) project was started in response to disproportionately high HIV morbidity and mortality rates in inner-city Boston. In 1997, the mayor's office released statistics demonstrating rising incidence rates of HIV among poor black women in the four low-income communities of Roxbury, Mattapan, Dorchester, and Hyde Park. These disparities existed despite the fact that these women had insurance, had access to ART, and lived within walking distance of some of the world's premier medical institutions affiliated with Harvard Medical School.

Concerned community members and clinicians established PACT, a community-based peer health promotion program, to build on the life experiences of marginalized HIV-positive individuals and forge an effective community-based response to AIDS disparities. Using community-based participatory research (CBPR) and borrowing from the *accompagnateur* model used successfully by Partners In Health in the central plateau of Haiti, in which trained community health workers (CHW) deliver home-based care, PACT staff created a unique and complementary disease management model that has been under continuous growth and refinement since its inception.

PACT staff recognize that engagement in health care and adherence to antiretroviral therapy (ART) are dynamic phenomena that are affected profoundly by changing patient attitudes, health status, life events, and environmental and sociocultural factors. Therefore, effective health promotion and adherence interventions must be customized and flexible to accommodate a variety of participant needs over time. With the goal of excellent long-term adherence and health outcomes, CHWs stabilize health and social crises; provide peer-to-peer coaching in disease self-management, adherence, and self-efficacy; and improve communication and shared decision making within patient–provider relationships. CHWs tailor services according to each patient's unique context and his or her preferences. These CHWs are ethnically and linguistically diverse and come from the communities served by the project, the Roxbury, Dorchester, and Mattapan neighborhoods of Boston's inner-city, in which HIV is increasingly concentrated among African-Americans, Puerto Ricans, and Haitians.

PACT patients are referred by their medical and social providers because of their clinical vulnerability and long histories of poor adherence. They are ART-experienced individuals who have lived with HIV disease for more than 10 years. They have had difficulty taking their medications as prescribed, and many have significant viral resistance. They come to PACT with low CD4 counts and nonsuppressed viral loads, often despite prescription of ART regimens to which their virus is susceptible. More than half of PACT participants are female, and almost all are people of color (64% black; 33% Latino). Most have attained no more than an eighth-grade education and most are unemployed. The majority of patients meet criteria for clinical depression with more than 70% reporting a history of trauma and abuse. More than 70% claim social isolation, and are not able to cite individuals on whom they can consistently rely for social support or practical assistance. More than 50% of patients have a history of substance use with 33% actively using (mostly crack, heroin, and alcohol), and 14% of participants are unstably housed or homeless.

Once referred to the program, each participant is assigned a CHW. CHWs are optimal change agents for the following reasons:

- They have an intimate understanding of the life circumstances of their patients.
- They have similar cultural and linguistic backgrounds.
- They approach the patient's disease in a holistic manner, taking into account the patient's experience of his or her illness from a personal, family, and community perspective.
- They provide an important bridge between the patient and the health and social service system by translating treatment recommendations into realistic options for the patient and maintaining communication with office-based providers.
- They provide services that will likely prove cost-effective; build solidarity, and promote positive normative values within the community.
- They promote growth and empowerment of communities from the inside out.

From the beginning, PACT has relied on CBPR to better understand the HIV illness experience of our participants as well as to foster community and provider involvement in achieving better HIV health outcomes. The key resources in this process are the unique and intimate relationships that develop between CHWs and participants. Most of the health promoter–participant contact occurs within the home and community, thus eliminating the artificial and strained environment of the provider's office. In addition, the health promoter and participant are involved in an egalitarian relationship. As a consequence, trust is quickly established and the relationships between the health promoter and participant are deep and fruitful. CHWs are granted access to all parts of participants' lives and explanatory models. They experience, on an almost daily basis, the operations and experiences of their clients, their families, and their social networks. These intimate and productive partnerships have allowed the CHWs great success in engaging participants who have otherwise failed more traditional case management approaches. In addition, these long-term, organic relationships make qualitative analyses easier and more valid, as the evaluation subjects are well known to the team. Their one-time commentaries and suggestions within an interview or focus group can be interpreted within a rich and multifaceted context, the fabric of which has been woven over time by the CHWs and other PACT personnel.

These relationships have enabled PACT staff to have a holistic and centered understanding of the reasons for disparate HIV morbidity and mortality rates among our community. These reasons include late HIV diagnosis, poor access to and utilization of existing resources (due to individual, community, healthcare system, and societal barriers), and poor adherence to medications. In the summer of 2001, a PACT CBPR team (consisting of 20 HIV-positive participants, the CHWs, medical students, an evaluation specialist, and the medical director) convened to discuss the creation of an intensive adherence intervention. Review of literature, review of CHW progress notes, and interviews of CHWs were performed. In addition, focus groups were held with participants and CHWs. These data were compiled and used to design the health promotion program.

Design and Methodology of PACT's Health Promotion Initiative

Based on the focus group data and knowledge gained from 5 years of experience in the underserved HIV community of Boston, we designed an intervention to overcome adherence barriers, provide participant support, and improve self-efficacy and ability to engage in fruitful patient–doctor relationships and cope with the structural and environmental barriers to good health and healthcare utilization. The following paragraphs describe the theoretical framework and details of the health promotion initiative.

Theoretical Basis for Health Promotion and DOT-Plus Programs: PACT's health promotion initiative is fundamentally based on Craig Ewart's Social Action Theory (SAT), which is a comprehensive behavior change model grounded in public health and psychological principles and incorporates the complex interactions between patients' physical environments, social interactions, internal cognition, motivation, self-efficacy, and health outcomes.[102] In addition to SAT's emphasis on the role of beliefs, expectations, goals, and problem solving on behavior change, SAT stands out from many other models because of its focus on the environmental context of the individual. PACT intervenes to improve adherence at all three levels of the model: contextual influences, self-change processes, and health actions. At the contextual level, PACT CHWs help patients find stable housing, employment, and education, as well as access to physical and mental health services to which the patients are entitled. To facilitate self-change processes, CHWs model medication adherence, educate patients on ART and side effects, assist patients in the development of individualized routines, and provide positive reinforcement of adherence. At the health action level, CHWs encourage harm reduction and provide patients with a supportive social network, critical to the success of the intervention.

CHWs also work closely with healthcare providers to ensure that they have a clear understanding of the context in which patients are experiencing their disease and translate healthcare recommendations into language that matches the health literacy, social reality, and capacity of the patient. They also model best practice communication styles for the provider and thereby improve the cultural competence and efficacy of the therapeutic alliance.

The Health Promotion Initiative: At intake, the CHW evaluates the patient's needs and characteristics, adherence strengths and barriers, environmental and social context, and social support network. The assessment is completed over a 4-week period. Based on the initial interviews, a personalized service plan is structured. The patient is encouraged to identify personal goals and is taught how to work toward each goal through small, manageable steps and identify short-term, midterm, and long-term objectives. Although referring providers might identify goals of undetectable viral load and improved CD4 count, patient goals are often much different and may include functional status (e.g., ability to go dancing again), appearance (e.g., ability to gain weight and fit into clothes again), or social standing (e.g., ability to visit family without fear of being "outed" by appearance or symptoms.) The CHW ties these goals in with those of the referring provider and helps the patient see how improved medication adherence can lead to their desired outcomes. Patients are encouraged to play an active part in accomplishing their goals: each service plan details action steps that will be taken by either the health promoter or the patient. Service plans and progress made along each objective are reviewed on a quarterly basis and adjusted as needed.

During the initial assessment, patients' support networks are explored. If family or friends are willing and able to participate in the care of the participant, they are recruited, trained, and supported in this role. If there are no available human resources, CHWs work with patients to restore or build them. CHWs also facilitate referrals to service agencies providing assistance with financial, housing, or legal issues. Although they do not provide case management services, CHWs promote good and regular communication between the patient and case manager, help the patient navigate the complex social system structure, and teach the patient how to advocate for him or herself in receiving services for which he or she is eligible. These activities are critical, as CHWs quickly discover that structural and system barriers commonly interfere with the patient's ability to practice health promotion and harm reduction.

The core of the health promotion intervention is the patient health promotion and harm reduction curriculum. This curriculum is composed of 20 modules that are delivered by the CHW two to three times per month over a 6–9 month period. The curriculum is informed by cognitive-behavioral therapy and motivational interviewing techniques. Modules build knowledge ("HIV 101," or "The Importance of Adherence") and skills ("Getting Your Prescriptions Filled" or "Communicating Effectively with Your Provider"). Modules also address social support ("Building Resources and Supports"), self-efficacy ("Embracing your HIV Disease and Taking Charge"), and harm reduction as it pertains to sex, drug use, and domestic violence. Modules are delivered by the CHW in the patient's home and require 1 hour for completion. Modules are designed for low health literacy and are primarily diagram based. Patients are given workbooks to keep track of progress (CD4/viral load charts), record new insights (diary of progress along meeting objectives) or record exercises (social support wheels), and share with their providers (previsit preparation sheets and postvisit summaries).

Another key health promoter intervention is patient "accompaniment" during which patients are accompanied to key medical and social provider appointments. Prior to each appointment, the patient is encouraged to complete a previsit preparation sheet. With the help of the health promoter, the patient identifies questions and issues he or she wishes to raise with the provider. During the visit, the health promoter advocates for the patient and shares insights with the provider about patient progress. After the visit, the patient, provider, and CHW complete a postvisit summary with goals for completion between then and the next visit. The CHW reviews the visit findings and goals with the patient after the visit and helps translate recommendations from the hypothetical into the context of the patient's life.

Adherence to medications and medical appointments is a special focus of the health promoter intervention. CHWs ask about adherence on a weekly basis and review pillboxes at least twice per month. Those patients who require more intensive adherence support are enrolled in the directly observed therapy (DOT) program, where in addition to receiving health promotion services from their health promoter CHW, they receive a daily visit (Monday through Friday) from an additional CHW (called a DOT specialist) who helps them take their medications. Approximately 30% of patients require entry into DOT between 3 and 6 months postenrollment in order to improve their adherence. On the other hand, 10% of PACT patients quickly respond to the standard weekly intervention and require only monthly visits in order to maintain their adherence to medications and outpatient appointments.

At any time, clients can cross between PACT's three tiers (monthly, weekly, and daily services) based on predetermined criteria. This three-tiered model is represented as seen in Figure 12-1.

Results to date have been promising. Most patients remain in the PACT program for 13 months with a 70% retention rate at 12 months. After 12 months of participation in the PACT health promotion and DOT programs, patients have an increase in median CD4 count from 145 cells/μl to 220 cells/μl (which is clinically significant as a CD4 count >200 cells/μl means patients no longer have AIDS and are at significantly reduced

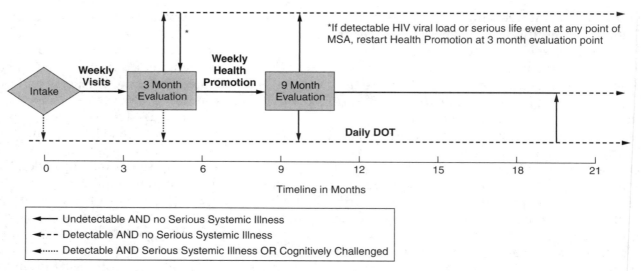

FIGURE 12-1   The PACT Model
Source: **Author created**

Susan

By the time Susan was referred to PACT, she was quite sick and depressed. She was on dialysis. She had had a below-the-knee amputation and a heart attack. Her CD4 count had dropped to 4 cells/μl and she weighed 84 pounds. Leon had left her. She didn't see the point in taking her meds on a regular basis, although she sometimes took them for Zachary. The pills made her tired and sick to her stomach. The diarrhea was awful. The pills did not seem to work well anyway: the doctor kept telling her that her numbers were no good. She stayed mostly to herself, as everyone talked about her. Leon had probably told everyone she had AIDS. She stopped going to church. Her mother saw her infrequently, and Zachary was out of control.

After Susan ended up in the hospital with pneumonia, a social worker referred her to PACT. She met Jeannette, a young Haitian woman her age, who told her she would be her health promoter. When she was discharged from the hospital, Jeannette helped her get home and cooked their dinner that night. She was positive and really seemed to care about Susan. Susan was suspicious at first, but she began to look forward to her weekly home visits. Jeannette helped her get to her appointments and helped her get insurance benefits and home meal delivery. She convinced Susan to accept DOT, and for a time, Susan had a daily visit from Sharon, her DOT specialist. Sharon helped her work through her nausea and taught her how to take Imodium for her diarrhea. Within 9 months, her viral load had dropped to undetectable, and her CD4 count was up to 120. She had gained almost 30 pounds and was stronger, though she continues to need support.

risk of opportunistic illness and hospitalization). Overall, patients experience a decrease in median viral load from 30,641 copies/ml to 421 copies/ml. Forty-eight percent of patients achieve a sustained undetectable viral load at 1 year. Participants have also shown a significant improvement in their healthcare utilization patterns. We analyzed the 2006 hospital billing records of 40 patients 1 year pre- and postenrollment in PACT. The analysis revealed a 35% decrease in inpatient days and a 50% decrease in hospitalization costs from an average cost of $22,443 per patient to $12,926 per patient. Additional analyses of data provided by Medicaid on overall medical costs demonstrated a 40% reduction in emergency room visits and hospitalizations among 19 patients enrolled in PACT for 24 months.

We believe that the PACT health promotion program is a cost-effective complementary model of health care. On average, PACT expends $5500 per patient per year. Yet with this expenditure, the medical costs of patients whose CD4 count increase from <50 cells/μl to >200 cells/μl (a common PACT outcome) can be reduced by close to $30,000 annually.[103]

Conclusion

As biomedical advances have defined a new standard of care and HIV-infected people are living longer, publicly funded HIV programs must rise to meet the challenge. More and more, the individuals suffering from HIV are members of historically disadvantaged groups who rely heavily on the public sector for financing their livelihood and care. Several scholars have argued that we have the resources to provide care for all HIV-infected individuals. However, it is the political will to restructure and refinance the healthcare system that is lacking.

I would further argue that the HIV epidemic is not strictly a public health crisis that can be addressed through a restructuring of the healthcare system. A quick glance through the CDC HIV/AIDS surveillance data will show that the HIV epidemic is most prominent among socially and economically excluded urban populations. Poor, undereducated, and sociopolitically unheard young men and women of color are experiencing the highest rates of infection and HIV/AIDS death. Young black women of the South, perhaps the poorest and most sociopolitically vulnerable group in the United States, are the newest population to make headlines in terms of HIV incidence and mortality. Contending with unemployment, poor housing conditions, inadequate education, poor social capital, gender inequality, and racism, they are the same people who fall through the cracks of a system that does not give universal coverage or provide the infrastructure needed to facilitate long-term, effective relationships with healthcare providers.

For these reasons, HIV is not only about public health, but is also about development. The political emphasis on expanding drug access or ensuring universal health coverage is important but ignores the basic problem. HIV is inextricably linked to poverty and marginalization. To address the HIV crisis at its most fundamental level, we must address the deeply rooted social and economic bases of poverty and prioritize the problems of the historically disenfranchised. The design and implementation of programs to strengthen and maintain capacity within these communities is critical. Even if some affluent and powerful people would argue against mobilization of resources on a pseudo-ethical basis, practically we have no choice. As is becoming apparent in other parts of the world, HIV topples economies, destroys generations of youthful workers, and quickly crosses class and race lines to become an omnipresent and formidable foe.

As the HIV epidemic in the United States changes—as women, injection drug users, people of color, and people of poverty increasingly bear the brunt of the disease—we are faced with a real crisis that must be met at both societal and individual levels. What can we do? At a minimum, we should support the notion that everyone should have health coverage and access to drug therapy. We should also accept that prejudices diminish access to health care for certain patients. With increasing humility, we are learning that we do treat our poor, female, black, mentally ill, or drug-using patients differently than their mainstream white male counterparts. Our challenge is to acknowledge and embrace the complexity of HIV and be leaders of developmental change, on personal, community, and societal platforms.

DISCUSSION QUESTIONS

1. What is the value of using race as a marker for health status? What are the potential problems of this approach?

2. How can a physician or healthcare worker address structural factors that increase the risk of HIV/AIDS infection, illness, or death?

3. How do you define *cultural competency*? What role might cultural competency play in mitigating risks for HIV infection and morbidity?

4. What are some ways in which the healthcare system can incentivize collaborations and more comprehensive disease management for complex HIV/AIDS patients?

5. Assuming that one believes that health is a human right, whose responsibility is it to ensure this right is enforced? What are the roles and duties of each player?

REFERENCES

1. Centers for Disease Control and Prevention. *HIV/AIDS Surveillance Report, 2006*. Vol. 18. Atlanta, GA: U.S. Department of Health and Human Services; 2008. http://www.cdc.gov/hiv/topics/surveillance/resources/reports/2006report/pdf/2006SurveillanceReport.pdf. Accessed June 23, 2008.

2. Glynn MK, Rhodes P. Estimated HIV prevalence in the United States at the end of 2003. Paper presented at: The National HIV Prevention Conference; June 2005; Atlanta, GA.

3. Kaiser Family Foundation. Women and HIV/AIDS in the United States. May 2008. http://www.kff.org/hivaids/upload/6092_05.pdf. Accessed June 15, 2008.

4. Kaiser Family Foundation. Women and HIV/AIDS in the United States. July 2007. http://www.kff.org/hivaids/upload/6092-04.pdf. Accessed June 11, 2008.

5. Centers for Disease Control and Prevention. *HIV/AIDS Surveillance in Adolescents and Young Adults (through, 2006)*. Atlanta, GA: U.S. Department of Health and Human Services; 2008. http://www.cdc.gov/hiv/topics/surveillance/resources/slides/adolescents/slides/Adolescents.pdf. Accessed June 2, 2008.

6. Thomas JC, Thomas KK. Things ain't what they ought to be: social forces underlying racial disparities in rates of sexually transmitted diseases in a rural North Carolina county. *Soc Sci Med*. 1999;49:1075-1084.

7. Gómez CA. Marín BV. Gender, culture, and power: barriers to HIV-prevention strategies for women. *J Sex Res*. 1996;33:355-362.

8. Berry DR. The emerging epidemiology of rural AIDS. *J Rural Health*. 1993;9:293-303.

9. Lam NS, Liu K. Spread of AIDS in rural America, 1982–1990. *JAIDS*. 1994;7:485-490.

10. Wortley PM, Fleming PL. AIDS in women in the United States: recent trends. *JAMA*. 1997;278:911-916.

11. U.S. Department of Health and Human Services. Women and HIV/AIDS in the United States. http:hab.hrsa.gov/history/women. Accessed October 23, 2007.

12. Wingood GM, DiClemente RJ. Application of the theory of gender and power to examine HIV-related exposures, risk factors, and effective interventions for women. *Health Educ Behav*. 2000;27:539-565.

13. Padian N, Marquis L, Francis DP, et al. Male-to-female transmission of human immunodeficiency virus. *JAMA*. 1987;258:788-790.

14. De Vincenzi I. A longitudinal study of human immunodeficiency virus. *JAMA*. 1987;331:341-346.

15. Hook EW III, Handsfield HH. Gonococcal infections in the adult. In: Holmes KK, Mardh PA, Sparling PF, et al., eds. *Sexually Transmitted Diseases*. 2nd ed. New York, NY: McGraw-Hill; 1990:149-165.

16. U.S. Census Bureau, Housing and Household Economic Statistics Division. Poverty 2006 highlights. http://www.census.gov/hhes/www/poverty/poverty06/pov06hi.html. Accessed June 22, 2008.

17. Sawhill IV. Poverty in the United States, the concise encyclopedia of economics. http://www.econlib.org/Library/Enc/PovertyintheUnitedStates.html. Accessed May 10, 2008.

18. Kondratas SA. Poverty in America: what the data reveal. The Heritage Foundation. December 26, 1985. http://www.heritage.org/Research/Welfare/bg475.cfm. Accessed June 1, 2008.

19. Tillerson K. Explaining racial disparities in HIV/AIDS incidence among women in the U.S.: a systematic review. *Stat Med*. 2008;June 12. [Epub ahead of print.]

20. Davidson OG. *Broken Heartland: The Rise of America's Rural Ghetto*. Iowa City: University of Iowa Press; 1996.

21. United States District Court for the District of Columbia. *Civil Action No. 97-1978, Timothy Pigford, et al., v. Dan Glickman, Secretary, U.S. Dept. of Agriculture*. http://lw.bna.com/lw/19981020/971978.htm. Accessed June 3, 2008.

22. Laumann EO, Gagnon JH, Michael RT, Michaels S. *The Social Organization of Sexuality*. Chicago, IL: University of Chicago Press; 1994.

23. Stratford D, Ellerbrock TV, Chamblee S. Social organization of sexual-economic networks and the persistence of HIV in a rural area in the USA. *Culture Health Sex*. 2007;9:121-135.

24. Institute of Medicine (IOM). *Health Literacy: A Prescription to End Confusion*. Washington DC: National Academies Press; 2004.

25. Osborn CY, Paasche-Orlow MK, Davis TC, Wolf MS. An overlooked factor in understanding HIV health disparities. *Amer J Prev Med*. 2007;33:374-378.

26. Jemmott LS, Jemmott JB, Hutchinson MK, Cenderbaum JA, O'Leary A. Sexually transmitted infection/HIV risk reduction interventions in clinical practice settings. *JOGNN*. 2008;37:137-145.

27. DiClemente RJ, Wingood CM, Harrington KF, et al. Efficacy of an HIV prevention intervention for African American adolescent girls. *JAMA*. 2004;292:171-179.

28. Jemmott JB, Jemmott LS, Braverman PK, Fong GT. HIV/STD risk reduction interventions for African American and Latino adolescent girls at an adolescent medicine clinic. *Arch Pediatr Adolesc Med*. 2005;159:440-449.

29. Cohen D, Scribner R, Bedimo R, Farley TA. Cost as a barrier to condom use: the evidence for condom subsidies in the United States. *Am J Public Health*. 1999;89:567-568.

30. Fenton KA, Peterman TA. HIV partner notification: taking a new look. *AIDS*. 1997;11:1535-1546.

31. Giesecke J, Ramstedt K, Granath F, et al. Efficacy of partner notification for HIV infection. *Lancet*. 1991;338:1096-1100.

32. Rutherford GW, Woo JM, Neal DP, et al. Partner notification and the control of human immunodeficiency virus infection: two years experience in San Francisco. *Sex Transm Dis*. 1991;18:107-110.

33. Wykoff RF, Heath Jr CW, Hollis SL, et al. Contact tracing to identify human immunodeficiency virus infection in a rural community. *JAMA*. 1988;259:3563-3566.

34. Pavia AT, Benyo M, Niler L, Risk I. Partner notification for control of HIV: results after 2 years of a statewide program in Utah. *Am J Public Health.* 1993; 83:1418-1424.

35. Pattman RS, Gould EM. Partner notification for HIV infection in the United Kingdom: a look back on seven years experience in Newcastle upon Tyne. *Genitourin Med.* 1993;69:94-97.

36. Wells KD, Hoff GL. Human immunodeficiency virus partner notification in a low incidence urban community. *Sex Transm Dis.* 1995;22:377-379.

37. Hoffman RE, Spencer NE, Miller LA. Comparison of partner notification at anonymous and confidential HIV test sites in Colorado. *J Acquir Immune Defic Syndr Hum Retrovirol.* 1995;8:406-410.

38. Fenton K, Adler M, Giesecke J, et al. HIV partner notification in England: results of a national evaluation programme. Paper presented at: XI International Conference on AIDS; July 1996; Vancouver, BC.

39. Peterman TA, Toomey KE, Dicker LW, Zaidi AA, Carolina.J. HIV partner notification: cost and effectiveness data from a multicenter randomised controlled trial. Paper presented at: XI International Conference on AIDS; July 1996; Vancouver, BC.

40. Fenton KA, Peterman TA. HIV partner notification: taking a new look. *AIDS.* 1997;11:1535-1546.

41. Normand J, Vlahov D, Moses LE. *Preventing HIV Transmission: The Role of Sterile Needles and Bleach.* Washington, DC: National Academies Press; 1995.

42. Koester SK. Copping, running, and paraphernalia laws; contextual and needle risk behavior among injection drug users in Denver. *Hum Org.* 1994;53:287-295.

43. Rich JD, Dickinson BP, Case P, et al. Strict syringe laws in Rhode Island are associated with high rates of re-using syringes and HIV risks among IDUs [letter]. *J Acquir Immune Defic Syndr Hum Retrovirol.* 1998;18(suppl 1):S140.

44. Case P, Meehan T, Jones TS. Arrests and incarceration of injection drug users for syringe possession in Massachusetts: implications for HIV prevention. *J Acquir Immune Defic Syndr Hum Retrovirol.* 1998;18(suppl 1):S71-S75.

45. Lurie P, Drucker E. An opportunity lost: HIV infections associated with lack of a national needle-exchange programme. *Lancet.* 1997;349(9052):604-608.

46. McFarland W, Chen S, Hsu L, Schwarcz S, Katz M. Low socioeconomic status is associated with a higher rate of death in the era of highly active antiretroviral therapy, San Francisco. *JAIDS.* 2003;33:96-103.

47. McGinnis KA, Fine MJ, Sharma RK, et al. Understanding racial disparities in HIV using data from the veterans aging cohort 3-site study and VA administrative data. *Am J Public Health.* 2003;93:1728-1733.

48. Muir KW, Santiago-Turla C, Stinnett SS, et al. Health literacy and adherence to glaucoma therapy. *Am J Ophthalmol.* 2006;142:223-226.

49. Boston Public Health Commission. Health of Boston Report, 2001; data extrapolation from neighborhood-specific AIDS mortality rates provided by Mary Yamate.

50. Shapiro MF, Morton SC, McCaffrey DF. Variations in the care of HIV-infected adults in the United States: results from the HIV Cost and Services Utilization Study. *JAMA.* 1999;281:2305-2315.

51. Levi J. Can access to care for people living with HIV be expanded? *AIDS Pub Pol J.* 13(2):56-74.

52. Kaiser Family Foundation. Financing HIV/AIDS care: a quilt with many holes [HIV/AIDS Policy Issue Brief]. May 2004. http://www.kff.org/hivaids/upload

/Financing-HIV-AIDS-Care-A-Quilt-with-Many-Holes.pdf. Accessed July 12, 2008.

53. Kaiser Family Foundation. Medicare and HIV/AIDS. HIV/AIDS policy fact sheet. Oct 2006. http://www.kff.org/hivaids/upload/7171-03.pdf. Accessed July 12, 2008.

54. U.S. Federal Funding for HIV/AIDS: The FY 2009 budget request. HIV/AIDS policy fact sheet. April 2008. http://www.kff.org/hivaids/upload/7029-041.pdf. Accessed July 12, 2008.

55. Guinan ME. Black communities' belief in "AIDS as genocide." A barrier to overcome for HIV prevention. *Ann Epidemiol*. 1993;3(2):193-195.

56. Montoya ID, Trevino RA, Kreitz DL. Access to HIV services by the poor. *J Comm Health*. 1999;24(5):331-346.

57. Peruga A, Rivo M. Racial differences in AIDS knowledge among adults. *AIDS Educ Prev*. 1992;4(1):52-60.

58. Aruffo JF, Coverdale JH, Vallbona C. AIDS knowledge in low-income and minority populations. *Pub Health Rep*. 1991;106(2):115-119.

59. Mays VM, Cochran SD. Acquired immunodeficiency syndrome and black Americans: special psychosocial issues. *Pub Health Rep*. 1987;102(2):224-231.

60. Johnson PA, Lee TH, Cook EF, Rouan GW, Goldman L. Effect of race on the presentation and management of patients with acute chest pain. *Ann Intern Med*. 1993;118:593-601.

61. Maynard C, Litwin PE, Martin JS, et al. Characteristics of black patients admitted to coronary care units in metropolitan Seattle: results from the Myocardial Infarction Triage and Intervention Registry (MITI). *Am J Cardiol*. 1991;67:18-23.

62. Peterson ED, Wright SM, Daley J, Thibault GE. Racial variation in cardiac procedure use and survival following acute myocardial infarction in the Department of Veterans Affairs. *JAMA*. 1994;271(15).

63. Schulman KA. Berlin JA. Harless W, et al. The effect of race and sex on physicians' recommendations for cardiac catheterization. *N Engl J Med*. 1999; 340(8):618-626.

64. Moore RD, Bone LR, Geller G, et al. Prevalence, detection and treatment of alcoholism in hospitalized patients. *JAMA*. 1989;261:403-407.

65. Ifudu O, Dawood M, Iofel Y, et al. Delayed referral of black, Hispanic, and older patients with chronic renal failure. *Amer J Kidney Dis*. 1999;33(4):728-733.

66. Ayanian JZ, Cleary PD, Weissman JS, Epstein AM. The effect of patients' preferences on racial differences in access to renal transplantation. *N Engl J Med*. 1999;341:1661-1669.

67. Hershman D, McBride R, Jacobsen JS, et al. Racial disparities in treatment and survival among women with early-stage breast cancer. *J Clin Oncol*. 2005; 23(27):6639-6646.

68. Shavers VL, Brown ML. Racial and ethnic disparities in the receipt of cancer treatment. *J Nation Cancer Instit*. 2002;94(5):334-357.

69. Montoya ID, Trevino RA, Kreitz DL. Access to HIV services by the poor. *J Comm Health*. 1999;24(5):331-346.

70. Piette JD, Mor V, Mayer K, et al. The effects of immune status and race on health service use among people with HIV disease. *Amer J Pub Health*. 1993; 83(4):510-514.

71. Shapiro MF, Morton, SC, McCaffrey DF et al. Variations in the care of HIV-infected adults in the United States. *JAMA*. 1999;281(24):2305-2315.

72. Turner BJ, Cunningham WE, Duan N, et al. Delayed medical care after

diagnosis in a US national probability sample of persons infected with human immunodeficiency virus. *Arch Intern Med*. 2000;160(17):2614-2622.

73. Moore RD, Stanton D, Gopalan R, Chaisson RE. Racial differences in the use of drug therapy for HIV disease in an urban community. *N Engl J Med*. 1994;330:763-768.

74. Cunningham WE, Markson LE, Andersen RM, et al. Prevalence and predictors of highly active antiretroviral therapy use in patients with HIV infection in the United States. *JAIDS*. 2000;25:115-123.

75. McNaghten A, Hanson D, Dworkin M; Differences in prescription of HAART persist in 1999 [abstract 494]. 8th Conference on Retroviruses and OIs; February 2001, Atlanta, GA.

76. Sorvillo F, Kerndt P, Odem S, Castillon M, Carruth A, Contreras R. Use of protease inhibitors among persons with AIDS in Los Angeles County. *AIDS CARE*. 1999;11(2):147-155.

77. Andersen R, Bozzette S, Shapiro M, et al. Access of vulnerable groups to antiretroviral therapy among persons in care for HIV disease in the United States. *Health Serv Res*. 2000;35(2):389-416.

78. Wong MD, Cunningham WE, Shapiro MF, et al. Disparities in HIV treatment and physician attitudes about delaying protease inhibitors for nonadherent patients. *J Gen Intern Med*. 2004;19(4):366-374.

79. Ciesla JA, Roberts JE. Meta-analysis of the relationship between HIV infection and risk for depressive disorders. *Am J Psychiatry*. 2001;158(5):725-730.

80. Leserman J, Petitto JM, Gu H, et al. Progression to AIDS, a clinical AIDS condition, and mortality: psychosocial and physiological predictors. *Psychol Med*. 2002;32:1059-1073.

81. Ickovics JR, Hamburger ME, Vlahov D, et al. Mortality, CD4 cell count decline, and depressive symptoms among HIV-seropositive women: longitudinal analysis from the HIV epidemiology research study. *JAMA*. 2001;285:466-474.

82. Cook JA, Grey D. Depressive symptoms and AIDS-related mortality among a multisite cohort of HIV-positive women. *Amer J Pub Health*. 2004;94(7):1133-1140.

83. Patterson TL, Shaw WS, Semple SJ, et al. Relationship of psychosocial factors to HIV disease progression. *Ann Behav Med*. 1996;18(1):30-39.

84. Hartzell JD, Janke IE, Weintrob AC. Impact of depression on HIV outcomes in the HAART era. *J Antimicrob Chemo*. 2008;62(2):246-255.

85. Ironson G, O'Cleirigh C, Fletcher MA, et al. Psychosocial factors predict CD4 and viral load change in men and women with human immunodeficiency virus in the era of highly active antiretroviral treatment. *Psychosom Med*. 2005;67:1013-1021.

86. Pence BW, Ostermann J, Kumar V, et al. The influence of psychosocial characteristics and race/ethnicity on the use, duration, and success of antiretroviral therapy. *JAIDS*. 2008;47(2):194-201.

87. Parienti JJ, Massari V, Descamps D, et al. Predictors of virologic failure and resistance in HIV-infected patients treated with nevirapine- or efavirenz-based antiretroviral therapy. *Clin Infect Dis*. 2004;38:1311-1316.

88. Anastos K, Schneider MF, Gange SJ, et al. The association of race, sociodemographic, and behavioral characteristics with response to highly active antiretroviral therapy in women. *J AIDS*. 2005;39(5):537-544.

89. Mugavero M, Ostermann J, Whetten K, et al. Barriers to antiretroviral adherence: the importance of depression, abuse, and other traumatic events. *AIDS Patient Care STDS*. 2006;20:418-428.

90. Leserman J, Pence BW, Whetten K, et al. Relation of lifetime trauma and depressive symptoms to mortality in HIV. *Am J Psychiatry*. 2007;164:1707-1713.

91. Pence BW, Miller WC, Gaynes BN, Eron JJ Jr. Psychiatric illness and virologic response in patients initiating highly active antiretroviral therapy. *J Acquir Immune Defic Syndrome*. 2007;44:159-166.

92. Jackson PB, Mustillo S. I am woman: the impact of social identities on African American women's mental health. *Women Health*. 2001;32(4):33-59.

93. Israelski DM, Prentiss DE, Lubega S, et al. Psychiatric co-morbidity in vulnerable populations receiving primary care for HIV/AIDS. *AIDS Care*. 2007;19(2): 220-225.

94. Wingood GM, Diclemente RJ, Mikhail I, et al. HIV discrimination and the health of women living with HIV. *Women Health*. 2007;46(2-3):99-112.

95. Williams DR. Race, socioeconomic status, and health: the added effects of racism and discrimination. *Ann NY Acad Sci*. 1999;896:173-188.

96. Williams DR, Williams-Morris R. Racism and mental health: the African American experience. *Ethnic Health*. 2000;5:243-268.

97. Safren SA, Otto MW, Worth JL, et al. Two strategies to increase adherence to HIV antiretroviral medication: life steps and medication monitoring. *Behav Res Therapy*. 2001;39:1151-1162.

98. Ickovics JR, Meisler AW. Adherence in AIDS clinical trials: a framework for clinical research and clinical care. *J Clin Epidemiol*. 1997;50:385-391.

99. Simoni JM, Frick PA, Pantalone DW, Turner BJ. Antiretroviral adherence interventions: a review of current literature and ongoing studies. *Topics HIV Med*. 2003;11:185-198.

100. Friedman SR, Maslow C, Bolyard M, et al. Urging others to be healthy: "intravention" by injection drug users as a community prevention goal. *AIDS Educ Prev*. 2004;16:250-263.

101. Wilson BD, Miller RL. Examining strategies for culturally grounded HIV prevention: a review. *AIDS Educ Prev*. 2003;15:184-202.

102. Ewart CK. Social action theory for a public health psychology. *Am Psychol*. 1991;46:931-946.

103. Gebo K, Fleishman J, Conviser R, et al. Contemporary costs of HIV health care in the HAART era [abstract 537]. Presented at: 13th Conference on Retroviruses and Opportunistic Infections; February 5-8, 2006; Denver, Colorado.

CHAPTER 13

INTRODUCTION

Cardiovascular Disease in Women: Risk Factors and Risk Reduction

Cardiovascular disease (CVD) accounted for 30% of an estimated 58 million deaths in the world from all causes in 2005.[1] Furthermore, CVD is the leading cause of death among women worldwide and accounts for one third of all deaths among them. In the United States, CVD is the number one cause of death and disability in women. Recent estimates from the Centers for Disease Control and Prevention (CDC) show that more than one third (38%) of the deaths of US women are related to coronary artery disease (CAD). This translates to more than a quarter million women who die from CAD and related causes, and this does not include stroke and other important cardiovascular diseases that are largely or entirely caused by atherosclerosis. The death toll from CVD is expected to increase further with the aging of the population.[2-4] Women have considerably lower age-specific rates of CAD as compared to men, with death rates from heart disease in women comparable to men 10 years younger until well past age 70. In contrast, death rates from cerebrovascular disease are much more similar between men and women across the age groups. Interestingly, women have similar total prevalence of both CAD and prior stroke as compared to men, because women more frequently survive to older ages than men, and because both CAD and stroke prevalence increase markedly with age.[5,6]

*Eliot A. Brinton, MD;**

Paul N. Hopkins, MD, MSPH;

Gopal Sankaran, MD, DrPH

Eliot A. Brinton, MD, is in the department of Cardiovascular Genetics at the University of Utah School of Medicine, Salt Lake City, Utah.

Paul N. Hopkins, MD, MSPH, is in the department of Cardiovascular Genetics at the University of Utah School of Medicine, Salt Lake City, Utah.

Gopal Sankaran, MD, DrPH is in the College of Health Sciences for the West Chester University of Pennsylvania, West Chester, PA.

Women's Knowledge About Their Risk for Coronary Artery Disease

Do women know that they are at risk for CVD? In the United States, surveys conducted by the American Heart Association[7] found that among women, awareness that heart disease is their leading cause of death increased from 30% in 1997 to 46% in 2003. Despite this progress, African-American and Hispanic women were barely half as likely as Caucasian women to be aware that heart disease is their leading cause of death (30% versus 27% versus 55%, respectively). Even more distressing is the fact that a US telephone survey of

* Dr. Brinton acknowledges a grant from the Aurora Foundation in support of this work.

1000 households in 1997 found that only 8% of women considered heart disease to be their foremost health concern.[8] A lack of knowledge about the true risk of heart disease was not only noted among women themselves, but also among their healthcare providers. A study of physician awareness and adherence to CVD prevention guidelines, conducted in 2004 in the United States, showed that less than one in five physicians knew that more women die every year from CVD than men.[9] Such gaps in awareness may disadvantage women in terms of diagnosis, treatment, and prevention of CVD. For example, women are reported to be 55% less likely than men to participate in cardiac rehabilitation.[10]

The fact that women have substantially lower CAD risk than men at any given age may lead to a common misperception among patients and even among clinicians that CAD is of little consequence for women.[11] This misperception has led both to underdiagnosis and undertreatment of CAD in women (as noted earlier), as well as a lack of research into CAD in women until the last two decades. An anecdote serves to illustrate.

In approximately 1989, a 42-year-old female patient with familial hypercholesterolemia consulted one of the authors (PNH) by telephone. She related a very clear history of angina, with chest pain brought on consistently by moderate exertion such as raking leaves or carrying groceries into the house. This was relieved promptly within 5–10 minutes by rest. She was advised to go to the emergency room since the pattern seemed to be increasing in frequency and she was currently having chest discomfort. At the emergency room she presented her history of extraordinarily elevated serum cholesterol (with multiple total cholesterol levels above 400 mg/dl prior to her recent start of lovastatin). She also related how her brother, with similarly elevated cholesterol, a poor diet, and a history of cigarette smoking had died of a myocardial infarction at age 25. Amazingly, she was told by the ER physician on duty that if she kept worrying about her cholesterol, she would end up giving herself a heart attack! This physician apparently had the mistaken impression that premenopausal women were immune to CAD. After further consultation with the author, the patient was referred for angiography where a 90% stenosis of the left anterior descending coronary artery was found and successfully treated with angio-plasty. Her symptoms were relieved and have not returned during the subsequent 19 years. Her lipids were aggressively treated with statin medication during this entire period as well.

Several key questions remain unclear in the minds of the vast majority of women and even most healthcare practitioners, and these questions still have not been adequately addressed in research studies:

1. Which women are at sufficiently high risk to warrant preventive measures?
2. Which CVD risk factors are important in women?
3. How do we best assess CVD risk and reduce it in women?

This chapter addresses our current state of knowledge and ignorance regarding these three questions, recommends a practical approach to CVD risk assessment and prevention, and also suggests top priorities for future research.

Cardiovascular Disease Risk Assessment in Women

Which Women Are at Risk?

All women may be considered at risk even though their risk is less than men of the same age. Indeed, considering all ages combined, as many or more women die of CAD and stroke in the United States as men, a frequently unappreciated fact.[8,9] This is because CVD incidence rises markedly with advancing age, and there are more women living at older ages than men. CAD mortality rates in women are approximately the same as men 10 years younger.[5,12]

The current evidence-based guidelines for cardiovascular disease prevention[13] in women (2007 update), based on a systematic review of the scientific literature by an expert panel, recommends a scheme for categorization of women into three risk groups—at high risk, at risk, or at optimal risk. This update of previous guidelines[14] noted some limitation of using the Framingham Global Risk scale, commented on the need to reduce through prevention the lifetime risk of CVD for women, and updated recommendations according to new clinical trial data. It also emphasized evidence that the presence of subclinical vascular disease greatly raises a woman's risk for CVD.[13] This is noteworthy as coronary artery calcium (CAC) in women, as well as in men, is a much stronger predictor of CAD events than is the Framingham Global Risk score.[15] Thus, while women have less coronary atherosclerosis than men by noninvasive screening (such as CAC), by coronary intravascular ultrasound (IVUS), and at autopsy, once atherosclerosis *is* present women are at similarly increased risk for clinical events as compared to men with similar extent of atherosclerosis.

Which CVD Risk Factors Are Important?

Generally, odds ratios associated with standard CVD risk factors are of a similar magnitude in men and women;[16,17] however, women do have an additional risk factor during menopause.[18] Sadly, the evidence that links CVD risk in women to most risk factors of interest tends to be poorer than the evidence in men.[19] Although much higher HDL-C in women explains a part of the lower age-corrected CVD risk in women versus men, none of the standard cardiovascular risk factors completely explain this difference.

In comparative research studies from 1960 through the 1990s, it became clear that although some risk factors were stronger on a relative basis in women than in men women still had lower absolute rates of CVD than men, at any given exposure to a particular risk factor. For example, in the Lipid Research Clinic follow-up, in both men and women, HDL-C levels were a powerful risk factor, but at any given level of HDL-C, women still had lower risk than men.[16]

Another interesting example of the lower CAD risk in women was angiographic data from the Cleveland Clinic of younger men and women.[15,20] Serum cholesterol was found to strongly predict significant (50% or greater) coronary stenosis in both men and women. However, at any given level of serum cholesterol, women still had less coronary stenosis than men, despite the women being 10 years older than the men. Some of the gender difference in coronary stenosis in this study may reflect, in part, the well-known phenomenon of angina without apparent obstructive disease in

epicardial coronary arteries (so-called metabolic syndrome; also known as syndrome X). According to the guidelines from the National Cholesterol Education Program Adult Treatment Panel (ATPIII),[14] any three of the following traits in a woman meets the criteria for metabolic syndrome:

- Abdominal obesity with a waist circumference of over 88 cm (35 inches)
- Fasting serum triglycerides of 150 mg/dL or greater
- HDL cholesterol of 50 mg/dL or lower
- Blood pressure of 130/85 mmHg or more
- Fasting blood glucose of 110 mg/dL or above

The NHLBI-sponsored Women's Ischemia Syndrome Evaluation (WISE) study reported that women with the metabolic syndrome had an intermediate risk between those with normal metabolic status and those with diabetes in terms of 4-year event-free survival rates (event-free survival refers to absence of death, nonfatal myocardial infarction, stroke, or congestive heart failure). However, in women with preexisting documented significant CAD, those with metabolic syndrome had a level of risk similar to those with diabetes and much lower survival rate than those with normal metabolic status. Thus, CVD risk in women with significant preexisting CAD is elevated by the presence of metabolic syndrome. In recent years, at least some of this angina has been attributed to small vessel endothelial dysfunction. Indeed, microvascular coronary disease may be more prevalent in women than in men and often may remain undetected by tests such as an angiogram.[21,95] The importance of diet and lifestyle in primary prevention of CAD has been studied using data from the World Health Organization Nurses' Health Study.[1,96] The researchers used a composite measure based on a diet made up of six dietary factors that was low in trans fat and glycemic load (i.e., how much the blood glucose levels are raised by the particular diet); high in cereal fiber, marine n-3 fatty acids, and folate; and with a high ratio of polyunsaturated to saturated fat. Researchers found a reduction in the incidence of CAD. Consumption of other dietary ingredients such as nuts, vitamin B_6, vitamin E, and linolenic acid, though not reported in this study, are also considered of value in the prevention of CAD.

Women are well known to have higher HDL-C than men (by about 10 mg/dL in most series). Most of this difference is in the form of larger HDL_2 particles, and this difference may be explained by the lower waist-to-hip ratio in women versus men.[22] The lower average waist-to-hip ratio in women, particularly premenopausal women, has been related to lower plasma triglycerides and lower blood pressure as well. Waist size (positively) and hip size (negatively) as well as waist-to-hip ratio have recently been clearly related to CAD risk in the very large INTERHEART case-control study.[18] Of note, in this study the odds ratios for most risk factors were rather similar between men and women.

In a study of female victims of early (age 55 and under) fatal myocardial infarction or CHD death, one of the authors (PNH) found an especially high prevalence of standard risk factors, especially smoking, hypertension, and positive family history.[23] A diagnosis in the medical chart of hyperlipidemia was probably underreported in this early study.[23] Several other studies, cited in that paper, had also reported an unusually high frequency of risk factors in women with early CAD. This suggests that, because of their relative protection from CAD, a high burden of atherogenic factors may be requisite to cause CAD in the average premenopausal woman and many older women as well. An unpublished observation in that study (as compared to an earlier reported but parallel study in males)[24] was an apparent high frequency of seemingly unrelated medical problems in women with early CAD compared to their male counterparts. Although this may have, in part, been related to the 10-year average greater age of the women, it might be due to a proatherogenic effect of autoimmune diseases, such as systemic lupus erythematosus (increased relative risk of CVD from 5 to 50 fold),[25-29] rheumatoid arthritis,[30] and systemic sclerosis.[31] As these diseases affect women far more often than men, women with earlier onset CAD may have had more medical problems potentially related to such autoimmune disorders. The overall effect on CAD and stroke of autoimmune disorders in women versus men has not been systematically studied to our knowledge.

Practical CVD Risk Assessment

Overall CAD risk is reasonably estimated by the Framingham Risk Calculator.[13,14] More recently, the Reynolds Score, which was developed in a large population of women and incorporates hsCRP, has been shown to be even more predictive.[32]

It is important to recognize that the presence of angina or of a positive exercise tolerance test are considerably less predictive of CAD in women than in men, and that considerable improvement in diagnostic accuracy for CAD is achieved by combining a stress test with various imaging modalities (including echocardiography, SPECT, or MRI).[2] Coronary artery calcium (CAC) measurement by CT scan seems to be similarly predictive of CAD event risk in men and women. Women have less CAC at all ages than men.[11,33-35] CAC scores greater than 300–400 are associated with greatly increased risk in both men and women.[34-37] Still, even elderly women may have somewhat better total survival at comparable CAC scores as compared to men.[38]

Cardiovascular Disease Prevention In Women

Background

According to current US guidelines (ATPIII), there is no substantial difference between the approach to treating men and women. The major difference is the lower estimated risk obtained from the Framingham Risk Calculator, and hence, generally lower LDL goals in women. What has been the major thrust in recent years is an urge to recognize more fully that women are susceptible to coronary disease and deserve similarly aggressive preventive efforts when warranted by ATPIII guidelines.[13,14] This section will therefore not focus on standard interventions such as lipid lowering, blood pressure control, and various lifestyle interventions.

Atherosclerosis seems to respond to aggressive treatment similarly in men and women. In the setting of intensive risk factor modification, there was no significant difference between genders with regard to the rates of plaque progression or regression.[39]

One area of continuing controversy and misunderstanding remains the effect of menopause and menopausal hormone replacement therapy on CVD risk. The remainder of this chapter will therefore focus on CVD prevention in postmenopausal women. CVD risk increases rapidly at menopause, independent of age,[40] suggesting that estrogen deficiency promotes atherosclerosis. In addition, observational studies consistently had found that postmenopausal women using menopausal hormone replacement therapy (MHT) are 40–50% less likely to have CHD than women who never took or discontinued MHT.[41]

Randomized Clinical Trials of MHT: Results and Their Misinterpretation

Until relatively recently, MHT was assumed to promote atheroprevention because of consistent apparent protection in numerous observational studies. Nevertheless, it was decided that testing in randomized trials was needed. Three large clinical endpoint trials were conducted to address this question, the Heart and Estrogen/progestin Replacement Study (HERS)[42] and the two MHT trials of the Women's Health Initiative (WHI).[43,44] Unexpectedly, all three trials showed no decrease, or even an increase in CVD with MHT, especially when consisting of estrogen plus progesterone (E+P), and especially during the first year of treatment. The consensus on MHT shifted immediately and dramatically. The HERS[42] and WHI reports[43,44] and accompanying editorials, as well as statements from the Food and Drug Administration (FDA), the American College of Obstetricians and Gynecologists (ACOG) and the American Heart Association (AHA), concluded that MHT should "not be initiated or continued"[45,46] for coronary heart disease prevention, and that MHT prescribed for symptoms of estrogen deficiency is recommended for use only for the "shortest possible duration."[44,47]

Was this seemingly obvious conclusion actually warranted? Surprisingly, the answer is a resounding no! Why not? The mandate of these trials was to test the effects of MHT in the typical pattern of clinical use, that is, MHT initiation early in the menopause, generally, although not exclusively, for estrogen-deficiency symptoms. Unfortunately, to facilitate the blinding of the trial, women with such symptoms were actively discouraged from enrolling in the trials. Even more unfortunately, to accelerate the accumulation of CVD events, women up to age 79 were allowed to enroll, and the average subject age at trial entry was in the mid-60s. Since most subjects had never taken MHT before trial entry, the HERS and WHI primarily studied a circumstance far removed from usual clinical practice, MHT initiation late in the menopause without any clinical reason for treatment. This striking disconnection between study design and clinical practice was ignored in the rush to judgment following the surprising and disappointing results. The lack of benefit or possible harm evident in *starting* MHT several years after menopause was incorrectly extrapolated to imply lack of benefit or possible harm from *continuing* MHT at the same general age. Thus, it was stated that short-term MHT was allowed for a few years for symptom relief, but then was mandated to *stop* before the age at which *starting* MHT was found to be harmful. Interestingly, neither the HERS nor WHI ever studied the consequences of early discontinuation of MHT, the action so adamantly recommended in their wake. Ironically, the only data regarding this approach, from observational studies, strongly suggest a rapid loss of benefit when MHT is discontinued after a few years of use.[48] Granted, observational studies cannot prove that early discontinuation of MHT is harmful, but we are aware of no studies showing any benefit from early discontinuation of MHT, despite its being a universally embraced guideline.

Evidence for Benefit of Early-Start MHT

Recent reanalyses of the WHI data and new WHI study results now strongly suggest that MHT can reduce atherosclerosis progression and clinical CHD events and total mortality, specifically when started within a few years of menopause. Importantly, this parallels the usual clinical pattern, in which MHT is started early in menopause for relief of estrogen-deficiency symptoms.

Subsequent to the initial report of the WHI trial, which used combined estrogen and progestin (E+P), analysis of centrally adjudicated coronary heart disease (CHD) event data from the WHI trial was done by years since menopause (at study entry). Instead of showing a consistent increase in CHD, there was a striking trend toward a more favorable CHD effect with fewer years since menopause (relative risk [RR] 0.89, 1.22, and 1.71 for < 10, 10–19 and ≥ 20 years, respectively),[46] a trend later shown to be statistically significant.[49] CHD effects of estrogen-only (E-only) in that part of the WHI trial were also found to vary directly by age (hazard ratio [HR] 0.63, 0.94, and 1.11 for women 50–59, 60–69, and 70–79, respectively, P value for interaction = .07). Despite these emerging data strongly suggesting CVD benefit when E+P or E-only were started in younger postmenopausal women, the AHA shortly thereafter issued a statement that "hormone therapy . . . should not be used for the primary prevention of CVD" without mentioning any variance by age at initiation.[13] Reanalysis of pooled CVD events in both the WHI E+P and E-only trials suggested CHD benefit from both types of MHT when started earlier after menopause or in younger women.[49] Total mortality showed the same trend and was significantly 30% lower in women starting MHT at ages 50–59 (HR 0.70, confidence interval [CI] 0.51–0.96 in pooled data and similarly for E+P and E-only separately).

Finally, E-only versus placebo started at ages 50–59 in WHI trial subjects caused a 32% lower mean CAC score (83.1 vs. 123.1, P = .02) and were more likely to have a low CAC (< 10 vs. > 300) (odds ratio [OR] 0.58, P = .03 by intention to treat; and OR 0.39, P = .004 with ≥ 80% adherence to study drug).[50] CAC greater than 300 (versus less than 10) predicts a several-fold increase in CHD risk over the next 3–5 years,[51] so just a few years of early-start MHT may extend CHD event reduction into the 7th and 8th decades. Unfortunately, there are no such data regarding the effects of continuation or discontinuation of MHT after 7 years.

A meta-analysis conducted recently involving 23 randomized trials of MHT that included more than 39,000 participants showed CHD benefit when MHT was begun within 10 years of menopause or before age 60 (OR 0.68, CI 0.48–0.96) while women more than 10 years postmenopausal or 60 and older had no net benefit (OR 1.03, CI 0.91–1.16).[52] Although more than 70% of the subjects were from the WHI trial, these results were similar to those from the WHI. A similar analysis of over 26,000 women by the same authors also showed decreased total mortality when MHT was started before age 60 (OR 0.61, CI 0.39–0.95), but not when initiated after age 60 (OR 1.03, CI 0.90–1.18).[53]

Analysis of early-start short-term MHT in 4065 women under 60 years of age in two additional randomized trials has suggested benefit similar to that seen in the above meta-analyses, there being 1.96 CVD events/1000 patient-years with various MHT regimens (mainly 0.625 mg/d CEE) versus 3.01 with placebo.[54] Although this difference was not statistically significant, due to the small numbers of events, a trend towards reducing the risk of CVD by one third is noteworthy since only the first year of treatment was analyzed and venous thrombotic events were included, both of which would be predicted to increase combined CVD events with MHT, especially in older women.[54]

Interestingly, one large observational cohort, the Nurses' Health Study, which has looked at time of initiation of MHT relative to the menopause, also has suggested the same effect.[55] CHD risk was reduced when MHT was started within 10 years of menopause, both for E-only (RR 0.66, CI 0.54–0.80) and for E+P (RR 0.72, CI 0.56–0.92). In contrast, MHT started 10 or more years after the menopause showed no such reduction.[55]

Potential Mechanisms of Differing MHT Effects by Timing of Initiation

Why might late-start MHT be harmful, when long-term continuation of MHT appears to be beneficial? Recent basic science studies indicate that estrogen may reduce early atherogenesis but precipitate clinical events at later stages and suggest mechanisms by which this may occur. When MHT is started before age 60, it is routinely reported to reduce many atherosclerosis risk factors.[56-63] The same appears to be true when MHT is started early after premature loss of estrogen from ovariectomy.[58]

One apparently proatherogenic effect of MHT, the increase in the proinflammatory factor C-reactive protein (CRP),[64] may in fact not truly increase CVD risk. CRP does not seem to be a true inflammatory factor but rather is a marker made in the liver in response to major systemic proinflammatory factors such as IL-6. MHT actually reduces the production of IL-6[65] and thus is likely anti-inflammatory.[66] The increase in CRP seen with MHT most likely just reflects the general increase in synthesis of many hepatic proteins caused by first-pass effects of oral MHT.[56]

There are, however, at least two effects of MHT that could increase the rates of CVD events. First, estrogen can stimulate production of matrix metalloproteinases by macrophages.[67] Second, MHT, especially in higher doses and when orally administered can promote thrombosis, probably largely by stimulating hepatic production of soluble coagulation factors.[68] It is important to realize that these two effects appear likely to increase arterial events only in the setting of late-stage atherosclerosis with advanced or vulnerable plaques. Matrix metalloproteinases seem to play a crucial role in the rupture of these plaques by eroding the fibrous cap.[57,69] Plaque rupture, in turn, appears to be the major stimulus for intra-arterial thrombosis, which causes abrupt total or near-total occlusion of the artery, hence leading to major CVD events such as unstable angina, acute myocardial infarction, or ischemic stroke. Thus, MHT appears to precipitate acute atherothrombotic events, especially in older women more likely to have advanced plaque. This mechanism is likely the major reason why only late-start MHT has been shown to increase CVD risk.[63] It is probably important that the prothrombotic effect of MHT is especially pronounced during the first year or so after MHT initiation.[42] Meanwhile, favorable lipid effects and anti-inflammatory and antioxidant effects should cause regression of advanced plaques over time, reducing macrophage content and thus decreasing the magnitude and impact of any increase in matrix metalloproteinase secretion. Thus, it is not surprising that the adverse effects of MHT on CVD events were concentrated in the first year or so of use and in the older women who presumably had more advanced atherosclerosis at the time of treatment initiation in the WHI and HERS.

Another mechanism that may contribute to the divergent effects of MHT on CVD events by age at initiation is the tendency for the numbers and activity of estrogen receptors to decrease during prolonged estrogen deficiency.[57] Coronary artery wall cells express estrogen receptors,[70] and when estrogen therapy is initiated immediately after surgical menopause in monkeys, atherosclerosis is subsequently reduced.[71,72] In contrast, when MHT initiation is delayed for a few years after surgical menopause in monkeys,[73] or natural menopause in women,[74] no reduction in atherosclerosis can be seen. Although this loss of effect may be caused by a loss or alteration of estrogen response, it might also be caused by changes in estrogen impact owing to progression of underlying atherosclerotic disease.

Clinical MHT Trials in Progress

The fact that many questions about estrogen effects on atherosclerosis remain unanswered has prompted two ongoing randomized clinical trials. The Kronos Early Estrogen Prevention Study (KEEPS; NCT00154180) is exploring effects of MHT (conjugated equine estrogen 0.45 mg/d vs. transdermal estradiol 50 micrograms/d vs. matching placebos) on change in carotid intima-media thickness (CIMT) by ultrasound in 720 women randomized 6 to 36 months past menopause.[75] Women posthysterectomy are excluded, and subjects receive oral micronized progesterone (200 mg/d) or matching placebo (in those not receiving estrogen) 12 days per month. The treatment period will be about 4 years. The Early versus Late Intervention Trial With Estradiol (ELITE; NCT00114517) is studying 504 women, roughly half being less than 6 years postmenopausal and half more than 10 years postmenopausal. They are randomized to receive oral estradiol 1 mg/d or matching placebo; with vaginal progesterone or placebo in subjects without a hysterectomy. Treatment is about 2 to 5 years, and the primary endpoint is change in CIMT. Thus, ELITE is testing early- versus late-start MHT, while KEEPS examines low-dose oral CEE vs. low-dose transdermal estradiol, both started early. Early-start ELITE subjects will be similar in most ways to KEEPS subjects, and the primary study endpoints of these trials are identical and are being read by the same central facility (University of Southern California Atherosclerosis Research Unit). Thus, pooling of results between the two studies should be possible and would help elucidate similarities and differences among various early-start MHT regimens, including oral estradiol versus oral CEE, and oral versus transdermal estradiol. An earlier study by Hodis et al. already showed reduced progression of CIMT in postmenopausal women with oral 17-beta estradiol.[76]

Key Unresolved Issues Regarding MHT in Postmenopausal Atheroprevention

An efficient way to catalog unresolved research questions regarding effects of MHT on CVD risk is to consider key aspects of MHT regimens: (1) timing of initiation (age and/or years since menopause), (2) medication type, (3) route of administration (oral versus transdermal versus other), (4) dose, (5) continuous versus monthly cycled administration, and (6) total duration of use. The first aspect of MHT noted above appears to be crucial in determining effects on CHD, as discussed in detail above. Regarding the second aspect, there is a possibility that estradiol (and perhaps other estrogen preparations) differs from CEE in its effects on atherosclerosis, but this seems unlikely, and the very limited data currently available do not strongly support this.[74,77] In contrast, oral MHT has much greater effect on lipids (generally but not completely favorable),[78-80] but a substantially greater procoagulant effect.[68,81]

Observational studies suggest that low-dose MHT (i.e., CEE 0.3 mg/d, or equivalent) may reduce CVD similarly to full-dose MHT (i.e., CEE 0.625 mg/d, or equivalent), for example, an RR of 0.58 (CI 0.37–0.92) was seen with CEE 0.3 mg/d versus an RR of 0.54 (CI 0.44–0.67) with 0.625 mg/d (both in comparison to no MHT) in the Nurses Health Study.[41] A slightly smaller benefit has been reported for carotid atherosclerosis, however.[82] With regard to osteoporosis, clinical trial data suggest nearly full benefit of lower MHT doses.[83] Importantly, lower doses are also reported to reduce adverse effects of MHT on thromboembolic disease[41] and stroke (RR 0.54, 95% CI 0.28–1.06 versus RR 1.35, CI 1.08–1.68, for CEE 0.3 mg versus 0.625 mg/d, respectively).[41] It seems unlikely that cyclicity versus continuity of MHT would alter effects on atherosclerosis, but this is unknown.

Sadly, the single most important practical issue in menopausal science has never been studied in a randomized human trial. The question is to what degree does early discontinuation of MHT differ in CVD effects from long-term if not lifelong MHT? More simply stated, what is the optimal duration of MHT use? After a woman has taken MHT for a few years for symptom relief (although the duration of estrogen deficiency symptoms varies from weeks to many years),[84] she is told categorically that it is harmful to continue further. The dogmatism of this guideline is distressing, given the fact that the HERS and WHI trials never addressed this question, and indeed there are very few or no clinical trial data in this regard. Ironically, the only available data, results from observational trials, strongly suggest that early discontinuation of MHT is harmful. Women taking low-dose MHT for estrogen-deficiency symptoms for up to 31 years

had lower CAC versus age-matched non-MHT-users.[85] Furthermore, in the large, observational Nurses' Health study, women who discontinued MHT had CHD mortality as high as never-users (RR 0.99, CI 0.75–1.30) while those who continued MHT had only half the CHD mortality (RR 0.47, CI 0.32–0.69 versus never-users).[48] Also, total CHD events are increased in women who discontinue MHT.[55] In addition, rapid bone loss is always induced by untreated estrogen deficiency, whether from menopause without MHT or from later MHT discontinuation.[86] Although these data are post hoc analyses from randomized trials or observational data, and therefore cannot prove that long-term continuation of MHT is beneficial, lacking any randomized data to the contrary, there is a strong case to be made that long-term MHT is better than early, arbitrary discontinuation. Despite all this, even recent guidance from the North American Menopausal Society[87] and from the WHI investigators[50] remains very conservative: "The current recommendations from many organizations that hormone therapy be limited to . . . the shortest duration necessary remain appropriate."[50]

What about other benefits or harms of long-term MHT? In addition to fewer osteoporotic fractures,[43,44] many other diseases appear to be reduced. These include diabetes mellitus incidence,[88] colon cancer diagnosis,[43] Alzheimer's disease,[89] breast cancer severity,[90] and mortality (RR 0.77, CI 0.59–1.00 in current- versus never-users).[91] Even total mortality appears to be reduced in long-term MHT users.[91] Although breast cancer incidence might increase with very long-term use, E-only MHT has been reported not to be associated with breast cancer, even when continued for 25 years or longer.[92]

Clear adverse risks of MHT include thromboembolic disease, but this probably can be reduced by use of lower doses, transdermal administration, and by screening to exclude women with a prior history or with a common genetic predisposition to thrombosis. Breast cancer diagnosis is increased in the near-term with MHT that contains systemic progestin[43] and may well be increased by long-term use of MHT with or without progestins;[93] however, long-term MHT compares favorably with other preventive measures in postmenopausal women.[62]

Although the lack of full utilization of traditional measures to reduce CHD risk in menopausal women, such as aspirin, statin therapy for cholesterol lowering, or treatment of blood pressure or diabetes, has been considered to argue against use of MHT for CHD prevention,[94] these other measures are likely complementary to MHT.[62]

Conclusion

Women have a far higher risk of CVD than generally appreciated by women themselves, or by their healthcare practitioners, especially in the estrogen-deficient postmenopausal state. Dogmatic overextrapolation of the HERS and WHI data has led to the near-universal belief that long-term MHT use increases CVD risk, and therefore has condemned postmenopausal women to early and certain estrogen deficiency.

Despite this, a strong case can now be made to individually consider in each woman the pros and cons of early-start MHT and its subsequent continuation or discontinuation, based on our current, incomplete, set of scientific data and the unique circumstances of each woman's personal situation. This can and must be done even while efforts are made to perform the additional research urgently needed to clarify the risks and benefits of long-term continuation versus early discontinuation of MHT and to compare effects of standard- versus low-dose oral CEE or transdermal estradiol (or possibly alternative MHT preparations).

In addition, given the data newly available since the original publications from the HERS and WHI, a thorough review of current MHT guidelines should be conducted, with special focus on the prevention of CHD, and with particular attention to the timing of its initiation and discontinuation.

[†] **Terms And Their Abbreviations:** HR: Hazard Ratio; OR: Odds Ratio; RH: Relative Hazard; RR: Risk Ratio

DISCUSSION QUESTIONS

1. Explain why it is necessary for women and their healthcare providers to be knowledgeable about the cardiovascular risks faced by women.

2. Discuss the role of menopausal hormone replacement therapy in women and the controversy surrounding its use.

3. What recommendations would you provide to women who want to reduce their risk of getting cardiovascular disease? How would you find the evidence necessary to support your recommendations?

REFERENCES

1. World Health Organization. *Preventing Chronic Disease: A Vital Investment*. Geneva, Switzerland: World Health Organization; 2005.

2. Bairey Merz N, Bonow RO, Sopko G, et al. Women's Ischemic Syndrome Evaluation: Current Status and Future Research Directions: Report of the National Heart, Lung and Blood Institute Workshop: October 2-4, 2002: Executive Summary. *Circulation*. 2004;109:805-807.

3. American Heart Association. Heart Disease and Stroke Statistics. Dallas, TX: American Heart Association; 2004. http://www.heart/107296940HSStats2004 Update.pdf. Accessed January 15, 2004.

4. Centers for Disease Control and Prevention. *Make Every Mother and Child Count*. Atlanta, GA: Centers for Disease Control and Prevention; 2005. http://www.cdc.gov/od/spotlight/nwhw/whlth05.htm. Accessed November 23, 2005.

5. National Center for Health Statistics. Health, United States, 2005, with Chartbook on Trends in the Health of Americans. Hyattsville, MD: National Center for Health Statistics; 2005. http://www.cdc.gov/nchs/data/hus/hus05.pdf. Accessed November 5, 2006.

6. Lerner DJ, Kannel WB. Patterns of coronary heart disease morbidity and mortality in the sexes: a 26-year follow-up of the Framingham population. *Am Heart J.* 1986;111:383-390.

7. Mosca L, Ferris A, Fabunmi R, Robertson RM. Tracking women's awareness of heart disease. An American Heart Association national study. *Circulation.* 2004;109:573-579.

8. Mosca L, Jones WK, King KB, Ouyang P, Redberg RF, Hill MN. Awareness, perception, and knowledge of heart disease risk and prevention among women in the United States. American Heart Association Women's Heart Disease and Stroke Campaign Task Force. *Arch Fam Med.* 2000;9:506-515.

9. Mosca L, Linfante AH, Benjamin EJ, et al. National study of physician awareness and adherence to cardiovascular disease prevention guidelines. *Circulation.* 2005;119:499-510.

10. Witt BJ, Jacobsen SJ, Weston SA, et al. Cardiac rehabilitation after myocardial infarction in the community. *J Am Coll Cardiol.* 2004;44:988-996.

11. Shaw LJ, Bairey Merz CN, Pepine CJ, et al. Insights from the NHLBI-sponsored Women's Ischemia Syndrome Evaluation (WISE) study: Part I: gender differences in traditional and novel risk factors, symptom evaluation, and gender-optimized diagnostic strategies. *J Am Coll Cardiol.* 2006;47:S4-S20.

12. Rosamond W, Flegal K, Friday G, et al. Heart disease and stroke statistics—2007 update: a report from the American Heart Association Statistics Committee and Stroke Statistics Subcommittee. *Circulation.* 2007;115:e69-171.© 2007 American Heart Association, Inc.

13. Mosca L, Banka CL, Benjamin EJ, et al. Evidence-based guidelines for cardiovascular disease prevention in women: 2007 update. *Circulation.* 2007;115:1481-1501.

14. Mosca L, Appel LJ, Benjamin EJ, et al. Evidence-based guidelines for cardiovascular disease prevention in women. *J Am Coll Cardiol.* 2004;43:672-693.

15. Welch CC, Proudfit WL, Sheldon WC. Coronary arteriographic findings in 1,000 women under age 50. *Am J Cardiol.* 1975;35:211-215.

16. Jacobs DR, Mebane IL, Bangdiwala SI, Criqui MH, Tyroler HA. High-density lipoprotein cholesterol as a predictor of cardiovascular disease mortality in men and women: The follow-up study of the Lipid Research Clinics Prevalence Study. *Am J Epidemiol.* 1990;131:32-47.

17. Ostlund RE Jr, Staten M, Kohrt WM, Schultz J, Malley M. The ratio of waist-to-hip circumference, plasma insulin level, and glucose intolerance as independent predictors of the HDL2 cholesterol level in older adults. *N Engl J Med.* 1990;322:229-234.

18. Yusuf S, Hawken S, Ounpuu S, et al. Effect of potentially modifiable risk factors associated with myocardial infarction in 52 countries (the INTERHEART study): case-control study. *Lancet.* 2004;364:937-952.

19. Grady D, Chaput L, Kristof M. Results of Systematic Review of Research on Diagnosis and Treatment of Coronary Heart Disease in Women [Evidence Report/Technology Assessment No. 80]. Rockville, MD: Agency for Healthcare Research and Quality; 2003. AHRQ Publication No. 03-0035.

20. Welch CC, Proudfit WL, Sones FM Jr, Shirey EK, Sheldon WC, Razavi M. Cinecoronary arteriography in young men. *Circulation*. 1970;42:647-652.

21. Bugiardini R, Bairey Merz CN. Angina with normal coronary arteries: a changing philosophy. *JAMA*. 2005;293:477-484.

22. Ostlund RE Jr, Staten M, Kohrt WM, Schultz J, Malley M. The ratio of waist-to-hip circumference, plasma insulin level, and glucose intolerance as independent predictors of the HDL2 cholesterol level in older adults. *N Engl J Med*. 1990;322:229-234.

23. Hunt SC, Blickenstaff K, Hopkins PN, Williams RR. Coronary disease and risk factors in close relatives of Utah women with early coronary death. *West J Med*. 1986;145:329-334.

24. Hopkins PN, Williams RR, Hunt SC. Magnified risks from cigarette smoking for coronary prone families in Utah. *West J Med*. 1984;141:196-202.

25. Jonsson H, Nived O, Sturfelt G. Outcome in systemic lupus erythematosus: a prospective study of patients from a defined population. *Medicine* (Baltimore). 1989;68:141-150.

26. Manzi S, Meilahn EN, Rairie JE, et al. Age-specific incidence rates of myocardial infarction and angina in women with systemic lupus erythematosus: comparison with the Framingham Study. *Am J Epidemiol*. 1997;145:408-415.

27. Asanuma Y, Oeser A, Shintani AK, et al. Premature coronary-artery atherosclerosis in systemic lupus erythematosus. *N Engl J Med*. 2003;349:2407-2415.

28. Roman MJ, Shanker BA, Davis A, et al. Prevalence and correlates of accelerated atherosclerosis in systemic lupus erythematosus. *N Engl J Med*. 2003;349:2399-2406.

29. Frostegard J. Systemic lupus erythematosus and cardiovascular disease. *Lupus*. 2008;17:364-367.

30. Roman MJ, Moeller E, Davis A, et al. Preclinical carotid atherosclerosis in patients with rheumatoid arthritis. *Ann Intern Med*. 2006;144:249-256.

31. Khurma V, Meyer C, Park GS, et al. A pilot study of subclinical coronary atherosclerosis in systemic sclerosis: coronary artery calcification in cases and controls. *Arthritis Rheum*. 2008;59:591-597.

32. Ridker PM, Buring JE, Rifai N, Cook NR. Development and validation of improved algorithms for the assessment of global cardiovascular risk in women: the Reynolds Risk Score. *JAMA*. 2007;297:611-619.

33. Newman AB, Naydeck BL, Sutton-Tyrrell K, Feldman A, Edmundowicz D, Kuller LH. Coronary artery calcification in older adults to age 99: prevalence and risk factors. *Circulation*. 2001;104:2679-2684.

34. LaMonte MJ, FitzGerald SJ, Church TS, et al. Coronary artery calcium score and coronary heart disease events in a large cohort of asymptomatic men and women. *Am J Epidemiol*. 2005;162:421-429.

35. Hopkins PN, Ellison RC, Province MA, et al. Association of coronary artery calcified plaque with clinical coronary heart disease in the National Heart, Lung, and Blood Institute's Family Heart Study. *Am J Cardiol*. 2006;97:1564-1569.

36. Lakoski SG, Greenland P, Wong ND, et al. Coronary artery calcium scores and risk for cardiovascular events in women classified as "low risk" based on Framingham risk score: the multi-ethnic study of atherosclerosis (MESA). *Arch Intern Med*. 2007;167:2437-2442.

37. Detrano R, Guerci AD, Carr JJ, et al. Coronary calcium as a predictor of coronary events in four racial or ethnic groups. *N Engl J Med.* 2008;358:1336-1345.

38. Raggi P, Gongora MC, Gopal A, Callister TQ, Budoff M, Shaw LJ. Coronary artery calcium to predict all-cause mortality in elderly men and women. *J Am Coll Cardiol.* 2008;52:17-23.

39. Nicholls SJ, Wolski K, Sipahi I, et al. Rate of progression of coronary atherosclerotic plaque in women. *J Am Coll Cardiol.* 2007;49:1546-1551.

40. Hu FB, Stampfer MJ, Manson JE, et al. Trends in the incidence of coronary heart disease and changes in diet and lifestyle in women. *N Engl J Med.* 2000;343:530-537.

41. Grodstein F, Manson JE, Colditz GA, Willett WC, Speizer FE, Stampfer MJ. A prospective, observational study of postmenopausal hormone therapy and primary prevention of cardiovascular disease. *Ann Intern Med.* 2000;133:933-941.

42. Hulley S, Grady D, Bush T, et al. Randomized trial of estrogen plus progestin for secondary prevention of coronary heart disease in postmenopausal women. Heart and Estrogen/progestin Replacement Study (HERS) Research Group. *JAMA.* 1998;280:605-613.

43. Rossouw JE, Anderson GL, Prentice RL, et al. Risks and benefits of estrogen plus progestin in healthy postmenopausal women: principal results from the Women's Health Initiative randomized controlled trial. *JAMA.* 2002;288:321-333.

44. Anderson GL, Limacher M, Assaf AR, et al. Effects of conjugated equine estrogen in postmenopausal women with hysterectomy: the Women's Health Initiative randomized controlled trial. *JAMA.* 2004;291:1701-1712.

45. Writing Group for the Women's Health Initiative Investigators. Risks and benefits of estrogen plus progestin in healthy postmenopausal women: principal results from the Women's Health Initiative randomized controlled trial. *JAMA.* 2002;288:321-333.

46. Manson JE, Hsia J, Johnson KC, et al. Estrogen plus progestin and the risk of coronary heart disease. *N Engl J Med.* 2003;349:523-534.

47. FDA updates hormone therapy information for postmenopausal women. 2004. http://www.fda.gov/bbs/topics/NEWS/2004/NEW01022.html. Accessed March 5, 2008.

48. Grodstein F, Stampfer MJ, Colditz GA, et al. Postmenopausal hormone therapy and mortality. *N Engl J Med.* 1997;336:1769-1775.

49. Rossouw JE, Prentice RL, Manson JE, et al. Postmenopausal hormone therapy and risk of cardiovascular disease by age and years since menopause. *JAMA.* 2007;297:1465-1477.

50. Manson JE, Allison MA, Rossouw JE, et al. Estrogen therapy and coronary-artery calcification. *N Engl J Med.* 2007;356:2591-2602.

51. Greenland P, Bonow RO, Brundage BH, et al. ACCF/AHA 2007 clinical expert consensus document on coronary artery calcium scoring by computed tomography in global cardiovascular risk assessment and in evaluation of patients with chest pain: a report of the American College of Cardiology Foundation Clinical Expert Consensus Task Force (ACCF/AHA Writing Committee to Update the 2000 Expert Consensus Document on Electron Beam Computed Tomography) developed in collaboration with the Society of Atherosclerosis Imaging and Prevention and the Society of Cardiovascular Computed Tomography. *J Am Coll Cardiol.* 2007;49:378-402.

52. Salpeter SR, Walsh JM, Greyber E, Salpeter EE. Brief report: coronary heart disease events associated with hormone therapy in younger and older women. A meta-analysis. *J Gen Intern Med.* 2006;21:363-366.

53. Salpeter SR, Walsh JM, Greyber E, Ormiston TM, Salpeter EE. Mortality associated with hormone replacement therapy in younger and older women: a meta-analysis. *J Gen Intern Med.* 2004;19:791-804.

54. Lobo RA. Evaluation of cardiovascular event rates with hormone therapy in healthy, early postmenopausal women: results from 2 large clinical trials. *Arch Intern Med.* 2004;164:482-484.

55. Grodstein F, Manson JE, Stampfer MJ. Hormone therapy and coronary heart disease: the role of time since menopause and age at hormone initiation. *J Womens Health* (Larchmt). 2006;15:35-44.

56. Mikkola TS, Clarkson TB. Estrogen replacement therapy, atherosclerosis, and vascular function. *Cardiovasc Res.* 2002;53:605-619.

57. Mendelsohn ME, Karas RH. Molecular and cellular basis of cardiovascular gender differences. *Science.* 2005;308:1583-1587.

58. Miller VM, Mulvagh SL. Sex steroids and endothelial function: translating basic science to clinical practice. *Trends Pharmacol Sci.* 2007;28:263-270.

59. Manson JE, Bassuk SS. Invited commentary: hormone therapy and risk of coronary heart disease—why renew the focus on the early years of menopause? *Am J Epidemiol.* 2007;166:511-517.

60. Salpeter SR, Walsh JM, Ormiston TM, Greyber E, Buckley NS, Salpeter EE. Meta-analysis: effect of hormone-replacement therapy on components of the metabolic syndrome in postmenopausal women. *Diabetes Obes Metab.* 2006;8:538-554.

61. Sherwood A, Bower JK, McFetridge-Durdle J, Blumenthal JA, Newby LK, Hinderliter AL. Age moderates the short-term effects of transdermal 17beta-estradiol on endothelium-dependent vascular function in postmenopausal women. *Arterioscler Thromb Vasc Biol.* 2007;27:1782-1787.

62. Hodis HN, Mack WJ. Postmenopausal hormone therapy in clinical perspective. *Menopause.* 2007;14:944-957.

63. Hodis HN, Mack WJ. Postmenopausal hormone therapy and cardiovascular disease: making sense of the evidence. *Current Cardiovascular Risk Reports.* 2007; 1:138-147.

64. Ridker PM, Hennekens CH, Rifai N, Buring JE, Manson JE. Hormone replacement therapy and increased plasma concentration of C-reactive protein. *Circulation.* 1999;100:713-716.

65. Straub RH, Hense HW, Andus T, Scholmerich J, Riegger GA, Schunkert H. Hormone replacement therapy and interrelation between serum interleukin-6 and body mass index in postmenopausal women: a population-based study. *J Clin Endocrinol Metab.* 2000;85:1340-1344.

66. Hodis HN, St John JA, Xiang M, Cushman M, Lobo RA, Mack WJ. Inflammatory markers and progression of subclinical atherosclerosis in healthy postmenopausal women. *Am J Cardiol.* 2007.

67. Zanger D, Yang BK, Ardans J, et al. Divergent effects of hormone therapy on serum markers of inflammation in postmenopausal women with coronary artery disease on appropriate medical management. *J Am Coll Cardiol.* 2000;36:1797-1802.

68. Canonico M, Oger E, Plu-Bureau G, et al. Hormone therapy and venous thromboembolism among postmenopausal women: impact of the route of estrogen administration and progestogens: the ESTHER study. *Circulation.* 2007;115:840-845.

69. Hwang J, Hodis HN, Hsiai TK, Asatryan L, Sevanian A. Role of annexin II in estrogen-induced macrophage matrix metalloproteinase-9 activity: the modulating effect of statins. *Atherosclerosis.* 2006;189:76-82.

70. Diano S, Horvath TL, Mor G, et al. Aromatase and estrogen receptor immunore-activity in the coronary arteries of monkeys and human subjects. *Menopause.* 1999;6:21-28.

71. Clarkson TB, Anthony MS, Morgan TM. Inhibition of postmenopausal athero-sclerosis progression: a comparison of the effects of conjugated equine estrogens and soy phytoestrogens. *J Clin Endocrinol Metab.* 2001;86:41-47.

72. Adams MR, Register TC, Golden DL, Wagner JD, Williams JK. Medroxyproges-terone acetate antagonizes inhibitory effects of conjugated equine estrogens on coronary artery atherosclerosis. *Arterioscler Thromb Vasc Biol.* 1997;17:217-221.

73. Williams JK, Anthony MS, Honore EK, et al. Regression of atherosclerosis in fe-male monkeys. *Arterioscler Thromb Vasc Biol.* 1995;15:827-836.

74. Hodis HN, Mack WJ, Azen SP, et al. Hormone therapy and the progression of coronary-artery atherosclerosis in postmenopausal women. *N Engl J Med.* 2003; 349:535-545.

75. Harman SM, Brinton EA, Cedars M, et al. Estrogen in the prevention of athero-sclerosis. A randomized, double-blind, placebo-controlled trial. *Ann Intern Med.* 2001;135:939-953.

76. Hodis HN, Mack WJ, Lobo RA et al.

77. Clarke SC, Kelleher J, Lloyd-Jones H, Slack M, Schofiel PM. A study of hormone replacement therapy in postmenopausal women with ischaemic heart disease: the Papworth HRT atherosclerosis study. *BJOG.* 2002;109:1056-1062.

78. Writing group for the PEPI Trial Effects of estrogen or estrogen/progestin regi-mens on heart disease risk factors in postmenopausal women. The Post-menopausal Estrogen/Progestin Interventions (PEPI) Trial. *JAMA.* 1995;273: 199-208.

79. Sendag F, Karadadas N, Ozsener S, Bilgin O. Effects of sequential combined trans-dermal and oral hormone replacement therapies on serum lipid and lipoproteins in postmenopausal women. *Arch Gynecol Obstet.* 2002;266:38-43.

80. Zegura B, Guzic-Salobir B, Sebestjen M, Keber I. The effect of various meno-pausal hormone therapies on markers of inflammation, coagulation, fibrinolysis, lipids, and lipoproteins in healthy postmenopausal women. *Menopause.* 2006;13:643-650.

81. Scarabin PY, Oger E, Plu-Bureau G. Differential association of oral and transder-mal oestrogen-replacement therapy with venous thromboembolism risk. *Lancet.* 2003;362:428-432.

82. Ostberg JE, Storry C, Donald AE, Attar MJ, Halcox JP, Conway GS. A dose-response study of hormone replacement in young hypogonadal women: effects on intima media thickness and metabolism. *Clin Endocrinol* (Oxf). 2007;66:557-564.

83. Lindsay R, Gallagher JC, Kleerekoper M, Pickar JH. Effect of lower doses of con-jugated equine estrogens with and without medroxyprogesterone acetate on bone in early postmenopausal women. *JAMA.* 2002;287:2668-2676.

84. Blumel JE, Castelo-Branco C, Binfa L, et al. Quality of life after the menopause: a population study. *Maturitas.* 2000;34:17-23.

85. Ge Q, Tian Q, Tseng H, Naftolin F. Development of low-dose reproductive hor-mone therapies in China. *Gynecol Endocrinol.* 2006;22:636-645.

86. Lindsay R. The menopause: sex steroids and osteoporosis. *Clin Obstet Gynecol.* 1987;30:847-859.

87. Smith TW, Uchino BN, Berg CA, et al. Hostile personality traits and coronary ar-tery calcification in middle-aged and older married couples: different effects for self-reports versus spouse ratings. *Psychosom Med.* 2007;69:441-448.

88. Kanaya AM, Herrington D, Vittinghoff E, et al. Glycemic effects of post-menopausal hormone therapy: the Heart and Estrogen/progestin Replacement Study. A randomized, double-blind, placebo-controlled trial. *Ann Intern Med.* 2003;138:1-9.

89. LeBlanc ES, Janowsky J, Chan BK, Nelson HD. Hormone replacement therapy and cognition: systematic review and meta-analysis. *JAMA.* 2001;285:1489-1499.

90. Schuetz F, Diel IJ, Pueschel M, et al. Reduced incidence of distant metastases and lower mortality in 1072 patients with breast cancer with a history of hormone replacement therapy. *Am J Obstet Gynecol.* 2007;196:342 e1-e9.

91. Grodstein F, Stampfer MJ, Colditz GA, et al. Postmenopausal hormone therapy and mortality [comment]. *N Engl J Med.* 1997;336:1769-1775.

92. Gloyn AL, Weedon MN, Owen KR, et al. Large-scale association studies of variants in genes encoding the pancreatic beta-cell KATP channel subunits Kir6.2 (KCNJ11) and SUR1 (ABCC8) confirm that the KCNJ11 E23K variant is associated with type 2 diabetes. *Diabetes.* 2003;52:568-572.

93. Chen WY, Manson JE, Hankinson SE, et al. Unopposed estrogen therapy and the risk of invasive breast cancer. *Arch Intern Med.* 2006;166:1027-1032.

94. Mendelsohn ME, Karas RH. HRT and the young at heart. *N Engl J Med.* 2007;356:2639-2641.

95. Marroquin OC, Kip KE, Kelley DE, et al. Metabolic syndrome modifies the cardiovascular risk associated with angiographic coronary artery disease in women: a report from the Women's Ischemia Syndrome Evaluation. *Circulation.* 2004;109:714-721.

96. Stampfer MJ, Hu FB, Manson, JE, Rimm EB, Willett WC. Primary prevention of coronary heart disease in women through diet and lifestyle. *N Engl J Med.* 2000:343:16-22.

CHAPTER 14

The Global Scourge of the 21st Century: Diabetes and Worse, for Women

INTRODUCTION

The current discourse on global health fails to appreciate a growing epidemic of chronic disease—especially diabetes—and its cost to society at all levels. Currently, 246 million people live with diabetes, a figure that is expected to increase 50% by the year 2025.[1,2] Diabetes is also no longer only a problem in developed countries. In fact, a majority of the 1 to 3 million yearly deaths due to diabetes occurs in low- and middle-income countries.[3] An ageing world population, increased urbanization, and changing lifestyle and dietary habits contribute to the expected increase in diabetes as a major cause of death globally.

Interestingly, women constitute approximately 10% more of current and future predicted diabetes cases than men,[4] and our review of this subject has generally revealed worse manifestations of diabetes in women. In many cases this is related to unknown pathophysiologic mechanisms such as the relatively poorer survival in women with diabetes compared with men with diabetes, or the greater mortality rate of myocardial infarction (MI) in diabetic women versus men. In other cases it may be related to gender-specific differences in treatment or in prevention of the same complication, such as coronary artery disease. Although there has been documentation of some gender differences in access to medical care, such studies are few and occasionally document worse access for men. In the end we conclude that current studies of access and treatment are insufficient, and future studies in diabetes must collect the gender-specific data necessary to better inform us. Thus, this chapter will discuss differences in morbidity and mortality as experienced by women and men with diabetes—with many manifestations worse for women.

Diabetes is a chronic disease characterized by either absolute or relative insulin deficiency with concomitant increases in serum glucose. Type 1 diabetes accounts for 5–10% of North American adult diabetes patients[5] and is an autoimmune form of the disease in which the rather sudden destruction of pancreatic beta cells results in little or no insulin production producing the acute complications of severe hyperglycemia, dehydration, and

Dima Yeshou, MD;
Michelle R. Detwiler, MA;
Donald A. Smith, MD, MPH

Dima Yeshou, MD, is in the Department of Endocrinology at Mt Sinai School of Medicine located in New York, NY.

Michelle R. Detwiler, MA, is a Consultant based in Houston, TX.

Donald A. Smith, MD, MPH is an Associate Professor of Medicine and Community Medicine in the Mount Sinai School of Medicine, New York, NY.

ketoacidosis. The much more prevalent type 2 diabetes is a disorder that develops slowly and because of the lack of acute symptoms seen in type 1, often has an unknown date of onset, resulting in many individuals being unaware of having the disease.

Generally the presence of insulin resistance leading to type 2 diabetes has genetic roots with increasing insulin resistance demanding higher insulin levels at the onset. Increasing age, central abdominal obesity, and lack of physical activity increase the insulin resistance associated with a steady, slow loss of insulin production by the beta cells eventually resulting in hyperglycemia, the presence of which establishes the diagnosis. Both types of diabetes may lead to the microvascular problems of retinopathy, nephropathy, and neuropathy and to the macrovascular problems of stroke, heart attack, and peripheral vascular disease. Given the much greater public health problem created by the sheer number of persons with type 2 diabetes compared with those with type 1, we shall focus in this chapter on the global problems associated with type 2 diabetes. Certainly when considering endocrine or metabolic disorders that will have the greatest impact on global women's health, nothing comes close to the devastating effects of increasing overweight/obesity and the secondary increase in maturity-onset, or type 2, diabetes.

Increased Prevalence of Diabetes in All Parts of the World: Women More So Than Men

Globally, diabetes is the most common noncommunicable metabolic disease. Currently, approximately 246 million people, or 6.0% of the adult population worldwide have diabetes—and those numbers are growing. By 2025, the International Diabetes Federation estimates that 380 million people worldwide will have diabetes.[1] With large populations, China and India are home to the highest absolute number of people living with diabetes in the world, 35.5 and 23.8 million respectively—and those numbers are estimated to double by 2025 (Figure 14-1).

While diabetes has a somewhat well-known presence in more developed regions of the world, many developing and newly industrialized countries are experiencing near epidemic upsurges. In fact, developing countries in general will see the largest increase in diabetes prevalence over the next 20 years.[4] The prevalence rate in countries of the Middle East and Eastern Mediterranean (EMME) region already exceeds that of North America (NA) and Europe (EUR) (see Figure 14-2).

Of the overall top 10 countries with highest prevalence rates, four are situated in the Persian Gulf: United Arab Emirates, Bahrain, Kuwait, and

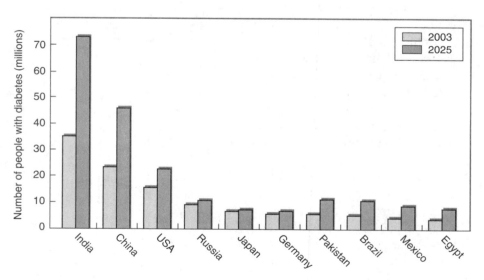

FIGURE 14-1 Top 10 Countries. Estimated number of ppl. with diabetes (age 20–79)
Source: Data from: Diabetes Atlas, 2nd edition. International Diabetes Federation, 2003.

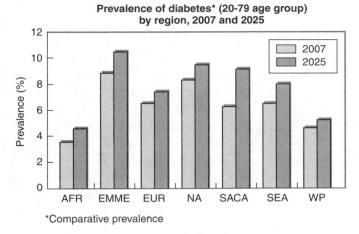

Prevalence of diabetes* (20-79 age group) by region, 2007 and 2025

*Comparative prevalence

FIGURE 14-2   Top 10 Countries. Prevalence of diabetes* (age 20–79), 2007 and 2025
Source: **Diabetes Atlas Third Edition, International Diabetes Federation, 2006.**

Oman (see Figure 14-2). A prevalence of 10% among adults older than 35 years old and 35% among those older than 65 years old reveals a huge public health problem in this area.[6] Such increases are of special concern for women, in part because more women around the world will have diabetes than men. There is a female predominance in the estimates of the number of persons with diabetes for both 2003 and 2025 by approximately 10%, and impaired glucose tolerance—the precursor for diabetes—also affects approximately 20% more women than men. Gestational diabetes is also a unique concern for women. It complicates pregnancies in 2.5–4% of women in the United States, for example, putting them at greater risk for infections, preeclampsia, and Cesarean section. Women with gestational diabetes also have up to a 63% risk of developing type 2 diabetes later in life.

Diabetes prevalence between ethnic groups can also vary widely within a country. In the United States for example, the prevalence of type 2 diabetes is at least 2–4 times higher among African-Americans, Hispanic, and Asian/Pacific Islander women than among white women. It is also a leading cause of death among Alaska natives and American Indians. Two-thirds of Pima Indian women age 45–64 years have diabetes, as do an estimated 41% of Navajo women in this age group. The highest prevalence rates of diabetes occur among native Hawaiian women and Yacqui Indian women.[7]

Increased Diabetic Complications in Women

In the Framingham Heart Study, women with diabetes had an 8.2 years shorter life expectancy than women without diabetes.[8] This shorter life expectancy, like that of 7.5 years in males with diabetes, most likely represents the cardiovascular complications associated with diabetes. Social, economic, and political barriers may also block high-quality care and easy access to health care for women with diabetes.[8]

Even when no symptoms are present, chronic elevation of blood glucose will eventually lead to tissue damage. Although tissue damage can occur in many organs, the kidneys, eyes, peripheral nerves, and vascular tree manifest the most significant diabetic complications. The elderly are at greater risk of developing diabetic complications such as heart disease, stroke, kidney disease, and blindness. Elderly women with diabetes are at particularly high risk for heart disease, visual problems, hyperglycemia or hypoglycemia, and depression.[2]

The mechanism by which diabetes leads to these complications involves the direct toxic effects of high glucose levels, along with the effect of often-associated elevated blood pressure, abnormal lipid levels, increased thrombotic and decreased fibrinolytic parameters, increased inflammation, and both functional and structural abnormalities of small blood vessels.[2]

Mortality Worsened in Those with Diabetes

Cardiovascular disease is the major cause of death in diabetic patients. People with diabetes without previous heart attacks have as high a risk of heart attacks as have nondiabetic patients with previous myocardial infarction.[9] The risks associated with heart disease are more serious among women than men. Women with diabetes who have a heart attack have lower survival rates and a poorer quality of life than men.[10] In the United States, diabetes is a leading cause of death among middle-aged women: fifth among white women, fourth among black and American Indian women, and third among Hispanic women aged 45–64 years. African-American, American Indian, and Hispanic women all have higher diabetes mortality rates than white women. Compared with elderly white women, elderly black women have twice the rate of death from diabetes, and elderly Mexican-American women have almost four times the rate.[11]

While all-cause mortality rates measured in the National Health and Nutritional Exam Survey (NHANES) follow-up studies in the United States from 1970 through 2001 decreased similarly among nondiabetic and diabetic men aged 35–74 years by 32% and 39% respectively, rates in nondiabetic women dropped 12% but increased by 31% in diabetic women. Furthermore, cardiovascular mortality rates have drastically decreased 45% in diabetic men but declined only 11% in diabetic women. The decline in heart disease mortality in the general US population has been attributed to better control of cardiovascular risk factors and improvement in treatment of heart disease. The smaller declines in cardiovascular mortality for diabetic women in the present study indicate that these changes may have been less effective for diabetic women.[12]

Previous studies have looked at the possible explanations of poor outcomes in diabetic women compared to men. Over the last three decades, diabetic women showed less improvement in cardiovascular disease risk factors than men.[13] Over the last two decades, hypertension control has improved for men but remained unchanged for women.[14] In addition, aspirin use was lower among women compared with men.[15] Only 35% of women with a history of diabetes were taking statin drugs compared to 45% in men. Overall 40% of women achieved total serum cholesterol levels of less than 200 mg/dL ($\leq$5 mmol/L) compared to 61% of men.[16]

Fewer women undergo cardiac catheterization or coronary bypass surgery despite their reports of symptoms consistent with greater functional disability from angina. Physicians are less aggressive in the management of coronary disease in women than in men.[17] Sex differences in the pathophysiology of coronary heart disease have been proposed, including a greater tendency for women to have more diffuse and more severe coronary atherosclerosis with higher prevalence of three-vessel disease.[18]

Increased Mortality Post-MI

In a study of approximately 2000 patients (124 diabetic patients) aged 25–64 years with a first-ever MI in the hospitals in Kaunas, Lithuania, in 1983–1992, 28-day and 1-year recurrent MI rates were the same in diabetic and nondiabetic patients, but 28-day and 1-year mortality rates following acute MI in diabetic subjects were approximately double those in nondiabetic patients. An earlier meta-analysis of eight prospective studies also showed that the multivariate-adjusted odds ratio for death in diabetic patients post-MI was 2.3 for men and 2.9 for women.[19] In the Kaunas study, 48% of diabetic patients with acute MI were female while in the nondiabetic population only 21% were female. Diabetic patients with their first MI had double the rates of hypertension, obesity, and acute congestive heart failure of nondiabetic patients. In the diabetic population, female versus male gender was associated with a 30-fold increased risk of death during the following 28 days, and a trend toward a 2.8-fold increase in 1-year death ($P = .09$). In the nondiabetic population, however, female gender held no increased risk for 28-day death, and was associated with reduced 1-year death rates of 34% ($P = .04$). Such discrepant outcomes post-MI for men and women with diabetes demands that metabolic and treatment differences associated with these mortality differences must be better understood if diabetic women are going to increase their survival post-MI.[10]

Increased Leg Amputations

The most common manifestation of diabetic neuropathy is sensory loss in the feet. Neuropathy can sometimes lead to severe pain, but it is often silent. Even in the absence of symptoms, neuropathy increases the risk of foot ulceration and amputation.[2] Foot ulceration affects 15% of diabetic patients during their lifetime.[20] A study of new diabetic foot ulcers in Germany, Tanzania, and South Africa showed foot ulcerations to be much more common in men than women.[21] More than half of diabetic patients with a history of neuropathy and foot ulceration develop recurrent foot ulcers.[22] There is a poor awareness regarding the need for foot care among diabetic patients.[23] Several social and cultural practices such as barefoot walking, inadequate facilities for diabetes care and education, and poor socioeconomic conditions play a role in the increased burden of the diabetic foot. In one study, patients without foot problems spent 9.3% of their total income on treatment, while patients with foot problems had to spend up to 32.3% of their total income.[24] While peripheral neuropathy was a common risk condition among patients, there is a wide discrepancy between Western countries and those in developing countries in peripheral vascular disease and amputation rate. Despite a lesser prevalence of peripheral vascular disease, subcontinent Indians have a higher prevalence of amputation rate when compared to those in Western countries—likely due to progressive infection.[21]

Increased Proliferative Retinopathy

Diabetic retinopathy remains the most important cause of visual loss in the developed world. Despite being the most characteristic, easily identifiable, and treatable complication of diabetes,[25] a significant number of people, even in developed countries, have retinopathy at the time of diagnosis since type 2 diabetes often remains undiagnosed for several years.[26] In one study, while the prevalence of diabetic retinopathy varied from 29% in persons who had diabetes for less than 5 years to 78% in persons who had diabetes for 15 or more years, the rate of proliferative diabetic retinopathy varied from 2% in persons who had

diabetes for less than 5 years to 16% in persons who had diabetes for 15 or more years.[27] Significantly, the risk of proliferative retinopathy is higher for girls, and women are at greater risk of blindness from diabetes than men.[11]

Causes of Increased Diabesity

Because of the close association of increasing abdominal obesity and the onset of type 2 diabetes, the term *diabesity* has been coined and serves to emphasize the management and prevention of obesity as a means to controlling the current upsurge in the prevalence of diabetes.

Obesity—Background

Increasing abdominal obesity and the onset of type 2 diabetes are closely associated. Figure 14-3 illustrates that for most regions of the world 50–90% of all cases of diabetes are attributable to weight gain, especially for women. Females with increased weight are more prone to develop

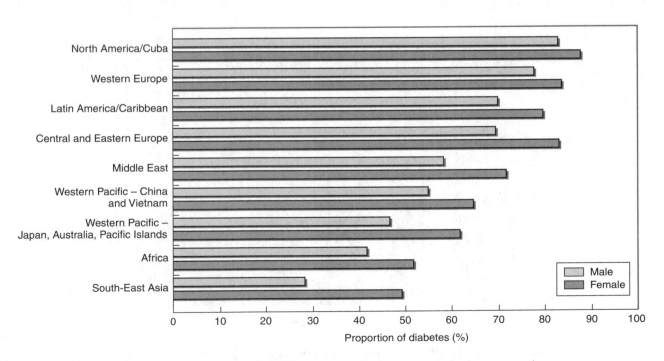

FIGURE 14-3   Proportion of diabetes (%) attributable to weight gain by region (30+ Years)
Source: **Diabetes Atlas second edition, International Obesity Task force, 2003.**

diabetes than men, especially in the regions of Central and Eastern Europe, the Middle East, Western Pacific, and Southeast Asia.

The World Health Organization defines obesity using the body mass index (BMI)—defined as weight in kilograms divided by height in meters squared. Persons are generally considered overweight if BMI is greater than 25.0–29.9 kg/m², obese if BMI is greater than 30 kg/m,² and morbidly obese if BMI is equal to or greater than 40 kg/m.²

Rates of overweight and obesity have increased rapidly worldwide over the last few decades with increased caloric consumption of high-simple-carbohydrate, high-fat diets and decreased levels of physical activity. Approximately 320 million people in the world are obese, and more than 1.1 billion people are overweight.² The levels of overweight and obesity are extremely high in the countries of the Middle East and the Eastern Mediterranean, particularly among women in countries such as Egypt and Saudi Arabia. Most countries in Europe report obesity rates of more than 10% while the rate of obesity in women in South and Central America is up to 36%.[28] Because of the relationship between weight gain and developing diabetes, high and increasing rates of obesity around the world as seen above increase the epidemic of diabetes in adults.

Regrettably, the world is also facing an increased prevalence of obesity among children that puts them at increased risk of developing diabetes at an early age. See Figure 14-4.

Genetic and Intrauterine Influences on Adult Obesity and Diabetes

The global epidemic in obesity and diabetes has generated many genetic and environmental hypotheses to help understand and thus modify the problem. A first explanation, the "thrifty gene hypothesis" offered by Neel in the 1960s suggested that a gene selected for its ability to increase survival in famine by promoting energy conservation and fat accumulation in times of sufficient food would lead to obesity and insulin resistance in times of excess nutrient supply.[29]

Hales and Barker then extended this genetic concept to a "thrifty phenotype" hypothesis based on their finding in the United Kingdom of lower human birth weight being associated with later development of obesity and insulin resistance in midlife.[30] This suggested that fetal exposure to malnutrition could lead to permanent programming of the organism to maximally conserve energy resulting in obesity and insulin resistance in times of excess nutrient supply. The association of

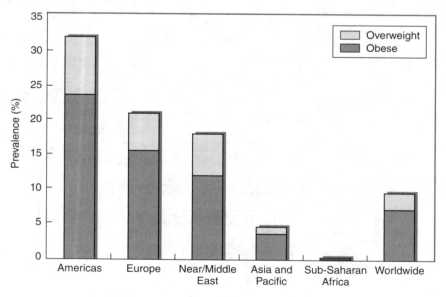

FIGURE 14-4   Overweight and obesity among school-age children (5–17 years)
Source: **Diabetes Atlas second edition, International Obesity Task force, 2003.**

low birth weight and the later development of obesity and metabolic syndrome has been found in other settings as well.[31-33] The calorically deprived fetus and later child responds by the development of a thrifty phenotype that hoards calories as an environmental adaptation. According to this hypothesis, the intrauterine growth retardation and low birth weight common to babies in developing countries may establish populations of adults susceptible to obesity and insulin resistance. Most importantly from the public health point of view, this hypothesis suggested that if a specific gestational, maternal dietary pattern could be proven to program an offspring's lifelong susceptibility to obesity and insulin resistance, then gestational dietary interventions could potentially have a major beneficial global impact on the growing diabetes epidemic.

On the other hand, maternal gestational overnutrition can also have negative biological responses that may foster later problems for both mother and child. Maternal insulin resistance during pregnancy may protect against fetal malnutrition by preferentially driving available calories toward the fetus; such a tendency poses an increased risk of developing diabetes for the mother later in life.[32] In settings of excess calories during pregnancy, typical of urban settings of the late 1900s, maternal insulin resistance has also been associated with high birth weight, which itself correlates with later obesity and diabetes in the offspring.[34] The field is extraordinarily complex, however, and such statements are not universal when studies are compared even among countries in Asia.[32]

Other Gestational and Infancy Risk Factors for Obesity

In a 1958 British birth cohort, maternal smoking during pregnancy was associated with lower birth weight in offspring but with an increased risk of being in the heaviest decile of BMI at ages 7 through 33 years.[35] In a study of 13,500 Bavarian children entering school, length of exclusive breastfeeding was associated in a dose-response fashion with a reduction in being overweight (>90th percentile) or obese (>97th percentile) not attributable to differences in social class or lifestyle.[36] Do these two findings represent other examples of fetal and infant imprinting or programming?[37] If so, and if such epidemiologic studies could be replicated, this type of information would provide extremely important public health tools to assist in reversing the global diabesity epidemic.

Increased Urbanization and Migration

Urbanization and migration in response to poverty and lack of employment negatively affect people's weight. Obesity among immigrants becomes increasingly likely as time passes after migration.[38-40] The prevalence of diabetes in multiple ethnic groups entering more high-calorie, low-activity environments increases about 20 years after immigration.[41]

There is a wide range of type 2 diabetes prevalence within the same or similar ethnic groups, when living under different conditions. Many of the differences between these rates reflect underlying behavioral and environmental and social risk factors, such as diet, level of obesity, and physical activity. Higher rates of type 2 diabetes are usually found in migrant or urbanized populations within the same ethnic groups. The rate of urbanization in India has doubled over the last 50 years. The lowest rates are generally found in rural communities where people have the highest level of physical activity. However, even in rural areas of India there has been a threefold increase in the prevalence of diabetes over the 14-year period ending in 2003 related to increases in physical inactivity and abdominal fat as economic and working conditions have improved and manual labor jobs have decreased.[42] Some studies of diabetes in rural India have also shown prevalence rates of diabetes similar to those in Delhi and London, and thus surveillance studies must be encouraged to keep track of the severity of the growing problem.[43]

Physical Inactivity

In the southern Indian city of Chennai, the prevalence of both metabolic syndrome and coronary heart disease were more than double in those with light versus heavy activity.[44] Prentice, in studies in the United Kingdom, concluded that it is inactivity created by the technological revolution, and particularly television watching, that was the dominant factor in the obesity epidemic reported in the mid-1990s.[45] He felt that physical inactivity was the basis of population susceptibility to obesity while the individual's inability to decrease calories to match the lowered activity level was the key individual determinant.[46]

A linear graded relationship was observed between physical inactivity and diabetes, with diabetes higher among those engaging in light exercise compared to moderate and heavy activities. Numerous modern occupational, lifestyle, and environmental changes such as machine-driven jobs, computers and Internet access, television, urban absence of places for children to play or for youth and adults to practice sports aggravate the global problem of obesity and diabetes.

Increased Dietary Fat and Simple Sugars

As populations increase income and urbanization, they change dietary habits and enter a stage called the "nutrition transition."[47] Diets high in complex carbohydrates are replaced by diets higher in fat, saturated fat, and sugars—all leading to an increase in obesity.[37] In the past, socioeconomic status has been consistently positively associated with obesity. More recently there has been a negative association of socioeconomic status and obesity in developed countries when socioeconomic status is defined by education and occupation, meaning those wealthy by higher education and occupational status tend to be the thinnest. In poorer developing countries the positive association between socioeconomic status, defined by income and material possessions, and obesity is still maintained, meaning those with more material wealth are the most obese.[48]

In many cultures larger physical size means more power, wealth, health, and higher social standing.[48] A fat baby is a healthy baby in societies where poverty and hunger are still realities. A skinny adult or one who is losing weight is thought likely to die, often from a stigmatized disease like tuberculosis or acquired immunodeficiency syndrome. The image of the big, strong, powerful, and healthy adult lingers in the collective imagination even among educated adults with stable food supplies. In such cultures, extra weight may be seen as attractive or sexually appealing.[49] Hispanic and African-American adults are more

likely than white adults to perceive their current overweight status as closer to an ideal body size. In general, African-Americans are more likely to perceive obesity as acceptable, desirable, or sexually attractive.[50-54]

Since the acceleration of obesity in the United States in 1980, the ingredient most increased in the American diet has been high fructose corn syrup mostly found in soft drinks and fruit juices. Consumption of milk with its accompanying calcium is down.[37] One study has demonstrated that higher soft drink consumption in adolescents not only was associated with higher baseline BMI, but also with an increase in BMI over a 2-year period.[55] Fat intake has also increased to a level of 30% of daily caloric consumption, mostly now in the form of vegetable oils, such as corn and soybean oils, with a decrease in butter intake. In animal studies increased fat intake has increased weight, and in human studies fat consumption has been associated with obesity.[56] But decreases in dietary fat using cognitive measures (self-restraint) have not been as successful in weight loss as partially replacing absorbable fat with a nonabsorbable, sucrose polyester fat substitute.[57]

The success of multinational fast-food vendors and changes in the availability of fats and sugars in developing countries has changed the patterns of food preference.[58] The low cost of high-fructose corn syrup and vegetable oils, aided by American governmental subsidies for corn and soybean crops, makes the calories from sweetened beverages and fats extremely cheap.[59] But the global switch to increased fat and sugar has been too great to be accounted for solely by American and multinational vending of fast foods. Surveys of changes in the diets of China and Japan during their nutritional transition showed increases in diversity of foods with increases in nutritional value and in fat.[60] There may be human innate sensory preferences, which previously assuaged in the form of animal fat, dairy products, and sugar in wealthier persons, and are now satisfied in the form of cheaper vegetable oils and high-fructose corn syrup in those with lesser means.[60]

Despite possible human innate sensory preferences to certain nutrients, public health legislation and lobbying interests play important roles in the societal determination of food choices, such as in-school meal programs.[61] In Scandinavia, taxation and import tariffs and public education policies have had a salutary effect on dietary choices and on public health.[62] When WHO recommended tighter restrictions on the use of junk food internationally in 2004 and tighter restrictions on food advertising to children, the United States and other sugar-producing countries opposed its release, illustrating the huge economic considerations at work in world nutrient supply and the growing obesity epidemic.[63,64]

Worldwide Ageing

Populations in most countries around the world are ageing. In developed countries, approximately one-third of the population will exceed age 60 by the year 2050. Older persons will constitute 20% of the population of less developed regions—a marked increase from the present 8%.[65] Because people are living longer (the average lifespan in India has increased 15 years in recent decades), and type 2 diabetes tends to disproportionately affect older persons, the demographic shift of a growing elderly population is likely to dramatically increase rates of diabetes over the next few decades.[66] In general, women live longer than men. In the United States for example, women live an average of 7 years longer than men.[11] Worldwide, elderly women with diabetes are therefore expected to outnumber elderly men with diabetes.

Causes of Increased Complications of Diabetes

Poor Control of Diabetes

A diabetes supplementary questionnaire associated with the 1989 National Health Interview Study (NHIS) was administered to approximately 2200 adults in the United States over the age of 18 with a physician-given diagnosis of diabetes. Even though the frequency of diabetes care was similar among non-Hispanic whites, African-Americans, and Mexican-Americans, there were major differences in the methods of glycemic control and patient education. African-Americans were more likely to be treated with insulin (52%) than non-Hispanic whites (36%) and Mexican-Americans (46%). Among insulin-treated subjects, African-

Americans were less likely to use multiple daily insulin injections and were less likely to self-monitor their blood glucose at least once per day (14% versus 30% of non-Hispanic whites and Mexican-Americans). The rates of visits to specialists for diabetes complications, testing of blood glucose, and screening for hypertension, retinopathy, and foot problems were not substantially different among the three racial/ethnic groups. A higher proportion of African-Americans (43%) than non-Hispanic whites (32%) and Mexican-Americans (26%) had received patient education, but the median number of hours of instruction was lower for African-Americans.[67]

Using data from approximately 1500 adults with type 2 diabetes in the third National Health and Nutrition Exam Survey (NHANES III) of 1988–1994, it was found that many patients with type 2 diabetes in the United States have poor glycemic control, placing them at high risk for diabetic complications. Use of multiple daily insulin injections was more common in whites. HbA1c values in the nondiabetic range were found in 26% of non-Hispanic whites, 17% of non-Hispanic blacks, and 20% of Mexican-Americans. Poor glycemic control (HbA1c > 8%) was more common in non-Hispanic black women (50%) and Mexican-American men (45%) compared with the other groups.[68]

Poor Control of Risk Factors

The 8-year Steno-2 Study randomly assigned individuals with type 2 diabetes and persistent microalbuminuria to intensive multifactorial intervention—tight glucose regulation and the use of renin-angiotensin system blockers, aspirin, and lipid-lowering agents—or conventional treatment. Intensive intervention resulted in a 50% reduction in cardiovascular events and 60% reductions in nephropathy, retinopathy, and autonomic neuropathy.[69] Subjects were then followed for another 6 years in an observational study, and those originally assigned to intensive intervention were found to have reduced risk of cardiovascular events, all cause and cardiovascular mortality, end-stage renal disease, and retinal photocoagulation.[69,70,71] This study has reasonably set the standards by which glucose and risk factor management in patients with diabetes may be evaluated.

Unfortunately in the United States, data from the National Health and Nutritional Exam Survey from 1999–2000 (NHANES 1999–2000) demonstrated that only 37% of participants achieved the target goal of HbA1c level less than 7%, and 37% of participants were above the recommended "take action" HbA1c level of greater than 8.0%. Only 36% of participants achieved the target of systolic blood pressure (SBP) less than 130 mm Hg and diastolic blood pressure (DBP) less than 80 mm Hg, and 40% had hypertensive blood pressure levels (SBP $\geq$ 140 or DBP $\geq$ 90 mm Hg). Worse yet, the above percentages for glucose and blood pressure control had not changed significantly from NHANES III conducted from 1988 to 1994. Although only 48% of the participants in NHANES 1999–2000 had total cholesterol levels at the recommended level of less than 200 mg/dL (5.18 mmol/L), at least this was not as bad as the 34% in the earlier NHANES III. In total, only 7% of adults with diabetes in NHANES 1999–2000 attained all three recommended goals for the prevention of coronary heart disease.[71] Such poor results juxtaposed by the enormous proven benefit of intense glucose and risk factor control cries out for intensified efforts to improve both glucose and risk factor control.

Issues of Access to Care

Part of the poor data on glucose and risk factor control from NHANES 1999–2000 might relate to issues of access to care. Women experience barriers in access to health care around the world. Challenges can be, among others, institutional, financial, cultural, political, geographic, and socioeconomic. A 2007 report to the WHO Commission on Social Determinants of Health cites barriers to care for women including discriminatory user fee structures, unequal human rights status, and lack of participation in health policy making as compared to men.[72] The WHO Department of Gender, Women, and Health finds that for some health issues, women around the world have less knowledge about possibilities for care, less social support, unequal access to family financial resources, and fewer travel options to seek care than do men.[73] While women in general experience challenges, to our knowledge, investigations on gender-specific access to type 2 diabetes care are

few. As detailed below, studies that do exist reveal varied results.

A population-based questionnaire study of general medicine practices in the former Trent Region of the United Kingdom concludes that women suffer more obstacles in accessing diabetes care than do men.[74] To explore why diabetic women experience more morbidity and mortality than men and in recognition of the importance of early control of blood glucose and blood pressure, a random selection of 1673 diabetic patients from 33 primary care practices were sent questionnaires to measure barriers to access to health care. Diabetic women in this study—more often than diabetic men—reported being housebound and having difficulties in finding transport and making convenient appointments. Women were also less likely than men to have talked to a doctor or nurse about their diabetes in the past 12 months. The study points largely to physical access as a significant barrier to care for women in this region.

While the United Kingdom study reveals gender limitations to accessing care, such inequities—because of differences in locality-specific circumstances—are not always biased against women. A study of barriers and facilitators to diabetes care in Tunisia reveals that diabetic men experience greater challenges to accessing initial care.[75] In fact, more women—62% of diabetes patients—attended healthcare facilities than men despite similar prevalence rates of diabetes. A recent study in Krakow, Poland, also found more previously undiagnosed men than women with diabetes in primary health clinics throughout the municipality.[76,77] Because of the many cultural and social complexities of "accessing" care, sensitivities to gender are crucial to delivering quality care for both women and men.

Where access to care is equitable for women and men, outcomes of care could remain uneven. Because women with diabetes have a higher mortality rate from cardiovascular disease than men, outcomes after access to care are particularly important. A review of Swedish population-based studies and statistics published between the years 1990 and 2000 found that diabetic women reported less patient satisfaction and a lower health-related quality of life than diabetic men.[77] If women's self-reported perceptions of care parallel measurable outcomes of care, there is true concern about correcting inequalities.

Similarly, a medical review of over 2000 patients with diabetes throughout Tunisia suggests that outcomes of diabetes care for women and men may be unequal.[78] In this study, women waited longer than men between medical appointments and were less likely to have results of their care recorded in disease-specific medical records that have been linked to better quality of care. A recent study in the United States also suggests that doctors may not be fully informed about women's health issues.[79] Health leaders in this study were largely unaware of the risk of cardiovascular disease for women despite the significant mortality burden.

Unfortunately, little is currently known about the effects of gender on diabetes care in part because investigators have not collected sufficient gender-specific data. A 2006 review of current literature on gender and diabetes care revealed female-specific epidemiological differences, greater prevalence of physiological risk factors, and an increased risk for developing cardiovascular disease for women.[80] However, because most studies on diabetes have been performed on men, the review identified few implications of gender on health outcomes of diabetes care. Drawing conclusions about care based on gender is further impractical because historically, clinical trials have included more male than female participants. Certainly, diabetes diagnosis and care will be improved for women and men where gender-specific barriers within and outside the healthcare system are identified and addressed.

While inequities in access to care do not universally affect women, gender-specific studies to improve opportunities for women's access will be particularly important where the diabetes burden is significant and increasing for women, where women are poised to positively influence societal health, and where cultural barriers acutely influence care for women. Because health inequities exist within and outside the healthcare system, recent studies acknowledge the need to study women's health issues within the social, political, and economic circumstances of women's lives.[81] Reviews of current literature suggest that improving women's health will require cultural change at the household level and institutional acknowledgment of the daily limitations in women's lives. Certainly sensitivity to this complexity should apply to exposing and improving gender-specific challenges to the prevention and delivery of care for women with type 2 diabetes around the world.

Efforts to Prevent Diabetes and Its Complications

Multiple diverse trends in the world are increasing obesity and the onset of type 2 diabetes that will unquestionably demand more and more national health resources. Prevention can be categorized into three different efforts: primary, secondary, and tertiary.

Primary Prevention

Primary prevention aims to prevent or delay the onset of diabetes in women. Undoubtedly the most efficacious way to prevent diabetes is to reverse the global epidemic of obesity. As discussed previously, it is very possible that influences on fetal and early childhood nutrition may affect long-term predisposition to obesity, insulin resistance, and diabetes. Educational programs to improve gestational and early childhood nutrition with neither deficient nor excess calories may be very important. Smoking during pregnancy, which has been associated with smaller newborn size and increased incidence of obesity starting in childhood, should be aggressively discouraged. Breast-feeding should be encouraged if one believes that the Bavarian cross-sectional study proves causality as opposed to association of exclusive breast-feeding and lower weights at ages 5–6. With the growing diabesity epidemic how long can one wait for more historical cohort or interventional confirmatory studies before acting in the public health sphere? Certainly more basic and epidemiologic research should be encouraged in the area of fetal and early childhood nutrition.

From the community point of view, there must be involvement in improving nutrition and activity in schools. Parent–teacher associations, educational administrations, and future teachers must begin to understand how school district policies involving school meals and physical education impact children's health. Educators must become increasingly wary of taking financial gifts from food vendors without specific restrictions on types and caloric content of foods to be vended. Physicians must work with educators and parents to establish advocacies that can foster legislative action for the benefit of children's health. In the United States,

California removed sugared beverages from their public schools following a statewide advocacy program including both physicians and community-minded individuals. Research into the best methodologies for promoting healthy change must be fostered. The National Institutes of Health in the United States is funding a school-based intervention program, the Healthy Study, involving 10,000 children in the sixth to eighth grades aimed at increasing physical activity, improving food service by decreasing calories—especially from fats—and increasing dietary fiber, and marketing an education program designed to help kids buy into a healthier lifestyle.

For adults, industries and corporations must become more involved in promoting programs for increased activity and decreasing caloric intake in the workplace. Policies that forbid the constant display and availability of foods to employees, although dictatorial in concept, could potentially help those individuals less able to constantly refuse such snacks. Architectural plans with more accessible stairways and employee policies encouraging small periods of time for activity may help though more occupational research is desperately needed to study methodologies and evaluate outcomes of increasing work time physical activity.[82]

The epidemiologic data in developed countries showing that higher socioeconomic status measured by education and occupation is associated with decreased prevalence of obesity is hopeful. Just as the highest prevalence of coronary heart disease in the post-World War II era in the upper social stratum has been reversed to the lowest prevalence in the last part of the 1900s, so perhaps can global education targeted to the prevention of obesity, metabolic syndrome, and diabetes change habits resulting in a slow reversal of the current upward trend. This will most likely have to involve legislation requiring the advertisement of food to be accompanied by caloric information, and thus will require the greatest effort by public-health-minded individuals.

Secondary Prevention

Individuals must become more aware when they are at risk of developing diabetes. The simple five-item definition of the metabolic syndrome in the United States and similar definitions in Europe have helped epidemiologists measure the societal extent of the problem and helped physicians more easily inform patients when they are in the "prediabetic stage" in order to allow the motivated patient to begin the 7% weight loss and increased moderate physical activity (150 minutes per week) program that has been shown to reduce onset of overt diabetes from 11% to 4.8% per year, a reduction of 58%.[83] In one study, abdominal diameter index—sagittal abdominal diameter (SAD) (height of abdomen from the table in the reclining position (Figure 14-5) divided by thigh circumference 10 cm proximal to the superior border of the patella—has been shown to be the most powerful anthropometric measure in predicting prevalence of coronary heart disease in male toll workers in New York City, equivalent to the Framingham Risk Score, and still significant when adjusted for the Framingham Risk Score.

Its predictive risk becomes nonsignificant after adjusting for the presence of diabetes and triglyceride levels, suggesting that it might be an anthropometric substitute for the biochemical measures of hyperglycemia and hypertriglyceridemia in global studies where the latter are unavailable.[84] Because we know that the central distribution of body fat is associated with a metabolic profile characterized by higher plasma insulin levels,[85] a

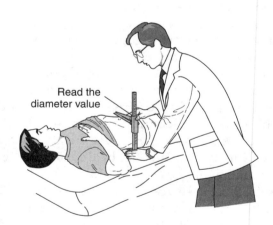

Read the diameter value

FIGURE 14-5 Measuring the sagital abdominal diameter (SAD) index
Reprinted from The American Journal of Cardiology, 78/8, Henry S. Kahn, Eduardo J. Simoes, Mark Koponen and Randy Hanzlick, The Abdominal Diameter Index and Sudden Coronary Death in Men, 1996, with permission from Elsevier.

greater degree of insulin resistance as measured by glucose clamp studies,[86] a higher prevalence of diabetes,[87] and premature coronary artery disease,[88] educating healthcare providers worldwide to universally measure abdominal diameter index—and funding its use—could be a simple and cost-effective preliminary tool to screen for risk of type 2 diabetes in women and men.

Globally, the institution of population-wide fingerstick glucose screening will be the only way to find and inform those with asymptomatic, new-onset type 2 diabetes that they have the disease so they may start earlier to take the necessary steps to prevent complications. In countries where adolescent obesity is increasing, this should begin in secondary schools. Certainly screening for diabetes as early as feasibly possible in pregnancy would reduce the complications of pregnancy for the mother and lower the risk of malformations in the offspring.

Tertiary Prevention

Tertiary prevention aims to eliminate, or at least delay and reduce, the onset and severity of complications and disability caused by diabetes once it has developed, such as cardiovascular disease (heart attacks, congestive heart failure, and strokes), neuropathy, lower limb amputations, blindness, and kidney failure.

The most studied tertiary prevention approaches have been control of glucose, blood pressure, cholesterol, and the use of aspirin to prevent not only the most common and life-threatening cardiovascular outcomes, but the microvascular complications as well. Almost all studies have used pharmacologic agents that fortunately are old enough that generically equivalent, less expensive formulations may be used. Wald and Law first explored the public health benefits of combining a moderate lipid-lowering statin (atorvastatin 10 or simvastatin 40), half doses of three antihypertensives (hydrochlorthiazide, a beta blocker, and an angiotensin-converting enzyme inhibitor), folic acid 0.8 mg/d, and aspirin 75 mg. They predicted such a polypill would decrease ischemic cardiovascular disease by 88% and strokes by 80% if given to all persons age 55 and over and to those younger if they already had experienced cardiovascular disease.[89] The polypill approach created con-

troversy concerning side effects, cost, efficacy, but it did point to the important issue of combining proven cardiovascular preventive agents into one less costly pill. The potential value of using an inexpensive polypill containing a statin, an angiotensin-converting enzyme inhibitor, and aspirin in high-risk patients such as those with diabetes and other risk factors, has been recognized by the Combination Pharmacotherapy and Public Health Research Working Group, WHO, and the World Heart Federation. It is hoped such a recommendation will assist in efforts to develop and test such a pill—combined with lifestyle interventions—as a global preventive strategy for ischemic cardiovascular disease.[90] Such an approach to control the microvascular complications of diabetic hyperglycemia will certainly be necessary as well.

National and International Efforts

Mitigating the global diabetes epidemic will require a broad, organized international effort that promotes research, education, and financing for the numerous problems relating to diabetes. The unanimous adoption of the 2006 UN Resolution on diabetes is one important step in that direction. Resolution 61/225 recognizes the costs of diabetes locally and globally, designates World Diabetes Day as a United Nations Day, and calls on governments to develop national policies targeting the prevention and care of diabetes. Recent response to the resolution includes a joint statement by health ministers from the United Arab Emirates, Bahrain, Kuwait, and other Persian Gulf countries to implement national strategies to alleviate risk factors and improve management and care of diabetes. We hope that other health ministries around the world will also make this a top priority.

Because of the disproportionate effects of diabetes on women, national and international organizations will also have a particularly important role to play in raising awareness and further highlighting women's health issues in this area.

The Centers for Disease Control and Prevention—the public health agency of the US Department of Health and Human Services—called particular attention to diabetes as a women's health issue with the publication of a 2001 report titled *Diabetes & Women's Health Across the Life Stages: A Public Health Perspective*.[11] We have drawn heavily on that report in this paper. Coming out of that report, the CDC cosponsored a National Public Health Initiative on Diabetes and Women's Health. The initiative created action plans on diabetes and women's health with input from a broad range of stakeholders and produced informational articles and radio and television broadcasts. National agenda goals established in the third phase of the initiative could provide a strong framework for other countries. Recognized goals include the need for increased local, state, and federal funding and increased awareness among families and communities of women at risk for developing diabetes. Other priorities include promoting research to better advocate for the prevention and care of diabetes as a women's health issue.

The American Diabetes Association is another US organization working to provide diabetes information and advocacy. The Government Affairs and Advocacy division works to improve access to quality care, eliminate discrimination, increase the federal government's financial commitment to diabetes research and programs, and to incorporate gestational diabetes into legislation being considered in Congress.

At the international level, the World Health Organization is particularly poised to advocate for further research on the gender specificities of diabetes. The WHO maintains multiple offices working on diabetes including the WHO Diabetes Program and the Department of Chronic Disease and Health Promotion. The WHO Global InfoBase also maintains country-specific data on some indicators of diabetes. Further, existing gender analysis work on health issues by the WHO is commendable. A joint study on gender and type 2 diabetes between the WHO Department of Gender, Women, and Health and the WHO Diabetes Program would do much to identify gender inequities where they exist and inform health policy in those areas.

The International Diabetes Federation (IDF) is a global alliance of diabetes associations in over 160 countries. IDF priorities include raising global awareness and advocating prevention and care of diabetes. Through its broad international network, IDF could also be a critical factor in raising awareness about diabetes as a women's health issue. Current gender-neutral efforts by IDF include the creation of diabetes education modules, promo-

tion of World Diabetes Day, and publication of the *Diabetes Atlas*. The *Diabetes Atlas* examines the scope of the current diabetes problem and projected rates of diabetes for 2025 in seven multinational areas of the globe where IDF has its branches (www.diabetesatlas.org).[1,2] The atlas also addresses differences in regional preventive emphasis in differing socioeconomic areas and draws attention to action plans that have been fostered in five regions of the world by a consortium of organizations interested in the problem: Europe (the St. Vincent Declaration, 1989); North, South, and Central America (Declaration of the Americas on Diabetes, 1996, www.dota.org); western Pacific (China, Japan, Singapore, Australia, New Zealand) (Western Pacific Declaration on Diabetes, 2000, www.wpdd.org); Eastern Mediterranean and Middle East region (the Declaration of the Eastern Mediterranean and Middle East Region, 2001).

Fortunately more than 90% of IDF member organizations cooperate with national health authorities on the prevention of type 2 diabetes. One such organization is the World Diabetes Foundation, an independent fund registered in Denmark that currently supports 120 projects in developing countries promoting education, care, and diabetes prevalence studies, among others.

Conclusion

Type 2 diabetes is a rapidly growing global health epidemic. In the coming decades, regions of the world experiencing rapid urbanization and ageing populations should consider implementation of comprehensive primary, secondary, and tertiary prevention programs. Where appropriate, a new sharing of policy priority and public health spending on infectious and chronic diseases such as type 2 diabetes may also be necessary.

Because diabetes is more prevalent in women and adversely affects them more so than men, building on existing initiatives and international networks to incorporate diabetes as a women's health issue could be increasingly important to global public health. While there is currently a tremendous deficiency of knowledge related to the basic pathophysiology of obesity, diabetes, and its complications in women and how it affects their offspring, we do know that women have a unique gestational ability to determine the nutritional environment of the fetus. As mothers of growing children, their understanding of nutrition and personal health is not only of great importance to themselves but to a future generation as well. In addition, gender-specific medical access problems have been minimally studied and in only a few global settings. Efforts to study all of these problems must be strongly encouraged in all regions. If unchecked this epidemic will eventually, and in the not so distant future, produce adverse public health and economic outcomes.

DISCUSSION QUESTIONS

1. A recent study by the University of Colorado Denver reveals that maternal diabetes and obesity influence the onset of type 2 diabetes in offspring.[91] Devise one program that you as the Minister of Health would institute to encourage behavioral change in women desiring pregnancy who are obese or have type 2 diabetes.

2. India has the largest number of current and future predicted persons with type 2 diabetes in the world. Develop a 10-year plan recommending progressive changes in India's healthcare infrastructure that could mitigate economic impacts on families and national income due to direct medical expenditures as well as lost productivity from disability and premature deaths from diabetes. Consider the fact that women constitute approximately 10% more of current and future predicted diabetes cases than men.

3. Assume the role of a small nongovernmental organization and devise an innovative peer-to-peer educational program to combat cultural stigma in a local community where women with diabetes receive inequitable access to diagnosis and care as compared to men.

4. It is a little known fact that most deaths from type 2 diabetes occur in low- and middle-income countries. Create a media campaign to increase awareness of the consequences of type 2 diabetes on global health, comparing the magnitude of the problem to better-known diseases.

REFERENCES

1. International Diabetes Federation. *Diabetes Atlas*. 3rd ed. Brussels, Belgium: International Diabetes Federation; 2006.
2. Diabetes Atlas Committee. *Diabetes Atlas*. 2nd ed. Brussels, Belgium: International Diabetes Federation; 2003.
3. WHO. *Diabetes Fact Sheets No. 312*. Geneva, Switzerland: WHO; 2006.
4. International Diabetes Federation. *Diabetes Atlas*. 2nd ed. Executive Summary. Brussels, Belgium: International Diabetes Federation; 2003.
5. Harris MI, Robbins DC. Prevalence of adult-onset IDDM in the U.S. population. *Diabetes Care*. 1994;17:1337-1340.

6. Thanopoulou A, Karamanos B, Angelico F, et al. Epidemiological evidence for the non-random clustering of the components of the metabolic syndrome: multicentre study of the Mediterranean group for the study of diabetes. *Eur J Clin Nutr.* 2006;60:1376-1383.

7. Williams DR. Racial/ethnic variations in women's health: The social embeddedness of health. *Am J Public Health.* 2002;92:588-597.

8. Franco OH, Steyerberg EW, Hu FB, Mackenbach J, Nusselder W. Associations of diabetes mellitus with total life expectancy and life expectancy with and without cardiovascular disease. *Arch Intern Med.* 2007;167:1145-1151.

9. Haffner SM, Lehto S, Ronnemaa T, Pyorala K, Laakso M. Mortality from coronary heart disease in subjects with type 2 diabetes and in nondiabetic subjects with and without prior myocardial infarction. *N Engl J Med.* 1998;339:229-234.

10. Jancaityte L, Rastenyte D. Short-term and one-year prognosis of diabetic patients with a first-ever myocardial infarction. *Medicina (Kaunas).* 2007;43:555-561.

11. Beckles GLA, Thompson-Reid PE. *Diabetes and Women's Health Across the Life Stages: A Public Health Perspective.* Atlanta, GA: Center for Disease Control and Prevention. http://www.cdc.gov/diabetes/pubs/pdf/women.pdf. Accessed May 12, 2008.

12. Gregg EW, Gu Q, Cheng YJ, Narayan KM, Cowie CC. Mortality trends in men and women with diabetes, 1970 to 2000. *Ann Intern Med.* 2007;147:149-155.

13. Imperatore G, Cadwell BL, Geiss L, et al. Thirty-year trends in cardiovascular risk factor levels among US adults with diabetes: national health and nutrition examination surveys, 1971-2000. *Am J Epidemiol.* 2004;160:531-539.

14. Ostchega Y, Dillon CF, Hughes JP, Carroll M, Yoon S. Trends in hypertension prevalence, awareness, treatment, and control in older U.S. adults: Data from the national health and nutrition examination survey 1988 to 2004. *J Am Geriatr Soc.* 2007;55:1056-1065.

15. Persell SD, Baker DW. Aspirin use among adults with diabetes: Recent trends and emerging sex disparities. *Arch Intern Med.* 2004;164:2492-2499.

16. Tonstad S, Rosvold EO, Furu K, Skurtveit S. Undertreatment and overtreatment with statins: the Oslo health study 2000-2001. *J Intern Med.* 2004;255:494-502.

17. Steingart RM, Packer M, Hamm P, et al. Sex differences in the management of coronary artery disease. Survival and ventricular enlargement investigators. *N Engl J Med.* 1991;325:226-230.

18. Walden CE, Knopp RH, Wahl PW, Beach KW, Strandness E Jr. Sex differences in the effect of diabetes mellitus on lipoprotein triglyceride and cholesterol concentrations. *N Engl J Med.* 1984;311:953-959.

19. Kanaya AM, Grady D, Barrett-Connor E. Explaining the sex difference in coronary heart disease mortality among patients with type 2 diabetes mellitus: a meta-analysis. *Arch Intern Med.* 2002;162:1737-1745.

20. Mayfield JA, Reiber GE, Sanders LJ, Janisse D, Pogach LM, American Diabetes Association. Preventive foot care in people with diabetes. *Diabetes Care.* 2003;26(suppl 1):S78-S79.

21. Morbach S, Lutale JK, Viswanathan V, et al. Regional differences in risk factors and clinical presentation of diabetic foot lesions. *Diabet Med.* 2004;21:91-95.

22. Vijay V, Narasimham DV, Seena R, Snehalatha C, Ramachandran A. Clinical profile of diabetic foot infections in south India—a retrospective study. *Diabet Med.* 2000;17:215-218.

23. Viswanathan V, Shobhana R, Snehalatha C, Seena R, Ramachandran A. Need for education on foot care in diabetic patients in India. *J Assoc Physicians India.* 1999;47:1083-1085.

24. Shobhana R, Rao PR, Lavanya A, Vijay V, Ramachandran A. Cost burden to diabetic patients with foot complications—a study from southern India. *J Assoc Physicians India.* 2000;48:1147-1150.

25. Rahmani B, Tielsch JM, Katz J, et al. The cause-specific prevalence of visual impairment in an urban population. The Baltimore Eye Survey. *Ophthalmology.* 1996;103:1721-1726.

26. Davis TM, Stratton IM, Fox CJ, Holman RR, Turner RC. U.K. prospective diabetes study 22. Effect of age at diagnosis on diabetic tissue damage during the first 6 years of NIDDM. *Diabetes Care.* 1997;20:1435-1441.

27. Klein R, Klein BE, Moss SE, Davis MD, DeMets DL. The Wisconsin Epidemiologic Study of Diabetic Retinopathy. III. Prevalence and risk of diabetic retinopathy when age at diagnosis is 30 or more years. *Arch Ophthalmol.* 1984;102:527-532.

28. Filozof C, Gonzalez C, Sereday M, Mazza C, Braguinsky J. Obesity prevalence and trends in Latin-American countries. *Obes Rev.* 2001;2:99-106.

29. Neel JV. Diabetes mellitus: A "thrifty" genotype rendered detrimental by "progress"? *Am J Hum Genet.* 1962;14:353-362.

30. Hales CN, Barker DJ. Type 2 (non-insulin-dependent) diabetes mellitus: The thrifty phenotype hypothesis. *Diabetologia.* 1992;35:595-601.

31. Levitt NS, Lambert EV. The foetal origins of the metabolic syndrome—a South African perspective. *Cardiovasc J S Afr.* 2002;13:179-180.

32. Yajnik CS. Early life origins of insulin resistance and type 2 diabetes in India and other Asian countries. *J Nutr.* 2004;134:205-210.

33. Ozanne SE, Fernandez-Twinn D, Hales CN. Fetal growth and adult diseases. *Semin Perinatol.* 2004;28:81-87.

34. Dyck RF, Klomp H, Tan L. From "thrifty genotype" to "hefty fetal phenotype": The relationship between high birthweight and diabetes in Saskatchewan registered Indians. *Can J Public Health.* 2001;92:340-344.

35. Power C, Jefferis BJ. Fetal environment and subsequent obesity: a study of maternal smoking. *Int J Epidemiol.* 2002;31:413-419.

36. von Kries R, Koletzko B, Sauerwald T, et al. Breast feeding and obesity: Cross sectional study. *BMJ.* 1999;319:147-150.

37. Bray GA. The epidemic of obesity and changes in food intake: the fluoride hypothesis. *Physiol Behav.* 2004;82:115-121.

38. Kaplan MS, Huguet N, Newsom JT, McFarland BH. The association between length of residence and obesity among Hispanic immigrants. *Am J Prev Med.* 2004;27:323-326.

39. Cairney J, Ostbye T. Time since immigration and excess body weight. *Can J Public Health.* 1999;90:120-124.

40. Goel MS, McCarthy EP, Phillips RS, Wee CC. Obesity among US immigrant subgroups by duration of residence. *JAMA.* 2004;292:2860-2867.

41. Diamond J. The double puzzle of diabetes. *Nature.* 2003;423:599-602.

42. Ramachandran A, Snehalatha C, Baskar AD, et al. Temporal changes in prevalence of diabetes and impaired glucose tolerance associated with lifestyle transition occurring in the rural population in India. *Diabetologia.* 2004;47:860-865.

43. Rao PV, Ushabala P, Seshiah V, Ahuja MM, Mather HM. The Eluru survey: prevalence of known diabetes in a rural Indian population. *Diabetes Res Clin Pract.* 1989;7:29-31.

44. Mohan V, Gokulakrishnan K, Deepa R, Shanthirani CS, Datta M. Association of physical inactivity with components of metabolic syndrome and coronary artery

disease—the Chennai urban population study (CUPS no. 15). *Diabet Med*. 2005;22:1206-1211.

45. Prentice AM, Jebb SA. Obesity in Britain: Gluttony or sloth? *BMJ*. 1995;311:437-439.
46. Prentice AM. Obesity and its potential mechanistic basis. *Br Med Bull*. 2001;60:51-67.
47. Popkin BM. The nutrition transition in low-income countries: an emerging crisis. *Nutr Rev*. 1994;52:285-298.
48. McLaren L. Socioeconomic status and obesity. *Epidemiol Rev*. 2007;29:29-48.
49. Nullis C. Africa faces growing obesity problem. November 29, 2006. http://www .pubmedcentral.nih.gov/articlerender.fcgi?artid=2094018. Accessed March 27, 2007.
50. Lynch E, Liu K, Spring B, Hankinson A, Wei GS, Greenland P. Association of ethnicity and socioeconomic status with judgments of body size: the Coronary Artery Risk Development in Young Adults (CARDYA) study. *Am J Epidemiol*. 2007;165:1055-1062.
51. Bennett GG, Wolin KY. Satisfied or unaware? Racial differences in perceived weight status. *Int J Behav Nutr Phys Act*. 2006;3:40.
52. Juarbe TC. Cardiovascular disease-related diet and exercise experiences of immigrant Mexican women. *West J Nurs Res*. 1998;20:765-782.
53. Davidson M, Knafl KA. Dimensional analysis of the concept of obesity. *J Adv Nurs*. 2006;54:342-350.
54. Becker DM, Yanek LR, Koffman DM, Bronner YC. Body image preferences among urban African Americans and whites from low-income communities. *Ethn Dis*. 1999;9:377-386.
55. Ludwig DS, Peterson KE, Gortmaker SL. Relation between consumption of sugar-sweetened drinks and childhood obesity: a prospective, observational analysis. *Lancet*. 2001;357:505-508.
56. Bray GA, Paeratakul S, Popkin BM. Dietary fat and obesity: A review of animal, clinical and epidemiological studies. *Physiol Behav*. 2004;83:549-555.
57. Roy J, Lovejoy J, Windhauser M, Bray GA. Metabolic effects of fat substitution with olestra [Abstract]. *FASEB*. 1997;11:A358.
58. Candib LM. Obesity and diabetes in vulnerable populations: Reflection on proximal and distal causes. *Ann Fam Med*. 2007;5:547-556.
59. Flannery T. We're living on corn! *New York Rev Books*. 2007;54:26-28.
60. Drewnowski A, Popkin BM. The nutrition transition: new trends in the global diet. *Nutr Rev*. 1997;55:31-43.
61. Hobbs SH, Ricketts TC, Dodds JM, Milio N. Analysis of interest group influence on federal school meals regulations 1992 to 1996. *J Nutr Educ Behav*. 2004;36:90-98.
62. Milio N. Toward healthy longevity. Lessons in food and nutrition policy development from Finland and Norway. *Scand J Soc Med*. 1991;19:209-217.
63. WHO/FAO. Diet, nutrition and the prevention of chronic diseases. Geneva, Switzerland: WHO; 2003.
64. Dyer O. US government rejects WHO's attempts to improve diet. *BMJ*. 2004;328:185.
65. United Nations Department of Economic and Social Affairs, Population Division. World population ageing 2007, executive summary. http://www.un.org/esa /population/publications/WPA2007/ES-English.pdf. Accessed June 27, 2008.
66. Diderichsen B. Diabetes in developing countries. In: Serageldin I, El-Faham M, Massoud A, eds. *Changing Lives*. Egypt: Bibliotheca Alexandrina; 2006:180-213.

67. Cowie CC, Harris MI. Ambulatory medical care for non-Hispanic whites, African-Americans, and Mexican-Americans with NIDDM in the U.S. *Diabetes Care*. 1997;20:142-147.

68. Harris MI, Eastman RC, Cowie CC, Flegal KM, Eberhardt MS. Racial and ethnic differences in glycemic control of adults with type 2 diabetes. *Diabetes Care*. 1999;22:403-408.

69. Gaede P, Vedel P, Larsen N, Jensen GV, Parving HH, Pedersen O. Multifactorial intervention and cardiovascular disease in patients with type 2 diabetes. *N Engl J Med*. 2003;348:383-393.

70. Gaede P, Lund-Andersen H, Parving HH, Pedersen O. Effect of a multifactorial intervention on mortality in type 2 diabetes. *N Engl J Med*. 2008;358:580-591.

71. Saydah SH, Fradkin J, Cowie CC. Poor control of risk factors for vascular disease among adults with previously diagnosed diabetes. *JAMA*. 2004;291:335-342.

72. Sen G, Östlin P, George A. Unequal, unfair, ineffective and inefficient gender inequity in health: why it exists and how we can change it. Final report to the WHO Commission on Social Determinants of Health. Women and Gender Equity Knowledge Network. Geneva, Switzerland: WHO; 2008.

73. Courtright P. *Gender and Blindness*. Geneva, Switzerland: WHO, World Health Organization, Department of Gender and Women's Health: 1998.

74. Hippisley-Cox J, Yates J, Pringle M, Coupland C, Hammersley V. Sex inequalities in access to care for patients with diabetes in primary care: Questionnaire survey. *Br J Gen Pract*. 2006;56:342-348.

75. Alberti H, Boudriga N, Nabli M. Primary care management of diabetes in a low/middle income country: a multi-method, qualitative study of barriers and facilitators to care. *BMC Fam Pract*. 2007;8:63.

76. Szurkowska M, Szafraniec K, Gilis-Januszewska A, et al. Prevalence of the glucose metabolism disturbances in screening of adult inhabitants of Krakow. *Przegl Lek*. 2006;63:728-732.

77. Jonsson PM, Sterky G, Gafvels C, Ostman J. Gender equity in health care: the case of Swedish diabetes care. *Health Care Women Int*. 2000;21:413-431.

78. Alberti H. Sex inequalities. *Br J Gen Pract*. 2006;56:628.

79. Liewer L, Mains DA, Lykens K, Rene AA. Barriers to women's cardiovascular risk knowledge. *Health Care Women Int*. 2008;29:23-38.

80. Legato MJ, Gelzer A, Goland R, et al. Gender-specific care of the patient with diabetes: review and recommendations. *Gend Med*. 2006;3:131-158.

81. Moss NE. Gender equity and socioeconomic inequality: a framework for the patterning of women's health. *Soc Sci Med*. 2002;54:649-661.

82. Jackson SD. The TODAY study. *Curr Diab Rep*. 2007;7:379-380.

83. Knowler WC, Barrett-Connor E, Fowler SE, et al. Reduction in the incidence of type 2 diabetes with lifestyle intervention or metformin. *N Engl J Med*. 2002;346:393-403.

84. Smith DA, Ness EM, Herbert R, et al. Abdominal diameter index: a more powerful anthropometric measure for prevalent coronary heart disease risk in adult males. *Diabetes Obes Metab*. 2005;7:370-380.

85. Snehalatha C, Ramachandran A, Mohan V, Viswanathan M. Insulin response in obese and nonobese offspring of conjugal Indian diabetic parents with increasing glucose intolerance. *Pancreas*. 1986;1:139-142.

86. Laws A, Jeppesen JL, Maheux PC, Schaaf P, Chen YD, Reaven GM. Resistance to insulin-stimulated glucose uptake and dyslipidemia in Asian Indians. *Arterioscler Thromb*. 1994;14:917-922.

87. McKeigue PM, Shah B, Marmot MG. Relation of central obesity and insulin resistance with high diabetes prevalence and cardiovascular risk in south Asians. *Lancet.* 1991;337:382-386.

88. McKeigue PM, Miller GJ, Marmot MG. Coronary heart disease in south Asians overseas: a review. *J Clin Epidemiol.* 1989;42:597-609.

89. Wald NJ, Law MR. A strategy to reduce cardiovascular disease by more than 80%. *BMJ.* 2003;326:1419.

90. Fuster V, Sanz G. A polypill for secondary prevention: time to move from intellectual debate to action. *Nat Clin Pract Cardiovasc Med.* 2007;4:173.

91. Dabelea D, Mayer-Davis EJ, Lamichhane AP, et al. Association of Intrauterine Exposure to Maternal Diabetes and Obesity with Type 2 Diabetes in Youth. *Diabetes Care.* 2008;31:1422-1426.

Neurological Disorders in Women

Gender differences are present in many aspects of neurological health and illness.[1] Differences in brain development between the sexes leads to differences in susceptibility to disease, with women being much more affected by several neurological conditions, including migraines, multiple sclerosis, and systemic lupus erythematosis.

Gayatri Devi, MD

Gayatri Devi, MD, is the Director of The New York Memory and Healthy Aging Services and an attending Physician in the Depts. of Medicine (Neurology) & Psychiatry at Lenox Hill Hospital. He is also a Clinical Associate Professor for the Depts. of Neurology & Psychiatry and New York University School of Medicine, New York, NY.

Migraine

Epidemiology

Migraine affects nearly two to three times as many women as men, with prevalence rates between 8% and 18% worldwide.[2-4] The incidence of migraine in women peaks after puberty, in contrast to men where the peak is at age 5.[5] Migraines typically worsen during the first trimester of pregnancy and then improve, perhaps because of sustained high estrogen levels.[6]

Pathogenesis

Migraine is caused by the interplay of genetic and environmental factors and is most likely caused by abnormal activity of nerve cells in the brain's trigeminal system, with the headache pain secondary to changes in the intracranial and extracranial blood supply.[7-9] This hypothesis is supported by the observed rise in levels of a substance called calcitonin gene-related peptide, which causes blood vessels to dilate and is released by the trigeminovascular system.[9,10]

Migraines generally present as headaches with or without nausea, vomiting, and light sensitivity (photophobia). A migraine "aura" precedes the headache in 12–88% of patients (*classic* migraine) and may be any neurological symptom, but most commonly is visual (99% of auras), with patients experiencing flashing lights or "fortification spectra".[11,12] Some patients develop a transient focal neurological deficit before, during, or after the attack. Triptan and ergot medications are avoided in these patients because of the risk of precipitating stroke.[13] Migraine without aura is also known as *common* migraine.

Treatment

Acute therapies terminate attacks, while chronic treatments prevent recurrence. Analgesics such as acetaminophen and aspirin treat mild attacks, while drugs such as dihydroergotamine and triptans (sumatriptan was the first drug in this class) target the trigemino-cerebrovascular system, and are used to treat more severe migraines.[9,14] Combination treatment with drugs such as acetaminophen, aspirin, ibuprofen, and caffeine may also be effective.[15] Triptans have the advantage of administration through multiple routes, including subcutaneous, intranasal, and oral routes. Less expensive treatments for acute attacks include prochlorperazine (10 mg) or magnesium sulfate (1 gm in 10 cc of normal saline) given intravenously by slow push.[16] Menstrual migraines in women may be helped with oral contraceptive use.[17]

Preventive therapies for migraine include amitriptyline, divalproex sodium, topiramate, and beta-blockers such as propranolol and timolol. Calcium channel blockers (verapamil), fluoxetine, oral magnesium, feverfew, and vitamin B_2 are also effective.[18] Botulinum toxin type A injected into muscles of the neck, jaw, and forehead benefit intractable cases.[19] Eliminating diet and environmental triggers such as excessive caffeine intake is important.[20]

Seizures and Epilepsy

Epidemiology

The lifetime prevalence of seizures is 3–5%, while 0.5–1% of the population has "active epilepsy," a chronic disorder where there are unprovoked recurrent seizures.[21] One-third to two-thirds of women with epilepsy experience changes in seizure activity related to their menstrual cycle and their reproductive lives.[22]

Pathogenesis

Seizures, a symptom, must be distinguished from epilepsy, a disease. It is important to accurately categorize seizures and epilepsy for appropriate treatment. Seizures may be focal (beginning in one area of the brain and confined to one hemisphere) or generalized (beginning in both hemispheres) at onset. A focal seizure may be a simple focal seizure, a partial complex seizure (with some alteration of consciousness, commonly arising in the temporal or frontal lobe), or become secondarily generalized, spreading to the other hemisphere with attendant loss of consciousness. Generalized seizures include generalized tonic-clonic seizures, absence *petit mal* seizures, and myoclonic seizure types and are characterized by bilateral, simultaneous onset of epileptic discharges on an electroencephalogram (EEG). The diagnosis of epilepsy is invariably clinical, as the EEG is normal in 25–50% of patients with generalized tonic-clonic epilepsy and an even higher proportion of patients with partial epilepsy.[23] Epilepsy is a chronic disease that results from predisposition to recurrent seizures and is caused by an underlying structural change in the brain. It is generally always treated to prevent more seizures. Seizures are symptomatic of brain excitability and may occur in a number of conditions and may not require chronic treatment if the underlying cause is treated, for example in the treatment of alcohol withdrawal seizures.

Ovarian steroid hormones affect neuronal excitability, particularly in the temporal and frontal lobes, affecting seizures.[24] Estrogen may be a potent proconvulsant, while progesterone may prevent seizures.[25,26] Catamenial epilepsy involves seizures correlated with the menstrual cycle.[27]

Treatment

Antiepileptic drugs (AEDs) reduce nerve cell excitability through various pathways.[28] When using AEDs in combination to achieve better seizure control when monotherapy is not sufficient, it is best to use AEDs with different mechanisms of action for a synergistic effect. Common AEDs include diphenytoin (active metabolite fosphenytoin) and valproic acid for generalized epilepsy and carbamazepine (active metabolite oxcarbazepine), levetirecetam, gabapentin, and lamotrigine in focal epilepsy. The use of active metabolite drugs reduces side effects associated with the prodrug.[29] Up to one-third of patients are unresponsive to medication and would benefit from epilepsy surgery, an underutilized option.[30]

Phenytoin is generally best avoided in women as chronic use causes the cosmetic disfigurements of hirsutism and gingival hyperplasia. During pregnancy, the best AED to use is the one that best controls the patient's seizures.[31,32] While there is a risk for fetal malformation with the use of AEDs, especially during the first trimester, the general consensus is that the risk to the mother and fetus from uncontrolled seizures is more harmful than the risk posed by the AED. These risks need to be discussed with women of childbearing age on AEDs. There may be a higher risk of congenital malformations with AED polytherapy than monotherapy.[33] For women with catamenial epilepsy, cyclic progesterone supplements and gonadotropin-releasing hormone analogues is of benefit.[34]

Alcohol withdrawal seizures are always generalized and do not require chronic AED treatment.[35] If a patient suspected of having withdrawal seizures has a focal onset, the seizures are not related to alcohol withdrawal. Finally, monitoring drug levels of AEDs is important for ascertaining compliance and bioavailability but *not* for determining toxicity.[35,36] Toxicity is a clinical diagnosis and may occur at any level, although it most often occurs at higher doses.

Stroke

Epidemiology

Stroke is the third leading cause of death in the developed world, and a major cause of long-term disability.[37,38] Two thirds of stroke deaths worldwide occur in developing countries and the incidence continues to rise.[39] Women have a higher lifetime stroke risk than men.[40] Strokes in men are more likely to be associated with ischemic heart disease and diabetes while those in women are more likely associated with hypertension and atrial fibrilla-

tion.[41] Women are also more likely to have stress-associated hypertension and stroke than men.[42]

Pathogenesis and Presentation

Stroke is a focal neurologic disturbance lasting more than 24 hours that is due to loss of blood supply to a brain region secondary to either the rupture (hemorrhagic stroke) or the blockage (ischemic stroke) of a blood vessel supplying an area of the brain.[43] Because any area of the brain may be involved, strokes can clinically present in numerous ways, with paralysis, loss of language or vision, or a change in mental acuity being just a few of the many symptoms.

Ischemic strokes may be thrombotic (due to a clot in a local blood vessel), embolic (a clot breaking off from the heart or from a larger vessel and clogging a smaller blood vessel leading into the brain) or due to reduced blood flow to the brain caused by hemodynamic instability. While 5–10% of strokes present with seizures, hemorrhagic strokes are more likely to do so, with recurrent seizures occurring in 2.5%.[44] Strokes are best detected very early on by special sequencing on MRI.[45] A stroke workup should ascertain the source of the stroke so that treatment may be targeted.

Historically, oral contraceptive pills (OCPs) were linked to strokes, but current low-dose OCPs do not appear to increase stroke risk in women without risk factors.[46] Smoking, hypertension, age over 35, obesity, diabetes, and prior history of thrombotic events may increase stroke risk in women on OCPs.[47] Mutations in certain genes such as the prothrombin gene and Factor V Leiden gene increase risk for cerebral venous thrombosis in patients on OCPs, increasing risk for stroke.[48]

The association between hormone replacement therapy (HRT) and stroke risk is inconclusive, with some studies finding an increased risk and others finding no such change.[49-59] Even in the latter studies however, there was no increase in the risk of stroke *mortality* in women on HRT.[50] HRT may reduce severity of strokes and subsequent morbidity and mortality, even if the frequency is not affected.[60] HRT may especially benefit women with high cholesterol and other risk factors, particularly with early treatment. The Women's Health

Initiative Study found that there was a slight increased risk in stroke among women who were on conjugated equine estrogens and progesterone, but these women began HRT later in life.[61,62] Further research is needed to clarify the association between stroke and HRT.

Treatment

Heparin is often used in the acute treatment of ischemic, nonhemorrhagic strokes, especially when a stroke evolves or an embolic cause is suspected, although the efficacy of heparin remains unproven.[63] In patients requiring protracted anticoagulation, such as those with persistent, paroxysmal atrial fibrillation, chronic treatment with warfarin (Coumadin) is indicated.[64,65]

Recent advances in stroke treatment have been exciting. Tissue plasminogen activator (tPA), intravenously and intra-arterially, is used in the first few hours after a stroke to dissolve clots and restore function.[66] Mechanical clot removal using fine intra-arterial catheters is also effective. These treatment modalities have dramatically altered acute stroke management and recovery.[67] For evolving strokes, acute anticoagulation with heparin is necessary, especially if tPA or clot removal facilities are not available.

For effective primary prevention of stroke and to prevent recurrence, risk factors have to be well controlled using antihypertensive agents, statins, and antiplatelet therapies.[68] Warfarin remains a mainstay for prevention of embolic strokes. Antiplatelet therapies, such as aspirin, clopidogrel, or aspirin in combination with dipyridamole, are effective in reducing stroke recurrences.[69] Exercise, weight loss, and other lifestyle modifications are also important.

Superior Sagittal Sinus Thrombosis (SSST)

Epidemiology

Superior sagittal sinus thrombosis (SSST) is the most common form of cerebral vein thrombosis (CVT), with increased risk during pregnancy.[70] CVT is thought to be responsible for about 0.5–1.0% of all strokes, with women affected three times more than men.[71] Pregnancy, oral contraceptive use, and mutations in the prothrombin gene and Factor V Leiden gene increase CVT risk.[48,72]

Pathogenesis and Presentation

SSST presents with headache in 70–90% of patients.[73] Intracranial hypertension, vein distension, and venous infarction alone, or in combination, cause the symptoms of SSST. Signs include papilledema, brain hemorrhage, seizures, and focal neurologic deficits. However, many patients may present with headaches alone, making diagnosis challenging. Clinical suspicion should be high in pregnant women presenting with headaches. Diagnosis is confirmed by MR venography or CT with contrast showing lack of blood flow through the sagittal sinus.[74,75]

Treatment

Heparin is used acutely to treat SSST.[63] Patients with noninfectious cause of thrombosis may have an indolent course even without therapy, with eventual recanalization of the sinus or development of collaterals.

Eclampsia

Epidemiology

Eclampsia is the end stage of preeclampsia (toxemia of pregnancy), and presents with seizures and coma. Preeclampsia occurs after the 20th week of pregnancy, with new-onset hypertension, protein in the urine, and edema, along with confusion, headaches, and visual disturbances.[76] Preeclampsia occurs in approximately 3% of all pregnancies, and remains a major cause of maternal and perinatal mortality and morbidity, particularly in developing countries.[77,78]

Pathogenesis and Presentation

During pregnancy a number of changes, including changes in immunity along with vasodilatation due to prostaglandin release, release of proinflammatory cytokines, and increased responsiveness to circulating catecholamines all combine to cause the clinical picture.[79] The brain then loses its ability to maintain an internal perfusion pressure independent of the blood pressure (cerebral autoregulation). This causes blood products to seep into the perivascular spaces leading to microhemorrhages and, if left untreated, large hemorrhages and strokes.[80] Postpartum, the risk for stroke remains elevated. Imaging may reveal reduced perfusion in the watershed areas between arterial zones in the brain.[81]

Treatment

Treatment of hypertension is especially important to prevent end-organ damage and restore cerebral autoregulation.[82] Seizure control is achieved by controlling blood pressure as well as with magnesium sulfate (superior to diazepam and phenytoin in controlling and preventing seizures in eclampsia).[83,84] Magnesium works by blocking or reducing neuronal excitability.[85] Low-dose aspirin may help prevent eclampsia.[86]

Tumors

Epidemiology

Both primary and metastatic tumors affect the central nervous system, and while metastatic tumors are the most common of all brain tumors, gliomas are the most common *primary* brain tumors, accounting for more than 70% of all such tumors.[87] Neuronal tumors are very rare as neurons are not mitotic.

While variable availability of neuroimaging makes comparisons across nations difficult, ethnicity may play a role in susceptibility to gliomas.[88] For example, gliomas are half as frequent in Japan as in the United States.[89] Caucasians are most affected by primary brain tumors, with glioblastomas and germ-cell tumors being 3.5 times more frequent in this population than among blacks in the United States.[90]

Women may be at lower risk for developing gliomas than men, particularly during the childbear-

ing years, suggesting a protective role for estrogen.[90] Naturally menopausal, nonhysterectomized women may be more at risk for gliomas and acoustic neuromas than menstruating women.[91]

Pituitary adenomas account for 5–8% of intracranial tumors and commonly present in women during childbearing years.[92] Because of the frequent association with infertility, adenomas rarely present during pregnancy, but when they do, there is an increased risk for tumor growth and hemorrhage.[93]

Meningiomas account for 13–26% of all primary brain tumors and are two to three times as common in women as in men.[94] Progesterone and estrogen receptors are present in meningiomas, and this, in addition to higher blood volume, may account for increasing size of meningiomas during pregnancy.[95]

Pathogenesis and Presentation

Gliomas may be astrocytomas, oligodendrogliomas, or mixed oligoastrocytomas, with pathological classification—using nuclear atypia, presence of mitotic figures, endothelial proliferation, and necrosis—to grade malignancy. Low-grade gliomas (grade I) have none of these criteria while grade IV gliomas (glioblastoma multiforme [GBM]) have necrosis and are synonymous with aggressive growth and poor prognosis.[96] Unfortunately, GBMs are the most common type of glioma and account for nearly 60% of primary brain tumors. Oligodendrogliomas are tumors whose cells resemble immature oligodendrocytes of the nervous system. Oligoastrocytomas have characteristics of both astrocytomas and oligodendrogliomas, and have an annual incidence of 9–19% of gliomas.[97]

Genes such as the tumor suppressor gene *p53* play a critical role in glioma pathogenesis.[98] Mutations of this gene are found in more than 65% of low-grade astrocytomas, anaplastic astrocytomas, and secondary glioblastomas.[99,100] Meningiomas are associated mutations on chromosome 22, home of the neurofibromatosis type-2 gene.[101]

Ovarian steroid hormones may play a role in tumor pathogenesis.[102,103] Estrogen reduces glutamate (the excitatory neurotransmitter) toxicity in glial cells and speeds up repair after brain trauma.[104,105] Women with an earlier age at menarche have a longer lifetime estrogen exposure, especially in youth with attendant accelerated brain development, possibly shortening the period of increased susceptibility to neurocarcinogens.[103]

Symptoms of tumors of the nervous system are primarily caused by the local effect of the mass on brain or spinal cord structures and can range from headaches and confusion to paralysis and coma. Pituitary adenomas may be nonsecreting, causing neurological symptoms primarily due to mass effect, or functional, secreting excess pituitary hormones causing systemic symptoms. Tumors are diagnosed by neuroimaging.

Treatment

Pathological evaluation of the tumor guides management options, which may include radiation and chemotherapy.[106] Surgical resection remains a mainstay for most types of primary brain tumor. In very low-grade gliomas, surgery has not been evaluated specifically in any randomized study, although it is widely practiced to prevent malignant transformation.[107] Even with high-grade gliomas, surgical resection improves survival.[108,109] The use of brain mapping and prior embolization of vascular tumors using interventional radiology techniques has improved outcome after tumor surgery.

Radiation therapy is commonly used in conjunction with surgery and chemotherapy in individuals with malignant gliomas.[106,110] However, despite these aggressive therapies, long-term survival in highly malignant gliomas like GBMs remains poor, with 2-year survival rates rarely exceeding 15%.[111]

Bromocriptine and cabergoline are effective in treating secreting pituitary adenomas and may obviate need for surgery, reducing or arresting tumor growth in most patients.[112]

Idiopathic Intracranial Hypertension (Pseudotumor Cerebri)

Epidemiology

This condition, characterized by symptoms of increased intracranial pressure without evidence of a focal mass lesion (hence *pseudo*tumor), is now called idiopathic intracranial hypertension (IIH). Ninety percent of patients are obese young women.

IIH is associated with pregnancy, use of oral contraceptives and hypercoaguable states, and is caused by reduced resorption of cerebrospinal fluid (CSF).[113,114] Cerebral venous thrombosis can mimic symptoms of IIH and must be ruled out. Laboratory evaluation for protein C and S deficiency, antiphospholipid antibody syndrome, and essential thrombocythemia is needed.[115] Systemic conditions such as thyroid abnormalities and Addison's disease may be associated with IIH.[113] Drugs such as penicillin, tetracycline, steroids, indocin, oral contraceptives, and high intake of vitamin A are associated with IIH.[116]

Pathogenesis and Presentation

All idiopathic and secondary cases of IIH are due to the interference with the venous outflow of the blood from the central nervous system, causing increased intracranial pressure with its attendant features. Clinically, IIH is associated with headache and other signs of increased intracranial pressure, including visual blurring and papilledema, as well as nausea and vomiting.[117] Many women have menstrual irregularities. The greatest risk of IIH is permanent loss of vision. An MR venogram is needed to rule out central venous thrombosis and to confirm presence of tell-tale slitlike ventricles in IIH.[117]

Treatment

A spinal tap often relieves symptoms of headache and visual obscurations and confirms the diagnosis. For IIH caused by a known etiology, treatment of the underlying condition is warranted. Idiopathic IIH is treated by reducing intracranial pressure by serial spinal taps, weight reduction (7–10% weight reduction can lead to resolution of papilledema), acetazolamide, and steroids.[118,119] Acetazolamide is a carbonic anhydrase inhibitor that reduces CSF production. In doses of 1 g daily, acetazolamide can ameliorate symptoms within hours.[120] Furosemide and diuretics work transiently by dehydrating the patient.[121] Systemic steroids may be of benefit in the acute treatment of IIH.[118] Shunting is fraught with problems in these obese patients and is reserved for patients who are not responsive to medical treatment.[122] Optic nerve sheath fenestration is one way of relieving pressure around the optic nerve and preventing blindness.[123]

Pregnancy-Related Neurological Complications of Systemic Infections

Estrogens are likely responsible for gender differences in immunity, with differential activation of T lymphocytes. During pregnancy, maternal immune tolerance of the fetal and placental antigens is mediated both by physical separation and changes in the composition of maternal hormones, ultimately increasing maternal susceptibility to infections, including tuberculosis, listeriosis, and malaria.[124-126]

Nearly a third of infections with *Listeria monocytogenes* occur during pregnancy, especially during the third trimester.[125] Neurologic manifestations include headaches and altered consciousness and can progress to seizures and focal deficits.[127] Infections such as tuberculosis are more severe during pregnancy as atypical presentations may lead to delay in diagnosis and treatment.[128]

Falciparum malaria is particularly lethal in pregnancy, being the largest cause of maternal mortality during pregnancy in Thailand, for example.[126] *Plasmodium falciparum*, with its propensity for cerebral involvement, can cause headaches, progressive mental status changes culminating in coma as well as seizures.[129] High levels of placental plasmodia along with maternal hypoglycemia increase fetal morbidity and mortality. The quinine used to treat the malaria may further exacerbate hypoglycemia, which behooves careful blood sugar monitoring in pregnant women with malaria.[129] Treatment is with choloroquine, although resistant strains of plasmodia are rising across endemic areas.[129,130]

The following four sections discuss infectious diseases affecting the central nervous system.

Meningitis

Epidemiology

Meningitis, due to inflammation of the meninges, may be secondary to an infectious (viral, bacterial, or fungal), malignant, or inflammatory cause. Bacterial meningitis continues to be associated with high rates of morbidity and mortality, although these rates are declining.[131] Epidemics of meningitis (*Neisseria meningitides*), with high mortality rates, occur in the "meningitis belt" of sub-Saharan Africa, extending from Mali and the Ivory Coast to Sudan and Ethiopia.[131]

In developed countries, current mortality rates for meningococcal meningitis (from *Neisseria meningitides*) is 10%, for *Haemophilus influenzae* meningitis around 5%, and for pneumococcal meningitis (from *Streptococcus pneumoniae*) about 20%.[132] *N. meningitides* is a normal inhabitant of the human nasopharyngeal mucosa, with approximately 10% of the world's population harboring meningococci in their nose at any given time.[133] Still, invasive disease is rare and occurs with change in strain virulence and break in mucosa.

Spirochete-related meningitis includes Lyme disease and syphilis. Lyme borreliosis-related meningitis is on the rise in endemic areas of the United States.[134] Syphilitic meningitis is also on the rise worldwide due to the increasing prevalence of HIV disease.[135]

Fungal meningitis is more common in immunocompromised patients. Cryptococcus, Coccidioides, and Candida are the three most common causes of fungal meningitis, with cryptococcal meningitis having the best prognosis of the three.[136,137]

Viral meningitis, such as West Nile meningitis, is endemic to parts of the United States, while other viral meningitis like Herpes simplex (HSV) meningitis occur worldwide. In adults, 80% of viral meningitis is caused by enteroviruses.[138] Second to enteroviruses, HSV and varicella zoster virus are common causes of the disease. The human immunodeficiency virus (HIV) and Epstein-Barr virus may also cause meningitis.[139]

Among adults with aseptic or sterile meningitis, often no cause is identified, although many patients have been found to be on nonsteroidal anti-inflammatory drugs (Mollaret's meningitis).[140,141]

Pathogenesis and Presentation

The most common presentation of meningitis in adults is headache and neck stiffness, along with photophobia. An urgent spinal tap for spinal fluid analysis is crucial in reducing morbidity, particularly in bacterial meningitis, where delay in treatment may rapidly lead to mental status changes, seizures, coma, and death. Lyme and sarcoid meningitis may present with cranial nerve involvement as the initial symptom.

Treatment

There is no specific antiviral treatment available for viral meningitis caused by enteroviruses.[138] However, new antiviral agents that inhibit viral replication have shown promise.[142] In patients with herpes simplex virus meningitis, antiviral treatment with acyclovir or a similar agent is helpful.[143]

Early initiation of appropriate antibiotic treatment for bacterial meningitis is crucial in reducing morbidity and mortality.[144] Stroke may occur as the result of meningeal inflammation irritating cerebral blood supply, causing vasospasm.[145] Steroids may be helpful in this instance, concurrent with antibiotic administration.[146]

Currently, there is a vaccine available for the prevention of meningococcal meningitis against four common strains (A, C, Y, W135).[147] This vaccine offers protection to individuals over 2 years old and has been successful in controlling large outbreaks of meningitis, particularly in the African meningitis belt.[148] Newer conjugated vaccines are currently in development. These vaccines would potentially be more effective in children under 2 years of age and in inducing immunological memory.

Cysticercosis

Epidemiology

Cysticercosis is the most common parasitic disease worldwide, with over 50 million people infected. It is endemic throughout the developing world.[149,150] Neurocysticercosis is the most prevalent infection of the brain worldwide[151] and the disease has become one of the leading causes of adult-onset seizures.[152-154]

Pathogenesis

Cysticercosis is caused by the pork tapeworm, *Taenia solium*, often present in undercooked pork.[155] When ingested by humans, *T. solium* larvae attach themselves to the human gut and grow into adult tapeworms, which shed eggs into human feces. Fecal-oral transmission occurs via infected food handlers with improperly washed hands, or by fruit and vegetables fertilized with contaminated human waste. Therefore, even individuals who do not eat pork can become infected with cysticercosis.[156]

The clinical presentation of cysticercosis depends on the location of the cysts and the overall cyst burden.[152] Brain cysts are the most common and are present in 60–90% of all cases.[152] Neurocysticercosis commonly causes seizures, but can also cause encephalopathy especially when the adult worm that is the nidus of the cyst dies, often as the result of treatment, causing surrounding inflammation and brain edema.[151] Rarely, cysts within the spinal column cause radicular pain and paresthesias.[152]

Treatment

Cysticercosis is treated with albendazole or parziquantel. In patients with seizures or brain edema, steroids may be administered with anticonvulsants in the acute phase of treatment with cysticidals.[152] Treatment of subarachnoid and intraventricular neurocysticercosis is more complicated and may require larger doses of albendazole or very rarely, if in a strategic location, surgery.[157,158] Cysticidal drug therapy has been shown to reduce seizures and increase the resolution of lesions in parenchymal neurocystercercosis.[159]

Schistosomiasis

Epidemiology

Chronic schistosomiasis is one of the world's most prevalent infectious diseases, with an estimated 200 million people infected worldwide.[160] Schistosomiasis rates are particularly high in sub-Saharan Africa (280,000 deaths annually) and parts of Asia. In China, prevalence rates range from 0.06–3.8%.[161]

Pathogenesis and Presentation

This disease is caused by schistosomes, or blood-dwelling fluke worms,[160] with the *Schistosoma mansoni* strain accounting for most human infections. The pathogenesis of schistosomiasis varies depending on the specific parasite causing the infection and the region of the body that is infected.[160] Neuroschistosomiasis results from an inflammation around ectopic worms or eggs in the cerebral or spinal venous plexus. This inflammation can evolve to irreversible fibrotic scars if left untreated.[162] Infections resulting from *S. mansoni* and *S. haematobium* can cause inflammation of the spinal cord, presenting as transverse myelitis, a complication of acute schistosomiasis in travelers.[163] *S. japonicum* is associated with cerebral granulomatous lesions, leading to epilepsy, paralysis, and meningoencephalitis.[162]

Treatment

Praziquantel is the drug of choice.[160] In neuroschistosomiasis, corticosteroids and anticonvulsants may be added.[162]

Leishmaniasis

Epidemiology

The global burden of disease of leishmaniasis is similar to schistosomiasis,[160] with over 2 million new cases each year. It is endemic in over 60 countries, including parts of southern Europe.[164]

Pathogenesis

Leishmaniasis results from the bite of a female sand fly that was infected by ingesting blood of an infected mammalian host. Peripheral neuropathy is present in a majority of cases.[165] Central nervous system involvement is uncommon, except as direct extension (e.g., through the paranasal sinuses) and can cause meningitis and cranial nerve involvement.[166,167]

Treatment

Treatment includes miltefosine, sodium stibogluconate, or amphoteriocin B lipid complex.[168] Amphotericin B lipid complex is a first line of therapy for HIV-infected individuals, although chronic suppressive therapy is recommended to prevent relapse.[169]

Systemic Lupus Erythematosus

Epidemiology

Many autoimmune diseases exhibit an overwhelmingly female preponderance, including Takayasu arteritis (9:1), Sjogren's syndrome (9:1), rheumatoid arthritis (4:1), scleroderma (15:1), and lupus (9:1).[170,171] However, systemic lupus erythematosus (SLE) is most likely to be associated with neurologic symptoms and will be discussed here.

Ninety percent of patients with SLE are women, suggesting a role of female hormones in promoting the disease or a protective role for male hormones.[170] Antecedent infections, particularly with the Epstein-Barr virus, and the use of certain drugs such as procainamide and quinidine may be associated with the onset of SLE.[171] Ultraviolet radiation may exacerbate lupus.

Pathogenesis and Presentation

Lupus is a prototypical autoimmune disease and has been linked to genes of the major histocompatibility complex (MHC).[172] T lymphocytes recognize antigens presented together with an MHC peptide on the surface of antigen-presenting cells such as B cells, macrophages, and dendrites.[173] Certain MHC genotypes may therefore increase risk of immune response to self-antigens. Affected organs generally show inflammation and deposition of complement-antibody complexes.[174] Autoantibodies to double-stranded DNA, a normal component of the body, are present in 70–80% of lupus patients and less than 0.5% of normal persons or persons with other autoimmune diseases.[175] Antinucleosome antibodies are present in 50–90% of patients.[176] Antiphospholipid antibodies, associated with hypercoagulable states are present in 20–40% of patients, while anti-NMDA receptor antibodies, specific to brain involvement, are present in 33–50% of patients.[177]

Cytokines such as tumor necrosis factor-alpha may have a protective effect in lupus, as noted by the positive effects of agents such as the anti-TNF-alpha-antibody drug infliximab.[178] Interleukin-10 and interferon levels are high in lupus and are an index of disease activity, the blocking of which may reduce autoantibody production.[179]

Neurological manifestations of lupus include cognitive dysfunction, headaches, mood disorders, seizures, strokes, transverse myelitis, and polyneuropathy in decreasing order of frequency.[180,181] Over 80% of patients present will exhibit neurologic dysfunction at some time during the course of disease.[182] Death is generally due to infection, stroke, or myocardial infarction.[183]

MRI and PET scans may find evidence of involvement of specific brain areas, showing reducing focal metabolic activity or stroke in some patients. In most cases, the brain MRI in neurologic lupus is normal.[184]

Treatment

Treatment is aimed at reducing autoantibody levels to reduce disease progression, with additional treatment of specific symptoms when needed. General immunosuppressive agents such as corticosteroids azathioprine, cyclophosphamide, and mycophenolate mofetil are commonly used.[185] Rituximab is a nonspecific antibody against CD20 found on the surface of all mature B cells.[186] Abetimus sodium is more specific.[187] Other treatments are directed against individual symptoms, for example anticonvulsants to treat seizures, and anticoagulants in the event of a hypercoagulable state causing a stroke.[188]

Multiple Sclerosis

Epidemiology

Multiple sclerosis (MS) affects individuals in temperate regions, with the incidence and prevalence of MS increasing with latitude, both north and south of the equator.[189] Interestingly, the lifetime risk for MS is determined by the region where one spends the first 14–15 years of life, implicating possible viral (HSV, EBV) or bacterial (spirochete) triggers during formative years predisposing to later development of the condition.[190] Women are affected more than men, with a female-to-male ratio between 1.5 and 2.5, and a lifetime risk for women of approximately 1 in 200.[191,192] The age at onset follows a relatively constant pattern across different regions, with incidence being low in childhood, increasing after adolescence, reaching a peak between 25 and 35 years, and then slowly declining.[189] Risk of MS is approximately 30 times higher among siblings of affected individuals than in the general population.[193] Environmental stressors such as exposure to excessive heat and infections may trigger attacks.[194]

Pathogenesis and Presentation

Multiple sclerosis is a demyelinating, autoimmune disease, hypothesized to be caused by infiltrating lymphocytes interacting with myelin proteins.[195] Inflammatory plaques from brains of MS patients contain an inflammatory cellular infiltrate, dominated by T cells and macrophages.[196] These plaques also contain areas of axonal demyelination, gliosis, and loss of axons and oligodendrocytes. MS patients most commonly present with relapsing or remitting MS (RRMS), primary progressive MS, or secondarily progressive MS, where RRMS is transformed into an inexorably progressive disease without remissions.[197]

MS pathogenesis is complex, with familial aggregation studies showing larger contributions from genes than the environment. So far, however, only the HLA-DRB1 locus has been firmly linked to MS risk.[198] Other genes linked to MS have been shown to be more common in females than in males.[199] There may be a relationship between MS and polymorphisms in the estrogen gene receptor.[200] Furthermore, the genotype may alter expression of the condition, with MS patients of Asian origin, for example, being more likely to exhibit optic nerve and spinal cord involvement.[201]

Schumacher's clinical criteria for diagnosing MS include lesions separated in space and time without another cause, involving primarily white matter.[202] Currently, diagnosis and follow-up may be made using MRI and the attendant McDonald criteria, which specify dispersed white matter lesions greater than 3 mm in size, with variable contrast enhancement attesting to dissemination in time.[203] Symptoms are based on area of the central nervous system affected. Fatigue, depression, and cognitive impairment are common generalized symptoms in MS.

There are differences in magnetic resonance imaging (MRI) between males and females with MS further suggesting that sex hormones may modulate brain damage in MS.[204] Low testosterone levels in women, for example, may correlate with a greater number of gadolinium concentrations and brain damage-enhancing lesions on MRI.[205] MRI studies also show that global white matter water content is higher in women when compared to men and in MS lesions as compared to normal white matter, which may have implications in MS pathogenesis.[204,206]

As with many autoimmune diseases, changes in hormone levels are considered to affect MS.[204] Symptoms may improve during pregnancy and fluctuate throughout the menstrual cycle.[204,207] Pregnancy reduces risk of attacks, although some MS symptoms, such as fatigue, bladder dysfunction, and spasticity, may worsen.[204,207] The relapse risk rises after delivery to nearly 40%.

Treatment

Based on the presumed autoimmune pathogenesis of MS, treatment for the past several decades has focused on anti-inflammatory strategies.[208] Older treatments with more broad-based anti-inflammatory and immunosuppressive drugs have yielded to newer, more targeted interventions.

Even so, steroids (intravenous methylprednisolone, 1 gm daily for 3–5 days) remain the mainstay in treating acute relapses and shortening the duration and severity of the relapse.[209] Several immunomodulators have disease-modifying effects and are helping to change the landscape of this chronic condition by reducing relapse rates, time between relapses, delaying time to eventual disability, and reducing lesions on MRI. These include glatiramer acetate, interferon-B1b and two types of interferon B1a, all given either subcutaneously or intramuscularly.[210,211] Immunosuppressive drugs, such as azathioprine, methotrexate, and particularly the newer mitroxantrone, may be of benefit in aggressive forms of MS.[211] Mitroxantrone reduces relapse rates and slows disease progression in such patients, but because of concerns of cardiotoxicity, there is a cap on cumulative lifetime exposure.[212]

These drugs may have as yet unknown deleterious effects on fetuses, requiring women of childbearing age to concomitantly use contraception. Menstruation may be affected with interferon use.

Myasthenia Gravis

Epidemiology

Myasthenia gravis (MG) is characterized by progressive muscle weakness with repetitive or sustained activity, affecting primarily the highly active eye muscles, pharyngeal muscles, and limb musculature.[213] High levels of antibodies to the acetylcholine receptor (AchR) in the skeletal muscles are the hallmark of the condition and found in 70–90% of patients.[214] Thymomas are present in 10–15% of MG patients, and 70% of patients have some thymic hyperplasia.[214] The condition is particularly common in adult women (14:1 female-to-male ratio) and is more severe in women.[215] Exacerbations of MG are more likely to occur just before onset of menses, although pregnancy is not consistently associated with change in disease activity.[216,217] However, pregnant myasthenic women require special considerations; magnesium sulfate is contraindicated as it worsens muscle weakness, and if any procedure is necessary, regional anesthesia is preferable to general anesthesia in these patients.[218]

Pathogenesis and Presentation

Patients may present with trouble swallowing, ptosis, or other symptoms of muscle weakness, worsening as the day progresses. Diagnosis is made using the edrophonium chloride test, where 1–10 mg is given intravenously with transient improvement in muscle weakness.[219] Single-fiber EMG is abnormal in 98% of patients showing abnormal repetitive firing.[220]

Treatment

Antiacetylcholinesterase agents reduce acetylcholine breakdown across the neuromuscular junction and improve symptoms. Pyridostigmine, with fewer side effects than other drugs in the class, is the preferred agent, given every 2–4 hours.[221] Immune suppressive therapy with the use of steroids, azothioprine, and cyclosporine is sometimes used.[222] Steroids can cause initial worsening of symptoms, with such patients requiring close monitoring.[222,223] Thymectomies are associated with discernible improvement in two-thirds of patients, although improvement may continue gradually over many years.[224] Plasmapheresis to remove circulating antibodies to the acetycholine receptor is indicated in severe cases.[225]

Menopause-Related Memory Disorders

Epidemiology

The association between menopause and cognitive loss is controversial with some studies finding an increased risk and others finding no such effects. Even so, several studies from around the world have reported rates of menopause-related cognitive loss as ranging from 35% to 65%, similar to the prevalence of hot flashes.[226]

Pathogenesis and Presentation

Women present with complaints of memory loss, word-finding difficulties, trouble with mental math, and recalling recent events and a reduction in verbal fluency. These symptoms may begin several years before actual cessation of periods and continue through and past the menopausal transition.[227] About 20% of women continue to experience changes in their cognitive function well past menopause although the association, if any, with the development of dementia in this subgroup is unknown. Estrogen levels drop precipitously during the years leading up to menopause and are extremely low after menopause. Estrogen plays a critical role in memory and cognitive processing through its effects on the neurotransmitter systems of the brain as well as through direct effects on neuronal receptors.[228-230] Whereas a century ago, the life expectancy of the average woman coincided with the onset of menopause, women now live a third to a half of their lives without estrogen.[231] The effects of such long-term deprivation on the brain of this essential hormone are unknown.

Treatment

Hormone replacement (HRT) is effective in treating cognitive and other symptoms of menopause. However, because of fear of its debatable long-term effects, including risk for breast cancer, HRT is no longer widely used. Early initiation of HRT after menopause may be more beneficial than later treatment, explaining discrepancies in benefits of treatment from various studies.[228,232] The type of estrogen used, whether conjugated equine estrogen or the bioidentical estradiol, is also important. Nonhormonal treatment of cognitive loss using donepezil, a cholinesterase inhibitor used in dementia treatment, was partially effective.[233]

Dementia

Epidemiology

Over 24 million people worldwide suffer from dementia, with over 4 million new cases every year,[234] and this number is expected to double every 20 years.[235] Currently, 60% of people with dementia live in developing countries. In India, China, and other Asian and Pacific countries, the prevalence of dementia is expected to increase by over 300% by 2040 and is often under diagnosed.[236] Of the many illnesses that cause dementia, Alzheimer's disease (AD) is the most common.[237] Women are more likely than men to develop Alzheimer's, even after controlling for their greater longevity.[238,239]

Infectious causes of dementia include the slow viral, transmissible spongiform prion diseases such as Creutzfeld-Jakob disease. Spirochetes such as syphilis and borrelia can cause a dementia.[240] As the HIV/AIDS pandemic grows, so has HIV-associated dementia. Of the nearly 40 million HIV-infected people worldwide, half will suffer from dementia prior to death.[241] With the advent of combination antiretroviral therapy, the overall incidence of HIV-associated dementia has decreased.

However, the prevalence of less severe HIV-associated neurocognitive impairment continues to increase.[242] Women are particularly affected as they make up one of the fastest growing groups of incident HIV cases.[243]

Pathogenesis

Dementia is defined as progressive, irreversible cognitive loss with functional impairment caused by nerve cell death. Common noninfectious causes of dementia include Alzheimer's, vascular dementia, and dementia due to Lewy-body disease.

Alzheimer's dementia (AD) may occur prior to age 60 (early-onset AD) or later in life (late-onset AD). Early-onset AD accounts for fewer than 5% of cases worldwide and is inherited in an autosomal dominant fashion and caused by mutations on chromosomes 1, 14, or 21.[244,245] Late-onset AD is felt to be multifactorial in etiology with both genetic and environmental risk factors (such as head trauma, early menopause or hysterectomies) playing a role in the disease development.[246,247] The E4 isoform of the apolipoprotein E (apoE) gene is associated with a significantly increased risk for late-onset AD.[248]

AD pathology is characterized by the deposition of insoluble extracellular senile plaques within the brain, beginning in the temporal cortex and spreading to other brain areas.[249,250] In addition, intracellular neurofibrillary tangles are found in AD. All known genetic mutations, in both early and late onset AD, cause increased plaque burden.

Studies have found risk reductions in AD development with the use of statins, estrogen replacement, or NSAIDs at high doses.[251] However, treatment with any of these agents is ineffective when one already has the disease.

Multi-infarct or vascular dementia (vD) is caused by strokes causing brain tissue destruction, leading ultimately to cognitive impairment.[252] A single stroke in an eloquent region of the brain or multiple progressive strokes both can cause dementia.[253] The commonly used Hachinski Rating Scale determines the likelihood of the dementia being secondary to multiple infarcts based on aspects of the history including stepwise deterioration.[254] However, neuroimaging is now generally preferred to help diagnose vD.

Dementia due to Lewy bodies (DLB) may well be the second most common dementia and is associated with the deposition of Lewy bodies within the nerve cells.[255] While vD is often thought to be more common, DLB may in fact be underdiagnosed. The condition is associated with early onset of psychiatric features, particularly visual hallucinations and depression, as well as neuroleptic sensitivity, frequent falls, Parkinsonian features, and fluctuations in level of consciousness.[255]

Dementia due to HIV infection may be either an indirect or a direct consequence of the infection itself.[256] Direct neuropathology includes HIV encephalitis, HIV leucencephalopathy, cerebral vasculitis, neuronal loss, and dendritic and synaptic damage. Indirect neuropathology is generally a result of opportunistic infections affecting the HIV-seropositive individual.

Treatment

Currently available dementia treatments are primarily symptomatic and do not alter underlying pathology. For the most common neurodegenerative dementias such as AD and DLB, as well as for vD, two major categories of drugs are used: cholinesterase inhibitors (donepezil, galantamine, rivastigmine) and N-methyl-D-aspartate glutamate receptor antagonists (memantine).[257-260] These drugs are not disease modifiers, but they do slow progression of symptoms over time and may be used synergistically. Current research on treatment is focused on drugs that modify deposition of amyloid and may thus have a disease-modifying effect. Effective treatments for psychiatric symptoms of dementia include antidepressants and antipsychotic medications. The atypical antipsychotic neuroleptic drugs (clozapine, quetiapine, olanzapine) are preferred for treating hallucinations in DLB as these patients are particularly prone to the extrapyramidal side effects of neuroleptics.[261]

For the treatment on HIV-associated dementia, antiretroviral therapies are generally used, based on viral load. Unfortunately, because of drug resistance and difficulty in maintaining adherence, only about half of patients achieve full success, while the remainder show only partial or no benefit.[262]

Conclusion

The risk of many neurological conditions varies between genders, with women bearing the greater burden in several diseases. Common neurological conditions in women were discussed in this chapter, with a particular emphasis on role of gender in the epidemiology, pathogenesis, and response to treatment.

Acknowledgements

Emiliya Zhivotovskaya, BA, was invaluable in her assistance with the editing and referencing of this chapter.

DISCUSSION QUESTIONS

1. What neurological conditions are women at risk for?
2. What are possible genetic, biological, and environmental factors that contribute to this differential risk?
3. Does gender predicate different treatment approaches to neurologic disease?

REFERENCES

1. Amatniek J, Frey L, Hauser A. Gender differences in diseases of the nervous system. In: Kaplan PW, ed. *Neurologic Disease in Women.* 2nd ed. Demos Med Pub; 2005:3-13.
2. Wang SJ. Epidemiology of migraine and other types of headache in Asia. *Curr Neurol Neurosci Rep.* 2003;3(2):104-108.
3. Lipton RB, Bigal ME. Migraine: epidemiology, impact, and risk factors for progression. *Headache.* 2005;45(suppl 1):S3-S13.
4. Lipton RB, Stewart WF, Diamond S, et al. Prevalence and burden of migraine in the United States: data from the American Migraine Study II. *Headache.* 2001; 41:646-657.
5. Stewart WF, Linet MS, Celentano DD, Van Natta M, Ziegler D. Age and sex-specific incidence rates of migraine with and without visual aura. *Am J Epidemiol.* 1991;134:1111-1120.
6. Silberstein S, Merriam G. Sex hormones and headache (menstrual migraine). *Neurology.* 1999;53(4 suppl 1):S3-S13.
7. Arulmozhi DK, Veeranjaneyulu A, Bodhankar SL. Migraine: current therapeutic targets and future avenues. *Curr Vasc Pharmacol.* 2006;4(2):117-128.
8. Longoni M, Ferrarese C. Inflammation and excitotoxicity: role in migraine pathogenesis. *Neurol Sci.* 2006;27(suppl 2):107-110.
9. Link AS, Kuris A, Edvinsson, L. Treatment of migraine attacks based on the interaction with the trigemino-cerebrovascular system. *J Headache Pain.* 2008;9(1):5-12.

10. Arulmani U, Maassenvandenbrink A, Villalon CM, Saxena PR. Calcitonin gene-related peptide and its role in migraine pathophysiology. *Eur J Pharmacol.* 2004;500(1-3):315-330.

11. Vincent MB, Hadjikhani N. Migraine aura and related phenomena: beyond scotomata and scintillations. *Cephalgia.* 2007;27(12):1368-1377.

12. Kirchmann M. Migraine with aura: new understanding from clinical epidemiologic studies. *Curr Opin Neurol* 2006;19(3):286-293.

13. Tietjen, GE. The risk of stroke in patients with migraine and implications for migraine management. *CNS Drugs.* 2005;19(8):683-692.

14. Ferrari MD, Goadsby PJ, Roon KI, Lipton RB. Triptans (serotonin, 5-HT1B/1D agonists) in migraine: detailed results of methods of a meta-analysis of 53 trials. *Cephalalgia.* 2002;22(8):633-658.

15. Derosier FJ, Kori SH. Acetaminophen, aspirin, and caffeine versus sumatriptan succinate in the early treatment of migraine: results from the ASSET trial–a comment. *Headache.* 2007;47(4):623-625.

16. Demirkaya S, Vural O, Dora B, Topçuoglu MA. Efficacy of intravenous magnesium sulfate in the treatment of acute migraine attacks. *Headache.* 2001; 41(2):171-177.

17. Ashkenazi A, Silberstein SD. Hormone-related headache: pathophysiology and treatment. *CNS Drugs.* 2006;20:125.

18. Ramadan MN, Silberstein SD, Freitag FG, et al. United States Headache Consortium. Evidence-based guidelines for migraine headache in the primary care setting: pharmacological management for prevention of migraine. *Amer Acad Neurology.* 2000.55;754-762.

19. Ashkenazi A, Silberstein S. Botulinum toxin type A for the treatment of headache: why we say yes. *Arch Neurol.* 2008;65(1):146-149.

20. Woolhouse M, Migraine and tension headache–a complimentary and alternative medicine approach. *Aust Fam Physician.* 2005;34(8):647-651.

21. Sridharan R. Epidemiology of epilepsy. Special section: recent advances in epilepsy. *Curr Science.* 2002;82(6):664-670.

22. Cramer JA, Gordon J, Schachter S, Devinsky O. Women with epilepsy: hormonal issues from menarche through menopause. *Epilepsy Behav.* 2007; 11(2):160-178.

23. Pillai J, Sperling MR. Interictal EEG and the diagnosis of epilepsy. *Epilepsia.* 2006;47(suppl 1):14-22.

24. Lofgren E, Mikkonen K, Tolonen U, et al. Reproductive endocrine function in women with epilepsy: the role of epilepsy type and medication. *Epilepsy Behav.* 2007;10:77-83.

25. Logothetis J, Harner R, Morrell F, Torres F. The role of estrogens in catamenial exacerbation of epilepsy. *Neurology.* 1959;9:352-360.

26. Herzog AG. Progesterone therapy in women with complex partial and secondary generalized seizures. *Neurology.* 1995;45:1660-1662.

27. Newmark NE, Penry JK. Catamenial epilepsy: a review. *Epilepsia.* 1980;21:281-300.

28. Bazil CW, Pedley TA. Clinical pharmacology of antiepileptic drugs. *Clin Neuropharmacol.* 2003;26(1):38-52.

29. Wilby J, Kainth A, Hawkins N, et al. Clinical effectiveness, tolerability and cost-effectiveness of newer drugs for epilepsy in adults: a systematic review and economic evaluation. *Health Technol Assess.* 2005;9(15):1-157.

30. Stefan H, Steinhoff BJ. Emerging drugs for epilepsy and other treatment options. *Eur J Neurol.* 2007;14(10):1154-1161.

31. Mattson RH, Cramer JA. Epilepsy, sex hormones, and antiepileptic drugs. *Epilepsia*. 1985;26 (1):S40-S51.

32. Battino D, Tomson T. Management of epilepsy during pregnancy. *Drugs*. 2007;67(18):2727-2746.

33. Tatum WO. Use of antiepileptic drugs in pregnancy. *Expert Rev Neurother*. 2006;6(7):1077-1086.

34. Herzog AG. Catamenial epilepsy: Definition, prevalence pathophysiology and treatment. *Seizure*. 2008;17(2):151-159.

35. Pugh CB, Garnett WR. Current issues in the treatment of epilepsy. *Clin Pharm*. 1991;10(5):335-358.

36. Glauser TA, Pippenger CE. Controversies in blood-level monitoring: reexamining its role in the treatment of epilepsy. *Epilepsia*. 2000;41(suppl 8):S6-S15.

37. Tegos T, Kalodiki E, Daskalopoulou, S, Nicolaides A. Stroke: epidemiology, clinical picture, and risk factors: part I of III. *Angiology*. 2000;51(10):793-808.

38. Kwan J. Clinical epidemiology of stroke. *CME J Geriatr Med*. 2001;3:94-98.

39. Christopher R, Nagaraja D, Shankar SK. Homocysteine and cerebral stroke in developing countries. *Curr Med Chem*. 2007;14(22):2393-2401.

40. Seshadri S, Beiser A, Kelly-Hayes M, et al. The lifetime risk of stroke: estimates from the Framingham Study. *Stroke*. 2006;37:345-350.

41. Wolf PA, Abbott RD, Kannel WB. Atrial fibrillation as an independent risk factor for stroke: the Framingham Study. *Stroke*. 1991;22:983-988.

42. O'Brien T, Nguyen TT. Lipids and lipoproteins in women. *Mayo Clin Proc*. 1997;72(3):235-244.

43. Tegos T, Kalodiki E, Daskalopoulou, S, Nicolaides A. Stroke: epidemiology, clinical picture, and risk factors: part I of III. *Angiology*. 2000;51(10):793-808.

44. Bladin CF, Alexandrov AV, Bellavance A, et al. Seizures after stroke: a prospective multicenter study. *Arch Neurol*. 2000;57(11):1617-1622.

45. Bisdas S, Donnerstag F, Ahl B, et al. Comparison of perfusion computed tomography with diffusion-weighted magnetic resonance imaging in hyperacute ischemic stroke. *J Comput Assist Tomogr*. 2004;28(6):747-755.

46. Chan WS, Ray J, Wai EK, et al. Risk of stroke in women exposed to low-dose oral contraceptives: a critical evaluation of the evidence. *Arch Intern Med*. 2004;164(7):741-747.

47. Siritho S, Thrift AG, McNeil JJ, et al. Risk of ischemic stroke among users of the oral contraceptive pill: The Melbourne Risk Factor Study (MERFS) Group. *Stroke*. 2003;34(7):1575-1580.

48. Ahmad A. Genetics of cerebral venous thrombosis. J Pak Med Assoc. 2006; 56(11):488-490.

49. Lobo RA. Menopause and stroke and the effects of hormonal therapy. *Climacteric*. 2007;10(2):27-31.

50. Bushnell CD. Stroke and the female brain. *Nat Clin Pract Neurol*. 2008;4(1): 22-33.

51. Bushnell CD, Hurn P, Colton C, et al. Advancing the study of stroke in women: summary and recommendations for future research from an NINDS-Sponsored Multidisciplinary Working Group. *Stroke*. 2006;37(9):2387-2399.

52. Bushnell CD, Goldstein LB. Ischemic stroke: recognizing risks unique to women. *Womens Health Primary Care*. 1999;2:788-804.

53. Wilson PW, Garrison RJ, Castelli WP. Postmenopausal estrogen use, cigarette smoking, and cardiovascular morbidity in women over 50. The Framingham Study. *N Engl J Med*. October 24 1985;313(17):1038-1043.

54. Lindenstrøm E, Boysen G, Nyboe J. Lifestyle factors and risk of cerebrovascular disease in women. The Copenhagen City Heart Study. *Stroke.* 1993;24(10): 1468-1472.

55. Lafferty FW, Fiske ME. Postmenopausal estrogen replacement: a long-term cohort study. *Am J Med.* 1994;97(1):66-77.

56. Grodstein F, Stampfer MJ, Colditz GA, et al. Postmenopausal hormone therapy and mortality. *N Engl J Med.* 1997;336(25):1769-1775.

57. Finucane FF, Madans JH, Bush TL, et al. Decreased risk of stroke among postmenopausal hormone users. Results from a national cohort. *Arch Intern Med.* 1993;153(1):73-79.

58. Falkeborn M, Persson I, Terént A, et al. Hormone replacement therapy and the risk of stroke. Follow-up of a population-based cohort in Sweden. *Arch Intern Med.* 1993;153(10):1201-1209.

59. Petitti DB, Sidney S, Quesenberry CP Jr, Bernstein A. Ischemic stroke and use of estrogen and estrogen/progestogen as hormone replacement therapy. *Stroke.* 1998;29(1):23-28.

60. Paganini-Hill A, Ross RK, Henderson BE. Postmenopausal oestrogen treatment and stroke: a prospective study. *BMJ.* 1988;297(6647):519-522.

61. Heiss G, Wallace R, Anderson GL, et al. Health risks and benefits 3 years after stopping randomized treatment with estrogen and progestin. *JAMA.* 2008; 299(9):1036-1045.

62. Rossouw JE, Anderson GL, Prentice RL, et al. Risks and benefits of estrogen plus progestin in healthy postmenopausal women: principal results from the Women's Health Initiative randomized controlled trial. *JAMA.* 2002;288(3):321-333.

63. Moonis M, Fisher M. Considering the role of heparin and low-molecular-weight heparins in acute ischemic stroke. *Stroke.* 2002;33(7):1927-1933.

64. McCabe DJ, Rakhit RD. Antithrombotic and interventional treatment options in cardioembolic transient ischaemic attack and ischaemic stroke. *J Neurol Neurosurg Psychiatry.* 2007;78(1):14-24.

65. Lip GY, Lim HS. Atrial fibrillation and stroke prevention. *Lancet Neurol.* 2007; 6(11):981-993.

66. Lewandowski CA, Frankel M, Tomsick TA, et al. Combined intravenous and intra-arterial r-TPA versus intra-arterial therapy of acute ischemic stroke: emergency management of stroke (EMS) bridging trial. *Stroke.* 1999; 30(12):2598-2605.

67. Kim D, Jahan R, Starkman S, et al. Endovascular mechanical clot retrieval in a broad ischemic stroke cohort. *Am J Neuroradiol.* 2006;27(10):2048-2052.

68. Phillips RA. A review of therapeutic strategies for risk reduction of recurrent stroke. *Prog Cardiovasc Dis.* 2008;50(4):264-273.

69. Bhatt DL, Fox KA, Hacke W, and CHARISMA Investigators. Clopidogrel and aspirin versus aspirin alone for the prevention of atherothrombotic events. *NEJM.* 2006;354:1706-1717.

70. Nakase H, Takeshima T, Sakaki T, et al. Superior sagittal sinus thrombosis: a clinical and experimental study. *Skull Base Surgery.* 1998;8(4):169-174.

71. Ferro JM, Canhao P. Cerebral venous and dural sinus thrombosis. *Practical Neur.* 2003;3;214-219.

72. Saadatnia M, Tajmirriahi M. Hormonal contraceptives as a risk factor for cerebral venous and sinus thrombosis. *Acta Neurol Scand.* 2007;115(5):295-300.

73. Alberti A, Venti M, Biagini S. Headache and cerebral vein and sinus thrombosis. *Neuroscience.* 2008;23:89-95.

74. Agid R, Shelef I, Scott JN, Farb RI. Imaging of the intracranial venous system. *Neurologist.* 2008;14(1):12-22.

75. Virapongse C, Cazenave C, Quisling R, et al. The empty delta sign: frequency and significance in 76 cases of dural sinus thrombosis. *Radiology.* 1987; 162(3):779-785.

76. Porapakkham S. An epidemiologic study of eclampsia. *Obstet Gynecol.* 1979; 54(1):26-30.

77. Villar J, Say L, Shennan A, et al. Methodological and technical issues related to the diagnosis, screening, prevention, and treatment of pre-eclampsia and eclampsia. *Int J Gynaecol Obstet.* 2004;85(1):S28-S41.

78. Conde-Agudelo A, Belizan JM. Risk factors for preeclampsia in a large cohort of Latin American and Caribbean women. *BJOG.* 2007;107:75-83.

79. Baumwell S, Karumanchi SA. Pre-eclampsia: clinical manifestations and molecular mechanisms. *Nephron Clin Pract.* 2007;106(2):c72-c81.

80. Sibai, BM. Diagnosis, prevention, and management of eclampsia. *Obstet Gynecol.* 2005;105(2):402-410.

81. Digre KB, Varner MW, Osborn AG, Crawford S. Cranial magnetic resonance imaging in severe preeclampsia vs eclampsia. *Arch Neurol.* 1993;50(4):399-406.

82. Editorial. Management of eclampsia. *Br Med J.* 1976;2:1485-1486.

83. The Eclampsia Trial Collaborative Group. Which anticonvulsant for women with eclampsia? Evidence from the Collaborative Eclampsia Trial. *Lancet* 1995; 45:1455-1463.

84. Lucas M, Leveno K, Cunningham G. A comparison of magnesium sulfate with phenytoin for the prevention of eclampsia. *N Engl J Med.* 1995;333:201-205.

85. Sadeh, M. Action of magnesium sulfate in the treatment of preeclampsia-eclampsia. *Stroke.* 1989;20(9):1273-1275.

86. CLASP (Collaborative Low-Dose Aspirin Study in Pregnancy) Collaborative Group. CLASP: a randomized trial of low-dose aspirin for the prevention and treatment of pre-eclampsia among 9,364 pregnant women. *Lancet.* 1994; 343:619-629.

87. Ohgaki H, Kleihues P. Epidemiology and etiology of gliomas. *Acta Neuropathol.* 2005;109(1):93-108.

88. Davis FG, McCarthy B, Jukich P. The descriptive epidemiology of brain tumors. *Neuroimaging Clin N Am.* 1999;9:581-594.

89. Kuratsu J, Takeshima H, Ushio Y. Trends in the incidence of primary intracranial tumors in Kumamoto, Japan. *Int J Clin Oncol.* 2001;6:183-191.

90. Davis FG, McCarthy B, Jukich P. The descriptive epidemiology of brain tumors. *Neuroimaging Clin N Am.* 1999;9:581-594.

91. Schlehofer B, Blettner M, Wahrendorf J. Association between brain tumors and menopausal status. *J Natl Cancer Inst.* 1992;84(17):1346-1349.

92. Gold EB. Epidemiology of pituitary adenomas. *Epidemiol Rev.* 1981;3:163-183.

93. Scheithauser BW, Sano T, Kovacs KT, et al. The pituitary gland in pregnancy: a clinicopathologic and immunohistochemical study of 69 cases. *Mayo Clin Proc.* 1990;65:461-474.

94. Fisher JL, Schwartzbaum JA, Wrensch M, Wiemels JL. Epidemiology of brain tumors. *Neurol Clin.* 2007;25(4):867-890.

95. Martuza RL, McLaughlin DR, Ojemann RG. Specific estradiol binding in schwannomas, meningiomas and beurofibromas. *Neurosurgery.* 1981;9:665.

96. Louis DN, Ohgaki H, Wiestler OD, et al. The 2007 WHO classification of tumours of the central nervous system. *Acta Neuropathol.* 2007;114(2):97-109.

97. Louis DN. Molecular pathology of malignant gliomas. *Annu Rev Pathol.* 2006; 1:97-117.

98. Sauvageot CM, Kesari S, Stiles CD. Molecular pathogenesis of adult brain tumors and the role of stem cells. *Neuro Clinics.* 2007;25(4):891-924.

99. Nozaki M, Tada M, Kobayashi H. Roles of the functional loss of p53 and other genes in astrocytoma tumorigenesis and progression. *Neuro Oncol.* 1999;1(2): 124-137.

100. Watanabe K, Sato K, Biernat W, et al. Incidence and timing of p53 mutations during astrocytoma progression in patients with multiple biopsies. *Clin Cancer Res.* 1997;3(4):523-530.

101. Zang KD. Cytological and cytogenetical studies on human meningioma. *Cancer Genet Cytogenet.* 1982;6(3):249-274.

102. Silvera SAN, Miller AB, Rohan TE. Hormonal and reproductive factors and risk of glioma: a prospective cohort study. *Int J Cancer.* 2006;118(5):1321-1324.

103. Hatch EE, Linet MS, Zhang J, et al. Reproductive and hormonal factors and risk of brain tumors in adult females. *Int J Cancer.* 2005;114(5):797-805.

104. Shy H, Malaiyandi L, Timiras PS. Protective action of 17beta-estradiol and tamoxifen on glutamate toxicity in glial cells. *Int J Dev Neurosci.* 2000;18:289-297.

105. Chowen JA, Azcoitia I, Cardona-Gomez GP, Garcia-Segura LM. Sex steroids and the brain: lessons from animal studies. *J Pediatr Endocrinol Metab.* 2000;13:1045-1066.

106. Asthagiri AR, Pouratian N, Sherman J, et al. Advances in brain tumor surgery. *Neurol Clin.* 2007;25(4):975-1003.

107. Keles GE, Lamborn KR, Berger MS. Low-grade hemispheric gliomas in adults: a critical review of extent of resection as a factor influencing outcome. *J Neurosurg.* 2001;95(5):735-745.

108. Ammirati M, Vick N, Liao YL, et al. Effect of the extent of surgical resection on survival and quality of life in patients with supratentorial glioblastomas and anaplastic astrocytomas. *Neurosurgery.* 1987;21(2):201-206.

109. Lacroix M, Abi-Said D, Fourney DR, et al. A multivariate analysis of 416 patients with glioblastoma multiforme: prognosis, extent of resection, and survival. *J Neurosurg.* 2001;95(2):190-198.

110. Lawson HC, Sampath P, Bohan E, et al. Interstitial chemotherapy for malignant gliomas: the Johns Hopkins experience. *J Neurooncol.* 2006;83(1):61-67.

111. Stark AM, Nabavi A, Mehdorn HM, Blömer U. Glioblastoma multiforme-report of 267 cases treated at a single institution. *Surg Neurol.* 2005;63(2):162-169.

112. Vilar L, Czepielewsh MA, Naves LA, et al. Substantial shrinkage of adenomas cosecreting growth hormone and prolactin with use of cabergoline therapy. *Endocr Pract.* 2007;13(4):396-402.

113. Giuseffi V, Wall M, Siegel PZ, Rojas PB. Symptoms and disease associations in idiopathic intracranial hypertension (pseudotumor cerebri): a case-control study. *Neurology.* 1991;41(2):239-244.

114. Goodwin J. Recent developments in idiopathic intracranial hypertension (IIH). *Semin Ophthalmol.* 2003;18(4):181-189.

115. Kesler A, Ellis MH, Reshef T, et al. Idiopathic intracranial hypertension and anticardiolipin antibodies. *J Neurol Neurosurg Psychiatry.* 2000;68(3):379-380.

116. Friedman DI. Medication-induced intracranial hypertension in dermatology. *Am J Clin Dermatol.* 2005;6(1):29-37.

117. Brazis PW, Lee AG. Elevated intracranial pressure and pseudotumor cerebri. *Curr Opin Ophthalmol.* 1998;9(6):27-32.

118. Binder DK, Horton JC, Lawton MT, McDermott MW. Idiopathic intracranial hypertension. *Neurosurgery*. 2004;54(3):538-551.

119. Celebisoy N, Gökçay F, Sirin H, Akyürekli O. Treatment of idiopathic intracranial hypertension: topiramate vs acetazolamide, an open-label study. *Acta Neurol Scand*. 2007;116(5):322-327.

120. Digre KB. Idiopathic intracranial hypertension. *Curr Treat Options Neurol*. 1999; 1(1):74-81.

121. Shin RK, Balcer LJ. Idiopathic intracranial hypertension. *Curr Treat Options Neurol*. 2002;4(4):297-305.

122. Abu-Serieh B, Ghassempour K, Duprez T, Raftopoulos C. Stereotactic ventriculoperintoneal shunting for refractory idiopathic intracranial hypertension. *Neurosurgery*. 2007;60(6):1039-1043.

123. Agarwal MR, Yoo JH. Optic nerve sheath fenestration for vision preservation in idiopathic intracranial hypertension. *Neurosurg Focus*. 2007;23(5):E7.

124. Hamadeh MA, Glassroth J. Tuberculosis and pregnancy. *Chest*. 1992;101:1114-1120.

125. McLauchlin J. Human listeriosis in Britain 1967-1985, a summary of 722 cases. Listeriosis during pregnancy and in the newborn. *Epidimiology Infect*. 1990; 104:181-190.

126. Khanavongs M. Maternal mortality rate at Phaholpolpayuhasena from 1970 to 1979. *Thai Med Council Bull*. 1980;9:877-881.

127. Bartt R. Listeria and atypical presentations of Listeria in the central nervous system. *Semin Neurol*. 2000;20(3):361-373.

128. Kingdom JCP, Kennedy DH. Tuberculous meningitis in pregnancy. *Br J Obstet Gynecol*. 1989;96:233-235.

129. Looareesuwan S, White NJ, Karbwang J, et al. Quinine and severe falciparum malaria in late pregnancy. *Lancet*. 1985;2:4-8.

130. Dilling WJ, Gemmell AA. A preliminary investigation of fetal deaths following quinine induction. *J Obst Gyn*. 1929;36:352-366.

131. Broutin H, Philippon S, Constantin de Magny G. Comparative study of meningitis dynamics across nine African countries: a global perspective. *Int J Health Geogr*. 2007;6:29.

132. Swartz MN. Bacterial meningitis—a view of the past 90 years. *NEJM*. 2004; 351(18):1826-1828.

133. Van Deuren M, Brandtzaeg P, Van der Meer JW. Update on meningococcal disease with emphasis on pathogenesis and clinical management. *Clin Microbiol Rev*. 2000;13(1):144-166.

134. Hoppa E, Bachur R. Lyme disease update. *Curr Opin Pediatr*. 2007;19(3):275-280.

135. Carmo RA, Moura AS, Christo PP, Morandi AC, Oliveira MS. Syphilitic meningitis in HIV-patients with meningeal syndrome: report of two cases and review. *Braz J Infect Dis*. 2001;5(5):280-287.

136. Perfect JR. Fungal Meningitis. In: *Infections of the Central Nervous System*. Scheld MW, Whitley RJ, Marra CM, eds. Lippincott, Williams and Wilkins. 2004;691-712, 939.

137. Prasad KN, Agarwal J, Nag VL, et al. Cryptococcal infection in patients with clinically diagnosed meningitis in a tertiary care center. *Neurol India*. 2003; 51(3):364-366.

138. Kupila L, Vuorinen T, Vainionpää R, Hukkanen V, Marttila RJ, Kotilainen P. Etiology of aseptic meningitis and encephalitis in an adult population. *Neurology*. 2006;66:75-80.

139. Logan SA, MacMahon E. Viral meningitis. *BMJ*. 2008;336(7634):36-40.

140. Hopkins S, Jolles S. Drug-induced aseptic meningitis. *Expert Opin Drug Saf.* 2005;4(2)285-297.

141. Wynants H, Taelman H, Martin JJ, Van den Ende J. Recurrence aspectic meningitis after travel to the tropics: a case of Mollaret's meningitis? Case report with review of the literature. *Clin Neurol Neurosurg.* 2000;102(2):113-115.

142. Sawyer, MH. Enterovirus infections: diagnosis and treatment. *Curr Opin Pediatr.* 2001;13(1):65-69.

143. Binetruy C, Deback C, Roubaud-Baudron C, et al. Herpes simplex virus meningitis in 11 patients. *Med Mal Infect.* 2008;9 (Epub ahead of print).

144. Schut ES, de Gans J, van de Beek D. Community-acquired bacterial meningitis in adults. *Pract Neurol.* 2008;8(1):8-23.

145. Roos KL. Acute bacterial meningitis. *Semin Neurol.* 2000;20(3):293-306.

146. van de Beek D, de Gans J, McIntyre P, Prasad K. Steroids in adults with acute bacterial meningitis: a systematic review. *Lancet Infect Dis.* 2004;4(3):139-143.

147. Lepow ML, Beeler J, Randolph M, et al. Reactogenicity and immunogenicity of a quadrivalent combined meningococcal polysaccharide vaccine in children. *J Infect Dis.* 1986;154:1033-1036.

148. Van Deuren M, Brandtzaeg P, Van der Meer JW. Update on meningococcal disease with emphasis on pathogenesis and clinical management. *Clin Microbiol Rev.* 2000;13(1):144-166.

149. Garcia HH, Del Brutto OH. Taenia solium cysticercosis. *Infect Dis Clin North Am.* 2000;14:97-119.

150. Sawhney IM, Singh G, Lekhra OP, et al. Uncommon presentations of neurocysticercosis. *J Neurol Sci.* 1998;154:94-100.

151. Garcia HH, Gonzalez AE, Evans CA, et al. Taenia solium cysticercosis. *Lancet.* 2003;362:547-556.

152. Hawk MW, Shahlaie K, Kim KD, Theis JH. Neurocysticercosis: a review. *Surg Neurol.* 2005;63:123-132.

153. Del Brutto OH, Santibanez R, Noboa CA, et al. Epilepsy due to neurocysticercosis: analysis of 203 patients. *Neurology.* 1992;42:389-392.

154. Ong S, Talan DA, Moran GJ, et al. Neurocysticercosis in radiographically imaged seizure patients in United States emergency departments. *Emerg Infect Dis.* 2002;8:608-613.

155. Kraft R. Cysticercosis: an emerging parasitic disease. *Am Fam Physician.* 2007;76(1):91-96.

156. Varma A, Gaur KJ. The clinical spectrum of neurocysticercosis in the Uttaranchal region. *J Assoc Physicians India.* 2002;50:1398-1400.

157. Gongora-Rivera F, Soto-Hernandez JL, Gonzalez Esquivel D, et al. Albendazole trial at 15 or 30 mg/kg/day for subarachnoid and intraventricular cysticercosis. *Neurology.* 2006;66:436-438.

158. Proano JV, Madrazo I, Garcia L, et al. Albendazole and praziquantel treatment in neurocysticercosis of the fourth ventricle. *J Neurosurg.* 1997;87:29-33.

159. Del Brutto OH, Santibanez R, Noboa CA, et al. Epilepsy due to neurocysticercosis: analysis of 203 patients. *Neurology.* 1992;42:389-392.

160. King CH, Dickman K, Tisch DJ. Reassessment of the cost of chronic helmintic infection: a meta-analysis of disability-related outcomes in endemic schistosomiasis. *Lancet.* 2005;365(9470):1561-1569.

161. Zhou XN, Guo JG, Wu XH. Epidemiology of Schistosomiasis in the People's Republic of China, 2004. *Emerg Infect Dis.* 2007;13(10):1470-1476.

162. Ferrari TC. Involvement of central nervous system in the schistosomiasis. *Mem Inst Oswaldo Cruz.* 2004;99:59-62.

163. Carod-Artal FJ. Neurological complications of Schistosoma infection. *Trans R Soc Trop Med Hyg.* 2008;102(2):107-116.

164. Murray HW. Kala-azar-progress against a neglected disease. *N Engl J Med.* 2002;22:347, 1793-1794.

165. Herwaldt BL. Leishmaniasis. *Lancet.* 1999;354(9185):1191-1199.

166. Hashim FA, Ahmed AE, el Hassan M, et al. Neurologic changes in visceral leishmaniasis. *Am J Trop Med Hyg.* 1995;52:149-154.

167. Mustafa D. Neurological disturbances in visceral leishmaniasis. *J Trop Med Hyg.* 1965;68:248-250.

168. Herwaldt BL. Leishmaniasis. *Lancet.* 1999;354(9185):1191-1199.

169. Laguna F. Treatment of leishmaniasis in HIV-positive patients. *Ann Trop Med Parasitol.* 2003;97(suppl 1):135-142.

170. Voulgari PV, Katsimbri P, Alamanos Y, Drosos AA. Gender and age differences in systemic lupus erythematosus. A study of 489 Greek patients with a review of the literature. *Lupus.* 2002;11:722-729.

171. Simard JF, Costenbader KH. What can epidemiology tell us about systemic lupus erythematosus? *Int J Clin Pract.* 2007;61(7):1170-1180.

172. Hirose S, Jiang Y, Nishimura H, Shirai T. Significance of MHC class II haplotypes and IgG Fc receptors in SLE. *Springer Semin Immunopathol.* 2006;28(2):163-174.

173. Tsokos GC. Lymphocytes, cytokines, inflammation, and immune trafficking. *Curr Opin Rheumatol.* 1994;6)5:461-467.

174. Rahman A, Isenberg DA. Systemic lupus erythematosus. *N Engl J Med.* 2008;358(9):929-939.

175. Childs SG. The pathogenesis of systemic lupus erythematosus. *Orthop Nurs.* 2006;25(2):140-145.

176. Gómez-Puerta JA, Burlingame RW, Cervera R. Anti-chromatin (anti-nucleosome) antibodies. *Lupus.* 2006;15(7):408-411.

177. Provenzale JM, Orel TL, Allen TB. Systemic thrombosis in patients with anti-phospholipid antibodies: lesion distribution and imaging findings. *Am J Roentgenol.* 1998;170:285-290.

178. Benucci M, Saviola G, Baiardi P, et al. Anti-nucleosome antibodies as prediction factor of development of autoantibodies during therapy with three different TNFalpha blocking agents in rheumatoid arthritis. *Clin Rheumatol.* 2008;27(1):91-95.

179. Rosado S, Perez-Chacon G, Mellor-Pita S, et al. Expression of human leukocyte antigen-G in systemic lupus erythematosus. *Hum Immunol.* 2008;69(1):9-15.

180. Bettero RG, Rahal MY, Barboza JS, Skare TL. Headache and systemic lupus erythematosus: prevalence and associated conditions. *Arg Neuropsiquatr.* 2007;65(48):1196-1199.

181. Alexa ID, Stoica MS, Paraschiv O, Rusu RI. Neuropsychiatric manifestations in systemic lupus erythematosus. *Rev Med Chir Soc Med Nat.* 2006;110(2):322-325.

182. Ainiala H, Loukkola J, Peltola J, et al. The prevalence of neuropsychiatric syndromes in systemic lupus erythematosus. *Neurology.* 2001;57:496-500.

183. Sarzi-Puttini P, Atzeni F, Carrabba M. Cardiovascular risk factors in systemic lupus erythematosus and in antiphospholipid syndrome. *Minerva Med.* 2003;94(2):63-70.

184. Jennings JE, Sundgren PC, Attwood J, et al. Value of MRI of the brain in patients with systemic lupus erythematosus and neurologic disturbance. *Neuroradiology.* 2004;46(1):15-21.

185. Pego-Reigosa JM, Isenberg DA. Systemic lupus erythematosus: pharmacological

developments and recommendations for therapeutic strategy. *Expert Opin Investig Drugs.* 2008;17(1):31-41.

186. Sfikakis PP, Boletis JN, Tsokos GC. Rituximab anti-B-cell therapy in systemic lupus erythematosus: pointing to the future. *Curr Opin Rheumatol.* 2005;17(5):550-557.

187. Mosca M, Baldini C, Bombardieri S. LJP-394 (abetimus sodium) in the treatment of systemic lupus erythematosus. *Expert Opin Pharmacother.* 2007;8(6):873-879.

188. Rhiannon JJ. Systemic lupus erythematosus involving the nervous system: presentation, pathogenesis, and management. *Clin Rev Allergy Immunol.* 2008.3 [Epub ahead of print].

189. Kurtzke JF. MS epidemiology world wide. One view of current status. *Acta Neurol Scand Suppl.* 1995;161:23-33.

190. Hogancamp WE, Rodriguez M, Weinshenker BG. The epidemiology of multiple sclerosis. *Mayo Clin Proc.* 1997;72(9):871-878.

191. Koch-Henriksen N, Hyllested K. Epidemiology of multiple sclerosis: incidence and prevalence rates in Denmark 1948-64 based on the Danish Multiple Sclerosis Registry. *Acta Neurol Scand.* 1988;78:369-380.

192. Hernán MA, Olek MJ, Ascherio A. Geographic variation of MS incidence in two prospective studies of US women. *Neurology.* 1999;53:1711-1718.

193. Compston A, Coles A. Multiple sclerosis. *Lancet.* 2002;359:1221-1231.

194. Ascherio A, Munger K. Epidemiology of multiple sclerosis: from risk factors to prevention. *Semin Neurol.* 2008;28(1):17-28.

195. Winquist RJ, Kwong A, Ramachandran R, Jain J. The complex etiology of multiple sclerosis. *Biochem Pharm.* 2007;74(9):1321-1329.

196. Frohman EM, Racke MK, Raine CS. Multiple sclerosis—the plaque and its pathogenesis. *NEJM.* 2006;354:942-955.

197. Siva A. The spectrum of multiple sclerosis and treatment decisions. *Clin Neurol Neurosurg.* 2006;108(3):333-338.

198. Sawcer S, Compston A. Multiple sclerosis: light at the end of the tunnel. *Eur J Hum Genet.* 2006;14:257-258.

199. Celius EG, Harbo HF, Egeland T, et al. Sex and age at diagnosis are correlated with the HLS-DR2, DZ6 haplotype in multiple sclerosis. *J Neurol Sci.* 2000;178:132-135.

200. Nino M, Kikuchi S, Fukazawa T, Yabe I, Tashiro K. Estrogen receptor gene polymorphism in Japanese patients with multiple sclerosis. *J Neurol Sci.* 2000;179:70-75.

201. Kira J. Multiple sclerosis in the Japanese population. *Lancet Neurol.* 2003;2(2):117-127.

202. Kurtzke JF. Clinical definition for multiple sclerosis treatment trials. *Ann Neurol.* 1994;36 (suppl):S73-S79.

203. Polman CH, Reingold SC, Edan G, et al. Diagnostic criteria for multiple sclerosis: 2005 revisions to the "McDonald Criteria." *Ann Neurol.* 2005;58:840-846.

204. Schwendimann N, Alekseeva N. Gender issues in multiple sclerosis. *Internat Review Neurobio.* 2007;79:377-392.

205. Tomassini V, Onesti E, Mainero C, et al. Sex hormones modulate brain damage in multiple sclerosis: MRI evidence. *J Neurol Neurosurg Psychiatry.* 2005;76(2):272-275.

206. Laule C, Vavasour IM, Moore GR, et al. Water content and myelin water fraction in multiple sclerosis. A T2 relaxation study. *J Neurol.* 2004;251(3):284-293.

207. Coyle PK. Gender issues. *Neural Clin.* 2005;23:39-60.

208. Hemmer B, Hartung HP. Toward the development of rational therapies in multiple sclerosis: what is on the horizon? *Ann Neurol*. 2007;62(4):314-326.

209. Beck RW, Cleary PA, Trobe JD, et al. The effect of corticosteroids for acute optic neuritis on the subsequent development of multiple sclerosis. The Optic Neuritis Study Group. *NEJM*. 1993;329:1764-1769.

210. Jacobs LD, Cookfair DL, Rudick RA, et al. Intramuscular iterferon beta-1a for disease progression in relapsing multiple sclerosis. The Multiple Sclerosis Collaborative Research Group (MSCRG). *Ann Neurol*. 1996;39:285-294.

211. Wingerchuk DM. Current evidence and therapeutic strategies for multiple sclerosis. *Semin Neurol*. 2008;28(1):56-68.

212. Le Page E, Leray E, Gregory T, et al. Mitoxantrone as induction treatment in aggressive relapsing remitting multiple sclerosis: treatment response factors in a 5-year follow-up observational study of 100 consecutive patients. *J Neurol Neurosurg Psychiat*. January 5 2008;79(1):52-56.

213. Vincent A, Palace J, Hilton-Jones D. Myasthenia gravis. *Lancet*. 2001;357(9274): 2122-2128.

214. García-Carrasco M, Escárcega RO, Fuentes-Alexandro S, et al. Therapeutic options in autoimmune myasthenia gravis. *Autoimmun Rev*. 2007;6(6):373-378.

215. Somnier FE. Myasthenia gravis. *Dan Med Bull*. 1996;43(1):1-10.

216. Keyes G. Obstetrics and gynaecology in relation to thyrotoxicosis and myasthenia gravis. *J Obstet Gynecol Brit Commonweal*. 1952;59:173-182.

217. Plauche WC. Myasthenia gravis in mothers and their newborn. *Clin Obstet Gynecol*. 1991;34:82-99.

218. Bashuk RG, Krendel DA. Myastenia gravis presenting as weakness after magnesium administration. *Muscle Nerve*. 1990;13:708-712.

219. Daroff RB. The office Tensilon test for ocular myasthenia gravis. *Arch Neurol*. 1986;43:843-844.

220. Benatar M. A systematic review of diagnostic studies in myasthenia gravis. *Neuromuscul Disord*. 2006;16(7):459-467.

221. Newsom-Davis J. Therapy in myasthenia gravis and Lambert-Eaton myasthenic syndrome. *Semin Neurol*. 2003;23(2):191-198.

222. Pascuzzi RM, Coslett HB, Johns TR. Long-term corticosteroid treatment of myasthenia gravis: report of 116 patients. *Ann Neurol*. 1984;15:291-298.

223. Miller RG, Milner-Brown HS, Mirka A. Prednisone-induced worsening of neuromuscular function in myasthenia gravis. *Neurology*. 1986;36:729-732.

224. Perlo VP, Arnason B, Poskanzer D, et al. The role of thymectomy in treatment of myasthenia gravis. *Ann NY Acad Sci*. 1971;183:308-315.

225. Trikha I, Singh S, Goyal V, et al. Comparative efficacy of low dose, daily versus alternate day plasma exchange in severe myasthenia gravis: a randomised trial. *J Neurol*. 2007;254(8):989-995.

226. Obermeyer CM, Reher D, Saliba M. Symptoms, menopause status, and country differences: a comparative analysis from DAMES. *Menopause*. 2007;14(4):788-797.

227. Devi G, Hahn K, Massimi S, Zhivotovskaya E. Prevalence of memory loss complaints and other symptoms associated with the menopause transition: a community survey. *Gend Med*. 2005;2(4):255-264.

228. Sherwin BB. Estrogen effects on cognition in menopausal women. *Neurology*. 1997;48:S21-S26.

229. Genazzani AR, Pluchino N, Luisi S, Luisi M. Estrogen, cognition, and female ageing. *Hum Reprod Update*. March-April 1 2007;13(2):175-187.

230. Hogervorst E, Williams J, Budge M, et al. The nature of the effect of female gonadal hormone replacement therapy on cognitive function in post-menopausal women: a meta-analysis. *Neuroscience.* 2000;101(3):485-512.

231. Gambacciani M, Pepe A. Menopause and related problems. *Minerva Med.* 2007;98(3):191-201.

232. Maki PM. Hormone therapy and cognitive function: is there a critical period for benefit? *Neuroscience.* 2006;138(3):1027-1030.

233. Devi G, Massimi S, Schultz S, Khosrowshahi L, Laakso UK. A double-blind, placebo-controlled trial of donepezil for the treatment of menopause-related cognitive loss. *Gend Med.* 2007;4(4):352-358.

234. Ferri CP, Prince M, Brayne C. Global prevalence of dementia: a Delphi consensus study. *Lancet.* 2005;366(9503):2112-2117.

235. Qiu C, De Ronchi D, Fratiglioni L. The epidemiology of the dementias : an update. *Curr Opin Psychiatry.* 2007;20(4):380-385.

236. Falagas ME, Vardakas KZ, Vergidis PI. Under-diagnosis of common chronic diseases: prevalence and impact on human health. *Int J Clin Pract.* 2007;61(9):1569-1579.

237. The Canadian Study of Healthy and Aging. Risk factors for Alzheimer's disease in Canada. *Neurology.* 1994;44:2073-2080.

238. Andersen K, Launer LJ, Deqey ME, et al. Gender differences in the incidence of AD and vascular dementia: The EURODEM studies. *Neurology.* 1999;53:1992-1997.

239. Ruitenberg A, Ott A, van Swieten JC, Hofman A, Breteler MM. Incidence of dementia: does gender make a difference? *Neurobio Aging.* 2001;22:575-580.

240. Almeida OP, Lautenschlager NT. Dementia associated with infectious diseases. *Int Psychogeriatr.* 2005;17:S65-S77.

241. Ances BM, Ellis RJ. Dementia and neurocognitive disorders due to HIV-1 infection. *Semin Neurol.* 2007;27:086-092.

242. Grant I. Neurocognitive disturbances in HIV. *Int Rev Psychiatry.* 2008;20(1):33-47.

243. Quinn TC, Overbaugh J. HIV/AIDS in women: an expanding epidemic. *Science.* 2005;308(5728):1582-1583.

244. Ertekin-Taner N. Genetics of Alzheimer's disease: a centennial review. *Neurol Clin.* 2007;25(3):611-667.

245. Levy-Lahad E, Tsuang D, Bird TD. Recent advances in the genetics of Alzheimer's disease. *J Geriatr Psychiatry Neurol.* 1998;11(2):42-54.

246. McDowell I. Alzheimer's disease: insights from epidemiology. *Aging.* 2001;13(3):143-162.

247. Chun MR, Mayeux R. Alzheimer's disease. *Curr Opin Neurol.* 1994;7(4):299-304.

248. Farrer LA, Cupples LA, Haines JL, et al. Effects of age, sex, and ethnicity on the association between apolipoprotein E genotype and Alzheimer disease. A meta-analysis. APOE and Alzheimer Disease Meta Analysis Consortium. *JAMA.* 1997;278(16):1349-1356.

249. Yaari R, Corey-Bloom J. Alzheimer's disease. *Semin Neurol.* 2007;27(1):32-41.

250. Hyman BT. New neuropathological criteria for Alzheimer disease. *Arch Neurol.* 1998;55:1174-1176.

251. Davies P, Maloney AJF. Selective loss of central cholinergic neurons in Alzheimer's disease. *Lancet.* 1976;2:1402-1406.

252. Erkinjuntti T. Vascular cognitive deterioration and stroke. *Cerebrovasc Dis.* 2007;24(suppl 1):189-194.

253. Erkinjuntti T. Diagnosis and management of vascular cognitive impairment and dementia. *J Neural Transm Suppl.* 2002;(63):91-109.

254. Pantoni L, Inzitari D. Hachinski's ischemic score and the diagnosis of vascular dementia: a review. *Ital J Neurol Sci.* 1993;14(7):539-546.

255. Geser F, Wenning GK, Poewe W, McKeith I. How to diagnose dementia with Lewy bodies: state of the art. *Mov Disord.* 2005;20(suppl)12:S11-S20.

256. Price RW. Management of AIDS dementia complex and HIV-1 infection of the nervous system. *AIDS.* 1995;9(suppl):S221-S236.

257. Tariot PN, Cummings JL, Katz IR, et al. A randomized, double-blind, placebo-controlled study of the efficacy and safety of donepezil in patients with Alzheimer's disease in the nursing home setting. *J Am Geriatr Soc.* 2001;49:1590-1599.

258. Winblad B, Engedal K, Soininen H, et al. A 1-year, randomized, placebo-controlled study of donepezil in patients with mild to moderate AD. *Neurology.* 2001;57:489-495.

259. Wolfson C, Oremus M, Shukla V, et al. Donepezil and rivastigmine in the treatment of Alzheimer's disease: a best-evidence synthesis of the published data on their efficacy and cost-effectiveness. *Clin Ther.* 2002;24:862-886.

260. Wilcock GK, Lilienfeld S, Gaens E. Efficacy and safety of galantamine in patients with mild to moderate Alzheimer's disease: multicentre randomised controlled trial. Galantamine International-1 study group. *BMJ.* 2000;321:1445-1449.

261. Frank C. Dementia with Lewy bodies. Review of diagnosis and pharmacologic management. *Can Fam Physician.* 2003;49:1304-1311.

262. Hinkin CH, Hardy DJ, Mason KI. Medication adherence in HIV-infected adults: effect of patient age, cognitive status, and substance abuse. *AIDS.* 2004;18(suppl 1):S19-S25.

CHAPTER 16

INTRODUCTION

Women's Musculoskeletal Health

Musculoskeletal disorders are a major source of pain and disability at all ages and in all regions of the globe. A study in the Netherlands found that those reporting musculoskeletal conditions scored worse on the Short-Form Health Survey (SF-36), especially in the areas of physical functioning and pain, than those without similar conditions. Scores were worse for those with multiple musculoskeletal complaints.[1] Although these conditions are common in both men and women, differences in incidence, presentation, and treatment outcomes have been identified between the sexes. These differences have been attributed to genetic, hormonal, environmental, and societal factors. Although musculoskeletal trauma and secondary infections have significant worldwide impact, because of different societal expectations and exposure, these are conditions seen more frequently among men in most regions. However, the most common bone and joint conditions—osteoporosis and osteoarthritis— have a significantly higher incidence among women.

With the continued and increasing societal demands on women regarding work both inside and out of the home, these bone and joint conditions can affect the ability of women to function in their expected roles, as well as impair their quality of life. In a survey of residents in Zimbabwe regarding sources of disability, Jelsma et al. found that among their subjects, who were primarily women aged 16 to 59, osteoarthritis was the second most common condition.[2] With life expectancy of most women improving, musculoskeletal conditions can be expected to take additional tolls with aging. In a survey of a cohort of older men and women in the United States to identify risk factors associated with physical functioning, Murtagh et al. found significantly greater limitations among the women, as well as a greater degree of disability.[3] The authors concluded that these differences were largely explained by differences in prevalence of disability-related health conditions. In addition to neurologic disease, the most commonly reported conditions were hip or lower extremity joint pain; fractures; back, neck, or shoulder pain; osteoarthritis; chronic back problems; and osteoporosis, again highlight-

Kimberley Templeton, MD

Kimberly Templeton, MD, is an Associate Professor of Orthopedic Surgery for the University of Kansas Medical Center in Kansas City, Kansas.

ing the effects of musculoskeletal conditions. In addition to the aging of the population in most regions, the increasing incidence of HIV will also affect the numbers of those with musculoskeletal conditions, as close to three-quarters of patients with HIV/AIDS exhibit one of these conditions at some point during the course of their illness.

Osteoporosis

The most common bone condition is osteoporosis. Although present in men, this condition is significantly more common in women. Until recently, this condition has been primarily described in the non-Hispanic White population; however, it is now recognized with increasing frequency in all races. This increase in incidence may be caused by the aging of the population, improved treatment of other health conditions leading to secondary osteoporosis, or increased awareness and diagnosis of the condition. With the aging of the population, the greatest rate of increase in osteoporosis and its associated fractures is predicted to occur in Asia in the coming decades.

In people with osteoporosis, the individual bone trabeculae are thinner, fewer in number, and less interconnected. This results in bone that is more prone to fracture, frequently during activities of daily living. Fractures secondary to osteoporosis typically occur with such low impact activities as lifting or a fall from standing height or less. In addition, however, as the older population or those with chronic illnesses remain more active, fractures as a result of more significant trauma may also occur more readily in those with osteoporosis. Unfortunately, osteoporosis is frequently not diagnosed until after the first fracture occurs, resulting in a significant risk of mortality, morbidity, alteration in independent lifestyles, and substantial cost to patients, families, and society.

The most common regions of fractures related to osteoporosis are the spine, hip, and wrist. Additional fractures occur at the shoulder and ankle. Osteoporosis-related fractures, especially those of the spine and hip, are related to a substantial increase in morbidity and mortality. Although the incidence of most osteoporosis-related fractures is known, the precise incidence of fractures of the spine, believed to be the most common site of fracture, is not known, as the most common presenting complaint is back pain; these fractures are often found in retrospect. Determination of the incidence of the remaining fractures in women is affected by access to health care, as well as the recognition by healthcare professionals of the role of osteoporosis in the development of fractures after more substantial trauma.

Various factors, such as genetics, hormones, exercise, nutrition, and other health conditions affect bone health, both in the development of peak bone mass as well as bone loss that occurs with aging. Peak bone mass typically develops during the first three decades of life, with the greatest increase in bone mass during the second decade. The sexes differ in the development of peak bone mass, both in timing as well as quantity of bone amassed, primarily through the different hormonal milieux: estrogen in both sexes acts primarily to control osteoclastic bone resorption, while testosterone stimulates osteoblastic bone formation. Women reach peak bone mass at an earlier age than men. An incremental loss of bone occurs in both sexes with aging, with greater loss occurring in periods of sex hormone deficiency, such as during menopause or medical hormone manipulation. Bone strength, or the ability of bone to resist fracture, is determined by bone quantity, typically approximated by bone density through the use of dual energy x-ray absorptiometry (DEXA), as well as bone quality and geometry. Research is in progress to develop accurate measures of bone quality or structure and connectivity. Three-dimensional bone geometry can be approximated utilizing DEXA or computed tomography, although the latter is primarily used for research purposes. Unfortunately, women frequently are not assessed for osteoporosis until the initial fracture occurs. In addition, evaluation and treatment for osteoporosis also varies by race. African American women have been reported to be evaluated and treated for osteoporosis significantly less often than Caucasians, even after a fracture and independent of demographic factors.[4] This bias may originate from the knowledge that African American women have a lower risk of osteoporosis; however, the incidence of osteoporosis is still significant in this population, especially in those who are older or who have other medical conditions. Access to technology such as DEXA is limited in underserved populations in industrialized and nonindustrialized nations, leading groups, such as the World Health Organization (WHO), to develop paradigms to estimate risk based on clinical parameters.

The genetic influence on bone health appears to primarily affect the development of peak bone mass, as well as the geometry of bone. Women of African descent tend to have thicker bone trabeculae and larger bones, decreasing their risk of osteoporosis and consequent fractures. This decreased risk, however, has led to the misperceptions among the medical and lay communities that women of African descent are not at risk of either osteoporosis or fractures. This is problematic as these women have an increased morbidity after sustaining fractures than do women of other races.

As mentioned, the greatest risk of increase in osteoporosis-related fractures is predicted to occur in Asia. However, this varies by country of origin, as the risk of osteoporosis, although high, is not the same for all women of Asian descent. In addition, the bone geometry and typically lower body mass index (BMI) of women from this group may place those with osteoporosis at lower risk of fracture compared to those of different races with similar bone strength.

In addition to the generalizations about osteoporosis risk related to race, individual risk is also influenced by family history. There is a significantly increased risk of developing osteoporosis among those with first-degree relatives with the condition. Although knowledge of the effect of genetics and family history on osteoporosis is important to better understand the condition, the roles of hormones, nutrition, and exercise in maintenance of bone health are those factors that can potentially be modified. As previously mentioned, estrogen acts as a modulator of osteoclastic bone resorption. Although bone resorption is necessary to allow remodeling of bone as it adapts to physical stresses, interference with hormonal control can lead to more rapid bone loss. Estrogen receptors have also been found to be one of the mediators of bone remodeling in response to mechanical stress.[5] Little bone loss is seen during pre- or early perimenopause. However, there is substantial bone loss during late perimenopause, resulting in an annual loss of 3–5% of bone mass during the first five years after the onset of menopause. Similar patterns of bone loss are since seen among women of all ethnicities. However, bone loss appears to be greatest among Japanese and Chinese, intermediate in non-Hispanic White, and slowest among women of African descent. In addition to genetic predisposition, there is some indication that these variations are due to body weight: loss of bone mineral density (BMD) is greatest among those in the lowest percentile of body weight,[6] perhaps reflecting differences in peripheral estrogen production.

Other alterations in estrogen metabolism, such as pregnancy, treatment for breast cancer, and endometriosis, can also lead to increased bone loss at an earlier age. Small degrees of bone loss occur throughout pregnancy, especially during the last trimester. This reflects hormonal changes, as well as alterations in calcium metabolism. Among those treated for breast cancer, Bruning et al. found that lumbar spine BMD was significantly decreased in premenopausal women who received chemotherapy in addition to mastectomy versus those women treated with mastectomy alone. [7] Seventy-one percent of those treated with chemotherapy became amenorrheic secondary to ovarian failure at the follow-up period, compared to 16% of the women undergoing mastectomy alone. Headley et al. found that premenopausal women who became amenorrheic during chemotherapy for breast cancer demonstrated a BMD 14% lower than those patients who remained eumenorrheic.[8] Somekawa et al. and Palomba, in independent studies, both demonstrated an approximately 5% decrease in BMD in premenopausal women with endometriosis treated with leuprolide for six months.[9,10] Makita et al. found similar bone loss early in treatment but that BMD recovered after 12 months of treatment.[11] The impact of oral contraceptives on bone health has not been clearly elucidated, but there is some data that use of this medication in young women may affect the development of peak bone mass.[12, 13] However, this effect may be reduced by other bone-enhancing behaviors, such as weight-bearing exercise.[14]

As the body's repository of calcium, bone requires adequate intake of dietary calcium as well as vitamin D, which is necessary for calcium absorption, for maintenance of structure and density. The recommended daily intake of calcium and vitamin D varies by age, with those in adolescence (during development of peak bone mass) and pregnant and lactating women requiring the highest levels of calcium intake. Unfortunately, most teenage and adult women do not take in enough calcium. Calcium intake is affected by social factors, such as traditional diet, which may not include dairy products or other sources of calcium. Intake of calcium is also affected by expectations of woman's appearance, affecting intake of sufficient calories and nutrients; access to dairy products; and lactose intolerance.

Teenage females, especially those in industrialized countries, are held to the ideal of being thin. This can lead to conditions such as anorexia nervosa or, in the athletic community, female athlete triad. The triad consists of eating disorders, amenorrhea, and osteoporosis. The eating disorder most frequently noted is anorexia nervosa, although the primary nutritional issue is an imbalance of calories consumed versus those expended.[15] The amenorrhea developed in this condition is caused by the development of hypothalamic hypogonadism. The resulting effect on bone mass was initially thought to be a reflection of decreased estrogen production, similar to that seen after menopause. However, it has since been found that bone loss occurs because of a negative calorie balance through a variety of hormones such as triiodothyronine, insulin-like growth factor 1, and dehydroepiandrosterone.[16] With reversal of this energy balance, serum markers of bone formation improve prior to resumption of menses,[17] although serum markers of bone resorption remain elevated. In addition, leptin, which is produced by adipocytes and is in lower concentrations in those with anorexia, may play a role in both fat metabolism as well as bone health through its regulation of osteoblast and osteoclast differentiation.[16] In anorexia nervosa alone, or in female athlete triad, decreased caloric intake as well as decreased calcium intake, affects bone health. These conditions are especially concerning as they may affect the development of peak bone mass, putting those affected at risk of stress fractures during their teenage years, as well as osteoporosis-related fractures at an earlier age.

A similar effect of the development of peak bone mass and the future risk of osteoporosis has been postulated to occur among women who have survived famine during the early years of their lives.[18] Among postmenopausal women in Hong Kong, those who had experienced famine as children were significantly more likely to have osteoporosis. However, the long-term effect of early famine on bone is most likely multifactorial.

Vitamin D is essential to the maintenance of bone health. Vitamin D insufficiency or deficiency is recognized in a significant percentage of women sustaining osteoporosis-related fractures. In a cross-sectional study of 2589 postmenopausal women from Northern, Central, and Southern Europe; the Middle East; Latin America; the Pacific Rim; and Asia, Rizzoli et al. found low levels of vitamin D in women from all regions.[19] [see Fig. 16-1] In addition, there was a significant difference between countries within the same region, implicating additional risk factors for vitamin D deficiency. Some of the risk factors identified were lack of adequate vitamin D supplementation, poor general health, and absence of discussion of the importance of vitamin D with a healthcare professional. The additional effect of vitamin D deficiency is that, not only does it lead to increased bone fragility, but it also leads to muscle weakness and an increased risk of falls.

Unlike calcium, which is readily available in several types of foods, especially dairy products, vitamin D is more difficult to obtain through nutritional sources. Certain types of fish, fortified dairy products, and egg yolks contain vitamin D. Young women, concerned about caloric consumption, frequently do not consume enough vitamin D. In addition, fortified dairy products are not readily available outside of industrialized nations. Even for those who have access to these products, those with lactose intolerance are at risk of vitamin D deficiency. This is most pronounced among those of African, Hispanic, and Aboriginal heritage. Women of African heritage have higher peak bone mass and lose bone more slowly after menopause than women from other genetic backgrounds, potentially delaying the effect of inadequate calcium and vitamin D intake. However, dietary deficiencies ultimately account for the majority of osteoporosis-related fractures in this group. Women of Hispanic and Aboriginal descent appear to have similar bone acquisition and loss profiles as do Caucasians; thus, the impact of calcium and vitamin D is more profound and affects bone earlier.

For women without access to these nutritional sources and not receiving vitamin D supplementation, the primary source of vitamin D is sunlight

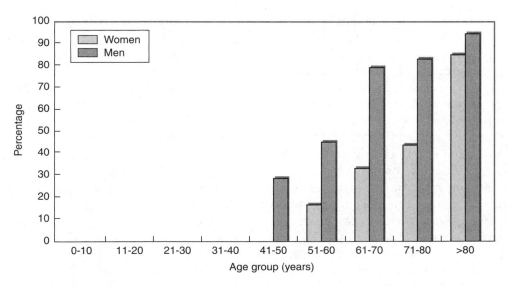

FIGURE 16-1 Age distribution by gender
Sodha S, Ring D, Zurakowski D, Jupiter J. Prevalence of osteoarthrosis of the trapeziometacarpal joint. *J Bone Joint Surg (Am)*. 2005; 87:2614–2618

exposure. The exposure to ultraviolet light B (UVB) transforms 7-dehydrochoesterol into vitamin D_3, which is hydroxylated at the 25-position in the liver and into the active 1,25 dihydroxy vitamin D_3 in the kidney. 25 hydroxyvitamin D is the primary storage form of the vitamin, while the formation of the more active 1,25 dihydroxyvitamin D is under control of the parathyroid hormone. The amount of production of vitamin D through sunlight exposure is determined by latitude and season, skin surface area, and duration of exposure, as well as by degree of skin pigmentation.

Vitamin D deficiency is common in people older than 50, when the concentration of substrate in the skin starts to decline. Although women living in equatorial countries would be presumed to have adequate sunlight exposure year round to produce sufficient amounts of vitamin D, changes in the production of vitamin D with aging make dietary intake even more important. In a study of older patients in Brazil, Saraiva et al. found that 42% of patients had insufficient serum vitamin D levels, and 15% of patients had deficient serum vitamin D levels.[20] In Brazil, food is not supplemented with vitamin D.

Increasing use of sunscreen or avoidance of the sun limits vitamin D production for people of all ages. Women living with societal expectations of having fair skin and thus avoiding direct sun exposure are at risk of vitamin D deficiency. In addition, for those living in inner-city or combat areas with limited safe exposure to outdoor activities, obtaining appropriate duration of sunlight exposure may be challenging.

For women in equatorial regions, the ability to make vitamin D through sun exposure is affected by skin pigmentation, as those with increased pigmentation produce less vitamin D with equivalent sun exposure. It can also be affected by cultural and societal expectations. Unfortunately, vitamin D status may be overlooked in these regions, based on the assumption that adequate sunshine exists to maintain vitamin D levels. However, traditional clothing worn in various countries, especially in the Middle East, limits exposure to the sun. Vitamin D deficiency has been found among women in countries such as India, Iran, Kuwait, Saudi Arabia, and Turkey. Up to 80% of the population of Iran is estimated to be deficient in vitamin D. In a study of premenopausal women in Turkey, serum 25 OH vitamin D concentrations were negatively correlated with the duration of being veiled.[21] Allali et al. found that the wearing of traditional clothing that conceals the arms, legs, and head was significantly related to the presence of osteoporosis among women in Morocco.[22] An additional risk factor identified was family history of fracture; this may reflect the genetic influence on bone mass development, traditional clothing wear among the generations, or a combination of both.

An additional factor affecting bone health and osteoporosis is weight-bearing exercise. As mentioned, excess exercise can lead to an increased risk of bone loss if not balanced with adequate caloric consumption. However, bone responds to mechanical loads, such as weight-bearing exercise. The effect of exercise, including the secondary strain placed on bone by adjacent muscle, may be modulated through estrogen receptor alpha.[5] The increasing incidence of osteoporosis among women of some cultures may be caused by prohibitions on physical activity. This not only limits potential sun exposure for vitamin D production but limits opportunities for weight-bearing exercise and consequent increase in lean tissue mass. Valdimarsson et al. noted an increase in bone mineral content and BMD among girls randomized to an exercise program.[22] Guzel et al. found that BMD at the lumbar spine was positively correlated with the degree of physical activity among premenopausal Turkish women.[21] Weight-bearing activity early in life affects the development of peak bone mass.[23] However, the long-term effect of early exercise is difficult to ascertain owing to inconsistent levels of activity in adults, as well as the variety of other factors that affect bone. However, lack of current weight-bearing exercise has been identified as a risk factor for osteoporosis in older adults.

As with osteoporosis, the incidence of fractures varies among ethnicities and countries. This variation is a reflection of differences in bone strength, anatomy, and risk of falls. In a study of postmenopausal Mayan women in Mexico, Beyenne et al. found a relatively low BMD, compared to non-Hispanic Whites.[24] However, the Mayan women demonstrated a low rate of osteoporosis-related fractures. This low rate of fractures may be caused by exposure to sunlight and maintenance of adequate vitamin D to prevent falls. However, in this culture, women are expected to perform strenuous household tasks from an early age. This may have led to development of improved bone quality, as well as the coordination and strength to prevent falls.

Educational levels have been found by some to be inversely related to the risk of developing osteoporosis.[25] Educational levels may reflect socioeconomic status and consequent access to adequate nutrition, health care, and family planning. However, education status in and of itself may affect lifestyle, such as dietary choices and risky behaviors. In a survey of postmenopausal women in Hong Kong, Wan Kin et al. found that those who had experienced famine at an early age were more likely to have a lower socioeconomic status and educational level, as well as a higher incidence of osteoporosis.[18] These women also had lower calcium intake and a higher risk of smoking at the time of the survey. Although the effect of famine on the development of peak bone mass was episodic and potentially reversible, the effect on education, socioeconomic levels, and consequent lifestyle factors was lifelong. In a survey of Turkish women, Ungan et al. found that approximately 40% of respondents could correctly identify calcium-rich foods and risk factors for osteoporosis.[26] Education level and a history of discussing osteoporosis with a physician, both potentially tied to socioeconomic status, were significantly correlated with knowledge of osteoporosis.

Unfortunately, even among women achieving higher levels of education, the knowledge of the importance of bone health and the factors affecting it is frequently poor. Women in Taiwan with first-degree relatives with osteoporosis—putting the subjects at increased risk of also having the condition—and at least a high school education, demonstrated an accuracy rate of about 50% on a survey to assess knowledge of osteoporosis.[27] In this group of women, knowledge about osteoporosis significantly affected the practice of healthy lifestyle behaviors. In a survey of middle-aged and elderly women in Hong Kong,[28] three-quarters of women surveyed had heard of vitamin D; however, only half recognized that vitamin D is good for bone health, and one-third knew the action of vitamin D. Unfortunately, substantially more women responded that they had acquired this information from the media rather than from discussion with a healthcare professional. Despite the high incidence of osteoporosis and substantial risk for subsequent fractures and their complications, women tend to rank levels of "worry" about this condition significantly lower than other conditions, such as breast cancer and cardiovascular disease. This area represents a significant opportunity for public health intervention and education, as well as increased involvement from the health-care community.

Arthritis

Arthritis is the most common joint disorder in both sexes. As with other inflammatory conditions, inflammatory arthritis, including rheumatoid arthritis, is primarily a condition for women. However, osteoarthritis, the predominant form of arthritis, is also more common in women than in men, especially over the age of 50. The development of osteoarthritis at various joints most likely has differing etiologies and risk factors, reflected in differing incidence rates between the sexes: osteoarthritis of the hip is more common in men, while women predominantly exhibit degenerative changes at the knee and base of the thumb. This female predilection is noted in all races and geographic locations. Osteoarthritis of the trapeziometacarpal joint occurs with such high frequency among aging women that it has been considered a part of aging[29] (see Figure 16-1).

In addition, symptoms of osteoarthritis occur earlier, progress more rapidly, and tend to be more debilitating in women.[30] The only exception to this sex-based variation is among those with HIV-related arthropathy. Up to one-third of patients with HIV/AIDS will experience joint pain at some during the course of their disease. However, unlike most of the other arthropathies, this HIV-related condition has equal prevalence between the sexes. Little is known about the pathophysiology of this condition. It is most likely an inflammatory arthritis, although it progresses more rapidly than the other inflammatory arthritides. There are few sex-based differences in presentation, other than a higher incidence of urogenital infections prior to onset in women as noted in one study.[31]

As with osteoporosis, the etiology of arthritis is multifactorial. Factors implicated in this condition include genetic factors, both in terms of specific triggers for the development of arthritis as well as sex-based differences in anatomy and neuromuscular development affecting the joints; sex hormone influences; injury; activity level; obesity; and societal factors. However, knowledge of differences in arthritis risk factors and presentation

among the races is by and large unknown, as most of the clinical research in this field has been conducted in industrialized countries with non-Hispanic White patients. The limited exploration of ethnic differences in the prevalence of osteoarthritis in Western countries has found that the condition appears to be more common among those of African and Aboriginal descent and less common among those of Asian origin.[32] A genetic predisposition leading to variable incidences of arthritis among various ethnicities has not been defined. This difference in incidence may reflect other factors, such as variable levels of obesity and socioeconomic status.

Twin studies have indicated a role for heritability of osteoarthritis; this role appears to be greater for women than for men. However, the precise mechanism of this genetic influence is not known. Articular cartilage has been found to express estrogen receptors; the genetic influence may act through inheritance of various estrogen receptor genotypes: Fytili et al. found a significant difference in distribution of estrogen receptor alpha and beta gene polymorphisms between patients undergoing total knee arthroplasty versus controls.[33] In addition, Ushiyama et al. demonstrated that women with the PpXx genotype of estrogen receptor alpha were more likely to demonstrate generalized osteoarthritis.[34]

The increased incidence of osteoarthritis in women may also be related to sex-based differences in anatomy as well as collagen metabolism. The latter is expressed in increased ligamentous laxity and has been described as one of the factors in the development of osteoarthritis at the base of the thumb. Both factors most likely influence development of osteoarthritis of the knee. Women are prone to developing arthritis of the pa-tellofemoral joint, presenting as anterior knee pain, exacerbated by sitting or stair use. The differential development of this condition appears to be related sex-based differences in anatomy and tissue laxity. Tracking of the patella within the femoral trochlea depends on quadriceps control. However, because of wider pelves in women, the Q-angle (the angle between the pelvis and tibia), which defines the direction of force of the patella, tends to lead to lateral translation of the patella. In addition, certain anatomic differences in women, such as the contour of the patella, increased incidence of femoral anteversion, and external tibia torsion all can contribute to lateral patella subluxation. Although men present more commonly with traumatic patella dislocations, women tend to develop recurrent subluxation. This subluxation is facilitated by the increased ligamentous laxity in women, most likely related to estrogen impact on collagen formation and matrix metalloproteinases, influential in tissue repair. This repetitive subluxation eventually leads to chondromalacia of the patellofemoral articular cartilage and consequent degenerative joint disease. In addition, Sharma et al. have demonstrated increased varus-valgus laxity of the knee in women compared to men, especially among women diagnosed with osteoarthritis.[35] This increased ligamentous laxity and consequent abnormalities in joint mechanics may help to explain the finding by Ding et al. that articular cartilage defects of the knee, demonstrated by magnetic resonance imaging, are significantly related to a higher BMI in women but not in men.[36]

As mentioned, estrogen receptors have been found to be present on articular cartilage; this may help to explain the increased incidence of osteoarthritis among women after menopause. Estrogen may modulate the cytokine response of cartilage to damage, influences inflammatory response, chondrocyte proliferation, and cartilage matrix synthesis. Animal studies of the effect of estrogen administration on cartilage degradation have been inconsistent. However, Christgau et al. demonstrated elevated serum levels of collagen degradation products and knee cartilage erosion in ovariectomized rats; there was significant improvement in both parameters after treatment with estrogen for four weeks.[37] In the same study, postmenopausal women demonstrated a significant decrease in serum markers of collagen degradation after treatment with a selective estrogen receptor modulator in a dose-dependent fashion over three to six months of treatment. Ravn et al. demonstrated an effect on collagen degradation markers among women using both oral and transdermal estrogen replacement.[38]

The increased risk of osteoarthritis of the knee in women may also be explained in part by the higher incidence of knee injuries, especially anterior cruciate ligament (ACL) tears, in women. Although this injury is also common in male athletes, the injury in men tends to be a result of contact, while that in women tends to occur in noncontact situations, such as change in direction or landing from a jump. Anterior Cruciate Liga-

ment (ACL) injuries in women occur most commonly among athletes playing soccer and basketball. The etiology of noncontact ACL injuries in women is most likely multifactorial. As with other conditions mentioned above, the increased ligamentous laxity in women may contribute to increased translation of the tibia on the femur, placing the ACL under stress. In addition, estrogen and relaxin receptors have been located on the ACL, and estrogen is known to decrease collagen production. However, studies have not conclusively indicated the role of female hormones in this injury or an increased risk of injury during certain times of the menstrual cycle. Female lower extremity anatomy that places the patellofemoral joint at risk of subluxation can also increase the risk of ACL injury. However, the sex-based difference that has a substantial effect and can be addressed by appropriate training methods is neuromuscular control. Prior to puberty, boys and girls land from jumps in approximately the same way. However, after the onset of puberty, boys tend to land from jumps with their hips and knees flexed and on the balls of their feet. However, girls tend to land with hips and knee straight and in valgus alignment. This combination increases the forces across the ACL. At this age, women also tend to have stronger quadriceps than hamstrings, also firing the former faster than the latter. Men tend to have quadriceps and hamstrings of equal strength and speed of firing. This muscle firing results in the tibia translating anteriorly on the femur, stressing the ACL. This sex-based difference, if recognized, can be ameliorated by appropriate training methods in landing from jumps, stretching, and muscle-strengthening exercises. The results of ACL reconstruction are approximately the same between women and men. However, those who have suffered ACL injuries are at increased risk of consequently developing osteoarthritis, even with an adequate reconstruction, most likely because of injury to the articular cartilage at the time of the initial injury. With the increased emphasis in some countries on women participating in sports, especially during the teenage years, female-specific training interventions are needed to prevent an even greater increase in the incidence of women with osteoarthritis of the knee.

Other societal expectations, such as shoe wear, may affect the development of osteoarthritis or joint pain. Although the greater development of bunions in women has been attributed to the wear of narrow toe box shoes, shoe design, especially high heels, has also been implicated in the development and progression of osteoarthritis of the knee.

The development of osteoarthritis has substantial impact on level of function, including interference with activities of daily living. Involvement of the base of the thumb leads to decreased grip strength and pain with resisted motion, leading to difficulty in performing daily tasks[39] (see Figure 16-2).

In addition, women with osteoarthritis of the hand frequently also have arthritis of the joints in the lower extremities. Arthritis of the hand can limit use of assistive devices, such as canes or walkers, further limiting function or increasing the risk of falls. Arthritis of the knee can lead to pain, inter-

fering with walking, increasing the risk of falls, and negatively affecting quality of life. However, the effect on quality of life is difficult to measure globally because of differences in culture and societal expectations. The effect also varies based on educational levels, socioeconomic status, and coping strategies. Chacon et al. found that pain, older age, and lower socioeconomic status, especially the first, all led to a poor perception of quality of life among Venezuelan patients with osteoarthritis.[40] Among patients with osteoarthritis in Taiwan, women tended to report greater levels of current pain and overall pain intensity than did men.[41] However, this sex-based difference appeared to be mediated by the number of depressive symptoms, possibly resulting from the presence of chronic pain or activity limitations imposed by the condition.

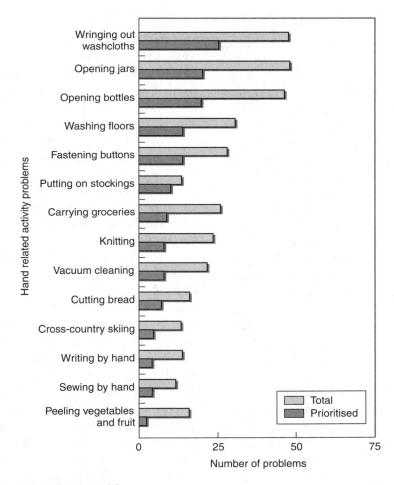

FIGURE 16-2   Hand related activity problems
Kjeken I, Dagfinrud H, Slatkowsky-Christensen B, Mowinckel P, Uhlig T, Kvien TK, Finset A. Activity limitations and participation restrictions in women with hand osteoarthritis: patients' description and associations between dimensions of functioning. *Ann Rheum Dis.* 2005;64:1633–1638

Women in most cultures tend to seek or receive treatment for osteoarthritis when they are substantially more disabled than men, including walking and negotiating stairs more slowly and demonstrating more difficulty arising from a chair.[42] In addition, women report less improvement in symptoms after corticosteroid or viscosupplementation treatment for knee osteoarthritis than do men, even for those with equivalent pretreatment levels of disease. The reason for this sex-based difference in outcome has not been elucidated.[43]

Numerous studies have demonstrated the safety and efficacy of total knee arthroplasty for patients with osteoarthritis not ameliorated by other modalities. Although total knee arthroplasty is performed more commonly in women, the incidence of the surgery is less than would be predicted based on the prevalence of disease. In a study of Canadian men and women over the age of 55,[44] women were found to have a higher incidence of osteoarthritis than men, based on examination and radiography, as well as worse symptoms and greater disability. However, they were less likely to have undergone total joint arthroplasty. Men and women in this study were equally likely to be willing to undergo surgery, but significantly fewer women reported discussing the possibility of joint arthroplasty with a healthcare professional. Women considering joint replacement surgery have also expressed concerns regarding recovery and may delay surgery owing to its potential impact on their family and societal roles.[45] In addition to the impact of sex on the likelihood of undergoing total knee arthroplasty, a difference has also been identified among the races in the United States.[46] African American and Hispanic women are significantly less likely to undergo total joint arthroplasty than are non-Hispanic White patients. However, unlike the situation among men, in whom similar race-based disparities were noted, the differences in care among the races of women could be explained by financial and geographic variables: African American women were more likely to receive a total joint arthroplasty if they lived in regions with less residential segregation; Hispanic women were as likely, and for some groups more likely, to receive a total knee arthroplasty than Caucasian women if they belonged to higher-income groups. This may reflect differences in overall health status, as the presence of a greater number of comorbidities in those in lower income strata may impact the decision for surgery. However, patient preferences for treatment and a lack of health insurance also play a role. It is not known if the women who decide not to undergo total knee arthroplasty are making an informed choice or, as in the Canadian study, this option for treatment is not discussed with them. Although improvements in pain and quality of life are typical after joint replacement surgery, the long-term outcome depends in part on preoperative function and disability. Women undergoing joint arthroplasty when they are significantly disabled or have substantially impaired joint function may have worse results than if they had had the surgery at an earlier stage.

Conclusion

Several musculoskeletal conditions have been found to have a higher incidence in women than in men. The etiology of these sex-based differences is in all instances multifactorial, including genetic, hormonal, and societal factors. A significant amount of research has been done in this area; however, the relative impact of these factors has not been elucidated.

Research up to this point has primarily focused on genetic and hormonal factors, especially in the non-Hispanic White community. However, societal factors are those through which most interventions could be targeted to decrease the incidence and impact of disease. Societal expectations, access to education, and limited financial resources may impact the availability of appropriate nutrition to maintain bone and joint health. The need to work outside of the home and/or to perform household tasks and care for family members can result in women seeking medical care at a late stage, leading to chronic pain and affecting their ability to perform activities of daily living, even with medical or surgical intervention. Additional information needs to be available to the public, patients, and healthcare professionals regarding the importance of musculoskeletal health, its impact on function, and the presence of sex-based differences. This awareness may help to promote prevention and to allow earlier diagnosis and treatment.

DISCUSSION QUESTIONS

1. What societal changes could potentially decrease the incidence of osteoporosis?
2. How could we address the disparities in treatment for women with osteoarthritis?
3. What is the impact of musculoskeletal conditions, such as osteoporosis and osteoarthritis, on women's quality of life, as well as their roles in the home and at work?

REFERENCES

1. Picavet HSJ, Hoeymans N. Health related quality of life in multiple musculoskeletal diseases: SF-36 and EQ-5D in the DMC3 study. *Ann Rheum Dis*. 2004;63: 723-729.
2. Jelsma J, Mielkes J, Powell G, De Weerdt W, De Cock P. Disability in an urban black community in Zimbabwe. *Disabil Rehab*. 2002;24:851-859.
3. Murtagh KN, Hubert HB. Gender differences in physical disability among an elderly cohort. *Am J Public Health*. 2004;94:1406-1411.
4. Mudano AS, Casebeer L, Patino F, et al. Racial disparities in osteoporosis prevention in a managed care population. *South Med J*. 2003;96:445-451.
5. Kitamura I, Ando F, Koda M, Okura T, Shimokata H. Effects of the interaction between lean tissue mass and estrogen receptor alpha gene polymorphism on bone mineral density in middle-aged and elderly Japanese. *Bone*. 2007;40:1623-1629.
6. Finkelstein JS, Brockwell SE, Mehta V, et al. Bone mineral density changes during the menopause transition in a multiethnic cohort of women. *J Clin Endocrinol Metab*. 2008;93:861-868.
7. Bruning PF, Pit MJ, deJong-Bakker M, van den Ende A, Hart A, van EnkA. Bone mineral density after adjuvant chemotherapy for premenopausal breast cancer. *Br J Cancer*. 1990;61:308-310.
8. Headley A, Theriault RL, LeBlanc AD, Vassilopoulou-Selin R, Hortobagyi GN. Pilot study of bone mineral density in breast cancer patients treated with adjuvant chemotherapy. *Cancer Invest*. 1998;16:6-11.
9. Somekawa Y, Chiguchi M, Ishibashi T, Wakana K, Aso T. Efficacy of ipriflavbone in preventing adverse effects of leuprolide. *J Clin Endocrinol Metab*. 2001;86: 3202-3206.
10. Palomba S, Orio Jr F, Morelli M, et al. Raloxifene administration in women treated with gonadotropin-releasing hormone agonist for uterine leiomyomas: effects on bone metabolism. *J Clin Endocrinol Metab*. 2002;87:4476-4481.
11. Makita K, Ishitani K, Ohta H, Horiguchi F, Nozawa S. Long-term effects on bone mineral density and bone metabolism of 6 months' treatment with gonadotropin-releasing hormone analogues in Japanese women: comparison of buserelin acetate with leuprolide acetate. *J Clin Endocrinol Metab*. 2005;23: 389-394.
12. Shoepe HA, Snow CM. Oral contraceptive use in young women is associated with lower bone mineral density than that of controls. *Osteoporosis Internat*. 2005;16:1538-1544.

13. Hartard M, Kleinmond C, Kirchbichler A, et al. Age at first oral contraceptive use as a major determinant of vertebral bone mass in female endurance athletes. *Bone*. 2004;35:836-841.

14. Burr DB, Yoshikawa T, Teegarden D, et al. Exercise and oral contraceptive use suppress the normal age-related increase in bone mass and strength of the femoral neck in women 18-31 years of age. *Bone*. 2000;27:855-863.

15. Stafford DEJ. Altered hypothalamic-pituitary-ovarian axis function in young female athletes: implications and recommendations for management. *Treatment Endocrinol*. 2005;4:147-154.

16. Jayasinghe Y, Grover SR, Zacharin M. Current concepts in bone and reproductive health in adolescents with anorexia nervosa. *BJOG*. 2008;115:304-315.

17. Heer M, Mika C, Grzella I, Heussen N, Herpertz-Dahlmann B. Bone turnover during inpatient nutritional therapy and outpatient follow-up in patients with anorexia nervosa compared to that in healthy control subjects. *Am J Clin Nutr*. 2004;80:774-781.

18. Wan Kin CF, Yeung Shan WS, Chi Shun LJ, Ping Chung L, Jean W. Experience of famine and bone health in post-menopausal women. *Internat J Epidemiol*. 2007;36:1143-1150.

19. Rizzoli R, Eisman A, Norquist J, et al. Risk factors for vitamin D inadequacy among women with osteoporosis: an international epidemiological study. *Int J Clin Pract*. 2006;60:1013-1019.

20. Saraiva GL, Cendoroglo MS, Ramos LR, et al. Influence of ultraviolet radiation on the production of 25 hydroxyvitamin D in the elderly population in the city of Sao Paulo, Brazil. *Osteoporosis Internat*. 2005;16:1649-1654.

21. Guzel R, Kozanoglu E, Guler-Uysal F, Soyupak S, Sarpel T. Vitamin D status and bone mineral density of veiled and unveiled Turkish women. *J Women's Health Gender-Based Med*. 2001;10:765-770.

22. Allali F, Aichaoui S El, Saoud B, Maaroufi H, Abouqal R, Hajjaj-Hassouni N. The impact of clothing style on bone mineral density among postmenopausal women in Morocco: case-control study. *BMC Public Health*. 2006;6:135-139.

23. Valdimarsson O, Linden C, Johnell O, Gardsell P, Karlsson MK. Daily physical education in the school curriculum in prepubertal girls during 1 year is followed by an increase in bone mineral accrual and bone width-data from the prospective controlled Malmo pediatric osteoporosis prevention study. *Calcif Tissue Internat*. 2006;78:65-71.

24. Beyene Y, Martin MC. Menopausal experiences and bone density of Mayan women in Yucatan, Mexico. *Am J Hum Biol*. 2001;13:505-511.

25. Kermat A, Patwardhan B, Larijani B, et al. The assessment of osteoporosis risk factors in Iranian women compared with Indian women. *BMC Musculoskeletal Disord*. 2008;9:28-37.

26. Ungan M, Tumer M. Turkish women's knowledge of osteoporosis. *Fam Pract*. 2001;18:199-203.

27. Chang S-F, Hong C-M, Yang R-S. Cross-sectional survey of women in Taiwan with first-degree relatives with osteoporosis: knowledge, health beliefs, and preventive behaviors. *J Nurs Res*. 2007;15:224-231.

28. Kung AWC, Lee K-K. Knowledge of vitamin D and perceptions and attitudes toward sunlight among Chinese middle-aged and elderly women: a population survey in Hong Kong. *BMC Public Health*. 2006;6:226-231.

29. Sodha S, Ring D, Zurakowski D, Jupiter J. Prevalence of osteoarthrosis of the trapeziometacarpal joint. *J Bone Joint Surg (Am)*. 2005;87:2614-2618.

30. Avci D, Bachmann GA. Osteoarthritis and osteoporosis in postmenopausal women: clinical similarities and differences. *J North Am Menopause Soc.* 2004;11: 615-621.

31. Njobvu P, McGill P. Human immunodeficiency virus related reactive arthritis in Zambia. *J Rheumatol.* 2005;32:1299-1304.

32. Canizares M, Power JD, Perruccio AV, Badley EM. Association of regional racial/cultural context and socioeconomic status with arthritis in the population: a multilevel analysis. *Arthritis Rheum.* 2008;59:399-407.

33. Fytili P, Giannatou E, Papanikolaou V, et al. Association of repeat polymorphisms in the estrogen receptors alpha, beta, and androgen receptor genes with knee osteoarthritis. *Clin Genetics.* 2005;68:268-277.

34. Ushiyama T, Ueyama H, Inoue K, Nishioka J, Ohkubo I, Hukuda S. Estrogen receptor gene polymorphism and generalized osteoarthritis. *J Rheumatology.* 1998;25:134-137.

35. Sharma L, Lou C, Felson DT, et al. Laxity I healthy and osteoarthritic knees. *Arthritis Rheum.* 1999;42:861-870.

36. Ding C, Cicuttini F, Scott F, Cooley H, Jones G. Knee structural alteration and BMI: a cross-sectional study. *Obes Res.* 2005;13:350-361.

37. Christgau S, Tanko LB, Cloos PA, et al. Suppression of elevated cartilage turnover in postmenopausal women and in ovariectomized rats by estrogen and a selective estrogen-receptor modulator (SERM). *Menopause.* 2004;11:508-518.

38. Ravn P, Warming L, Christgau S, Christiansen C. The effect on cartilage of different forms of application of postmenopausal estrogen therapy: comparison of oral and transdermal therapy. *Bone.* 2004;35:1216-1221.

39. Kjeken I, Dagfinrud H, Slatkowsky-Christensen B, et al. Activity limitations and participation restrictions in women with hand osteoarthritis: patients' description and associations between dimensions of functioning. *Ann Rheum Dis.* 2005;64:1633-1638.

40. Chacon JG, Gonzalez NE, Veliz A, et al. Effect of knee osteoarthritis on the perception of quality of life in Venezuelan patients. *Arthritis Rheum.* 2004;51:377-382.

41. Tsai Y-F. Gender differences in pain and depressive tendency among Chinese elders with knee osteoarthritis. *Pain.* 2007;130:188-194.

42. Pagura SMC, Thomas SG, Woodhouse LJ, Ezzat S, Marks P. Circulating and synovial levels of IGF-I, cytokines, physical function and anthropometry differ in women awaiting total knee arthroplasty when compared to men. *J Ortho Res.* 2005;23:397-405.

43. Leopold SS, Redd BB, Warme WJ, Wehrle PA, Pettis PD, Shott S. Corticosteroid compared with hyaluronic acid injections for the treatment of osteoarthritis of the knee. *J Bone Joint Surg (Am).* 2003;85:1197-1203.

44. Hawker GA, Wright JG, Coyte PC, et al. Differences between men and women in the rate of use of hip and knee arthroplasty. *N Engl J Med.* 2000;342:1016-1022.

45. Chang HJ, Mehta PS, Rosenberg A, Scrimshaw SC. Concerns of patients actively contemplating total knee replacement: differences by race and gender. *Arthritis Rheum.* 2004;51:117-123.

46. Skinner J, Weinstein JN, Sporer SM, Wennberg JE. Racial, ethnic, and geographic disparities in the rate of knee arthroplasty among Medicare patients. *N Engl J Med.* 2003,349:1350-1359.

Making Reproductive Rights a Reality

For decades global declarations have asserted the rights of women to control their sexual and reproductive health. This right is essential to furthering the well-being and opportunities of women and thus of their families, their communities, and their nations. Many global human rights protect and support reproductive health, including:

Rights to be free from all forms of discrimination

Rights to life, liberty, and security of the person

Rights to marry and found a family

Rights to private and family life

Rights regarding information and education

Rights to health care

Rights to the benefits of scientific progress

This chapter reviews three reproductive health issues—contraception, abortion, and sexually transmitted infections—from a human rights perspective. Each section covers the relevant rights that can be invoked to advocate for the highest standard of reproductive health care. For each issue, specific examples from communities and countries illustrate how the rights can be used to promote reproductive health.

A variety of international agreements put forth principles in support of reproductive health that signatory countries have agreed to abide by. Human rights are best used as tools for advocacy, to establish a case that certain minimum standards in reproductive health or other health areas should be met. Human rights are powerful approaches to defining and advancing the health and well-being of all people. International declarations supporting women's reproductive health include the following:

- Proclamation of Teheran (1968)
- Convention on the Elimination of All Forms of Discrimination Against Women (1979)
- International Conference on Population and Development (ICPD) Program of Action (1994)

CHAPTER **17**

Sexual and Reproductive Health: Women's Health Is Society's Wealth

Ushma D. Upadhyay, PhD, MPH
Padmini Murthy MD, MPH, MS, CHES

Ushma D. Upadhyay, PhD, MPH is a Research Specialist at the Baby Center for Global Reproductive Health, at University of California, San Francisco.

Padmini Murthy MD, MPH, MS, CHES, is an Assistant Professor in the Department of Health Policy and Management, as well as the Director of the Global Health Program at New York Medical School of Public Health in Valhalla, NY. She is the Medical Women's International Association NGO Representative to the United Nations, New York, and Robert F. Wagner Public Service Scholar, New York University.

- Beijing Platform for Action (1995)
- Beijing Plus Five (2000)
- Millennium Development Goals (2000)
- Beijing Plus Ten (2005)

In the years following the ICPD in Cairo, sexual and reproductive health topped government agendas around the world. By the mid 2000s however, these rights dropped down in priority. Sexual and reproductive health has dropped down the international development agenda and was omitted from the Millennium Development Goals (MDG) framework. Funding for sexual and reproductive health has decreased at the expense of increases in resources for HIV/AIDS, and comprehensive reproductive health services are increasingly being replaced by abstinence-only programs.[1] Nevertheless, reproductive health is affected by several of the eight MDG, including the promotion of gender equality and the empowerment of women, the reduction of child mortality, improving maternal health, combating AIDS, and ensuring environmental sustainability.[2] If governments hope to achieve these development goals, sexual and reproductive health must also remain a high priority.

Governments that sign international documents of principle make a commitment to act on these principles. The extent of government attention to such commitments and the amount of money allocated to implementing them, however, vary considerably around the world. Reproductive health advocates have urged that governments be held to their commitments, that people be encouraged to exercise their rights, and that healthcare providers respect these rights.

Human rights can be powerful tools in advocating for the expansion of reproductive health services. For example, ever since the city of Manila, Philippines, imposed a ban against the provision of modern contraceptives in 2000, local women's organizations have been appealing the order using rights-based arguments. Not only does the Philippines Constitution guarantee the right to health, equality, and various rights relating to family, but the government signed on to the Convention on the Elimination of All Forms of Discrimination against Women (CEDAW) and other covenants that obligate the government to provide access to family planning services and information.[3]

In Nepal where abortion had been illegal for decades, physicians and public health advocates, nongovernmental organizations, and eventually the Ministry of Health advocated for liberalized abortion laws. The overriding rationale for reforming the abortion law was to ensure safe motherhood—a right guaranteed by several human rights documents. As a result of these advocacy efforts, in 2002 parliament passed a liberal abortion law, and by 2004 the first government abortion services officially began at the Maternity Hospital in Kathmandu.[4]

Healthcare providers are in a unique position to effect change in the area of sexual and reproductive health rights. They have the medical expertise, the status, the credibility, and the commitment to improve health. They have great influence on opinion leaders and policymakers at local, national, and international levels.[5] Providers can use rights guaranteed by international agreements to protect, defend, and promote the sexual and reproductive health and rights of their patients and clients. As more medical, nursing, and other paramedical training programs incorporate reproductive rights (separate from reproductive health) into their curriculums, it is likely that healthcare providers will become more active in reproductive rights advocacy.[6]

Contraception

Women's rights to make their own choices about childbearing have long had their basis in international consensus statements, including the Proclamation of Teheran, issued at the 1968 International Conference on Human Rights.[7] Two fundamental human rights underlie women's decision-making about contraception: (1) the right to decide freely how many children to have and when to have them, and (2) the right of access to family planning information and services.

The ICPD Program of Action states that "the aim of family planning programs must be to enable couples and individuals to decide freely and responsibly the number and spacing of their children and to have the information and means to do so and to ensure informed choice and make available a full range of safe and effective methods."[8] National governments play the major role in developing and enforcing standards for health services in both the public and private sectors, including guidelines for service delivery.[8,9] In some countries, including Malaysia, Peru, and Zambia, laws explicitly protect men' and women's rights to make decisions about their reproductive health.[10]

National family planning guidelines are most accurate when they are based on international consensus documents such as the Medical Eligibility Criteria developed under the auspices of WHO.[9] Many of these new guidelines state that all people, regardless of their age or marital status, shall have the right and access to family planning information and services.[11,12]

Quality of Care and Informed Choice

Enjoying good-quality contraceptive services is a component of the right to health. According to one framework, good-quality services involve a choice of contraceptive methods, information given to clients, technical competence, interpersonal relations, mechanisms to encourage continuity, and an appropriate constellation of services.[13] Good quality of care takes into account the clients' perspective. When healthcare systems and healthcare providers put clients first, they offer services that not only meet technical standards of quality but also satisfy the client's need for other aspects of quality, such as respect, relevant information, access, and fairness.

All people have a right to education and information. Education and information empowers individuals to consider their sexual and reproductive health, to plan their families, and to consider whether they want to use contraception. If they decide to use contraception, individuals require information about a wide range of contraceptive methods, including the risks, benefits, and potential side effects. One study in Madagascar noted that gaps in knowledge about the range of available contraceptive methods and misinformation were primary barriers to the use of modern contraceptive methods.[14] In a study in East Azerbaijan, Iran, two thirds of family planning clients interviewed were not encouraged to ask questions or raise concerns, and 54% were not satisfied with the amount of information given.[15]

Healthcare providers are instrumental in providing information to patients and clients and respecting their autonomy to make informed choices for themselves. According to the Federation of Gynecology and Obstetrics (FIGO), professionals must respect women's and men's rights including the right to the highest available standard of health care for all aspects of their sexual and reproductive health; the right to decide matters related to their sexuality, without coercion, discrimination, or violence; the right to make choices about whether or not to reproduce; and the right to have access to legal, safe, effective, affordable, and acceptable methods of fertility regulation consistent with their choice.[16]

These principles support providing clients a choice of contraceptive methods and allowing women and men to choose the method that is best for them. Nevertheless, many providers think that they should make family planning decisions for their clients because they know what is best. Providers often have their own preferences and preconceived ideas about what contraceptive method is best for clients.[17]

The rights to liberty and security and to freedom from inhuman and degrading treatment empowers individuals to decide what can be done to their bodies and by whom. They protect individuals against coercive measures that affect their physical integrity. Thus, individuals should give fully informed consent to any medical or surgical procedure, including male or female sterilization.[10]

Providers sometimes erect barriers based on people's age, marital status, or other inappropriate criteria that are not based on scientific evidence.[18] In many countries providers commonly turn away women seeking contraception who are not menstruating at the time of their visit, for fear that they may be pregnant. Guidelines can be used, however to determine with reasonable certainly that they are not pregnant.[19] The principle of informed choice means that providers avoid bias and, instead, respect a client's preferences over their own—even if a client chooses a less effective contraceptive method, uses a method only sporadically, switches frequently from one method to another, or refuses any or all services.[10]

Contraceptive Security and Access

Offering widespread access to as many contraceptive methods as possible is key to ensuring that women can make choices about their reproductive health. As more methods become available, and as access to these methods increases, more people can find a method that suits them—initially, and later if they want to switch methods.[20] In sub-Saharan Africa, for example, after recent expansions in access to progestin-only injectables, they have become one of the most popular contraceptive methods due to their high effectiveness and suitability for discreet use.[21]

Although virtually every country provides at least a few methods, in many countries people have little or no access to certain methods.[20] An evaluation of reproductive health programs in public hospitals and primary healthcare centers in Buenos Aires, Argentina, found that while hormonal contraceptives, IUDs, and male condoms were mostly available, emergency contraception, female condoms, and other barrier methods were not.[22] Family planning programs should provide a variety of types of methods to meet the different needs of different individuals and couples, such as the following:

- Contraception options both for men and for women
- Temporary methods and permanent methods
- Hormonal methods and nonhormonal methods
- Supply methods and fertility awareness methods
- Provider-controlled methods and user-controlled methods
- Contraceptive options for breastfeeding women, including the Lactational Amenorrhea Method
- A method that can be used after sexual intercourse

Recent advances have been made in contraceptive technology, yet many people around the world cannot exercise their right to scientific progress. Many of the newer contraceptive methods are still hard to obtain. For example, the contraceptive patch and the vaginal ring offer new modes of hormonal delivery, making it ideal for women who can tolerate the contraceptive pill but have trouble remembering to take it every day.

An area where few advances have been made is in contraceptive choices for men. This is essential for women's equality so that the burden of family planning can be shared jointly. The right to nondiscrimination and equality provides the basis for advocacy for more contraceptives for men. Currently, except for vasectomy, no method is priced low enough to be financially viable for the majority of men in the world. Men are calling for more contraceptive choices, however. Many men and women in surveys, focus groups, and interviews say that they want to share the responsibility for contraception. Studies also suggest that many men are willing to take on the side effects and health risks of contraceptive use.[23,24] This interest is universal. A large survey of 9000 men in nine countries showed that, despite great country-to-country variation, in every country more than 57% of men would consider using a contraceptive method.[23]

Emergency Contraception

Emergency contraception has an important role in the range of contraceptive methods because it is the only contraceptive that can be taken after sexual intercourse. Women are guaranteed the right to the benefits of scientific progress, yet this innovation that can prevent millions of unintended pregnancies each year is still unavailable in many communities.[25]

Emergency contraception is provided as hormonal pills or as an intrauterine device. It works before conception and is not a form of abortion. It is most effective when taken as soon as possible but can prevent pregnancy up to five days after sexual intercourse.[26]

Dedicated emergency contraceptive products in the form of pills are still unavailable in Panama and Costa Rica due to pressure from the Catholic Church.[27] Where it is available, costs are often prohibitively expensive. At the same time, other countries recognize that emergency contraception is safe and effective and have taken great measures to increase its access. Over 30 countries including Cameroon, Malaysia, Tunisia, and Vietnam have made it available without prescription, substantially reducing barriers to its use.[25]

Emergency contraception is an essential component of compassionate care for rape victims and should be provided routinely in all cases of rape in all healthcare facilities. Every year rape results in thousands of unwanted pregnancies. A study of adolescents in Ethiopia found that among those who reported being raped, 17% became pregnant after the rape.[28] Of the 300,000 women who are raped in the United States each year, an estimated 32,000 become pregnant as a result, and about half of these women undergo an abortion.[29] With emergency contraception, these pregnancy rates could be drastically reduced.

In addition to rape, emergency contraception can help women avoid unintended pregnancy in a wide variety of circumstances. It is safe for all women, and therefore, there is no reason it should be denied to anyone who may have had unprotected sex. Emergency contraception can be used after such contraceptive mistakes as a broken or slipped condom, forgotten pills (three or more), a late contraceptive injection, or if an IUD comes out of place.[26]

Choices for Women with HIV

With access to family planning services, supportive care, and the information needed to make good choices, women with HIV in many cases can lead healthy sexual and reproductive lives.[30] Like all other women, women with HIV have the right to make their own decisions about their reproductive and sexual health.

Women with HIV may or may not want children, and these decisions deserve respect and support from healthcare providers.[31] Regardless of their fertility desires, many women with HIV are sexually active after learning of their infection. In a review of studies from developed and developing countries, it was found that 40–80% of women with HIV report sexual activity.[30] Healthcare programs and providers can help women with HIV and their partners make and carry out informed reproductive health decisions.

Many women with HIV who are sexually active want to prevent pregnancy. Some may decide not to have children to avoid the risk of transmission to a newborn and the potential health risks of pregnancy. Many of these women have an unmet need for family planning—that is, they are not using family planning despite wanting to avoid pregnancy, and thus they risk unintended pregnancy.[32,33]

Often, women with HIV may feel reluctant to seek family planning services, fearing stigma and discrimination. Research in many countries around the world shows that women often fear and actually experience HIV/AIDS-related stigmatization and discrimination in healthcare settings.[34] In a study in South Africa, the majority of men and women with HIV interviewed said they had never discussed their reproductive intentions with their HIV or general healthcare providers because they perceived healthcare provider attitudes to be disapproving and unsupportive of open discussion about reproductive options.[31] These men and women have the same rights as others to comprehensive sexuality and reproductive health services. Because of such barriers, there is a great need for explicit policies recognizing reproductive rights and choices for women with HIV.

Sexual Health Education and Services for Adolescents

Human rights—including sexual and reproductive rights—are guaranteed to adolescents just as they are to adults. These rights cannot be amended because of their age or the wishes of their parents or society.

Adolescence is the transitional period in human development between puberty and adulthood. Defined by WHO as those between the ages of 10 and 19. Adolescence in the developing world is gaining attention. There are 1.2 billion adolescents in the world today, more than ever before,[35] and making up almost 20% of the world's total population.[36] More and more adolescents are sexually active at younger ages.[37-40] Premarital sexual experience has become more common; as the age at first marriage has risen and the age at puberty has fallen.[41,42] Young people are particularly at risk of HIV and other sexually transmitted infections (STIs) as well as unintended pregnancies because of risky behavior, drug use, and lack of access to health information and services.

Abstinence-only education is clearly a violation of adolescents' rights.[43] Several studies have found that denying access to reproductive health information to adolescents does not reduce adolescent sexual activity.[44,45] Comprehensive education about sexuality and contraception works. Adolescents are more likely to make healthy choices about their sexual behavior when they can make informed decisions in an empowering, enabling environment.[46,47] As described by the Self-Aware sex education program in Venezuela, young people should be able to experience their sexuality in a "full, responsible, pleasurable, and just manner."[48]

Adolescent sexual behavior is not in itself risky. Countering the common belief that sexuality in adolescence is dangerous and problematic, sexuality should be considered a normal part of healthy adolescent development. While interventions should focus on reducing risks that young people face, all adolescent sexual activity must not be categorized as risky.[49] More threatening to young people is unplanned, unprotected, and unwanted sexual behavior which too often leads to unwanted births and STIs.

All adolescents need access to good quality, youth-friendly services provided by clinicians trained to work with young people.[50,51] Adolescents deserve and have the right to confidential, nonjudgmental, and respectful care no matter how young they are. They need open and honest discussions about sex and sexuality. Counseling and services do not encourage young people to have sex. Instead, they help young people protect their health. Sex education programs should offer accurate, comprehensive information while building skills for negotiating in sexual behavior. They have an important responsibility in helping to ensure that adolescents have the information, understanding, and ability to make well-informed voluntary decisions about their sexual and reproductive health.

Abortion

The language in human rights documents on the right to abortion is ambiguous, but safe abortion is instrumental to a woman's right to life and right to enjoy good health. Also, human rights declarations that guarantee the right to decide the number and spacing of children apply to the issue of abortion, and therefore can and should be used to advocate for legalization of abortion and access to safe abortion services. One of the MDGs is to reduce maternal mortality. Making abortion legal and safe would prevent 13% of all maternal deaths each year

and is one of the easiest and most cost-effective ways for governments to achieve that goal.[52]

Abortion remains a major cause of death among women in the developing world, particularly among young, poor, and rural women.[53] There are 42 million abortions each year, and half are unsafe—that is, done by people lacking the necessary skills or in an environment lacking the minimal medical standards, or both. Every year, nearly 70,000 women die from complications of unsafe abortion, and countless more suffer from infections, infertility, and debilitating injuries.[52,54,55]

In countries where abortion is legal only under certain circumstances, healthcare providers have enormous authority in determining whether a woman receives reproductive health services. In Chile where abortion is limited by law, medical professionals are required to report abortions to the authorities, but less than 1% of women in hospitals with abortion complications are reported. The remainder of abortions are disguised as a different procedure or reported as a spontaneous abortion in public hospitals.[56] In Nicaragua where only "therapeutic abortion" is legal, but is not defined, it is up to doctors to decide whether an abortion is permissible.

Ambiguity in the law leads to inconsistent access to legal abortions as well as decisions based on providers' personal beliefs, which may not be in their clients' best interests.[57] Some healthcare providers are adversarial toward women seeking an abortion. Often they do not respect women's choices, are judgmental or hostile toward women seeking abortion services, or exaggerate risks to dissuade women from having an abortion.[58,59] For example, in Rajasthan, India, facilities routinely refuse to perform abortions in certain circumstances, including if a woman presents alone, is married but has never had children, or is unmarried. Although not required by law, nearly three-quarters of facilities studied required a woman's husband's consent before performing an abor-tion.[60] Providers' responsibilities involve providing accurate information, listening to their clients, understanding their situations, encouraging them to decide what is best for themselves, and then to support their decisions.[5]

Women also need to know about where they can access safe and legal abortion services. In

South Africa, abortion is legal and available upon request up to 12 weeks gestation. Yet many women still have unsafe abortions either by self-inducing or by going to traditional healers because they are unaware of their rights to abortion or do not know of any legal facilities.[61]

Expanding Access to Medical Abortion

Even in cases where abortion is legal, it is often inaccessible because it is not provided by existing public health systems. Surgical abortion is expensive, and many healthcare providers, even qualified gynecologists, are not sufficiently trained in the techniques of vacuum aspiration or dilation and evacuation.

A woman's right to the benefits of scientific progress extends to developments in abortion. Advances in technology, including the development of safe, effective, and acceptable regimens for medical abortion can improve women's access to safe abortion and her chances for survival.

Medical abortion—first introduced in France in 1988—holds substantial promise for expansion of services into rural areas around the world.[62] This technique involves taking mifepristone orally, and then misoprostol 24 to 72 hours later to empty the uterus. It can be done up to 49 days gestation and is 92–98% effective depending on when the drugs are administered.[63]

Medical abortion has only recently become available in the global south, and physicians are slowly providing it more often. Medical abortion can be provided in a variety of settings, including practitioners' private offices. Medical abortion is sometimes available from pharmacists as well, with or without a prescription. South Africa and Tunisia have pioneered home administration of misoprostol, the second dose of the medical abortion regimen.[64,65] Studies have shown that many women may prefer home administration of medical abortion, which would make the procedure more convenient, accessible, and private.[66]

Expanding access and reducing barriers to medical abortion would allow women a full range of choices in the case of unintended pregnancy. Because a lower level of service provider is required to offer medical abortion than surgical abortion, it is the only way to offer safe services in remote areas. In such areas, unsafe abortion contributes substantially to maternal morbidity and mortality and is therefore all the more essential.

Even countries with restrictive abortion laws should provide medical abortion, as well as a variety of safe abortion methods for women legally entitled to terminate a pregnancy. Medical abortion is extremely safe and complications are rare.[67,68] Both mifepristone and misoprostol are on WHO's Model List of Essential Medicines, indicating that they should be "available at all times in adequate amounts and in appropriate dosage forms, at a price the community can afford."[69]

At a minimum, regardless of national policies on abortion, all countries that have signed on to the ICPD Program of Action are obligated to ensure that all women have access to postabortion care (PAC), because in many cases, it can be life-saving. PAC involves treatment for complications caused by incomplete or spontaneous abortion and provides family planning counseling and services to prevent future unplanned pregnancies. Such programs have become politically acceptable and more common since the 1994 ICPD Program of Action because they are developed with the objective of improving health and saving women's lives. They are usually acceptable even where abortion is illegal or limited by law.

Sexually Transmitted Infections

The right to the highest attainable standard of health suggests a right to counseling, care, and treatment for sexually transmitted infections (STIs). Universal access to prevention and treatment of STIs is mentioned in the ICPD Program of Action and the Beijing Platform for Action among other documents.[8,70] Additionally, combating HIV/AIDS is one of the MDGs, and thus international governments and institutions are committed to reducing this infection worldwide.

Political will is needed to prioritize resource allocation and to ensure collaboration between various programs within the ministry of health for STI control. But government and societal responses to STIs usually are affected more by moral judgments and social attitudes towards sexual behavior than the health consequences of the infections.[71]

Consequently, worldwide, STIs continue to be a major cause of morbidity and mortality. The most recent global estimates suggest that there are more than 340 million new cases of syphilis, gonorrhea, chlamydia, and trichomoniasis per year,[72] and STI prevalence rates continue to rise in most countries, including developed countries.[73]

The consequences of STIs are serious and extensive, affecting men, women, and infants. STIs are a major global cause of illness, long-term disability, and death, with severe medical and psychological consequences. In all countries, but especially developing countries, STIs result in substantial losses in productivity.[74]

Each year, STIs cause countless cases of pelvic inflammatory disease, infertility, chronic pelvic pain, ectopic pregnancy, cervical cancer, and liver disease.[73] Over time, HIV suppresses the immune system. STIs also greatly increase the chance of becoming infected with HIV.[75,76] Up to 4000 newborn babies become blind every year because of eye infections that are attributable to untreated maternal STIs.[77] Untreated syphilis is the cause of up to 1.5 million stillbirths and early neonatal deaths.[78]

STIs are caused by bacteria and viruses spread through sexual contact. Infections can be found in body fluids such as semen, on the skin of the genitals and areas around them, and some also in the mouth, throat, and rectum. Some STIs cause no symptoms. Others may cause discomfort or pain. STIs spread in a community because an infected person has sex with an uninfected person. The more sexual partners a person has, the greater his or her risk of either becoming infected with STIs or transmitting STIs.

Who Is at Risk of Contracting STIs?

STIs thrive for several reasons. First, on an individual level people lack information on how STIs are transmitted and how they can be prevented. On a community level, cultural norms and traditions can perpetuate transmission of infections. Gender inequities and power imbalances place women at higher risk than men. Sexually transmitted infections are predominantly a disease linked to poverty. STIs are more prevalent among the poor than the affluent, and women are more likely than men to live in poverty.[79]

Some women lack the power to ensure consistent and correct condom use. Relationships that subject women to coercion, violence, and dependency can make it difficult or impossible for them to negotiate condom use or to leave the relationship even though it puts their health at risk.[80,81] In Goa, India, married women who experienced sexual violence from their husbands were at significantly increased risk of becoming infected with an STI compared with women who didn't experience sexual violence.[82] Women who lack the power to ensure the use of condoms are at far greater risk than men because women are biologically more vulnerable to HIV and its consequences. The rate of transmission of HIV from men to women is at least two to eight times greater than the rate of transmission from women to men because during sex the vaginal epithelium is easily torn, and there is more HIV in semen than in vaginal secretions.[83-85]

Adolescent females probably are at greater biological risk for STIs than grown adults because the cervix is physiologically less mature and therefore more vulnerable to infection. Most young women have cervical ectopy, a normal condition of the cervix that changes with age. These cells are more vulnerable to infections such as chlamydia and gonorrhea.[86,87]

Several studies have found that people in certain occupations can be a significant risk factor for STIs—and most often it is those who are most economically disadvantaged.[88] An Indian case control study found that people in the STI group were 1.4 times as likely to be unskilled laborers and twice as likely to have a job that requires travel.[89] In another study in China almost 20% of long-distance truck drivers tested positive for at least one STI.[90]

Sex workers are often considered the most vulnerable and powerless to negotiate condom use. Empowered with knowledge and access to condoms, however, research finds they can protect themselves. Women in the Democratic Republic of Congo who knew that condoms prevent HIV and who had been exposed to voluntary counseling and testing and who had access to condoms were significantly more likely to be consistent condom users with their clients.[91]

STI Prevention

An evidenced-based strategy to reduce STI infections requires the scaling-up of STI diagnosis and treatment to primary point-of-care sites.[73] Such services would need to be available to all at subsidized fees or without charge for those unable to pay. Where laboratory testing is unavailable, syndromic management for people who present with STI symptoms has been demonstrated to be effective and should be offered at primary care facilities. Since many people with STIs do not have symptoms, screening individuals, particularly women, at high risk for STIs may be effective at reducing the burden among the most vulnerable.[74]

Among the most cost-effective strategies is early screening and treatment for syphilis among pregnant women, costing as little as US $1.[92] Many other STIs can also be cured with affordable antibiotics, including gonorrhea and chlamydia. Also important is the integration of STI, HIV, contraceptive, and other reproductive health services to increase patient access and efficiency. For example, incorporating syphilis screening into routine antenatal care services has shown to be efficient and effective in South Africa and elsewhere.[92,93]

Any screening program should be developed with substantial attention to ensuring confidentiality and client rights. In a study in Russia, despite the establishment of anonymous STI testing clinics, interviews with physicians revealed that physicians were confused about the concept of confidentiality, and retaining anonymity in standard clinics was difficult. The lack of prioritizing confidentiality dissuaded potential clients from being tested and treated.[94] It is clear that there is a real need for testing and treatment programs to place greater emphasis on respect and dignity for clients. Expansion of training among staff should review clients' rights.

Treatment of sex partners is a core component of STI testing and treatment; it prevents reinfection and prevents STIs from spreading throughout a community.[74] In the process of notifying partners, however, it is essential to protect clients. Even with a client's consent to contact a sexual partner, pro-

grams need to address power dynamics within sexual partnerships and be aware of the possibility of abandonment or abuse among their clients.

Conclusion

International law provides the basis needed to compel states to observe reproductive rights. Nevertheless, reproductive rights are without value where governments, organizations, and individuals fail to understand or recognize those rights. Governments must be held accountable to the commitments they make in international agreements by their own people, not just international bodies. International, national, and local organizations, as well as healthcare programs and providers all have a role to play in monitoring reproductive rights and advocating for rights where they are absent.

In addition to recognition, serious investments in sexual and reproductive health are needed to make these reproductive rights a reality. Advocacy is also needed to ensure that budgetary resources are allocated so that sexual and reproductive health services are provided for the most vulnerable and the neediest.

Fortunately, there are favorable trends throughout the world that hold promise for women's reproductive health and rights. There is an increased awareness and use of new reproductive health technologies and a desire to bring these technologies to every region of the world. There have been long-term improvements in the status of women and gender equity in every country. With a more integrated global economy, countries are less able to remain private and isolated, and with that, there is increased international pressure to respect human rights and an increased desire on the part of governments to be viewed favorably. Such improvements, along with increased advocacy, are likely to result in widespread gains in reproductive rights for all. Good reproductive health will be achieved only through popular and political mobilization of attention and resources. Reproductive health and reproductive rights are inherently tied, and it is only when we achieve both will individuals be able to enjoy the highest levels of well-being.

DISCUSSION QUESTIONS

1. Should governments be responsible for providing contraceptives free of charge for individuals who want them but cannot afford them? If so, which ones? What economic incentives or disincentives should governments consider?

2. What effect do you think accurate sexual health information and services might have on an adolescent's decisions about becoming sexually active?

3. What human rights can be invoked when advocating for more liberal abortion laws?

4. Where abortion is legal, how can legal systems balance the protection of women's rights to choose abortion and the enforcement of laws against sex-selective abortion?

5. How do programs that address gender inequities result in reduced rates of sexually transmitted infections?

REFERENCES

1. Glasier A, Gulmezoglu AM. Putting sexual and reproductive health on the agenda. *Lancet.* 2006;368(9547):1550-1551.
2. Singh S, Darroch JE, Vlassoff M, Nadeau J. Adding it up: the benefits of investing in sexual and reproductive health. *Issues Brief (Alan Guttmacher Inst).* 2004;4.
3. The Center for Reproductive Rights. Filipino women and men sue Manila mayor for ban on contraception. Jan. 30, 2008. http://www.reproductiverights.org/pr_08_0130FilipinoSueManila.html Accessed January 8, 2009.
4. Thapa S. Abortion law in Nepal: the road to reform. *Reprod Health Matters.* 2004;12(24 Suppl):85-94.
5. Briozzo L, Faundes A. The medical profession and the defense and promotion of sexual and reproductive rights. *Int J Gynaecol Obstet.* 2008;100(3):291-294.
6. Haslegrave M. Integrating sexual and reproductive rights into the medical curriculum. *Best Pract Res Clin Obstet Gynaecol.* 2006;20(3):433-445.
7. United Nations (UN). *Proclamation of Teheran.* International Conference on Human Rights. In: UN, ed. Teheran; 1968.
8. United Nations (UN). *Programme of Action of the International Conference on Population and Development,* 1994; Cairo, Egypt.
9. Peterson HB, Curtis KM. The World Health Organization's global guidance for family planning: an achievement to celebrate. *Contraception.* 2006;73(2):113-114.
10. Upadhyay UD. Informed choice in family planning. Helping people decide. *Population Reports, Series J.* Baltimore, MD: Johns Hopkins School of Public Health, Population Information Program; 2001:39.
11. World Health Organization (WHO). *Medical Eligibility Criteria for Contraceptive Use.* Geneva, Switzerland: WHO; 2004.
12. World Health Organization (WHO). *Selected Practice Recommendations for Contraceptive Use.* Geneva, Switzerland: WHO; 2005.
13. Bruce J. Fundamental elements of the quality of care: a simple framework. *Stud Fam Plann.* 1990;21(2):61-91.

14. Randrianasolo B, Swezey T, Van Damme K, et al. Barriers to the use of modern contraceptives and implications for woman-controlled prevention of sexually transmitted infections in Madagascar. *J Biosoc Sci.* 2008;16:1-15.

15. Alizadeh SM, Marions L, Vahidi R, Nikniaz A, Johansson A, Wahlstrom R. Quality of family planning services at primary care facilities in an urban area of East Azerbaijan, Iran. *Eur J Contracept Reprod Health Care.* 2007;12(4):326-334.

16. Federation of Gynecology and Obstetrics (FIGO). *Ethical Issues in Obstetrics and Gynecology.* London: FIGO; 2006.

17. Welsh MJ, Stanback J, Shelton J. Access to modern contraception. *Best Pract Res Clin Obstet Gynaecol.* 2006;20(3):323-338.

18. Stanback J, Twum-Baah KA. Why do family planning providers restrict access to services? An examination in Ghana. *Internat Fam Plan Perspec.* 2001;27(1):37-41.

19. Stanback J, Nanda K, Ramirez Y, Rountree W, Cameron SB. Validation of a job aid to rule out pregnancy among family planning clients in Nicaragua. *Rev Panam Salud Publica.* 2008;23(2):116-118.

20. Sullivan TM, Bertrand JT, Rice J, Shelton JD. Skewed contraceptive method mix: why it happens, why it matters. *J Biosoc Sci.* 2006;38(4):501-521.

21. Adetunji J. Rising popularity of injectable contraceptives in sub-Saharan Africa. Annual meeting of the Population Association of America. 2006; Los Angeles, California.

22. Petracci M, Ramos S, Szulik D. A strategic assessment of the reproductive health and responsible parenthood programme of Buenos Aires, Argentina. *Reprod Health Matters.* 2005;13(25):60-71.

23. Heinemann K, Saad F, Wiesemes M, White S, Heinemann L. Attitudes toward male fertility control: results of a multinational survey on four continents. *Hum Reprod.* 2005;20(2):549-556.

24. Weston GC, Schlipalius ML, Bhuinneain MN, Vollenhoven BJ. Will Australian men use male hormonal contraception? A survey of a postpartum population. *Med J Austral.* 2002;176(5):208-210.

25. Center for Reproductive Rights. *Governments Worldwide Put Emergency Contraception into Women's Hands: A Global Review of Laws and Policies.* New York, NY: Center for Reproductive Rights; 2004.

26. World Health Organization Department of Reproductive Health and Research (WHO/RHR), Johns Hopkins Bloomberg School of Public Health, Center for Communication Programs (CCP), INFO Project. *Family Planning: A Global Handbook for Providers.* Baltimore, MD, and Geneva, Switzerland: CCP and WHO; 2007.

27. Faundes A, Tavara L, Brache V, Alvarez F. Emergency contraception under attack in Latin America: response of the medical establishment and civil society. *Reprod Health Matters.* 2007;15(29):130-138.

28. Mulugeta E, Kassaye M, Berhane Y. Prevalence and outcomes of sexual violence among high school students. *Ethiop Med J.* 1998;36:167-174.

29. Holmes MM, Resnick HS, Kilpatrick DG, Best CL. Rape-related pregnancy: estimates and descriptive characteristics from a national sample of women. *Am J Obstet Gynecol.* 1996;175(2):320-324; discussion 324-325.

30. Richey C, Setty V. *Family Planning Choices for Women With HIV.* Baltimore: INFO Project, Johns Hopkins Bloomberg School of Public Health; 2007. Series L, No. 15.

31. Cooper D, Harries J, Myer L, Orner P, Bracken H, Zweigenthal V. "Life is still going on": reproductive intentions among HIV-positive women and men in South Africa. *Soc Sci Med.* 2007;65(2):274-283.

32. de Bruyn M, Njoko M, Odhiambo D, Paxton S. *HIV/AIDS, pregnancy and abortion-related care: A preliminary inquiry.* Chapel Hill, NC: Ipas; 2002.

33. Shelton JD, Peterson EA. The imperative for family planning in ART therapy in Africa. *Lancet.* 2004;364(9449):1916-1918.

34. de Bruyn M. Women, reproductive rights, and HIV/AIDS: issues on which research and interventions are still needed. *J Health Popul Nutr.* 2006;24(4):413-425.

35. Brown A, Jejeebhoy S, Shah I, Yount K. *Sexual Relations Among Young People in Developing Countries: Evidence from WHO Case Studies.* Geneva, Switzerland: World Health Organization (WHO); 2001.

36. Population Division of the Department of Economic and Social Affairs of the United Nations Secretariat. World Population Prospects: The 2006 Revision and World Urbanization Prospects. http://esa.un.org/unpp. Accessed September 20, 2007.

37. Han S, Choe MK, Lee MS, Lee SH. Risk-taking behavior among high school students in South Korea. *J Adolesc.* 2001;24(4):571-574.

38. Zulkifli SN, Low WY. Sexual practices in Malaysia: determinants of sexual intercourse among unmarried youths. *J Adolesc Health.* 2000;27(4):276-280.

39. Blanc AK, Way AA. Sexual behavior and contraceptive knowledge and use among adolescents in developing countries. *Studies Fam Plan.* 1998;29(2):106-116.

40. Isarabhakdi P. Factors associated with sexual behavior and attitudes of never-married rural Thai youth. *J Population Soc Studies.* 1999;8(1):21-44.

41. Wellings K, Collumbien M, Slaymaker E, et al. Sexual behaviour in context: a global perspective. *Lancet.* 2006;368(9548):1706-1728.

42. Bearinger LH, Sieving RE, Ferguson J, Sharma V. Global perspectives on the sexual and reproductive health of adolescents: patterns, prevention, and potential. *Lancet.* 2007;369(9568):1220-1231.

43. Kelly PJ, Schwartz LR. Abstinence-only programs as a violation of adolescents' reproductive rights. *Int J Health Serv.* 2007;37(2):321-331.

44. Ott MA, Santelli JS. Abstinence and abstinence-only education. *Curr Opin Obstet Gynecol.* 2007;19(5):446-452.

45. Kirby DB, Laris BA, Rolleri LA. Sex and HIV education programs: their impact on sexual behaviors of young people throughout the world. *J Adolesc Health.* 2007;40(3):206-217.

46. Pachauri S, Santhya KG. Reproductive choices for Asian adolescents: a focus on contraceptive behavior. *Internat Fam Plan Perspec.* 2002;28(4):186-195.

47. Talashek ML, Norr KF, Dancy BL. Building teen power for sexual health. *J Transcult Nurs.* 2003;14(3):207-216.

48. Muñoz M. Self-aware sex education: a theoretical and practical approach in Venezuela. *Reprod Health Matters.* 2001;9(17):146-152.

49. Chilman CS. Promoting healthy adolescent sexuality. *Fam Relat.* 1990;39:123-132.

50. Cook RJ, Erdman JN, Dickens BM. Respecting adolescents' confidentiality and reproductive and sexual choices. *Int J Gynaecol Obstet.* 2007;98(2):182-187.

51. Sundby J. Young people's sexual and reproductive health rights. *Best Pract Res Clin Obstet Gynaecol.* 2006;20(3):355-368.

52. World Health Organization (WHO). *Unsafe Abortion: Global and Regional Estimates of Incidence of Unsafe Abortion and Associated Mortality in 2003.* 5th ed. Geneva, Switzerland: WHO; 2007.

53. Fawcus SR. Maternal mortality and unsafe abortion. *Best Pract Res Clin Obstet Gynaecol.* 2008;22(3):533-548.

54. Sedgh G, Henshaw S, Singh S, Ahman E, Shah IH. Induced abortion: estimated rates and trends worldwide. *Lancet.* 2007;370(9595):1338-1345.

55. Ahman E, Shah I. Unsafe abortion: worldwide estimates for 2000. *Reprod Health Matters.* 2002;10(19):13-17.

56. Shepard BL, Casas Becerra L. Abortion policies and practices in Chile: ambiguities and dilemmas. *Reprod Health Matters.* 2007;15(30):202-210.

57. McNaughton HL, Mitchell EM, Blandon MM. Should doctors be the judges? Ambiguous policies on legal abortion in Nicaragua. *Reprod Health Matters.* 2004;12(24 Suppl):18-26.

58. Tangmunkongvorakul A, Kane R, Wellings K. Gender double standards in young people attending sexual health services in Northern Thailand. *Cult Health Sex.* 2005;7(4):361-373.

59. Puri M, Ingham R, Matthews Z. Factors affecting abortion decisions among young couples in Nepal. *J Adolesc Health.* 2007;40(6):535-542.

60. Barge S, Bracken H, Elul B, Kumar N, Khan W. *Formal and Informal Abortion Services in Rajasthan, India: Results of a Situation Analysis.* New Delhi, India: Population Council; 2004.

61. Jewkes RK, Gumede T, Westaway MS, Dickson K, Brown H, Rees H. Why are women still aborting outside designated facilities in metropolitan South Africa? *BJOG.* 2005;112(9):1236-1242.

62. International Consortium for Medical Abortion. Medical abortion: expanding access to safe abortion and saving women's lives. *Reprod Health Matters.* 2005; 13(26):11-12.

63. American College of Obstetricians and Gynecologists. ACOG practice bulletin. Clinical management guidelines of obstetrician-gynecologists. Number 67, October 2005. Medical management of abortion. *Obstet Gynecol.* 2005;106(4):871-882.

64. Hajri S, Blum J, Gueddana N, et al. Expanding medical abortion in Tunisia: women's experiences from a multi-site expansion study. *Contraception.* 2004; 70(6):487-491.

65. Ipas. *Medical Abortion: Implications for Africa.* Chapel Hill, NC: Ipas; 2003.

66. Newhall EP, Winikoff B. Abortion with mifepristone and misoprostol: regimens, efficacy, acceptability and future directions. *Am J Obstet Gynecol.* 2000;183 (2 Suppl):S44-53.

67. Grimes DA. Risks of mifepristone abortion in context. *Contraception.* 2005; 71(3):161.

68. Berer M. Medical abortion: issues of choice and acceptability. *Reprod Health Matters.* 2005;13(26):25-34.

69. World Health Organization (WHO). *WHO Model List of Essential Medicines.* Geneva, Switzerland: WHO; 2007.

70. United Nations. The Beijing Declaration and The Platform for Action: Fourth World Conference on Women; September 4-15, 1995; Beijing, China.

71. Low N, Broutet N, Adu-Sarkodie Y, Barton P, Hossain M, Hawkes S. Global control of sexually transmitted infections. *Lancet.* 2006;368(9551):2001-2016.

72. World Health Organization (WHO). *Global Prevalence and Incidence of Curable STIs.* Geneva, Switzerland: WHO; 2001.

73. World Health Organization (WHO). *Global Strategy for the Prevention and Control of Sexually Transmitted Infections, 2006-2015.* Geneva, Switzerland: WHO; 2006.

74. Mayaud P, Mabey D. Approaches to the control of sexually transmitted infections in developing countries: old problems and modern challenges. *Sex Transm Infect.* 2004;80(3):174-182.

75. Cohen MS. HIV and sexually transmitted diseases: lethal synergy. *Top HIV Med.* 2004;12(4):104-107.

76. Fleming DT, Wasserheit JN. From epidemiological synergy to public health

policy and practice: the contribution of other sexually transmitted diseases to sexual transmission of HIV infection. *Sex Transm Infect.* 1999;75(1):3-17.

77. Schaller UC, Klauss V. Is Crede's prophylaxis for ophthalmia neonatorum still valid? *Bull World Health Organ.* 2001;79(3):262-263.

78. Schmid GP, Stoner BP, Hawkes S, Broutet N. The need and plan for global elimination of congenital syphilis. *Sex Transm Dis.* 2007;34(7 Suppl):S5-10.

79. Aral SO, Mann JM. Commercial sex work and STD: the need for policy interventions to change societal patterns. *Sex Transm Dis.* 1998;25(9):455-456.

80. Jewkes RK, Levin JB, Penn-Kekana LA. Gender inequalities, intimate partner violence and HIV preventive practices: findings of a South African cross-sectional study. *Soc Sci Med.* 2003;56(1):125-134.

81. Wang Y, Li B, Song DM, Ding GY, Cathy E. Power relation and condom use in commercial sex behaviors. *Biomed Environ Sci.* 2007;20(4):302-306.

82. Weiss HA, Patel V, West B, Peeling RW, Kirkwood BR, Mabey D. Spousal sexual violence and poverty are risk factors for sexually transmitted infections in women: a longitudinal study of women in Goa, India. *Sex Transm Infect.* 2008; 84(2):133-139.

83. European Centre for the Epidemiological Monitoring of AIDS. Comparison of female to male and male to female transmission of HIV in 563 stable couples. European Study Group on Heterosexual Transmission of HIV. *BMJ.* 1992;304(6830): 809-813.

84. Nicolosi A, Correa Leite ML, Musicco M, Arici C, Gavazzeni G, Lazzarin A. The efficiency of male-to-female and female-to-male sexual transmission of the human immunodeficiency virus: a study of 730 stable couples. Italian Study Group on HIV Heterosexual Transmission. *Epidemiology.* 1994;5(6):570-575.

85. Padian NS, Shiboski SC, Glass SO, Vittinghoff E. Heterosexual transmission of human immunodeficiency virus (HIV) in northern California: results from a ten-year study. *Am J Epidemiol.* 1997;146(4):350-357.

86. Lee V, Tobin JM, Foley E. Relationship of cervical ectopy to chlamydia infection in young women. *J Fam Plann Reprod Health Care.* 2006;32(2):104-106.

87. Arya OP, Mallinson H, Goddard AD. Epidemiological and clinical correlates of chlamydial infection of the cervix. *Br J Vener Dis.* 1981;57(2):118-124.

88. Pant B, Chaturvedi M, Bansal R, Tiwari R, Parashar P. A study on clinico-social factors for sexually transmitted diseases among urban males. *Indian J Public Health.* 2007;51(4):244-245.

89. Shendre MC, Tiwari RR. Role of occupation as a risk factor for sexually transmitted disease: A case control study. *Indian J Occupat Environ Med.* 2005 2005;9(1):35-37.

90. Chen XS, Yin YP, Gong XD, et al. Prevalence of sexually transmitted infections among long-distance truck drivers in Tongling, China. *Int J STD AIDS.* 2006; 17(5):304-308.

91. Kayembe PK, Mapatano MA, Busangu AF, et al. Determinants of consistent condom use among female commercial sex workers in the Democratic Republic of Congo: implications for interventions. *Sex Transm Infect.* 2007;84(3):202-206.

92. Conway JH. Recognizing and reducing the global burden of congenital syphilis: the time is now. *Sex Transm Dis.* 2007;34(7 Suppl):S2-4.

93. Blandford JM, Gift TL, Vasaikar S, Mwesigwa-Kayongo D, Dlali P, Bronzan RN. Cost-effectiveness of on-site antenatal screening to prevent congenital syphilis in rural eastern Cape Province, Republic of South Africa. *Sex Transm Dis.* 2007;34 (7 Suppl):S61-S66.

94. Platt L, McKee M. Observations of the management of sexually transmitted diseases in the Russian Federation: a challenge of confidentiality. *Int J STD AIDS.* 2000;11(9):563-567.

CHAPTER 18

The Impact of Chronic Kidney Disease on the Girl-Child

Guillermo Hidalgo, MD

Guillermo Hidalgo, MD, is an Assistant Professor of Pediatrics at the University of Illinois, Chicago, IL.

INTRODUCTION

In 1945, the United Nations Charter created the groundwork for the Convention on the Rights of the Child (CRC) by urging nations to promote and encourage respect for human rights and fundamental freedoms "for all." The Universal Declaration of Human Rights followed three years later, further highlighting that "motherhood and childhood are entitled to special care and protection" and referring to the family as "the natural and fundamental group unit of society." Several declarations on the rights of the child were agreed to during the 1900s, as in 1959 "recognizing that mankind owes to the child the best that it has to give."

Declarations are statements of moral and ethical intent, but they are not legally binding instruments. The international human rights framework has been built therefore to contain covenants (or conventions) that involve and carry the weight of international law. In 1976, the first two covenants—the International Covenant on Civil and Political Rights and the International Covenant on Economic, Social, and Cultural Rights—became binding on states. Both covenants used the foundation of the rights and principles in the Universal Declaration of Human Rights, thus providing a legal as well as a moral obligation for countries to respect the human rights of each individual.

In 1978, a working group within the United Nations collaborated and revised a draft that finally became the articles of the CRC.

United Nations member states final approval came when the UN General Assembly unanimously adopted the text of the CRC on November 20, 1989. The Convention then became legally binding in September 1990, after 20 states had ratified it. Many countries ratified the convention very soon after it was adopted, and others continued to ratify or accede to it, making it the most widely ratified human rights treaty. As of December 2005, nearly all states are parties. Somalia and the United States have not yet ratified the convention but have signed it, indicating their support.

The 1993 World Conference on Human Rights recognized that the human rights of children constitute a priority for action within the United Nations system. In May 2002, the UN Special Session of the General Assembly on Children focused attention on making progress for children and investing in them as keys to building global peace and security. At the 2005 Special Session on Children, member states committed themselves to improving the situation of children.

Children's Rights in the Context of Human Rights Work

The CRC encompasses the rights that must be realized for children to develop their full potential, protected, free from hunger and want, neglect, and abuse. It reflects a new vision of the free child. Children are neither the property of their parents nor are they helpless objects of charity; they are human beings and are the subject of their own rights. The convention offers a vision of the child as an individual *and* as a member of a family and community, with rights and responsibilities appropriate to his or her age and stage of development. By recognizing children's rights in this way, the convention firmly sets the focus on the whole child.

The convention and its acceptance by so many countries have heightened recognition of the fundamental human dignity of all children and the urgency of ensuring their well-being and development. The convention makes clear the idea that a basic quality of life should be the right of all children, rather than a privilege enjoyed by a few. The convention establishes and delineates in its Article 24 the framework of health provisions as part of the human rights of all children.

From Abstract Rights to Day-to-Day Realities

Despite the existence of rights, children, and in particular the girl-child, suffer from poverty, homelessness, abuse, neglect, preventable diseases—including a variety of causes of chronic kidney disease (CKD), and unequal access to health, education, and justice systems that do not recognize their special needs. These are problems that occur in both industrialized and developing countries.

The near-universal ratification of the convention reflects a global commitment to the principles of children's rights. By ratifying the convention, governments state their intention to put this commitment into practice. State parties are obligated to amend and create laws and policies to fully implement the convention; they must consider all actions taken in light of the best interests of the child. The task, however, must engage not just governments but all members of society. The standards and principles articulated in the convention can only become a reality when they are respected by everyone—within the family, in schools, hospitals, healthcare facilities and other institutions that provide services for children, in communities, and at all levels of administrations and governments. The convention establishes and delineates in its Article 24 the framework of health provisions as part of the human rights of all children and in such context this chapter will examine the impact of CKD on the health of the girl-child around the globe.

Chronic Kidney Disease

Worldwide and in the United States of America, the proportion of patients with chronic kidney disease (CKD) is reaching epidemic proportions. This is true especially in adults but also in children, although it remains significantly underdiagnosed. CKD is now being recognized as a major public health problem that is threatening the healthcare system and its financial support over the next decade.[1] In North America, up to 11% of the population (19 million) may have CKD,[2] and surveys in Australia, Europe, and Japan describe the prevalence of CKD to be 6–16% of their respective populations.[3,4,5]

In North America alone, more than 100,000 individuals entered end-stage renal disease (ESRD) programs in 2003.

The growing cost of treating patients with ESRD is substantial and poses a great financial challenge. The economic burden of North American ESRD programs reached $25.2 billion in 2002, an 11.5% increase over the previous year, and is expected to reach $29 billion by 2010.[1]

In contrast to adults, pediatric ESRD patients (less than 18 years of age) constitute a small proportion of the total ESRD population in the United States. However, their numbers are steadily rising and they pose unique challenges to families (especially to single-parent households), providers, and to the healthcare system. In North America, children and adolescents younger than 18 years of age account for less than 2% of the total US ESRD population, and the prevalence of patients aged 0–18 years has only grown a modest 32% since 1990. This is in sharp contrast to the 126% growth experienced by the entire ESRD population over the period of time.[6] Nonetheless, CKD in children is a devastating illness that, if caught early, can be modified to extend the native kidney life. The mortality rate for children with ESRD receiving dialysis therapy is between 30 and 150 times that of the general pediatric population. In fact, the expected remaining lifetime for a child 0–14 years of age and on dialysis is only 20 years.[7]

The diagnosis of ESRD for the vast majority of children living in the developing world stops short of being a death sentence. Governments that have ratified the CRC have failed to implement policies that would diagnose and treat pediatric CKD. Similarly, this is also true for a widening component of the populations that within developed countries continue to live within the settings of the developing world.

Access to Health Care and Diagnosis of CKD

North America

Within the United States there are at least 46 million uninsured of which 18 million are children and approximately half of those are girls. The majority of states have Medicaid programs that aim at universal pediatric coverage. However, because of multiple variables (e.g., lack of legal framework to enforce such coverage, Medicaid HMO policies, parental educational attainment, language barriers, or assimilation programs) children and families are increasingly becoming medically uninsured in the United States, the nation that has the largest gross domestic product in the world.

A review of the North American Pediatric Renal Trials Collaborative Studies (NAPRTCS) data

reveals that the majority of children with CKD are diagnosed late in the course of their disease.[8] They may also have had a late referral to a pediatric subspecialist or never received any preventive screening for CKD owing to lack of access. Therefore, if caught late in its course, a significant proportion of patients with pediatric CKD may have a more rapid progression to ESRD. Efforts to identify the causes, presentation, and progression of CKD in children are urgently needed not only in the United States but also worldwide.

Worldwide

In many parts of the world the main day-to-day struggle remains to be survival for life, efforts to defeat hunger, pursuit of clean water sources, and protection from violence and drugs. Among diseases that top the priority list of developing countries, malnutrition, diarrhea disease, and dehydration, as well as pneumonias and asthma relegate pediatric CKD, dialysis, and transplantation to lower health priorities. In the vast majority of less-developed countries, there is limited, sporadic, or no access to health care despite being an inherent human right of children. The reasons for limited or no access to health care are mainly structural and economic, including scarce financial resources, government negligence and poor planning, corruption scandals, and fraud. These perpetuate disastrous violations of children and girl-child health and human rights.

Direct Impact of Pediatric Chronic Kidney Disease

North America

Seen in its global perspective, two-thirds of the pediatric predialysis CKD and ESRD patients are males. As a whole, CKD in the 0–6 years of age affects more males than females because of the congenital and structural nature of CKD. Causes at this age include obstructive uropathy, dysplasia-hypoplasia, and reflux nephropathy.[8]

However, before six years of age, girls more often than boys are affected by congenital nephrotic syndrome, pyelonephritis, and interstitial nephritis. Notably, after one year of age, girls are three times more likely than boys to have urinary tract infections (UTIs). As childhood years go on until 5–7 years of age, the incidence and prevalence of UTIs continues to be higher in girls. Anatomic and functional reasons play a roll. Short urethra and its risk associated with perineal Enterobacteriacea colonization and invasiveness (*E. coli* in more than 80% of the time) and higher incidence of voiding dysfunction in girls play a major roll. Nonetheless, other risk factors may include vesico-ureteral reflux (VUR), poor genital hygiene, and any cause of incomplete bladder emptying as well as constipation. The importance of higher prevalence of UTIs and its prevention in girls is highlighted by the inherent risk of recurrent UTIs and renal scarring. Renal scars play a pivotal role in the later development of hypertension, proteinuria, and CKD leading to ESRD.

After six years of age, girls are more affected by systemic lupus erithematosus nephritis, idiopathic crescentic glomerulonephritis, and membranous nephritis.[6]

The family dynamics of minorities, immigrants, and low-income and single mother families are disproportionately affected by the burden of CKD. These families need support and orientation to pull their own resources together to overcome the burden of CKD.

A wide array of immunosuppressive medications (e.g., tacrolimus, mycophenolate mofetil), ACE inhibitors, and angiotensin receptor blockers alone or in combination can take a toll on adolescent girls and young adult women who are sexually active. Exposure to such drugs within their renal disease treatment may have a deleterious effect on their pregnancy, fetus, and infant. Aside from medications exposure, it is well known that pregnancy in adolescents and women with CKD and ESRD is associated with high rates of preterm and low birth weight infants with resultant increased risk of their neonatal morbidity and mortality.

Worldwide

The incidence and prevalence of childhood ESRD are influenced by a wide variety of factors. Factors such as ethnicity and race distribution, type of prevalent renal disease, and quality of medical care available for predialysis CKD patients have a significant effect on patient outcomes. There is an abysmal disparity in the prevalence of ESRD between developed and developing countries that largely stems from the financial capacity of different countries to afford the ever-growing cost of renal replacement therapies. In less developed countries, due mainly to structural causes, there is poor allocation and support for programs that provide preventive services of predialysis CKD and renal replacement therapies for children with ESRD.[1,3]

Comprehensive information on the etiology of ESRD from many developing countries is unavailable owing to poor data collection and the absence of renal registries.

In contrast to the experience within developed countries, many of these countries continue to suffer from the burden of preventable infectious diseases such as schistosomiasis, hepatitis B and C, malaria, and tuberculosis, with resultant infection-related glomerulonephritis. Nigeria, as is the case with many countries in Africa and Asia, has reported a variety of infectious glomerulopathies as the cause of renal failure in one-half of their patients.[9]

Human-immunodeficiency virus nephropathy (HIVN) in children is another entity that is notably underdiagnosed and underreported. HIVN is likely to increase along with the increasing incidence of HIV in Africa and Asia.

Hereditary disorders are more prevalent in countries where consanguinity is common. Among Middle Eastern countries up to one-third of children with CKD have been diagnosed with hereditary renal disorders such as polycystic kidney disease, primary hyperoxaluria, and congenital nephrotic syndrome (CNS).[10]

In contrast with structural and glomerulopathies causing the bulk of CKD in children, in many countries adult and pediatric CKD is still caused by pesticides. Due to a variety of economic reasons, non-US Environmental Protection Agency (EPA)-approved pesticides and insecticides produced by large multinational firms continue to be allowed into their markets.

Acute and chronic renal and nonrenal toxicities from all kinds of otherwise banned (e.g., organophosphates, paraquat, malathion) pesticides in the industrialized world are rampant in El Salvador and in many other countries of Central America.[11] Acutely, pesticide and insecticide toxicities cause significant morbidity and mortality. Pesticide and herbicide toxicities cause a severe impact in families—just as in war—killing predominately male workers in agriculture and leaving women as single parents of large families and leaving children with a single parent.

Chronically, in coastal rural areas of El Salvador where the chemical residues tend to accumulate, they are one of the most prevalent causes of CKD.[12]

The environmental nondegradable heavy metal accumulation and its toxicity is another silent but important cause of, not only renal, but multisystemic toxicity in children of resource-poor communities.[13] Lead toxicity is an important cause of developmental delay, seizure disorder, anemia, and CKD in such countries. In El Salvador, due to government neglect and flagrant corruption, only recently has it been revealed by "records" from a battery factory, the long standing, silent intoxication of hundreds of children. Due to liability issues and ongoing legal battles, only a few of the children have received proper chelating therapy, and almost none will have long-term follow up to assess the multisystemic long-term consequences of their exposure.

In developing countries and in any resource-poor communities, including underserved and uninsured populations of developed countries, poor hygienic conditions lead to high prevalence of parasitic infestations such as lice, pediculosis, cutaneous larva migrans, and scabies. *Sarcoptes scabeii* infestation in turn aggravated by itching and poor hand and nail hygiene leads to a higher incidence of pyoderma by *Staphylococcus* and *Streptococcus* species. This is particularly important because of its high prevalence of parasitic infestations and pyoderma in children.[14]

Group A streptococcus infections, especially in the form of cellulitis, erysipelas, and impetigo, has been associated with increased incidence and prevalence of postinfectious (streptococcal) glomerulonephritis (PIGN).[15] PIGN is, in the majority of cases, a self-limited disease. However, certain conditions such malnutrition and poor diagnosis and management may aggravate its evolution from an easily contained status to chronic glomerulonephritis and subsequent development of CKD. Pyoderma and parasitic skin diseases receive very little importance in the health agenda of many communities. As the global burden of poverty worsens around the globe, one may expect a rise in the postinfectious causes of CKD. There is a clear need for considerably more commitment from local health authorities, the research community, and healthcare workers than both of these disease associations currently receive. There is an urgent need to know the burden of disease in vulnerable populations, to identify individuals at risk for developing severe complications, and to develop methods to reduce parasitic skin disease and pyoderma leading to PIGN in impoverished populations.[12,14]

Access to Dialysis

North America

Dialysis in pediatric ESRD, although temporary, allows for survival. Thus, dialysis in pediatrics should be just a stepping stone before renal transplantation. However, in many states of the nation pediatric nondocumented immigrants have no ESRD coverage. This situation forces them to rely on emergency Medicaid and dialysis treatments alone rather than comprehensive management. If they decide to remain in the same location they need to reapply repeatedly for emergency Medicaid coverage. A different alternative is for families to move to a different state with an inclusive policy for nondocumented immigrants with pediatric ESRD. A review of the Cooperative Research Centre articles, the mandate, and the state policies that argue that it is legally viable to exclude such populations from full ESRD coverage does little, if anything, to clarify the coverage issue.

Worldwide

In Mexico, Guatemala, and El Salvador, the main dialysis modality is in-center peritoneal dialysis (PD). Due to difficulties in transportation and finances, in-hospital programs see themselves obligated to provide shelter for families who stay over 3–5 days while children receive continuous ambulatory PD, after which they return to their communities for a couple of weeks until it is time to return for another cycle of treatments. A vast majority of patients are underdialyzed and suffer from complications of ESRD. Others may be lucky enough to receive in-center hemodialysis (HD). Nonetheless, due to governments' budgetary restrictions and local hospitals' financial restraints, patients' families are asked to buy supplies for their children's HD treatments. Sometimes they are capable of affording treatments, but more often they cannot. Thus, every treatment day may become a gamble between prolongation of life, ESRD complications, or the need to convert to PD. The risk of death is significantly increased. In summary, these are all clear violations of children's human rights.

Access to Renal Transplantation

Pediatric ESRD patients who, for different causes, may remain in dialysis have a higher rate of complications and mortality. Renal transplantation is the treatment of choice for pediatric ESRD in order to avoid ESRD complications and death. Nonetheless, in the case of pediatric ESRD, patients in need of renal transplantation who do not have immigration documents that allow them to have insurance coverage for the transplantation package (hospital charges, operation and surgeons, medications, etc.) as well as posttransplant immunosuppressant coverage will not receive renal transplantation. They have to wait long periods of time without the possibility of a kidney transplant, sometimes until they have life-threatening complications and death. This is just as unjust as a jailed person without a day in court. It is noteworthy that dialysis is associated with an appreciably higher risk of death compared with renal transplantation; therefore, patients who experience a longer wait for transplantation are more likely to have a worse overall outcome.

Not only is the benefit of transplantation evident when one compares transplant recipients to patients deemed "not medically suitable" for trans-

plantation. This has been substantiated in a recent longitudinal study of 5961 pediatric patients, all of whom were placed on the deceased donor kidney transplant waiting list in the United States. Gillen et al. showed that transplanted children had a lower estimated mortality rate (13.1 deaths/1000 patient years) compared with patients on the waiting list (17.6 deaths/1000 patient years). Thus, pediatric renal transplantation is not only the most preferred modality of treatment for pediatric ESRD, but it may be the treatment of choice in order to reduce mortality.[13]

Similarly, the 2005 US Renal Data System reported that approximately 92% of children initiating therapy with a transplant survive five years compared with 81% of those receiving HD or PD. Finally, the expected remaining lifetime for children 0–14 years of age and on dialysis is only 18.3 years, whereas the prevalent transplant population of the same age has an expected remaining lifetime of 50 years.[6]

Conclusion

International as well as local efforts are necessary to ensure that children and the girl-child with ESRD have access to renal transplantation soon enough to limit complications. International surgical and physician teams, the World Transplant Fund, and other institutions share the goal of making it available and sustainable to all children in all nations.

It is essential for the global health community to realize the serious public health challenge CKD and ESRD pose to the health of the girl-child and women globally.

DISCUSSION QUESTIONS

1. Why are renal diseases such as chronic kidney disease and end-stage renal disease major public health challenges worldwide?

2. Discuss the barriers to access renal dialysis and transplantation facilities within a human rights context.

3. Discuss the role of public health practitioners in implementing measures to address the global burden caused by renal diseases.

REFERENCES

1. Lysaght MJ. Maintenance dialysis population dynamics: current trends and long-term implications. *J Am Soc Nephrol.* 2002;13:37-40
2. Coresh J, Astor BC, Greene T, Eknoyan G, Levey AS. Prevalence of chronic kidney disease and decreased kidney function in the adult US population: Third National Health and Nutrition Examination Survey. *Am J Kidney Dis.* 2003;41:1-12
3. El Nahas AM, Bello AK. Chronic kidney disease: the global challenge. *Lancet.* 2005;365:31-40.
4. Hallan SI, Coresh J, Astor BC, et al. International comparison of the relationship of chronic kidney disease prevalence and ESRD risk. *J Am Soc Nephrol.* 2006;17:2275-2284.
5. De Vecchi AF, Dratwa M, Wiedmann ME. Healthcare systems and end-stage renal disease: an international review—costs and reimbursement of ESRD therapies. *N Eng J Med.* 1999;14:31-41.
6. US Renal Data System (USRDS). Annual Data Report: Atlas of End-Stage Renal Disease in the United States. Bethesda, MD: National Institute of Diabetes and Digestive and Kidney Diseases; 2005.
7. US Renal Data System (USRDS). Annual Data Report: Atlas of End-Stage Renal Disease in the United States. Bethesda, MD: National Institute of Diabetes and Digestive and Kidney Diseases; 2004.
8. North American Pediatric Renal Transplant Cooperative Study (NAPRTCS). 2005 Annual Report. Rockville, MD: EMMES Corporation; 2005.
9. Anochie I, Eke F. Chronic renal failure in children: a report from Port Harcourt, Nigeria (1985–2000). *Pediatr Nephrol.* 2003;18:692-695.
10. Hamed RMA. The spectrum of chronic renal failure among Jordanian children. *J Nephrol.* 2002;15:130-135.
11. Wesseling C, Corriols M, Bravo V. Acute pesticide poisoning and pesticide registration in Central America. *Toxicol Appl Pharmacol.* 2005;207(2 Suppl):697-705
12. Gracia-Trabanino R, Domínguez J, Jansà JM, Oliver A. Proteinuria and chronic renal failure in the coast of El Salvador: detection with low cost methods and associated factors. *Nefrologia.* 2005;25(1):31-8.
13. Gillen DL, Smith J, Stehman-Breen CO, et al. The survival advantage of pediatric recipients of a first kidney transplant among children awaiting kidney transplantation. (Abstract). *J Am Soc Nephrol.* 2006;17:667A.
14. Currie BJ, Carapetis JR. Skin infections and infestations in aboriginal communities in northern Australia. *Australas J Dermatol.* 2000;41:139-143.
15. Feldmeier H, Chhatwal GS, Guerra H. Pyoderma, group A streptococci and parasitic skin diseases—a dangerous relationship. *Trop Med Internat Health.* 2005;10(8):713-716.

CHAPTER 19

INTRODUCTION

Breast Cancer in Women: A Public Health Perspective

Breast cancer is the most common cause of cancer-related death among women worldwide, with case fatality rates highest in low-resource countries.[1] There has been tremendous progress in the last 30 years in the treatment and early diagnosis of breast cancer making it one of the most researched and well-documented cancers in medicine. The development of treatment guidelines, preventive strategies, and interventions for early detection has made a significant difference in improving survival in breast cancer. However as pointed out by the World Health Organization (WHO), the guidelines defining optimal breast care and services have limited utility in resource-constrained countries.[1]

Breast cancer, a disease that overwhelmingly affects women, can be staged from I to IV depending on the size of the tumor and extent of spread within the body. The stage at the time of diagnosis determines the survival rate—the estimate being a 100% survival for stage I to only 20–30% for stage IV according to the American Cancer Society (ACS). Hence there is great emphasis for early detection and diagnosis of breast cancer. The cancers diagnosed in later stages are the most difficult, resource intensive, and expensive to treat. However, most of the cancers diagnosed in developing countries fall under this category.[2] Efforts aimed at early detection can reduce the stage at diagnosis, potentially improving the odds of survival and cure, and enabling simpler and more cost-effective treatment in these countries.[2]

The treatment of breast cancer includes diagnosis with a biopsy, surgical treatment supplemented by radiation, and chemotherapy or hormonal therapy. Local treatment of early-stage breast cancer involves either mastectomy or breast-conserving surgery followed by whole-breast irradiation.[3] Breast cancer care requires involvement of various specialties—such as primary care medicine or gynecology, surgery, hematology oncology, radiation oncology, pathology, genetics, and ancillary care specialties (see Figure 19-1). Even if these specialties are available in a developing country the local healthcare practices lack a teamwork approach for the treatment of the

Anitha Srinivasan, MD, MPH, FACS

Anitha Srinivasan, MD, MPH, FACS, is an Assistant Professor in the New York Medical College, and an Attending Surgeon at Metropolitan Hospital, New York, NY.

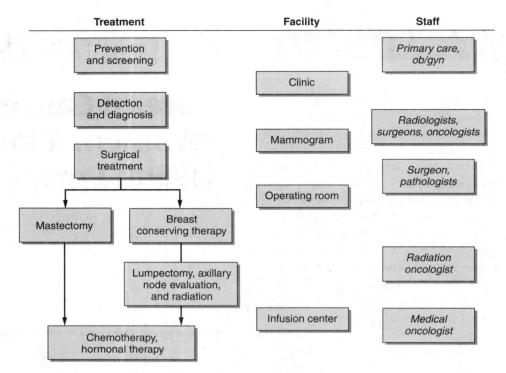

| Treatment | Facility | Staff |

Prevention and screening → Primary care, ob/gyn

Clinic

Detection and diagnosis

Mammogram → Radiologists, surgeons, oncologists

Surgical treatment

Operating room → Surgeon, pathologists

Mastectomy   Breast conserving therapy

Lumpectomy, axillary node evaluation, and radiation → Radiation oncologist

Infusion center → Medical oncologist

Chemotherapy, hormonal therapy

FIGURE 19-1   Standardized Diagnosis and Treatment of Breast Cancer

patient. This may be one of the arguments for considering cancer centers even in developing countries with emphasis on early diagnosis and prevention programs in the rural areas.

Breast cancer can be a valid reflection of the current state of women's health care within a country. Gender inequalities in health care are a consequence of resident inequalities between men and women in many societies.[4] In many cases, women do not have equal access to facilities for cancer prevention and treatment. The political will to assign funding for women's cancer programs may be low due to male-dominated societies. Frequently women are expected to continue their household duties despite cancer diagnoses and may be the only caregivers for their children. This makes access to timely treatment difficult. There may be cultural and social issues that prevent women from obtaining medical care necessary for prevention and early detection services of cancer.

Statistics

Each year, breast cancer is newly diagnosed in more than 1.1 million women, and these cases represent more than 10% of all new cancer cases.[1] By 2010, the majority of approximately 1.5 million annual new cases of breast cancer will be diagnosed in women in countries with limited resources.[5] With more than 410,000 deaths each year, the disease accounts for more than 1.6% of all female deaths worldwide.[1] Breast cancer is an urgent public health problem in high-resource regions and is becoming an increasingly urgent problem in low-resource regions, where incidence rates have been increasing by up to 5% per year.[1] Before 2010, the total annual number of cases in countries with limited resources will exceed the number in developed countries.[5] In countries with limited resources, at least half of the women have advanced or metastatic breast cancer at the time of diagnosis.[6] Because advanced breast cancer has the poorest survival rate and is the most resource intensive to treat, measures to reduce the stage at diagnosis are likely to have the greatest overall benefit in terms of both survival and costs.[7] More people die from cancer than from AIDS, malaria, and tuberculosis put together; 12.5% of all deaths each year are due to cancer globally. The numbers strongly support the need for increased attention to breast cancer as a global health problem rather than a disease of the western world.

Treatment of Breast Cancer— A Global Perspective

Globalization is rapidly happening in all fields including health care, aided by improvements in information technology and science. The treatment in the Western world for breast cancer has largely evolved based on clinical trials and research data. Clinical trials rightfully represent the most powerful strategy for improving cancer treatments.[8] However such trials and data may carry flaws with regards to representation of minorities and ethnically diverse populations even within the United States.[9] The data support standardized treatment guidelines and have largely contributed positively to increasing survival rates in breast cancer. However such guidelines may not be universally applicable for various reasons. This prompted the strategy of categorizing countries based on the resources available for breast cancer care and then finding the optimum standard of care within those resource limitations.[10]

The essentials of a basic breast care program include the following:

■ Prevention
■ Early detection
■ Optimal treatment

The breast care resource level of countries as stratified by the BHGI (Breast Health Global Initiative) is labeled:

■ Basic
■ Limited

■ Enhanced
■ Maximal

WHO categorizes the resource levels as low- and medium-resourced countries (LRC, MRC). The resources available once evaluated are maximally utilized to produce the best possible breast care program. Obstacles to improving cancer care can arise from multiple sources:

■ Deficits in public knowledge and awareness
■ Social and cultural barriers
■ Challenges in organizing health care
■ Insufficient resources

There are many variations to what is considered standard of care by the United States in these programs. For example a prevention and early detection program should include mammograms as a screening tool, which may not be a cost-efficient method in an LRC, and programs emphasizing self-breast exams (SBE) and clinical breast exams (CBE) may be more feasible. In analyzing the scientific literature there is lack of support that SBE and CBE improve detection rates and survival as opposed to mammograms that have shown to do so.[6] However it is important to remember that the initial data supporting mammography as recommended screening did not include the resource-strapped countries where SBE and CBE are used as primary screening tools.

The Difference in Cancer Care Among Developing and Western Countries

Breast cancer is one the few cancers that has undergone significant improvements in survival and early detection over the past few decades. While this has been largely true in the Western world, developing countries are now dealing with increasing incidence and diagnosis of advanced cancers while lacking a definite breast care program.

The example of mammograms for screening can be used to compare the breast care in the United States or other European nations to the developing countries. In the United States, it is recommended that once women turn 40 they should have a mammogram annually. This may differ slightly from the Canadian and European models where mammograms are recommended after age 50 and advised for every other year. However it is clear that serial mammograms detect early changes, and breast cancer can potentially be detected in its very early stages when it presents as an in-situ cancer. In fact the existence of DCIS (ductal carcinoma in situ) has been widely recognized and understood after the increased mammographic screening. The diagnosis of breast cancer as DCIS will lead to a 100% survival rate. Despite standardization of breast cancer care and aggressive screening within the United States there are still disparities in access for the underserved communities.[11]

There are key differences in treatment options as well with respect to the resource levels available in the country. Breast cancer can be treated surgically by two methods—a mastectomy, which does not require radiation therapy, or breast-conserving therapy (BCT), where radiation is an integral part of the treatment. It is obvious that the access to radiation in rural areas and in developing countries will result in higher mastectomy rates.[12] Here the protocols for treatment have to be adapted to suit the needs of the patients and their access to care and available resources. In many developing countries treatment methods and guidelines have been adapted to fit the local resource availability, such as BCT despite lack of mammographic screening in India,[13,14] or the use of radiation therapy in all stages for breast cancer.[15] Locally advanced breast cancer (LABC) accounts for at least half of all breast cancers in countries with limited resources and has a poor prognosis.[3] In these cases the chemotherapy protocol has been adapted to suit the stage of presentation and has shown good results.[3]

The role of data maintenance, cancer registries, SEER (surveillance, epidemiology, and end results) and large cohort studies such as the NSABP (the National Surgical Adjuvant Breast and Bowel Project) have contributed enormously to the development of standardized guidelines for breast cancer care within the United States. However there is poor data maintenance in developing countries,[12] and they tend to follow what has evolved in the United States as standardized treatment even if it may be impractical or inappropriate to do so.[5]

Cancer Care Programs in Developing Countries

Healthcare systems in countries with limited resources are generally overburdened, inadequately funded, and structurally challenged to meet their intended goals. Although 75% of the world's population lives in low- and middle-income countries, only 6% of the gross national expenditure in such countries is spent on health care.[16] Resource-constrained countries suffer from a lack of trained medical personnel, inadequate facilities, insufficient funding for equipment and supplies, and inequity of access to care between rural and urban populations.[16] The healthcare funding is usually allocated to healthcare crises, and cancer care is largely underrecognized as a public health need in these countries. In addition, public health policies are largely governmental and bureaucratic and not based on sound public health policy.[16] The nongovernmental organizations (NGOs) in these cases can be champions of change and help in increasing awareness and attracting attention to cancer care.[16] It is clear that most policies that affect local delivery of health services arise from the central governmental policy where there are financial constraints, understaffing for projects proposed, and most of all lack of recognition that cancer care is a public health necessity. There is no perfect healthcare system because a system must strike a compromise in meeting the many diverse health needs of the population it serves. Specifically, a healthcare system must achieve a balance among four primary healthcare system trade-offs: equity in access, scope of services, quality of care, and cost containment.[16]

The guidelines provided by the BHGI stratify the resource levels of the countries and then provide roadmaps for developing individual breast cancer care programs. These have to be individually tailored according to the countries' needs, social and cultural factors that play a vital role in the success of these programs, and the degree of staff coordination, training, and resource allocation necessary.[16] The program development guidelines as recommended by the BHGI emphasize record maintenance as an important part, aiming toward national cancer registries in developing countries. Such registries, if established, will be extremely useful in further strengthening the programs and providing vital information regarding cancer care internationally.

The Organizations Worldwide that Support Breast Cancer Prevention and Care

The women's health advocacy movement began during the second half of the 1900s. Organizations by and for patients with breast cancer that provide support and information for patients such as the Reach to Recovery by the ACS have been active since the 1950s.[17] In this program, survivors of breast cancer help women with the newly diagnosed disease. Members of Reach to Recovery, all of whom have had mastectomies, provide a support group for women who are undergoing mastectomies.[17] This organization continues today as an organization supporting women throughout the world. The awareness and attention for breast cancer care increased in the United States when well-known women such as Betty Ford, Nancy Reagan, Happy Rockefeller, and Shirley Temple Black began to speak out about their experiences with the disease in the 1970s and 1980s. As survivors and advocates, these American women helped raise public awareness about breast cancer and the need for early detection programs.[17] Women increasingly identified themselves publicly as survivors.

Breast cancer advocacy further developed as dedicated organizations such as Y-ME, the Susan G. Komen Breast Cancer Foundation, the National Alliance of Breast Cancer Organizations, and the National Breast Cancer Coalition added a political dimension to the provision of breast cancer information and support. Today, breast cancer advocacy movements are generally well established in North America and Western Europe. The movement in the United States, one of the most successful worldwide, provides a model of how the breast cancer advocacy movement has the power to improve breast health care.

Globally there are multiple organizations that contribute to breast cancer care. WHO's International Agency for Research on Cancer (IARC) is the sole United Nations research organization dealing with cancer on a global scale. BHGI, which is a part of the Fred Hutchinson Cancer Research Center, has evolved strategies to tackle breast cancer globally and hopes to encourage all countries to establish viable breast cancer care programs.

In the early 1990s, EUROPA DONNA, the European Breast Cancer Coalition, was formed. The emergence of breast cancer advocacy throughout Europe can be traced through the development of EUROPA DONNA, a coalition of affiliated groups in countries across Europe.[17] Reach to Recovery has an international network of survivor advocates that includes 84 groups in 50 countries.[17]

The Komen Foundation began to develop international affiliates in countries that were interested in implementing Komen activities, such as the Race for the Cure. Today the Komen Foundation has three international affiliates—in Germany, Italy, and Puerto Rico—that fund grants and carry out breast cancer education programs. In addition, the foundation has made grants to NGOs in more than 30 countries to support a range of breast cancer education, outreach, and support programs.[17]

The ACS and PACT, a program of the International Atomic Energy Agency (IAEA), worked for over 30 years in 110 developing countries to deploy sound radiotherapy programs, expending over $160 million on cancer-related assistance, while improving access to safe and effective cancer treatment.

Social Issues and Breast Cancer Care

The society and culture in a country set the tone for implementation and success of any program. With respect to breast cancer this is especially true, as it happens to be a disease that affects women. In countries where women are not culturally empowered with the right to health care, such programs, even if established, will not reach the public. In countries with devastating epidemics such as HIV/AIDS, women are the only breadwinners for their families and may not have time for accessing health care and prevention. In some cases it is noted that bundling of services such as simultaneous screenings for cervical cancer and breast cancer can encourage women to attend screening clinics.[18] Breast cancer survivor-advocates from countries with limited resources indicate that the commonality of the experience of breast cancer survivors leads to the development of support groups.[17] Survivors recounted the various taboos and beliefs in society that were deterrents to early cancer detection and care, such as belief that women who were diagnosed with cancer are thought to bring bad genes into the family; hence, these survivors did not want to get screened for cancer. The common belief in the developing world is that cancer is "incurable," means a death sentence, and must be accepted as "fate." Survivor-advocates also identified common themes related to the changes in body image associated with mastectomy.[17] In addition, they noted how women with breast cancer must assimilate into their lives the physical scars of treatment, emotional distress, and disruption in family relations. They identified the need for information about prostheses and the need for emotional support. Survivor-advocates, by virtue of their personal life experiences, possess unique insights regarding the complex sociocultural issues that may hinder the implementation of breast health awareness and early detection programs in countries with limited resources.[17] The practice of breast cancer advocacy has increasingly become international, with sustained, effective collaboration among groups. There is a role for advocacy groups to play an increasing role in raising awareness and encouraging early detection in resource-strapped countries.

Conclusion

Breast cancer is a disease that has to be acknowledged as a rapidly increasing cancer in the developing world. There is standardized treatment guidelines in the Western world that have managed to increase survival rates greatly and provide good quality of life to those affected. However the same cannot be applied to the developing countries. International organizations are working globally to develop programs that are best suited for each country according to the available resources. Such programs will be implemented in countries where awareness and education about breast cancer have been propagated by local organizations and NGOs. The governmental organizations, which fund these programs, have to recognize that early detection will decrease morbidity and save much-needed resources that are currently being spent on advanced disease with poor results. Breast cancer is a highly treatable cancer with great public awareness in the United States. Globally, however, the picture still shows a grossly underrecognized public health problem. To view breast cancer care from a developing world perspective means estimating cost benefits, survivals, and quality of life data as applied to a population as opposed to the highly individualized treatment that is available in the West. This perspective will facilitate self-sustaining programs for breast cancer care within low-resource countries.

DISCUSSION QUESTIONS

1. What is the key factor leading to high case-fatality rates of breast cancer in developing countries?
2. What is the UN organization that deals with breast cancer on a global scale?
3. Who are the most effective advocates in providing emotional support for breast cancer victims through advocacy groups?
4. What screening programs and preventive strategies can be implemented in developing countries to reduce morbidity and mortality as a result of breast cancer?

REFERENCES

1. Anderson BO, Carlson RW. Guidelines for improving breast health care in limited resource countries: The breast health global initiative. *J Natl Compr Canc Netw*. 2007;5:349-356.
2. Anderson BO, Braun S, Lim S, et al. Early detection of breast cancer in countries with limited resources. *Breast J*. 2003;9(Suppl 2):S51-S59.
3. Carlson RW, Anderson BO, Chopra R, et al. Treatment of breast cancer in countries with limited resources. *Breast J*. 2003;9(Suppl 2):S67-S74.
4. Anderson BO, Shyyan R, Eniu A, et al. Breast cancer in limited-resource countries: an overview of the breast health global initiative 2005 guidelines. *Breast J*. 2006;12(Suppl 1):S3-S15.
5. Love RR, Love SM, Laudico AV. Breast cancer from a public health perspective. *Breast J*. 2004;10:136-140.
6. Pisani P, Parkin DM, Ngelangel C, et al. Outcome of screening by clinical examination of the breast in a trial in the Philippines. *Int J Cancer*. 2006;118:149-154.
7. Anderson BO, Braun S, Carlson RW, et al. Overview of breast health care guidelines for countries with limited resources. *Breast J*. 2003;9(Suppl 2):S42-S50.
8. Newman LA, Griffith KA, Jatoi I, Simon MS, Crowe JP, Colditz GA. Meta-analysis of survival in African American and White American patients with breast cancer: ethnicity compared with socioeconomic status. *J Clin Oncol*. 2006;24: 1342-1349.
9. Newman LA, Lee CT, Parekh LP, et al. Use of the national cancer data base to develop clinical trials accrual targets that are appropriate for minority ethnicity patients: a report from the American College of Surgeons Oncology Group (ACOSOG) special population committee. *Cancer*. 2006;106:188-195.
10. Anderson BO. Breast healthcare and cancer control in limited-resource countries: A framework for change. *Nat Clin Pract Oncol*. 2006;3:4-5.
11. Bickell NA. Race, ethnicity, and disparities in breast cancer: victories and challenges. *Women's Health Issues*. 2002;12:238-251.
12. El Saghir NS, Khalil MK, Eid T, et al. Trends in epidemiology and management of breast cancer in developing Arab countries: a literature and registry analysis. *Int J Surg*. 2007;5:225-233.
13. Nadkarni MS, Gupta PB, Parmar VV, Badwe RA. Breast conservation surgery without pre-operative mammography—a definite feasibility. *Breast*. 2006;15:595-600.
14. Dinshaw KA, Sarin R, Budrukkar AN, et al. Safety and feasibility of breast conserving therapy in Indian women: two decades of experience at Tata Memorial Hospital. *J Surg Oncol*. 2006;94:105-113.
15. Bese NS, Kiel K, El-Gueddari B, et al. Radiotherapy for breast cancer in countries with limited resources: program implementation and evidence-based recommendations. *Breast J*. 2006;12(Suppl 1):S96-S102.
16. Anderson BO, Yip CH, Ramsey SD, et al. Breast cancer in limited-resource countries: health care systems and public policy. *Breast J*. 2006;12(Suppl 1):S54-S69.
17. Errico KM, Rowden D. Experiences of breast cancer survivor-advocates and advocates in countries with limited resources: a shared journey in breast cancer advocacy. *Breast J*. 2006;12(Suppl 1):S111-S116.
18. Kim JJ, Salomon JA, Weinstein MC, Goldie SJ. Packaging health services when resources are limited: the example of a cervical cancer screening visit. *PLoS Med*. 2006;3:e434.

CHAPTER 20

Cervical Cancer Mortality: A Preventable Tragedy

INTRODUCTION

Cervical cancer is the second most common cancer in women worldwide with an annual estimate of 510,000 newly diagnosed cases and 288,000 deaths.[1] Tragically, more than 80% of cervical cancer cases occur in developing countries. Millions of women worldwide never undergo cervical cancer testing and die as a result of a very preventable death,[1] despite the availability of low-cost and relatively simple techniques for cervical cancer early detection and treatment. Yet, even in the United States where widespread use of the Papanicolaou (PAP) smear test since the 1940s has drastically reduced the burden of cervical cancer there are cases of cervical cancer mortality. According to The American Cancer Society (ACS) the 2006 estimates for this disease indicated that as many as 9710 cases of invasive cervical cancer will be diagnosed in the United States, and 3700 women will succumb to this disease.[2]

Cervical cancer usually begins in the lower part of the uterus and it occurs most commonly in the transformation zone at the juncture between the endocervix and ectocervix, in an area most exposed to sexual trauma. About 80% of cervical cancers are of epithelial origin known as squamous cell carcinomas; the remaining 20% are adenocarcinomas, which can be more difficult to detect because of their physical location.[3] Some of the terms used to describe precancerous changes are *cervical intraepithelial neoplasia* (CIN), *squamous intraepithelial lesion* (SIL), and *dysplasia*. High-grade SIL (HSIL) or CIN2/3 are associated with a worse prognosis then low-grade SIL (LSIL) or CIN1.[4] According to estimates about 500,000 precancerous lesions (CIN) are diagnosed each year in the United States because of screening techniques.[1]

Absence of screening and/or follow-up treatment is one of the main reasons cervical cancer mortality is so high in developing countries where women present with advanced cases that are less responsive to treatment. A number of barriers have been identified to account for this high burden of cervical cancer worldwide. These include poverty, ignorance, lack of healthcare

Padmini Murthy, MD, MPH, MS, CHES;
Eric Li, BA;
Hala Azzam, PhD, MPH;
Aishwarya Narasimhadevara;
Marie Yezzo, MPH

Padmini Murthy MD, MPH, MS, CHES, is an Assistant Professor in the Department of Health Policy and Management as well as the Director of the Global Health Program at New York Medical School of Public Health in Valhalla, NY. She is the Medical Women's International Association NGO Representative to the United Nations, New York, and Robert F. Wagner Public Service Scholar, New York University.

Eric Li, BA, is affiliated with the New York Medical College School of Public Health.

Hala Azzam, PhD, MPH, is an Assistant Professor in the Department of Epidemiology of Preventive Medicine, School of Medicine, University of Maryland Baltimore, and the Emerging Pathogen Institute, College of Public Health, University of Florida.

Aishwarya Narasimhadevara is affiliated with Boston University, Boston, MA.

Marie Yezzo, MPH, is affiliated with Westchester Medical Centre, New York, NY.

access and belief in local myths, fear of using "Western treatments," lack of sufficient female healthcare providers, and discrimination. Countless women worldwide succumb to their disease without even being aware of why they were ill. This chapter will explore some of the causes for the high burden of this preventable disease with emphasis on developing countries.

Brief Historical Overview

Cancer of the uterine cervix had been described as early as 450 BC by Hippocrates, but it was not until the 1800s that the first inkling of probable risk factors for cervical cancer emerged when Rigoni-Stern, an Italian physician, observed that nuns did not present with symptoms of cervical cancer.[5] A series of epidemiological studies conducted from the 1950s to the 1970s identified sexual transmission as a key factor in the occurrence of this disease. Further research in the 1980s and the 1990s lead to the discovery of the human papillomavirus (HPV) as the main factor responsible for cervical cancer.[6]

Treatment and prevention measures for cervical cancer have been available before the epidemiology and understanding of cervical cancer risk factors became widespread among the scientific community and general population. In the late 1800s both surgery and X-rays were used to treat cervical cancer. This was followed by radiation in 1910 with the discovery of radium by Marie Curie. Prevention measures came later with the advent of the PAP smear test in 1930, a simple low-cost measure that allowed early detection of cellular abnormalities in the cervix and paved the way for early treatment and arrest of further progress of the disease.[7] Currently, treatment modalities include surgery, chemotherapy, and radiation. Prevention, which includes regular screening and understanding cervical cancer risk factors, is vital in addressing this devastating disease. The remainder of the chapter will focus on prevention and screening strategies being utilized in the United States and representative low- and middle-income countries.

Risk Factors for Cervical Cancer and the Human Papillomavirus (HPV)

HPVs, are a group of approximately 100 viral strains of which 13 subtypes (HPV 16, 18, 31, 33, 35, 39, 45, 51, 52, 56, 58, 59, and 66) have been shown to infect the genital tract and were classified as carcinogenic by WHO's International Agency for Research on Cancer (IARC) while others were considered probably carcinogenic or as yet undetermined due to lack of sufficient of data.[8,9] Existing data indicate that HPV 16 and 18 are among the most carcinogenic HPV subtypes and account for about 70% of the cervical cancer cases with the rest of the HPV subtypes accounting for about 20% of all cervical cancer cases.[10] Prevalence of HPV is high, and in the United States, it is estimated that over 6 million people are infected with HPV each year and an estimated 20 million (approximately 15% of the population), are currently infected with HPV.[1]

Other probable risk factors for cervical cancer include lack of screening, smoking, prolonged use of oral contraceptives, early onset of sexual activity, age, multiparity, diet which is deficient in fruits and vegetables, low socioeconomic status, usage of Diethylstilbestrol (DES), immunosuppressent conditions caused by diseases such as HIV/AIDS, and a family history of cervical cancer.[11] Studies have shown that infection from HPV leads to low- and high-grade cervical cancer lesions. Presence of HPV in the cervix does not automatically translate into cancer. Among 85% of newly HPV-infected women that have cytologic abnormalities only a small percent progress to cancer.[12] Thus about 1% of cervical intraepithelial neoplasia or CIN 1 cases, 5% of CIN2, and greater than 12% of CIN3 cases are thought to progress to invasive cancer.[13] Persistent infections (that last a year or more and become chronic) with high-risk HPV subtypes have been linked to a worse prognosis.[12] Because the early stages of cervical cancer are typically asymptomatic or present with minimal nonspecific symptoms such as intermenstrual spotting, bleeding, or an increase in vaginal discharge, regular screening becomes critical to detect and treat early onset of precancerous lesions.

Cervical Cancer: Prevention and Screening Strategies

Prevention of cervical cancer can be achieved by preventing infection initially or detecting and treating precancerous lesions at early stages. There are currently three methods for cervical cancer prevention: these include screening techniques such as the PAP smear, liquid-based cytology, or alternative technologies such as visual inspection with acetic acid (VIA); HPV vaccination; and condom use. HPV DNA testing can also be used for screening, but much discussion is underway to determine cost-benefits and efficacy. Each method has its own strengths and weaknesses, and efficacy varies according to available resources and cultural norms.[1,4]

Primary Prevention: Condoms and the HPV Vaccine

Primary prevention is key in cervical cancer prevention. This can be accomplished by empowering and educating women about the use of barrier methods, contraception, and safe sexual practices.[4,15] Condoms provide about 70% protection against HPV when used consistently and regularly. The usage of condoms helps prevent cervical cancer to an extent, but increased condom use can reduce the increasing rates of sexually transmitted infection. The U.S. Public Health Service has included increased condom use as part of *Healthy People 2000* and *Healthy People 2010*.[14]

Two prophylactic HPV vaccines have been recently developed: Gardasil, a quadrivalent vaccine against HPV 16, 18, 6, and 11, and Cervarix, a bivalent vaccine against HPV 16 and 18.[2] Vaccination using Gardasil was approved in the United States in 2006; however, currently there is little information regarding the duration of immunity conferred by the vaccine. Furthermore, the available vaccines do not completely protect a person against all types of HPV subtypes, nor do they protect women who have previously been exposed to HPV.[2] Additional research is needed to ensure the efficacy of HPV vaccines and to design and implement strategies for their availability in the developing world. Unfortunately, the prohibitive cost of these vaccines makes them unavailable for women who have low socioeconomic status and deprives them of protection against this deadly disease. Furthermore, while the HPV vaccines represent a major advance in protection against cervical cancer, frequent screening is required of all women and is one of the most important tools in prevention.[15] For further details on the HPV vaccine and its acceptance, the reader is referred to Chapter 24, "Vaccines and Women: Cultural and Structural Issues for Acceptability."

Papanicolaou Test (PAP Test)

Secondary prevention is achieved through screening and treatment once the precancerous lesions are found. There are several new types of screening methods that are either available or under development. The Papanicolaou test or PAP smear test is a screening procedure that permits diagnosis of preinvasive and early invasive cancer. A PAP smear test is a simple procedure where cells from the cervix are obtained and used for cervical cytology screening. PAP smears have been effective in early detection and prevention of cervical cancer and are generally reliable in identifying women who have precancerous cells as well as those who do not have abnormal cervical cytology. However, to be effective PAP smear screenings need to be conducted on a regular basis. It is recommended that women have their first PAP smear soon after becoming sexually active and to repeat the test every one to three years depending on the initial results. Unfortunately, effective and large-scale PAP smear programs in developing countries are expensive, and improper procedures of fixing and storing the smears and misinterpretations resulting in false negatives. A significant proportion of women in developing countries do not have access to PAP screening due to lack of infrastructure, awareness, and access to health care services.[16]

Visual Inspection with Acetic Acid (VIA)

The difficulties in organizing cytology screenings in developing countries have lead to alternative ways to screen women for cervical cancer. One such strategy is using a method called visual inspection with 30% acetic acid (VIA). It has been shown that VIA has an acceptable sensitivity in detecting CIN and is also very cost-effective. VIA detected abnormalities in 98.4% of patients assessed colposcopically as having an abnormal transformation zone, and it correctly identified 98.9% of normal cases.[17] One of the advantages of VIA testing is that it is done in real time as the results are reported immediately after the screening examination. Instead of the patient coming in for multiple checkups, everything is done in one day which allows planning for further investigation and treatment in the same session.[15] The test is also very reasonable for developing countries because it is a simple, inexpensive, low-technology test that requires minimal infrastructure for use.[15] VIA tests have similar results to cytology in detecting high-grade disease and it is possible to train workers to use VIA screening methods in a short period of time (one to two weeks).[18]

The Christian Fellowship Community Health Centre and the IARC conducted a trial to assess the efficacy of VIA screening to reduce cervical cancer incidence and mortality in a high-risk population in India.[19] In developing countries successful screening and early detection of precancerous cells can be instrumental in reducing the incidence of cervical cancer. It is not cost-effective and beneficial for women in developing countries to have multiple visits for cervical cancer screening. This study indicated that VIA is a simple, feasible, and cost-effective method for detection and early diagnosis of abnormalities, which can help to reduce the mortality rate associated with cervical cancer among deprived populations in both developing and developed countries.[17] One of the drawbacks associated with VIA screening programs is that there has to be high-quality training of providers, continuous quality assurance and monitoring, as well as making people aware of the benefits of availing themselves of such programs in the community.

HPV Detection

A new test known as the Hybrid Capture II test has been approved by the FDA. The test can detect DNA of 13 high-risk HPV types in vaginal or cervical smears and is clinically reliable.[20] It can identify women who already have cervical disease in addition to those who are at increased risk for developing it.[21] A review of 14 studies concluded that HPV DNA testing is particularly valuable in detecting high-grade precancerous lesions in women over age 30 because HPV infections in women under 30 are likely to be transient.[22] The disadvantages of HPV DNA testing are its high costs, requirement for a molecular diagnostic laboratory, and its low specificity in younger women and populations with significant rates of HIV seropositivity.[16] Also, the test results are not provided at the time of the visit because of the need to transport the specimens to a laboratory for analysis. A rapid low-cost test that can be used by low-resource countries is being developed by researchers in PATH and should be available soon for the detection of precancerous and cancerous lesions in the cervix .[22]

Cost-Effective Strategies

Ideally, the most effective screening method would be inexpensive, painless, simple to perform, socially and culturally acceptable, accurate, without adverse effects, and the ability to provide immediate results.[4,15] The Alliance for Cervical Cancer Prevention (ACCP) research in South Africa looked at the cost-effectiveness of different strategies for screening, diagnosis, and treatment of cervical abnormalities. ACCP estimated cancer incidence, life expectancy, lifetime costs, and the costs of three different screening strategies: visual inspection, PAP tests, and HPV tests. The research showed that a single lifetime screening of women ages 35 to 40 would reduce the incidence of cervical cancer in South Africa by at least 26%.[16] The cheapest strategy was visual inspection, followed by treatment with cryotherapy (cold therapy), and the most effective strategy in terms of lives saved was the use of a single lifetime HPV test, followed by cryotherapy for women who tested positive.[16]

Cervical Cancer Burden and Barriers to Cervical Cancer Screening: Case Studies

United States

Cervical cancer was the most common cause of death among women in the United States during the 1930s, but that declined by as much as 70% during the 1900s.[20] This is largely because of widespread use of screening tests, mainly the PAP smear. However, despite the success of the screening interventions, the rates of cervical cancer incidence and mortality have remained the same in the last decade or so. This is due in part to an increase in the number of sexual partners, which in turn has led to a higher incidence of HPV infections.[20] Adoption of the HPV vaccine may decrease the incidence of HPV and precancerous lesions, assuming vaccine acceptability, affordability, and good outreach within communities whose parents may be reluctant to vaccinate their teenage daughters. However, another significant cause of these unchanged cervical cancer rates reflects the lack of screening among vulnerable and poor communities in the United States. A recent report by the National Institute of Health (NIH) highlights the need to focus on these harder to reach communities including recent immigrants, African Americans, and Hispanics.[23] African American women have experienced a dramatic decline in cervical cancer incidence, but still suffer a 72% excess in incidence and 13% lower five-year survival rate compared with Caucasians.[24] Throughout the United States there are geographical variations on the occurrence of cervical cancer. The Midwest, South, and particularly Appalachia, have the highest cervical cancer mortality rates.[24] This can be mainly attributed to the socioeconomic factors and rural environment which contribute to a decrease in access to health care. A study carried out in the United States showed that low-income women living in metropolitan areas may be less likely to be screened for cancer than more prosperous women living in those areas.[25] Analyzation and study of cancer screening rates in the United States by measures of income, educational attainment, lack of access, and other factors may help health officials and policy makers better allocate their resources to areas where they are needed the most.

In a recent systematic review of immigrants and ethnic minorities, barriers to cervical cancer screening included lack of knowledge regarding cervical cancer, fatalistic attitudes about disease, misconception that only sick or married individuals needed screening, perceived lack of female providers, embarrassment by the test procedure, mistrust of the healthcare system, fear of being considered sexually immoral, and stigmatization by the community. For instance, among the Asian community there was a lack of understanding of the Western concept of prevention and the belief that cervical cancer was caused by wind, a more traditional medicine interpretation of disease.[26] It is important to note that knowledge of risk factors for cervical cancer is generally low among all women in the United States.[27] The ACS conducted a study in which over 1000 women attending a well-known women's clinic were asked if they were aware of what HPV infection was and the link between HPV and cervical cancer. The results were surprising since only 30% of them had heard of HPV.[2] Other studies both in the United States and abroad report similar findings. Hence it is important to educate adolescents and women about the importance of regular screening for cervical cancer and HPV detection.

Developing Countries

Cervical cancer has a major impact on the lives of women worldwide, but it has a greater impact on the women in developing countries. Estimates indicate that 83% of new cervical cancer cases detected are in developing countries, where screening programs are not well established or effective. According to a report released in 2004 by the Population Reference Bureau and Alliance for Cervical Cancer Prevention, there are an estimated 1.4 million women globally living with cervical cancer and another estimated 7 million women worldwide who may have undetected precancerous conditions that need to be confirmed and treated to prevent progression to cancer.[16] The mortality rates associated with cervical cancer in developing countries are reported to be 11.2 per 100,000 which is almost three times more than the death rate in developed countries. Unfortunately, more than 40% of the deaths in developing countries occur in countries such as India, Bangladesh, and Pakistan, indicating the poor healthcare status of women in these countries.[16]

The reason for the high number of cervical cancer in developing countries is that some women do not receive the healthcare that they need. Indeed, in many developing countries cervical cancer screening is practically nonexistent or available only to those who can afford it. This is often due to competing health priorities such as HIV, TB, and malaria in the face of limited budgets, poorly developed healthcare infrastructures, and lack of trained human resources, namely cytologists, pathologists, and colposcopists. Other challenges include lack of cancer registries and data to highlight the burden of disease, lack of education, and last but not least women disempowerment in male dominant societies.[28]

Where cervical cancer screening is available, women in the developing world face more inequities including poverty, socioeconomic discrimination, and lack of access to health care as well as stigma. With early screening measures and improved access to health care, wealthy women in poorer countries are likely to be better off than poor women in wealthier countries.[16] Another observed inequity is gender-based: cervical cancer is a disease specifically targeting women, and in many countries women are not allowed access to healthcare by their spouses or in-laws.[23] Often this leads to neglect, and the disease is only detected at an advanced stage; hence, the prevention of early detection of cervical cancer is a violation of women's human rights. The challenge many women in developing countries face is the fact that those discovered to have abnormalities cannot return to the clinic for management. Those who are discovered to have a high-grade of abnormalities should be followed annually for at least five years before they are returned to routine screening protocols.[16] WHO has continued to monitor the progress of cervical cancer screening in developing countries and continues to make recommendations about effective screening procedures.

However, the success of effective screening depends not only on the quality of the screening test but also on how well planned and implemented the screening programs are in order to achieve the maximum benefit in a community. It is important to define a target population by conducting a needs assessment in communities and implementing strategies to increase awareness and benefits of screening and then follow-up that population in order for screening programs to be effective.[16]

Ghana

In Ghana, many women lack access to cervical cancer prevention services. Johns Hopkins Program for International Education in Gynecology and Obstetrics (JHPIEGO), which partnered with the health ministry and Ghana Health Services, started to air information on cervical cancer on popular television programs. Soon hundreds of women flocked to hospitals nearby to get tested. JHPIEGO and the Ghana Health Services wanted to evaluate the approach that links low-cost visual screening with cryotherapy for those with abnormal cells. They tested a single-visit approach that enabled providers to offer treatment for abnormalities during the same visit to women with positive test results.[16] This approach helps to reduce the number of visits a woman must make to the health center and can drastically reduce the number of women who receive sporadic or no treatment at all since there are no follow-up appointments to miss. This project helped motivate women to get tested and to gain their husbands' support. The project highlighted the benefit of increasing awareness by educating women about seeking care in a timely fashion. This project also further illustrated that educational and counseling messages must be refined so that patients and male partners could better understand test results and the differences between cervical cancer and precancerous conditions.[16] Increasing the involvement of male partners is an effective strategy to improve outreach and creating an enabling environment for their decisions to seek treatment and follow-up care.

Nigeria

Cervical cancer is the most common genital cancer found in Nigerian women. The reported age-adjusted incidence rate is approximately 24.1 per 100,000.[29] There is a lack of awareness and a lack of programs in the country about cervical cancer. A descriptive case study conducted in Lagos, Nigeria, looked at cervical cancer screenings conducted in 503 healthcare facilities. The results of this study showed that screening services were more available in the urban than in the rural areas, yet cervical cancer screening was restricted to only a few urban research centers. Thus, cervical cancer screening practices and services in Lagos are inadequate, which is no different from other parts of Nigeria and sub-Saharan Africa.[25]

Sub-Saharan Africa

Part of the challenges facing many sub-Saharan and other developing countries is the absence of functional cancer registries. The reasons typically include incomplete medical records (making it hard to collect data), lack or scarcity of trained personnel for estimating disease burden, and lack of financial resources to maintain these registries. This, in turn, leads to underestimates of the true cancer burden with underrepresentation of rural areas, inadequate resource allocation for cervical cancer prevention programs, and an inability to evaluate the efficacy of these programs when they exist.

In sub-Saharan Africa, cervical cancer still remains a major burden on public health resources. Countries in this region have some of the World's highest death rates from cervical cancer: 67 per 100,000 people in Harare, Zimbabwe, and 40.8 per 100,000 in Kampala, Uganda.[30] In East, Central, and Southern African (ECSA) about 95% of the healthcare institutions had the basic infrastructure to carry out cervical screening, but only a small percentage of women were actually screened. The reason for this is because of the lack of policy guidelines, infrequent supply of basic materials, and a lack of qualified staff. Overall this shows that there is an urgent need for more investment (including human capital in the form of trained healthcare providers, social workers, and community activists) and monetary resources in the diagnosis and treatment of cervical cancer in ECSA countries. In this region and other countries with low resources, suitable screening programs should be established by the stakeholders in order to lower cervical cancer incidence rates.[27]

Cervical cancer screening services in many countries have failed to reach the majority of the population. There is a significant difference in the types of women who access and who do not access PAP smear services. Women who are underserved seem to be the older, poorer, less educated, and unemployed and were not empowered to make decisions regarding their lives, including seeking healthcare services. Typically these women do not know anyone else who has had a PAP smear or know exactly what a PAP smear test is. They probably have never sought care for other health ailments or usually ignore getting proper healthcare services. To make prevention programs effective and allocate the most effective resources, communities with the greatest concentration of marginalized women need to be targeted. These women need to be educated, empowered, and be provided with innovative programs to help them understand cervical cancer and the services that are available to them. Healthcare providers, policy makers, and other stakeholders should work to ensure that messages are culturally relevant and appropriate and are more focused on women's physical, mental, and emotional health.[15]

Cape Town, South Africa

A study conducted in areas around Cape Town, South Africa, educated 5045 patients about cervical cancer and its prevention.[15] They were offered a free PAP smear test in a fully equipped mobile clinic. The concept of using of using a mobile clinic was very effective in reaching out to women in areas where limited facilities are available. This onsite screening also helped to improve community outreach effectively, since the women who sought the services were instrumental in spreading the news about the benefits of such screening procedures.

Implementation of Screening Programs: Advantages and Challenges

Establishment of screening programs in developing countries has been helpful in the early detection of cervical cancer, and this can aid in early intervention and treatment that will improve the patient outcomes. The most clinically effective and cost-effective strategies found in developing countries are screening early detection and treatment, through either a reduced number of visits or improved follow-up. Therefore, there needs to be a mass screening program developed in low- and middle-income countries.[31] This is to be advocated with the most immediate emphasis on areas where the prevalence of cervical cancer is high. For this to come about, the availability of a proven method of screening and its advantages must be introduced.[28] In many African countries, there is currently no program for screening for detection of cervical pathology in women. Services are only available in family planning clinics that are located primarily in the teaching hospitals, and even where they are offered, screening services are not adequately utilized.[32] In some developing countries cervical screening is available, but the problem to providing adequate screening is that the follow-up is inadequate. This can result in failure of detection of recurrences. Hence it is crucial to emphasize the importance of regular follow-up and screening procedures in communities and on an individual case-by-case basis to improve the quality of life among these women.

It is a challenge to initiate screening programs in developing countries when there is no organized healthcare system that is capable of providing the diagnostic and treatment services as integrated components of screening. Initially these programs can be supported by funding from donor countries but have a slim chance of becoming self-sufficient if there is no political will, health policies, or decisions in place to support them by providing government funding.

Professional and public education, combined with the availability of treatment for early stages of invasive cancer of the cervix, has an important effect in reducing the morbidity and mortality associated with the disease.[16,20,25] It is important that the educational programs that are designed to teach women about cervical cancer be culturally sensitive and specifically designed to address the needs of the women in the targeted communities and country.

The goals of any cervical cancer prevention program should include achieving the highest coverage of the population at risk, to screen women with an accurate test as part of high-quality services, and to ensure that women with positive test results are properly managed and followed up as needed.[29] The lack of effective screening and treatment strategies is a major reason there is a much higher cervical cancer rate in developing countries. Without access to certain programs and basic health care, women from poor communities generally seek care only when they develop symptoms and become incapacitated. Women who are seeking help at an advanced stage of the disease would make it more challenging for healthcare professionals to provide effective treatment or improve their quality of life. Often healthcare providers are helpless and feel frustrated because they lack the facilities, including specialized forms of treatment, to treat these women. Other barriers to prevention and treatment may include a lack of awareness of cervical cancer progression and of ways to prevent the disease, difficulty in getting to clinics and hospitals, the need for multiple visits, and high costs associated with screening.[16,29]

Myths, misconceptions about the disease, suspicion of the treatments offered at healthcare facilities, distance and access to healthcare facilities, cultural barriers to screening, and high costs of vaccination or the screening tests are some of the universal challenges faced by women and other stakeholders in working to reduce the incidence of cervical cancer globally. In Kenya for example, women report being unable to convince their husbands to spend money and access healthcare facilities if they are feeling healthy.[33] The economic and social burden associated with cervical cancer can be devastating on individuals, families, communities, and the nation. Implementation of successful screening programs depends on providing training at all levels for healthcare professionals, social workers, and program managers, as well as increasing awareness among community elders and family members.[34]

Sociocultural barriers such as myths, taboos, and misconceptions about cervical cancer increase women's vulnerability to sexually transmitted diseases and cervical cancer. Certain cultural teachings in the developing world will contradict health education messages and certain interventions for women. Fear of stigmatization is also rampant. Many women believe that the test is meant to detect sexually transmitted diseases, and in South Africa and Kenya, women fear that a positive test for abnormal cervical cytology indicates the presence of HIV infection.[33] In Latin America and the Caribbean, women do not necessarily understand that cervical cancer is a preventable disease.[33] The existence of myths and misconceptions about sexual and reproductive health plays a vital role in influencing gender dynamics that render women less likely to seek services, contrary to the prevailing cultural norms and beliefs. Such norms and community practices, therefore, indirectly deter women's utilization of health services and thereby deny them access to health care.[31]

In developing countries efficient and high-quality laboratory services are rare. Small laboratories tend to use or interpret reporting systems inconsistently. Improper handling and storage of the histopathology and cytology specimens can lead to incorrect reporting. Sometimes these reports can be misinterpreted by clinical staff, which may explain why so many women are requested to return for unnecessary repeat smears.[30]

Future Strategies

Certain scientific advancements have made cervical cancer screening easier and available to women, but the costs are still high. It is important for the global community to increase access to these new technologies and make them affordable so that more women worldwide can benefit from them.[35] Women and their sexual partners need to be educated about ways to protect themselves from HPV and other sexually transmitted diseases. Even though condoms are not 100% effective against HPV, they are still the most effective way to prevent it and offer protection to the couple. Many women in developing countries do not receive regular PAP smear tests because of an inability to pay for services, a lack of knowledge, and a lack of support. The National Breast and Cervical Cancer Early Detection Program administered by the Center for Disease Control (CDC) is a program that provides free or low-cost PAP smear testing and diagnostic services for low-income and uninsured women.[18, 34] There is a great need for such programs like the National Breast and Cervical Cancer Early Detection Program to be established in developing countries. Such programs will help to increase awareness of this preventable disease by providing the necessary resources to women and their communities.

Conclusion

To design, implement, and ensure the sustainability of a successful screening program, a package of education, screening, and precancerous treatment options and services should be made available to all women in developing and developed countries. The various initiatives should complement each other; implementation of any one without the others would not be beneficial in reducing the morbidity and mortality associated with cervical cancer. Integration of cervical cancer screening programs within the context of primary care services will also help to increase the outreach of such programs.

Advocacy, male involvement, lack of gender discrimination, and policies beneficial for promoting women's health will go a long way to reduce the devastating effects of cervical cancer worldwide.

DISCUSSION QUESTIONS

1. Discuss the factors contributing to the high incidence of cervical cancer in the developing World.
2. Discuss policies, programs, and strategies that can be implemented to address the challenges faced by women and communities as a result of cervical cancer.

REFERENCES

1. Ferley J, Bray F, Pisani P, Parkin DM. GLOBOCAN 2002 cancer incidence: mortality and prevalence worldwide. *IARC Cancer Base*. 2004;5(version 2.0). Lyon, France: IARC.

2. Cancer Journal for Clinicians. American Cancer Society guidelines for human papillomavirus (HPV) vaccine use to prevent cervical cancer and its precursors. http://caonline.amcancersoc.org/cgi/content/full/57/1/7. Accessed July 23, 2008.

3. Wang SS,Sherman ME, Hildesheim A, et al. Cervical adenocarcinoma and squamous cell carcinoma incidence trends among White women and Black women in the United States for 1976-2000. Cancer. 2004;100(5):1035-1044.

4. American Cancer Society. Cervical Cancer. http://www.rho.org/files /ACS_CC_2007.pdf. Accessed July 19, 2008.

5. Ricci, J. V. (1945). One hundred years of gynaecology, 1800-1900; A comprehensive review of the specialty during its greatest century with summaries and case reports of all diseases pertaining to women. Philadelphia: The Blakiston company.

6. Nasca P. *Fundamentals of Cancer Epidemiology*. 2nd ed. http://www.jbpub.com /catalog/9780763736187/. Accessed July 29, 2008.

7. Rubin SC. Cervical cancer: successes and failures. *CA Cancer J Clin*. 2001;51(2): 89-91.

8. IARC. Monographs on the evaluation of carcinogenic risks to humans. *Hum Papilloma*. 2005;90:1-670.

9. Walboomers JM, Jacobs MV, Manos MM, et al. Human papillomavirus is a necessary cause of invasive cervical cancer worldwide. *J Pathol*. 1999;189(1):9-12.

10. Clifford GM, Smith J S, Plummer M, et al., Human papillomavirus types in invasive cervical cancer worldwide: a meta-analysis. *Br J Cancer*. 2003;88(1):63-73.

11. American Cancer Society. What are the risk factors for cervical cancer? http://www.cancer.org/docroot/CRI/content/CRI_2_4_2X_What_are_the_risk _factors_for_cervical_cancer_8.asp. Accessed July 27, 2008.

12. Gravitt PE, Jamshidi R. Diagnosis and management of oncogenic cervical human papillomavirus infection. *Infect Dis Clin North Am*. 2005;19(2):439-458.

13. Ostor AG. Natural history of cervical intraepithelial neoplasia: a critical review. *Int J Gynecol Pathol*. 1993;12(2):186-192.

14. Planned Parenthood. The truth about condoms. http://www.plannedparenthood.org/issues-action/birth-control/condoms-truth-6543.htm. Accessed July 29, 2008.

15. Mahone SM. Cervical cancer: what should we tell women about screening? http://www.ons.org/publications/journals/cjon/Volume10/Issue4/pdf/1004527 .pdf. Accessed July 23, 2008.

16. Alliance for Cervical Cancer Prevention. Preventing cervical cancer worldwide. http://www.path.org/files/RH_prp-accp_cervical_cancer_worldw.pdf. Accessed July 19, 2008.

17. Bradley J, Risi L, Denny L. Widening the cervical cancer screening net in a South African township: who are the underserved? http://www.ingentaconnect.com /content/routledg/uhcw/2004/00000025/00000003/art00003. Accessed October 12, 2008.

18. World Health Organization. Cervical cancer screening in developing countries. http://www.who.int/reproductive-health/cancers/cervical_cancer_screening _in_dev_countries.pdf. Accessed July 24, 2008.

19. Sankaranarayanan R. Effect of visual screening on cervical cancer incidence and mortality in Tamil Nadu, India: a cluster-randomised trial. http://www.ncbi.nlm.nih.gov/pubmed/17679017?ordinalpos=4&itool=EntrezSystem2.PEntrez.Pubmed.Pubmed_ResultsPanel.Pubmed_RVDocSum. Accessed July 23, 2008.

20. Castle P, Wheeler C, Solomon D, Schiffman M. Interlaboratory reliability of hybrid capture. *Am J Clin Pathol*. 2004;122: 238-245.

21. American Society for Colposcopy and Cervical Pathology. Consensus Guidelines. http://www.asccp.org/consensus.shtml. Accessed July 29, 2008.

22. PATH. Preventing cervical cancer: unprecented opportunities for improving women's health. http://www.rho.org/files/PATH_outlook23_1_web.pdf. Accessed July 19, 2008.

23. Freeman HP, Wingrove BK, eds. *Excess Cervical Cancer Mortality: A Marker for Low Access to Health Care in Poor Communities*. Rockville, MD: National Cancer Institute, Center to Reduce Cancer Health Disparities; 2005. NIH Pub. No. 05-5282.

24. Cancer Journal for Clinicians. Cervical cancer: prevention, diagnosis, and therapeutics. http://caonline.amcancersoc.org/cgi/reprint/51/2/92. Accessed July 22, 2008.

25. Coughlin SE, King J, Richards T, Ekwueme D. Cervical cancer screening among women in metropolitan areas of the United States by individual-level and area-based measures of socioeconomic status. http://cebp.aacrjournals.org/cgi/content/full/15/11/2154. Accessed July 23, 2008.

26. Johnson CE, et al. Cervical cancer screening among immigrants and ethnic minorities: a systematic review using the Health Belief Model. *J Low Genit Tract Dis*. 2008;12(3):232-241.

27. Tiro JA, Meissner, H, Kobrin, S. et al. What do women in the U.S. know about human papillomavirus and cervical cancer? *Cancer Epidemiol Biomarkers Prev*. 2007;16(2):288-294

28. Denny L, Quinn M, Sankaranarayanan R. Screening for cervical cancer in developing countries. *Vaccine*. 2006;24(Suppl 3):S71-S77.

29. Anorlu RI, Ribiu KA, Abudu OO, Ola ER. Cervical cancer screening practices among general practitioners in Lagos Nigeria. http://www.informaworld.com/smpp/content~content=a773287239~db=all~order=page. Accessed July 23, 2008.

30. Chirenje ZM, Rusakaniko S, Kirumbi L, et al. (2001). Situation analysis for cervical cancer diagnosis and treatment in East, Central, and Southern African countries. 79:127-132.

31. Adewole I, Benedet JL, Crain B, Follen M. Evolving a strategic approach to cervical cancer control in Africa. http://www.sciencedirect.com. Accessed July 23, 2008.

32. Bradley J, Barone M, Mahe C, Lewis R, Luciani S. Delivering cervical cancer prevention services in low-resource settings. http://ww.rho.org/files/IJGO_89_S2_2005_04.pdf. Accessed July 23, 2008.

33. Bingham A, Bishop, A. Patricia, C., Winkler, J., Bradley, J., Dzuba, Illana, Agurto, I. Factors affecting utilization of cervical cancer prevention services in low-resource settings. *Salud Publica Mex*. 2003;45(Suppl 3):S408-S416.

34. World Health Organization. Cervical cancer screening in developing countries. http://www.who.int/reproductive-health/cancers/cervical_cancer_screening_in_dev_countries.pdf. Accessed July 24, 2008.

35. Goldie S. Health economics and cervical cancer prevention: a global perspective. http://www.elsevier.com. Accessed July 24, 2008.

CHAPTER 21

Maternal Mortality: The Eye of the Storm

INTRODUCTION

The greatest unsolved public health issue of our time is the death of women due to pregnancy and childbirth complications. Each year there are over half a million maternal deaths around the globe, with 99% occurring in developing nations.[1] In fact, maternal mortality is the health indicator that demonstrates the greatest difference between developed and developing countries.[2] The most common measure of the magnitude of maternal mortality is known as the maternal mortality ratio (MMR), which is based on the number of maternal deaths per 100,000 live births in a given year. The countries with the highest MMRs (greater than 1000 maternal deaths per 100,000 live births) are in Africa, with the exception of Afghanistan.[1] A nation's MMR is a direct reflection of how well- or ill-functioning its health system is. From a gender equity perspective, the MMR is also a litmus test of the status of women and girls in a given society.

During the last few decades of the 1900s, child mortality rates fell dramatically in the developing world. The same rate of decline was not seen with maternal deaths. A landmark article in 1985 refocused international attention on maternal mortality by asking "Where is the *M* in *MCH?*" (i.e., where is the *maternal* in *maternal-child health?*)[3] The Safe Motherhood Initiative was subsequently launched in 1987, a concerted 15-year effort lead by United Nations agencies to reduce maternal deaths. During these years, a strong focus on the potential role of traditional birth attendants (TBAs) and improved prenatal care failed to achieve the results desired.[4] This is largely because most maternal deaths arise from complications that occur around the time of labor and delivery and are, for the most part, unpredictable. Most complications cannot be adequately treated by TBAs; rather they require timely access to well-understood medical interventions, such as transfusion for excessive bleeding, antibiotics for infection, and caesarean section for obstructed labor. Among the many lessons learned from the Safe Motherhood Initiative was the need for a clear, defined strategy and sustained funding to create changes in health—as well as economic and political—systems. The Millennium Development

Anne Foster-Rosales, MD, MPH, FACOG

Anne Foster-Rosales, MD, MPH, FACOG, is the Chief Medical Officer of Planned Parenthood Golden Gate, located in San Francisco, CA. Dr. Foster-Rosales is also an Assistant Clinical Professor in the Department of Obstetrics, Gynecology, and Reproductive Sciences for the University of California, San Francisco. She is a Kellogg Scholar in health disparities.

Goals (MDGs), set forth by the United Nations in 2000, embrace a set of eight broadly stated goals of social and economic development. They include a specific goal, MDG5, to improve maternal health. MDG5 is further delineated into two main components: MDG5A seeks to reduce the MMR by three-quarters between 1990 and 2015; MDG5B aims to achieve universal access to reproductive health by 2015.[5] Since the MDGs are essentially a negotiated political document, they steer governments to a renewed focus on reducing maternal mortality, while at the same time making the critical linkage between development and reproductive health.

The Magnitude of the Problem

Every minute of every day, a woman dies from complications of pregnancy or childbirth. This translates to 10 million women dying per generation.[6] In many developing regions deaths from pregnancy and childbirth among reproductive age women account for more premature deaths and illness than any other cause.[7] A maternal death is defined as one which occurs during pregnancy or up to 42 days after delivery (or the end of the pregnancy after miscarriage or abortion). Eighty percent of maternal deaths are caused by conditions directly related to pregnancy, such as severe bleeding after delivery, complications of pregnancy-related hypertensive diseases (known as preeclampsia/eclampsia), infection, or obstructed labor. Also included are deaths from complications of abortion (usually due to bleeding and infection from unsafe conditions), which are very difficult to measure as abortion is still legally restricted in most countries. MMRs also include indirect deaths in which the pregnancy aggravates an underlying medical problem such as malaria, tuberculosis, or HIV/AIDS. Not included in the ratio are deaths due to accidents, homicides, or suicides.

While the death of a woman owing to complications of pregnancy and delivery is tragic, the impact extends not only to her family, but also to her community where she is often a key economic producer. Of note, her surviving children are 10 times more likely to die within 2 years of their mother's death.[8] It is also important to note that for every woman who dies, there are at least 30 more who suffer maternal morbidity or serious injury and disability that may impact the rest of their lives.[9] The study of severe complications or the "near miss" maternal death has gained attention over the last few years. Cases of near miss are those in which the woman develops a potentially life-threatening complication during pregnancy, delivery, or during the postdelivery period, but who survives by chance or through appropriate medical care.[10] The study of near misses can be useful in evaluating the quality of obstetric care, particularly in areas when accurate numbers of maternal deaths cannot be estimated by surveillance systems, or in areas where the absolute number of maternal deaths is very small.

One obstetrical complication in particular has devastating social consequences—obstetrical fistulas. A fistula can develop during a long and obstructed labor when the pregnant woman does not have timely access to a cesarean section. It forms when prolonged pressure on the birth canal from the fetal head causes a hole to form between the vagina and bladder or rectum. The subsequent disability, chronic leaking of urine and/or stool from the vagina, is a huge social stigma that often leads to the woman being shunned by her family and community.[11] While fistulas are preventable and easily correctable with surgery, it is still a well-known phenomenon in many African nations.

Why Maternal Mortality Is Unique

Maternal mortality is unique among health indicators because exposure to the primary risk factor, pregnancy, can occur repeatedly throughout a woman's reproductive life. This is different from child mortality, which is a risk each human being faces only once when passing through childhood. Although much progress has been made in reducing child mortality, little progress has been observed in reducing newborn mortality. Newborn and maternal health outcomes are closely linked. Of the 6.5 million newborn deaths each year (98% in developing nations), 50% occur within the first

24 hours, and 75% occur within the first week.[12] Adequate obstetrical care for the mother translates to significant reduction in newborn mortality, thus the importance of strategies that ensure services benefit both the mother and the infant.

Unlike many communicable diseases, such as measles, there is no vaccine to prevent a maternal death, no single intervention that will protect a woman as she experiences each subsequent pregnancy in her lifetime. While most pregnancies and deliveries occur without serious problems, it is a biological truth that 10–15% of pregnant women will develop a complication. This complication, if not recognized in a timely fashion and managed correctly, may result in the death of the mother. The Three Delays Model has been applied widely around the world in the design of maternal mortality reduction programs, and takes into account cultural, economic, and institutional barriers that contribute to maternal deaths.[13] First, a woman or her family may delay the decision to seek care once a complication, such as a postpartum hemorrhage, occurs, leading to her death. Secondly, once the decision to seek care is made, there may be a delay in accessing a facility because of lack of transport, causing her to die in transit. Thirdly, when care is accessed, she may not receive appropriate interventions, owing to lack of blood products or because of inadequately trained healthcare providers.

The Skilled Birth Attendant

From a medical point of view, the single most important factor in maternal death reduction is to guarantee a skilled birth attendant is present at every birth. A skilled attendant is a clinically trained and certified provider, such as an obstetric nurse, professional midwife, or physician. In fact, as a general rule, the higher the percentage of births attended to by skilled attendants, the lower the MMR in a given area. A comparison of Egypt to Sri Lanka in the 1960s, when these nations' gross national products were similar, reveals that Egypt had an MMR that was 10-fold higher than Sri Lanka. The difference is that in Egypt only about 50% of births were attended by a skilled birth attendant, versus about 95% of women in Sri Lanka.[14] Experience in the Goma Refugee camp during the 1990s provides a recent example of the importance of skilled birth attendants and timely access to emergency obstetric care, such as cesarean section, transfusion, and antibiotics. The MMR was noted to be approximately 10-fold lower in this camp of Rwandan refugees than the surrounding rural Zaire population. Among the camp population, the MMR was noted to be 60 maternal deaths/100,000 live births, compared to 600/100,000 in the surrounding population, which relied primarily on TBAs and had limited access to emergency obstetric care.[15]

Although the presence of a skilled birth attendant is critical in maternal death reduction, accountability for the quality of care given in institutions is also key. For example, simply moving most births to a hospital setting is not a guaranteed solution to reducing maternal deaths. In the Dominican Republic the vast majority of births occur in a hospital setting, yet the MMR continues to be high. This appears to be due to the poor quality of care in hospitals, insufficient number of skilled attendants, inadequate supervision of staff, and the overmedicalization at birth leading to excess complications.[16] Likewise, when hospital maternal deaths in Surinam were closely examined, a significant number were identified as preventable and caused by substandard care by hospital staff.[17]

Contraception Is Prevention

There is no doubt that prevention is the key to maternal death reduction. Avoiding a pregnancy when it is not desired removes a key risk factor that can lead to a woman's death. Wide access to family planning, including contraception and safe abortion services when pregnancy is undesired, decreases mortality by reducing the overall number of pregnancies and deliveries during a woman's lifetime. The World Bank estimates that 100,000 maternal deaths could be avoided each year if all women who said they want no more children were able to stop childbearing.[18]

One way to assess women's access to contraception is to compare total fertility rates (TFT), an estimate of the total number of children a woman will have during her reproductive years. The TFT in Angola is 6.75 (live births per woman), 4.60 in

Guatemala, 2.37 in Indonesia, 2.04 in the United States, and 0.84 in Hong Kong. The percentage of women in a given country using modern contraceptives is generally inversely related to fertility rates and MMRs. For example, Canada has a TFT of 1.51, an MMR of 6/100,000, and 73% of married women of childbearing age report using a modern method of contraception. In comparison, Mozambique has a TFT of 5.51, an MMR of 1000/100,000, and only 5% of married women of childbearing age use a modern method of contraception.[19]

Who Chooses? The Political Football of Abortion

Although the MMR in the United States declined dramatically by the 1960s, it was not until the legalization of abortion that the last major decline in the MMR was achieved.[20]

In fact, no industrialized nation has been able to achieve its current low levels of maternal mortality without access to both contraception and safe abortion care. In the United States, Canada, and most European nations, abortion is legal, safe, and widely accessible by women, irrespective of their financial means. In countries such as Chile where abortion is legally restricted, the procedure is fairly accessible to women of financial means, under the guise of physicians providing the woman "other" gynecological services. As such, Chile's MMR in 1995 was 16/100,000.

In countries where women are denied both contraception and safe abortion, high maternal mortality is guaranteed. This was the situation in Romania during Ceausescu's rule when, in 1966, both contraception and abortion were outlawed. Afterward, the MMR rose to a level 10 times greater than any other European nation. After the laws were repealed in 1989, the MMR dropped by two-thirds.[21] It is sobering to think that in some nations, up to half of maternal deaths are attributed to complications of unsafe abortions. Legal restrictions to abortion are both irresponsible and irrational as a public health policy, and result in profound economic and social costs to society. Unfortunately, a number of countries still refuse to address the legal restriction of abortion, yet state that reducing maternal mortality is a national priority.

Health Disparities and Human Rights

As noted earlier in this chapter, the disparity in maternal death ratios between higher-income and lower-income countries is striking. Estimates from 2005 show a 50-fold difference in the MMR between developing and developed regions. The average MMR for developing regions is 450 maternal deaths per 100,000 live births, whereas for developed regions it is 9/100,000.[1] This disparity can also be clearly seen when examining the lifetime risk of maternal death, which averages 1 in 75 for developing regions, but only 1 in 7300 for developed regions. About 86% of global maternal deaths occur in sub-Saharan Africa (270,000) and South Asia (188,000), and India is the country with the largest single number of maternal deaths (117,000).[1] The actual changes in MMR for various regions of the world between 1990 and 2005 can be seen in Table 21-1.

Recent studies have focused on inequities within individual countries as well. For example, the burden of maternal mortality is generally concentrated among women in the lowest income quintiles, suggesting that programs that aim to reduce maternal deaths should direct poverty alleviation efforts to the poor, especially the rural poor.[22] Conversely, wealthy women, and particularly urban women, in poor nations have maternal mortality ratios equivalent to women in developed nations. For example, the MMR in Buenos Aires, Argentina, was 9/100,000 live births in 2002, but in the poorer area of Jujay it was 197/100,000.[23] However, the poorest quintile in Tanzania shows an MMR of 816/100,000 live births, whereas the richest quintile has an MMR of 374/100,000, a further reflection of this nation's low development index.[24]

As Gwatkin has noted, "The availability of good medical care tends to vary inversely with the need for it in the population served."[22]

Given that maternal mortality is the medical manifestation of deep-rooted socioeconomic, gender, and cultural inequities, a human rights framework can be applied. Freedom from illness and access to health care is a core concept in social justice efforts. Health systems are truly "core social institutions that function at the interface between people and the structures of power that shape their broader society."[25]

Table 21-1

Region	MMR (maternal deaths per 100,000 live births)	Number of maternal deaths	Lifetime risk of maternal death:[1] 1 in:
WORLD TOTAL	400	536,000	92
Developed regions[2]	9	960	7300
Developing regions	450	533,000	75
Africa	820	276,000	26
Northern Africa[3]	160	5700	210
Sub-Saharan Africa	900	270,000	22
Asia	330	241,000	120
Eastern Asia	50	9200	1200
South Asia	490	188,000	61
Southeastern Asia	300	35,000	130
Western Asia	160	8300	170
Latin America and the Caribbean	130	15,000	290
Oceania	430	890	62

Estimates of MMR, Number of Maternal Deaths, Lifetime Risk by United Nations MDG Regions, 2005

Notes: [1]The MMR and lifetime risk have been rounded.

[2]Includes Albania, Australia, Austria, Belgium, Bosnia and Herzegovina, Bulgaria, Canada, Croatia, Czech Republic, Denmark, Estonia, Finland, France, Germany, Greece, Hungary, Iceland, Ireland, Italy, Japan, Latvia, Lithuania, Luxembourg, Malta, Netherlands, New Zealand, Norway, Poland, Portugal, Romania, Serbia and Montenegro, Slovakia, Slovenia, Spain, Sweden, Switzerland, the former Yugoslav Republic of Macedonia, the United Kingdom, and the United States of America.

[3]Excludes Sudan, which is included in sub-Saharan Africa.

Source: Modified from WHO, 2007, reprinted with permission.

As a result, instead of serving to level the playing field and assuring equal access to care, health systems tend to reinforce and perpetuate inequities. Human rights can thus be seen as a system to reduce inequalities in health outcomes of any particular social group, in this case women, especially poor, rural women who bear most of the burden of maternal mortality around the world. A human rights framework can be effectively applied to promote accountability in a positive, not punitive fashion; it can serve as a guide for what governments, policy makers, health systems, health workers, and national and international communities ultimately do.[26]

Reducing Maternal Mortality: Poverty Is Not an Insurmountable Obstacle

Poverty is the primary social determinant driving maternal deaths. In Ireland, the MMR is 1/100,000,
in the United States it is 11/100,000, but in Sierra Leone it is estimated to be 2100/100,000.[1] However, there are clear exceptions that underscore that poverty alone is not an insurmountable barrier to reducing maternal deaths. Sri Lanka is an often-cited example, where MMR was reduced dramatically over a 50-year period to that of levels consistent with higher-income countries.[14] In the case of Sri Lanka, maternal care became a governmental and societal priority, with the establishment of birthing centers staffed by obstetric nurses. Deliveries moved from the home setting to these centers, and emergency obstetric care was accessible onsite or through transfer should complications arise. As a result, maternal mortality in Sri Lanka was halved about every 10 years.[14] Sadly, the current armed conflict in Sri Lanka has seriously affected the government's ability to assure quality maternity care in all areas of the country, underscoring that diversion of healthcare resources to support military interventions has an immediate impact on public health.

Cuba, Malaysia, and China are also examples where significant progress has been made in reducing maternal mortality. Despite very different cultural, political, and geographical realities, each country has successfully harnessed national political will to reduce maternal mortality by prioritizing maternal health services. Prior to the Cuban revolution some 50 years ago, maternal mortality was high and many births still occurred at home. One of the priorities of the healthcare system was to provide universal obstetric care to all women. Now, all women receive prenatal care, and 99% of infants are delivered in a hospital by an obstetrician. Despite these efforts, there were approximately 61 maternal deaths in 2005 in Cuba, equivalent to an MMR of 45/100,000.[1] Given the development index of this nation, this indicator is much better than other nations with similar development indices. Cuba also has an active Maternal Mortality Surveillance program, headed by a senior obstetrician. Despite the relatively low MMR, there is some room for improvement, particularly with preventing deaths due to severe hemorrhage or due to preexisting cardiac problems in the woman, and focused efforts are underway to address this.[27]

China, Malaysia, and a handful of other nations have demonstrated similar progress in reducing maternal deaths. The common thread in each of these nations is sustained political will at the highest levels of government, along with prioritization of maternal health with a focus on skilled birth attendants and access to emergency obstetric care, expanded access to contraception, and in some cases, access to safe abortion. This has also been coupled with significant strides in both the status and educational level of women in these nations.

In higher-income nations, the MMR declined dramatically throughout the 1900s. In 1900, the United States' MMR was approximately 700/100,000, but it has now been reduced nearly a hundred-fold to 11/100,000. However, the United States has not yet reached an irreducible minimum, due to the persistence of health disparities among ethnic and socioeconomic groups: African American women have a four-fold higher MMR than White women, while Hispanic women face nearly a two-fold increased risk.[28] There has been no significant decrease in the U.S. MMR over the last 20 years, and it is unlikely to fall unless pervasive social inequities are addressed.

Conclusion

Solving the dilemma of maternal mortality is perhaps the greatest sociopolitical test of our time; it is indeed the eye of the storm. It is unique among health indicators because of two specific issues: the fact that women face repetitive risk with each pregnancy, and the fact that gender inequity is pervasive in the very institutions that are responsible for eliminating maternal deaths. Yet experience has shown that when political will is mobilized, countries can rapidly reduce maternal mortality by half every decade, even in the midst of extreme poverty. The majority of maternal deaths are preventable with solutions that are well known and affordable when prioritizing the right services for the people that need them most. Despite the fact that the world has adopted the MDGs, and significant funding has been leveraged to focus intensively on the countries with the highest MMRs, we are far from achieving our goal. At the current rate of decline, it may take 100 years for countries with the highest levels of maternal mortality to achieve levels consistent with that of developed nations. What will it take for the world to reject this projection? Perhaps, it is most important to first answer: what is the value of a woman's life?

Acknowledgement

The author would like to acknowledge the contributions of Casey O'Bryan, BA, in the preparation of this chapter.

DISCUSSION QUESTIONS

1. What are the contributing factors to the alarming rates of maternal mortality in many countries?

2. Discuss how implementing a human rights framework can contribute to reducing maternal mortality worldwide.

3. What is the significance of *M* in *MCH* (i.e., where is the importance of *maternal* in *maternal–child health?*).

REFERENCES

1. *Maternal Mortality in 2005: Estimates Developed by WHO, UNICEF, UNFPA, and the World Bank*. Geneva, Switzerland: World Health Organization; 2007.

2. Cook R, Dickens B. Ethics, justice and women's health. *Int J Gynecol Obstet.* 1999;64(1):81-85.

3. Rosenfield A, Maine D. Maternal mortality—a neglected tragedy. Where is the M in MCH? *Lancet.* 1985;2(8446):83-85.

4. Freedman LP. Strategic advocacy and maternal mortality: moving targets and the millennium development goals. *Gender Dev.* 2003;11(1):97-108.

5. United Nations Millennium Declaration, 2000. Resolution of the General Assembly 55/2. September 18, 2000. New York, NY: UN. A/RES/55/2.

6. Unfortunate facts of life about maternal mortality. Women Deliver Web site. http://www.womendeliver.org/fact/Unfortunate_Facts_of_Life_factsheet_(A4).pdf. Accessed June 20, 2008.

7. AbouZahr C. Disability adjusted life years (DALYs) and reproductive health: a critical analysis. *Reprod Health Matters.* 1999;7(14):118-129.

8. Programming for safe motherhood. United Nations Children's Fund Web site. http://www.unicef.org/sowc01/references.html. 1999. Accessed June 20, 2008.

9. *Maternal Mortality Update 2002: A Focus on Emergency Obstetric Care*. New York, NY: UNFPA; 2003:6.

10. Souza JP, Cecatti JG, Parpinelli MA, Serruya SJ, Amaral E. Appropriate criteria for identification of near-miss maternal morbidity in tertiary care facilities: a cross sectional study. *BMC Pregnancy Child.* 2007;7:20.

11. Lewis G, De Bernis L, eds. *Obstetric Fistula: Guiding Principles for Clinical Management and Programme Development*. 2nd ed. Geneva, Switzerland: World Health Organization; 2006:3-5.

12. Maternal and newborn health. UNICEF Web site. http://www.unicef.org/health/index_maternalhealth.html. Accessed June 20, 2008.

13. Thaddeus S, Maine D. Too far to walk: maternal mortality in context. *Soc Sci Med.* 1994;38(8):1091-1110.

14. Pathmanathan I, Liljestrand J, Martins JM, et al. *Investing in Maternal Health: Learning from Malaysia and Sri Lanka*. Washington, DC: The World Bank; 2003.

15. Schopper D. *What Happens to the Health of Women in Crisis Situations*. Presented at XV FIGO World Congress of Gynecology and Obstetrics; August 4, 1997; Copenhagen, Sweden.

16. Reproductive health: maternal deaths in the Dominican Republic analyzed. Population Council Web site. http://www.popcouncil.org/publications/popbriefs/pb8(2)_3.html. Accessed June 23, 2008.

17. Mungra A, Van Roosmalen J, van Kanten RW, Kanhai HHH. *Substandard Care in Maternal Mortality in Surinam.* Presented at XV FIGO World Congress of Gynecology and Obstetrics August 7,1997; Copenhagen, Denmark http://www.ncbi.nlm.nih.gov/pubmed/9286171. Accessed November,14, 2008

18. Family planning saves lives and improves health. World Health Organization Web site. http://www.who.int/reproductive-health/publications/health_benefits_family_planning/FPP_95_11_chapter1.en.html. Accessed June 20, 2008.

19. United Nations statistics division—demographic and social statistics. United Nations Web site. http://unstats.un.org/unsd/demographic/products/socind/childbr.htm. Accessed June 19, 2008.

20. Meyer RE. Maternal mortality related to induced abortion in North Carolina: a historical study. *Fam Plan Perspect.* 1994;26:179-180,191.

21. Remez L. Romanian maternal death rate fell by two-thirds after the 1989 revolution. http://findarticles.com/p/articles/mi_qa3634/is_199511/ai_n8722997. November 1995. Accessed June 20, 2008.

22. Gwatkin D, Bhuiya A, Victoria C. Making health systems more equitable. *Lancet.* 2004;364(9441):1273-1280.

23. Medici A. Health trends and health goals in the region. Inter-American Development Bank Web site. http://www.iadb.org/biz/ppt/0715medici.ppt.#2561, healthtrendsandhealthgoalsintheregion. April 13, 2007. Accessed June 19, 2008.

24. Measuring Maternal Mortality, IMMPACT Fact Sheet, February 2007, Web site http://www.abdn.ac.uk/~wdu016/uploads/files/Immpact_Measuring%20Maternal%20Mortality.pdf Accessed Nov 14, 2008.

25. Freedman LP, Waldman R, de Pinho H, Wirth ME, Chowdry AMR, Rosenfeld A. Transforming health systems to improve the lives of women and children. *Lancet: UN Millennium Project.* 2005;365:997-1000.

26. Freedman LP. Using human rights in maternal mortality program: from analysis to strategy. *Internal J Gynecol Obstet.* 2001;75(1):51-60.

27. Cabezas A. *Jefe, Programa de Vigilancia de Mortalidad Materna, Republica de Cuba, 2000.* Presented at XVI FIGO World Congress of Gynecology and Obstetrics Washington DC, http://www.obgyn.net/women/women.asp?/page=/fig02000 Accessed November 16, 2008.

28. Hopkins FW, MacKay AP, Koonin LM, Berg CJ, Irwin M, Atrash HK. Pregnancy-related mortality in Hispanic women in the United States. *Obstet Gynecol.* 1999;94(5 Pt 1):747-752.

Women do not have to die from the postpartum hemorrhage (PPH). Whether they give birth with a skilled provider at home or in a facility, or even when they have to undergo childbirth without skilled care, most cases of PPH can be prevented using safe, low-cost, evidence-based practices. Knowing how to prevent PPH, however, is not enough. This knowledge must be translated into program actions when implementing essential maternal and newborn health care and basic emergency obstetric and newborn care interventions. Action means doing the following:

- Ensuring that national policies and clinical guidelines are in place to support the use of active management of the third stage of labor (AMTSL) at every birth attended by skilled providers, as well as supporting community distribution of oral uterotonic agents where births are likely to occur without skilled care.

- Incorporating the knowledge and skills needed to perform AMTSL into preservice education and providing in-service training for skilled providers, as well as training community health workers to safely distribute oral uterotonics for use by women at time of childbirth.

- Ensuring that supplies of uterotonics and other items needed for clean and safe birth are available.

- Bringing essential maternal and newborn health care and basic emergency obstetric and newborn care as close to the family as possible through community health workers and skilled providers.

- Mobilizing the community to help women and their families prepare for birth with a skilled provider and be ready for complications should they occur while at the same time preparing for the possibility of childbirth without skilled care.

CHAPTER 22

Ensuring a Woman's Right to Survive Childbirth: Preventing Mortality from Postpartum Hemorrhage*

Harshadkumar Sanghvi, MD;
Jaime Mungia, MPH

Harshadkumar Sanghvi, MD, is Vice President and Medical Director of Jhpiego, an affiliate of Johns Hopkins University, Baltimore, MD.
Jaime Mungia, MPH, is affliated with Jhpiego, an affiliate of Johns Hopkins University, Baltimore, MD.

* *Adapted with permission of authors from* Preventing Postpartum Hemorrhage. ACCESS Technical Brief. 2006. ACCESS Program: Baltimore, MD.

Epidemiology of Postpartum Hemorrhage (PPH)

Each year in developing countries, 14 million women experience PPH.[1] Hemorrhage accounts for over 25% of maternal deaths in Latin America and the Caribbean, 30.8% in Asia, and 39% in Africa.[2] Nearly half of all postpartum deaths are due to immediate PPH,[3] and millions of women suffer acute and chronic disability following immediate PPH.[4]

Uterine atony causes up to 70% of PPH. Other causes include ruptured uterus; lacerations of the cervix, vagina or perineum; and retained placenta or placental fragments. One unfortunate result of institutionalized births appears to be higher levels of lacerations of cervix, vagina, perineum, and of unneeded episiotomy. There also appears to be higher levels of PPH among institutional births as compared to home births even in relatively normal populations perhaps as a result of increased operative and nonoperative interventions.

Two thirds of PPH cases occur in women with no known risk factors.[5] Most women with factors that were traditionally thought to increase risk (preeclampsia, high parity, multiple pregnancy, previous PPH, etc.), do not, in fact, have PPH. Because we cannot predict who will experience PPH on the basis of risk factors, strategies to prevent PPH must reach *all* women. This is one reason why the high-risk approach to antenatal care that has been used in low-resource settings to determine which woman would best benefit from institutional births and which could undergo childbirth at home has been replaced with a greater emphasis on focused antenatal care including birth preparedness and complication readiness education, and on ensuring skilled care for all births.

Definition of PPH

The most commonly used definition of PPH is blood loss of 500 mL or more in the first 24 hours following childbirth; severe PPH is defined as blood loss of 1000 mL or more.[6] However, it is difficult to accurately assess the amount of blood that a woman has lost because it is mixed with amniotic fluid or dispersed on sponges or linens, in buckets, or on the floor. In addition, slow bleeding from an episiotomy or tear may go unnoticed. Clinical estimates of blood loss, where no special efforts are made to physically measure it, are generally thought to be underestimated by 34–50%.[7] Blood measurement systems suitable for facility and home births in low-resource settings are being tested, including the BRASSS-V drape used in PPH research in rural India. This is a plastic drape with a calibrated collection device that is placed under the woman after the birth of the baby. Since blood loss can be quantified objectively with this device, providers can intervene appropriately before life is threatened by hemorrhage.[8] One additional benefit of improved measures of postpartum blood loss is that the traditional definition of PPH is being challenged as most births that appear normal seem to have blood loss of around 300 mL or less. Another factor to be considered together with postpartum blood loss is the level of anemia. For a woman going into childbirth with severe anemia, even small amounts of postpartum bleeding may push her into serious morbidity. The implication of this is that any blood loss following childbirth needs to be minimized to prevent morbidity and mortality.

Because of the difficulty in accurately measuring blood loss, even in a clinical setting, work is being done to determine the best way to measure blood loss in the home setting where there is no skilled provider. In Tanzania, traditional providers were trained to recognize excessive bleeding using a local garment known as a *kanga*. In this study, it was determined that two kangas soaked with blood after birth of the baby indicated blood loss of slightly more than 500 mL.[9] Communities in Asia often refer to soaking of two sarongs (or sarees) as indicative of PPH.

Hemorrhage, if uncontrolled or untreated, can quickly lead to shock and death. Most deaths caused by PPH occur within the first seven days after childbirth.[3] One study in Egypt found that 88% of these deaths occur within the first 4 hours postpartum.[10] Death from severe PPH may occur within two hours of onset of hemorrhage. Many factors influence whether or not PPH is fatal. Anemia, estimated to affect half of all pregnant women in the world, contributes to the high death toll.[11] A woman who is anemic is unable to tolerate the amount of blood loss that a healthy woman can.[12]

Another important consideration is that 66% of births in the least developed countries occur in the home without a skilled provider.[13] The UN estimates that in the 15 years between 1990 and 2005, skilled attendance at birth increased from 43% to 57%, but in some countries such as Tanzania, it actually declined from 50% to 46%. *(UN 2007)

A woman may give birth alone or in the presence of an untrained birth attendant or family members. If a woman begins to hemorrhage, the birth attendant and family often do not recognize and handle the emergency. Long delays may occur in making the decision to seek help and in transporting the woman to a hospital or center equipped to treat PPH. And because any or all of these factors cause delay in instituting appropriate treatment, PPH that occurs at home has the worst prognosis.

Strategies for Prevention of Postpartum Hemorrhage

One of the most important prevention measures, therefore, is having a skilled provider present at birth. In addition to using the World Health Organization (WHO) partograph to monitor labor (to avoid prolonged labor or obstructed labor and thus uterine rupture), the appropriately trained skilled provider is less likely to perform procedures such as episiotomy or operative vaginal delivery without clear indications. Finally, the skilled provider can perform AMTSL in order to prevent uterine atony, the most common cause of immediate PPH.

Another important implication for preventing mortality and morbidity from PPH is to find better solutions for preventing PPH when births occur at home even where there are no skilled providers.

Understanding the Challenge: An Assessment of the Use of AMTSL in Ethiopia

In 2006, the Ethiopian Society of Obstetrics and Gynecology, with support from the U.S. Agency for International Development-funded Prevention of Postpartum Hemorrhage Initiative (POPPHI), conducted a national assessment on the use of AMTSL in healthcare facilities.[22] Key findings included the following:

- A uterotonic was used in 100% of births in health facilities: oxytocin was used in 68% and ergometrine was used in 28% (mostly after delivery of the placenta).
- Only 29% of facility births received AMTSL.
- Most ergometrine was stored inappropriately.
- Harmful practices in third stage of labor were prevalent in more than one-third of facility births.

Resulting from this assessment, concerted efforts are being made in Ethiopia to address policy, training, logistics, and monitoring of PPH interventions, including AMTSL. Tools used in this assessment and from other countries are available at http://www.pphprevention.org/files/EthiopiaSurveyFinalReport1-16-07.pdf.

Source: Facility-Based Management and Community Perceptions and Actions for PPH: Findings of a National Survey in Ethiopia.

Active Management of the Third Stage of Labor

To understand how to prevent uterine atony, it is necessary to understand the physiologic processes that occur during the third stage of labor (the period of time from the birth of the baby to delivery of the placenta).

Immediately after the birth of the baby, the muscles of the uterus contract and the placenta separates from the uterine wall as the surface of the uterus becomes smaller. At the end of a term pregnancy, 500–800 mL of blood flow through the blood vessels at the placental site every minute.[14] As the placenta separates, these vessels break and bleeding occurs. Continuous, coordinated contractions of the uterus compress these blood vessels to control bleeding at the placental site and allow formation of a retroplacental clot. When the uterus fails to have coordinated muscular contractions, it is said to be atonic; in this case, blood vessels at the placental site are not constricted and hemorrhage occurs.

Active management differs from physiologic or expectant management. In the latter, the placenta is allowed to deliver spontaneously, by gravity, or maternal effort. Four large-scale randomized controlled trials (RCTs) compared active and expectant management of the third stage of labor.[15-18] All four studies found that AMTSL resulted in up to a 70% decrease in PPH and a decrease in the length of the third stage. A 2003 Cochrane Review found that AMTSL was associated with an approximately 60% reduction in occurrence of PPH and severe PPH, decreased need for blood transfusion, decreased postpartum anemia (Hgb < 9 g/dl), and an approximately 80% reduction in the use of therapeutic drugs.[7]

Choice of Uterotonic Drug for AMTSL

Giving a uterotonic drug within one minute of birth is the component of AMTSL that has the greatest impact on the prevention of PPH.

Oxytocin and syntometrine (oxytocin plus ergometrine) are both effective in preventing PPH.[19] However, the use of syntometrine is consistently associated with an increased incidence of side effects such as nausea, vomiting, headache, and increased blood pressure. In addition, ergometrine cannot be given to women with hypertension (a common problem during pregnancy). Oxytocin is therefore the preferred drug for use in AMTSL performed by a skilled provider.

Oxytocin and syntometrine, although effective in preventing PPH, can have disadvantages. In addition to the side effects mentioned above, these drugs must be handled and stored properly. They are unstable when exposed to tropical conditions of temperature and light, although oxytocin is more stable than ergometrine and may be stored at room temperature for up to three months without losing potency.[20] For practical purposes, room temperatures exceeding 30°C for long periods of time, or storing the oxytocin near the sterilizer are not recommended. Storing oxytocin in clay water pots used for storage of HIV test kits can be a prac-

> ### Case Study: Ensuring Rapid Uptake of AMTSL in Bangladesh
>
> In 2004, a team of health professionals attended a regional meeting in Bangkok, Preventing Postpartum Hemorrhage: From Research to Practice, organized by the Jhpiego-led Maternal and Neonatal Health (MNH) program with support of the U.S. Agency for International Development (USAID). On their return, the Bangladesh team proposed specific actions to address PPH. With support from UNICEF, a team of three obstetricians and three midwives (MNH regional experts) were organized to visit 48 district hospitals to do the following:
>
> - Advocate for AMTSL
> - Train providers on models and on clients using competency-based methods
> - Develop action plans for addressing challenges in universal use of AMTSL
>
> An evaluation of 48 sites after 6 months revealed:
>
> - 93% of all cases (1870 births) in the month prior to visit had AMTSL
> - PPH cases decreased by 2.8%, down from 7.8% the previous year
> - No PPH related deaths occurred in any of the 48 sites
>
> The team concluded that with a limited investment, fairly simple interventions, sound training, occasional phone contact, and follow-up on action plans, it was possible for AMTSL to become the norm for all births in Bangladesh.
>
> *Source:* UNICEF internal report, Dr. Farhana Dewan, personal communication.

tical approach for "cool storage" in really hot environments (FHI 2008).

Furthermore, these drugs must be injected. This requires that the provider be trained and qualified to administer the injection, and have access to the drug and a readily available supply of sterile syringes and needles, which must be handled and disposed of properly.

In 2007, WHO published its recommendations for the prevention of PPH based on a stringent systematic review of all available evidence.[21] It is recommended that AMTSL be offered by skilled attendants to all women (strong recommendation, moderate quality evidence) and the drug of choice be oxytocin.

A skilled provider can perform AMTSL in the home. However, when the necessary supplies are not available to give an injection of oxytocin (e.g., at home birth, in a primary healthcare facility without electricity), misoprostol should be considered a useful alternative, even if it is less effective than injectable uterotonic drugs.[23]

Several studies have examined the role of misoprostol in preventing PPH (see Table 22-1). The efficacy of misoprostol in preventing PPH was demonstrated most convincingly by a carefully designed trial from India,[24] where either misoprostol or a placebo was given by auxiliary nurse midwives (lower-level providers with some midwifery skills) at home births. The study measured blood loss after delivery using a calibrated device and demonstrated a highly significant reduction in PPH with the use of misoprostol.

Common side effects of misoprostol are shivering and fever, but these are usually short lived and are less serious than the side effects usually seen with oxytocin (nausea, vomiting, and diarrhea). Lumbiganon et al.[30] documented that the side effects of misoprostol are dose-dependent and determined that the optimal dose of misoprostol for postpartum use is 600 mcg.

Based on the available data, Goldberg et al.[31] concluded in their review that when oxytocin is not available, use of misoprostol to prevent PPH should be considered a category A recommendation (i.e., good and consistent evidence to support the recommendation). The U.S. Pharmacopoeia Expert Advisory Panel has also recommended that prevention of PPH be considered an "accepted" indication for use of misoprostol.[32]

Most recently, WHO[21] recommended that, in the absence of AMTSL, a uterotonic drug (oxytocin or misoprostol) should be offered by a health worker trained in its use for prevention of PPH (strong recommendation, moderate quality evidence). It is important to note that WHO's definition of trained health workers—not to be confused with skilled attendants[†]—includes village mid-

---

[†] According to WHO, skilled attendants are health professionals who have been educated and trained to proficiency in skills needed to manage normal labour and delivery, recognize the onset of complications, perform essential interventions, start treatment, and supervise the referral of mother and baby for interventions that are beyond their competence or are not possible in the particular setting. Depending on the setting, healthcare providers such as auxiliary nurse-midwives, community midwives, village midwives, and health visitors may also have acquired appropriate skills, if they have been specially trained.

wives and health visitors. The implication of the efficacy of oral misoprostol and these recommendations is that PPH prevention is possible even where there are no skilled attendants.

Preventing PPH at Home Birth

Misoprostol may also offer a solution for home-births attended by a provider not qualified to perform AMTSL. The Maternal and Neonatal Health Program (1998–2004), funded by the U.S. Agency for International Development, established the safety of home- and community-based distribution of misoprostol for prevention of PPH through a study conducted in rural Indonesia.[33] Community health volunteers (*kaders*) were trained to provide counseling about the importance of giving birth with a skilled provider, the danger signs of PPH, and the need to seek care immediately should the woman experience severe bleeding. Counseling also included information about the timing and safe use of misoprostol and its side effects. Pregnant women participating in the study received packets of misoprostol tablets and a safety reminder card in their eighth month of pregnancy with instructions to take the misoprostol immediately after the birth of the baby. The community-based approach was found to be safe and acceptable to women studied. Based on the study's results, the government of Indonesia has implemented plans to scale up community-based distribution of misoprostol as an effective strategy for reducing the risk of PPH when skilled care is not available. In situations where this approach is used, a careful monitoring and evaluation component should be included in order to demonstrate the impact on public health.

Role of the Community Health Worker (CHW)
In implementing community-based distribution of misoprostol to prevent PPH, it is important to realize that the most vital role of the CHW is to educate the woman and her support persons. The CHW is trained to do the following:

■ Identify all pregnant women in her area. Where CHWs are illiterate, use of simple household mapping is an effective strategy to locate women.

TABLE 22-1

Summary of Evidence for Using Misoprostol to Prevent PPH		
Author, year, and location of study	**Study type**	**Key findings**
Bamigboye et al., 1998 Johannesburg, South Africa[25]	Randomized trial Misoprostol 400 mcg rectally (n = 241) vs. Syntometrine 1 ampoule IM (n = 250)	No significant differences in length of third stage of labor, postpartum blood loss, or postpartum hemoglobin levels Postpartum hypertension more common in women receiving Syntometrine (systolic blood pressure, $P = .00004$; diastolic blood pressure, $P = .00007$)
Hofmeyr et al., 1998 Johannesburg, South Africa[26]	Randomized, double-blind, placebo-controlled trial Misoprostol 400 mcg orally (n = 250) vs. placebo (n = 250)	Misoprostol decreased incidence of blood loss 1000 mL or more (6% vs. 9%; RR 0.65, 95% CI 0.35–1.22) Misoprostol decreased the need for therapeutic oxytocin (2.8% vs. 8.4%; RR 0.33, 95% CI 0.14–0.77)
Gülmezoglu et al., 2001 Argentina, China, Egypt, Ireland, Nigeria, South Africa, Switzerland, Thailand, and Vietnam[27]	Randomized, double-blind, placebo-controlled, multicenter trial Misoprostol 600 mcg orally (n = 9264) vs. oxytocin 10 IU given IV or IM (n = 9266)	Oxytocin decreased incidence of severe PPH ($\geq$ 1000 mL) (3% vs. 4%; RR 1.39, 95% CI 1.19–1.63, $P < .0001$) Oxytocin decreased need for therapeutic uterotonic (11% vs. 15%; RR 1.40, 95% CI 1.29–1.51, $P < .0001$) Authors concluded that when both drugs are available, oxytocin is preferred over misoprostol.
Hoj et al., 2005 Guinea Bissau[28]	Randomized, double-blind, placebo-controlled trial Misoprostol 600 mcg sublingual (n = 330) vs. placebo (n = 331)	Misoprostol decreased mean blood loss by 10.5% Misoprostol decreased incidence of blood loss >1000 mL (RR 0.66, 95% CI 0.45–0.98) Misoprostol decreased incidence of blood loss > 1500 mL (RR 0.28, 95% CI 0.12–0.64)
Derman et al., 2006 Four primary health centers in rural India[29]	Randomized, placebo-controlled trial Misoprostol 600 mcg orally (n = 812) vs. placebo (n = 808)	Misoprostol decreased incidence of PPH ($\geq$ 500 mL) 12% vs. 6.4% (RR 0.53, 95% CI 0.39–0.74, $P < .0001$) Misoprostol decreased incidence of severe PPH ($\geq$ 1000 mL) 1.2% vs. 0.2% (RR 0.20, 95% CI 0.04–0.91, $P < .0001$) Misoprostol decreased mean blood loss (262.3 mL vs. 214.3 mL, $P < .0001$) One case of PPH was prevented for every 18 women treated

Notes: RR = relative risk; CI = confidence interval

Ensuring a Woman's Right to Survive Childbirth: Preventing Mortality from Postpartum Hemorrhage

- Educate pregnant women and support persons about PPH during home visits through pictorial messages and reinforce by providing the same information to husbands, mother-in-laws, and other support persons.

- Distribute misoprostol when the woman is eight months pregnant: it is recommended not to distribute earlier than eight months gestation to reduce the likelihood that the drug is lost or misused. Before providing the misoprostol, the CHW is taught to once again ensure that the educational message is understood.

- Conduct postpartum home visits to determine maternal and newborn outcomes and retrieve any unused misoprostol.

The most important aspect of the process is the educational message which includes: (1) warning signs of dangerous bleeding; (2) what to do if hemorrhage occurs during or after delivery; (3) where to seek emergency medical care; and (4) the role of the midwife in providing AMTSL.

In addition to the information described above, women are also educated on the purpose, correct timing, and use of misoprostol to prevent PPH, the risks of taking misoprostol prior to delivery, common side effects of misoprostol, what to do if side effects occur, and where to go if PPH occurs *even* after taking medication.

Case Study: Bringing a Life-Saving Intervention Closer to the Home in Remote Populations

Afghanistan has one of the highest maternal mortality rates in the world estimated at 1600/100,000 births.[34] PPH is responsible for about 38% of the maternal deaths or approximately 7600 women per year. In addition to rebuilding midwifery services, which is a long-term solution, Afghanistan is also expanding prevention of PPH at homebirth. Eighty-one percent of births in Afghanistan are not attended by a skilled provider,[35] and there remains a critical dearth of skilled female health workers in the rural areas. Based on the model from Indonesia, the Afghan Ministry of Public Health undertook the following steps in collaboration with the USAID-funded ACCESS Program:

1. Policy decision to adopt both AMTSL and community-based distribution of misoprostol
2. Creation of national technical advisory group to oversee the safe introduction of community-based distribution of misoprostol
3. Qualitative study to determine women's perception and understanding about PPH, leading to development of appropriate pictorial educational materials and CHW training program
4. Field implementation in selected demonstration sites to understand operational challenges and establish safety, acceptability, feasibility, and program effectiveness required to take PPH prevention to the community.

CHWs who underwent five days of training distributed misoprostol to pregnant women and provided counseling on birth preparedness, complication readiness, and the correct use of the drug. CHWs were supervised by paid health supervisors who do this as part of implementing the basic healthcare package. Results showed high coverage is possible, even in some of the most challenging and remote areas of the world; CHWs provided the correct information on which women could act; and the intervention was acceptable both to the community and healthcare providers. The Ministry of Public Health is now planning to scale up the effort.

Minimizing Potential for Drug Misuse

One major concern all stakeholders have is the possibility of misuse of misoprostol for other purposes. To minimize any misuse, the following strategies have proven successful:

In the distribution system:

- Procurement is done centrally.
- Repackaging and branding are done in a way that it is clear that pills are for postpartum use only; a safety insert provides another visual reminder.

- Main drug stock is housed at the nearest health center under direct control of the nurse in charge.

- Tracking of the drug distribution is conducted systematically—on a weekly basis if possible.

- The CHW keeps only a small number of doses, to be replenished after recruitment information is submitted to the nurse in charge.

In the target population:

- Emphasis on educating clients and support persons
- Distribution at eight months gestation
- Package with safety information
- Retrieval of unused drug

Monitoring Framework for Preventing PPH at Homebirth There are a number of critical areas to monitor in a program with community-based distribution of misoprostol. A monitoring system should observe how well the program is operating and whether the program is being implemented as intended—including whether the intervention is being delivered to the intended recipients (often in underserved and hard-to-reach populations). Key areas of a monitoring system should include the following:

- Number of pregnant women in the target area
- Number of pregnant women enrolled in the program and number of women who actually took the drug

- Coverage of the messages and acceptance by the women and their families
- Community response and acceptance to the program
- Exposure and comprehension of messages about PPH and misoprostol and the woman's source of this information
- How well the CHWs are doing their job and reaching out to clients with the correct information
- Overall knowledge and competency of both the CHWs and the supervisory staff, including midwives
- Drug supply, drug distribution patterns, and any stock outs
- Postpartum outcomes within one week after delivery
- Women's reasons for taking or not taking misoprostol, referrals, and willingness to pay for misoprostol

Data collection can be achieved through various methods, such as review of the CHW forms, observation of client and CHW interaction by a supervisor, client exit interviews, and review of stock cards.

If it is a new or pilot program, then rigorous safety monitoring should carefully address (1) reporting of any complications; (2) monitoring adverse events; (3) monitoring the CHW and client interaction to ensure that complete messages are being provided; and (4) monitoring use of misoprostol by scrutinizing stock cards and records to ensure that the misoprostol was not misused, and that all packs of the drug that were distributed are accounted for.

Case Study: Integrating a Community-Based Intervention into the Public Health System in Nepal

The Nepal project to prevent PPH at home birth demonstrates how an intervention can be implemented at scale through integration into the public-sector health system. In the Banke district of Nepal, the project was designed for full integration within existing community-based maternal and child health program activities. Using the antenatal FCHV contact with women during the eighth month of pregnancy as a platform, the provision of oral misoprostol and counseling on correct use was provided to the target population. An early postnatal FCHV home visit was also conducted to counsel and recover unused misoprostol. Over the first 18 months the project successfully reached an estimated 11,000 pregnant women in Banke, translating to 70% of all pregnant women in the district. Results have indicated that this community-level approach to reducing the incidence of PPH can achieve high impact and coverage in the population and improve care-seeking and household practices.

Source: Hodgins S, Rajbhandari S. Global Health Conference Abstract, 2007.

Conclusion

PPH accounts for more maternal deaths than any other cause, and the primary cause of PPH is uterine atony. We cannot predict who will experience PPH on the basis of risk factors. PPH can be difficult to recognize and blood loss difficult to measure.

When you have a skilled attendant:

- AMTSL is the standard of care.
- Oxytocin (injection) is the preferred uterotonic.
- Ergometrine (injection or oral) and oral oxytocin are unstable and should be phased out.
- Misoprostol may be used if oxytocin is not available.

When you do not have a skilled attendant:

- Misoprostol used alone, without the other components of AMTSL, prevents PPH.

- Woman may also benefit from uterine massage.

Once PPH occurs, death can follow very rapidly. Expanding quality basic emergency obstetric care services will reduce unmet need for PPH treatment. Women, their support persons, TBAs, and community health volunteers can be taught to recognize PPH. AMTSL by skilled providers (using misoprostol when oxytocin is not feasible) and use of misoprostol by unskilled providers or the woman herself are life-saving interventions that can positively affect maternal mortality in low-resource settings.

DISCUSSION QUESTIONS

1. What areas should be addressed within a comprehensive national policy to reduce PPH in a low-resource setting? Who are the key stakeholders that should be involved in this policy development and endorsement?

2. What are the service delivery barriers that need to be addressed to ensure AMTSL for all?

REFERENCES

1. World Health Organization (WHO). *Mother-Baby Package: Implementing Safe Motherhood in Countries.* Geneva, Switzerland: WHO; 1998.
2. Khan KS, Wojdyla D, Say L, Gülmezoglu AM, Van Look PF. WHO analysis of causes of maternal death: a systematic review. *Lancet.* 2006;367(9516):1066-1074.
3. Li XF, Fortney JA, Kotelchuck M, et al. The postpartum period: The key to maternal mortality. *Int J Gynecol Obstet.* 1996;54:1-10.
4. Murray C, Lopez A (eds.). *Health Dimensions of Sex and Reproduction.* Vol. 3, Global Burden of Disease and Injury Series. Boston, MA: Harvard University Press; 1996.
5. Akins S. Postpartum hemorrhage. A 90s approach to an age-old problem. *J Nurse Midwifery.* 1994;39:123S-134S.
6. Prendiville W, Elbourne D. Care during the third stage of labor. In: Chalmers I, Enkin M, Keirse MJNC, eds. *Effective Care in Pregnancy and Childbirth.* Vol. 1. Oxford, UK: Oxford University Press; 1998:1145-1169.

7. Prendiville WJ, Elbourne D, McDonald S. Active versus expectant management in the third stage of labour (Cochrane Review). *Cochrane Library*. Issue 3. Chichester, UK: John Wiley and Sons, Ltd; 2003.

8. Patel A. *A New Approach for Collecting and Estimating Postpartum Blood Loss in Rural India.* Proceedings from the XVII FIGO World Congress of Gynecology and Obstetrics; November 2–7, 2003; Santiago, Chile.

9. Prata N, Mbaruku G, Campbell M, Potts M, Vahidnia F. Controlling postpartum hemorrhage after home births in Tanzania. *Int J Gynec Obstet*. 2005;90:51-55.

10. Kane TT, El Kady AA, Saleh S et al. Maternal mortality in Giza, Egypt: magnitude, causes, and prevention. *Stud Fam Plann*. 1992;23:45-47.

11. Brabin BJ, Hakimi M, Pelletier D. An analysis of anemia and pregnancy-related maternal mortality. *J Nutr*. 2001;131:604-615.

12. Tsu VD. Postpartum haemorrhage in Zimbabwe: a risk factor analysis. *Br J Obstet Gynaecol*. 1993;100:327-333.

13. Global, regional and sub-regional estimates of the proportion of births attended by a skilled health worker 2008. World Health Organization (WHO) http://www.who.int/reproductive-health/global_monitoring/data_regions.html. Accessed November 14, 2008

14. World Health Organization (WHO). *Third Stage of Labour: Physiology and Management.* Geneva, Switzerland: WHO; 1996:11–46. WHO/FRH/MSM/96.2.

15. Bagley C. A comparison of "active" and "physiological" management of the third stage of labour. *Midwifery*. 1990;6:3-27.

16. John IS, Wani S, Doherty T, Sibai B. Controlled cord traction versus minimal intervention techniques in delivery of the placenta: a randomized controlled trial. *Am J Obstet Gynecol*. 1997;177:770-774.

17. Prendiville W, Elbourne D, Chalmers I. The effects of routine oxytocin administration in the management of the third stage of labour: an overview of the evidence from controlled trials. *Br J Obstet Gynaec*. 1988;95:3-16.

18. Rogers, J., Wood, J., McCandlish., R., Ayers, S., Truesdale, A., Elbourne D. Active versus expectant management of third stage of labour: the Hinchingbrooke randomized controlled trial. *Lancet*. 1998;351:693-699.

19. McDonald SJ, Prendiville WJ, Blair E. Randomized controlled trial of oxytocin alone versus oxytocin and ergometrine in active management of third stage of labour. *Br Med J*. 1993;307:1167-1171.

20. World Health Organization (WHO). *Stability of Injectable Oxytocics in Tropical Climates. Results of Field Surveys and Simulation Studies on Ergometrine, Methylergometrine and Oxytocin.* Geneva, Switzerland: WHO; 1993. WHO/DAP/93.6.

21. World Health Organization (WHO). *WHO Recommendations for the Prevention of Postpartum Haemorrhage*. Geneva: WHO; 2007:14-15.

22. Getachew A, Muleta M, Mogessie F. et al. *Facility-Based Management of the Third Stage of Labor and Community Perceptions and Actions on Postpartum Hemorrhage: Findings from a National Survey in Ethiopia.* Washington, DC: Prevention of Postpartum Hemorrhage Initiative (POPPHI); 2006.

23. Darney PD. Misoprostol: A boon to safe motherhood . . . or not? [commentary]. *Lancet*. 2001;358:682-683.

24. Derman RJ, Kodkany B, Goudar S, et al. Oral misoprostol in preventing postpartum haemorrhage in resource-poor communities: a randomized controlled trial. *Lancet*. 2006;368:1248-1253.

25. Bamigboye AA, GJ, Merrell DA. Rectal misoprostol in the prevention of postpartum hemorrhage: a placebo-controlled trial. *Am J Obstet Gynecol*. 1998;179: 1043-1046.

26. Hofmeyr GJ, Nikodem VC, de Jager M, Gelbart BR. A randomized placebo controlled trial of oral misoprostol in the third stage of labour. *Br J Obstet Gynaecol.* 1998;105:971-975.

27. Gülmezoglu AM, Villar J, Ngoc NTN, et al. WHO multicentre randomized trial of misoprostol in the management of the third stage of labour. *Lancet.* 2001;358: 689-695.

28. Hoj L, Cardoso P, Nielsen BB, Hvidman L, Nielsen J, Aaby P. Effect of sublingual misoprostol on severe postpartum haemorrhage in a primary health centre in Guinea-Bissau: randomized double blind clinical trial. *BMJ.* 2005;331:723.

29. Derman RJ, Kodkany BS, Goudar SS, et al. Oral misoprostol in preventing postpartum haemorrhage in resource-poor communities: a randomized controlled trial. *Lancet.* 2006;368:1248-1253.

30. Lumbiganon P, Hofmeyr J, Gülmezoglu AM, Pinol A, Villar J. Misoprostol dose-related shivering and pyrexia in third stage of labour. WHO collaborative trial of misoprostol in the management of the third stage of labour. *Br J Obstet Gynaecol.* 1999;106:304-308.

31. Goldberg AB, Greenberg MA, Darney PD. Misoprostol and pregnancy. *N Engl J Med* 2001;344:38-47.

32. Carpenter JP. *Misoprostol for Prevention of Postpartum Hemorrhage: An Evidenced-Based Review by the US Pharmacopeia.* Rockville, MD: United States Pharmacopeia; 2000:28.

33. Winkjosastro G et al. Preventing postpartum hemorrhage in home births: The Indonesia experience. In Pfitzer A, Sanghvi H, eds. *Preventing Postpartum Hemorrhage: From Research to Practice.* Baltimore, MD: JHPIEGO/MNH Program; 2004.

34. Bartlett L, Mawji S, Whitehead S, Crouse C, Dalil S, Ionete D, Salama P, and the Afghanistan Maternal Mortality Study Team. Where giving birth is a forecast of death: maternal mortality in four districts of Afghanistan, 1999-2002. *Lancet.* 2005;365:864-870.

35. MOPH, 2006. Afghanistan Household Survey. Estimates of Priority Health Indicators for Rural Afghanistan. The Johns Hopkins University Bloomberg School of Public Health and the Indian Institute of Health Management Research. Unpublished.

The existence of involuntary childlessness in many developing countries has been known for decades. Colonial powers first noted low birth rates in certain regions of Central Africa in the beginning of the last century, being highly alarmed about a shrinking population base for labor and Christianity.[1] Several reasons for this phenomenon, such as new diseases being brought in by Europeans, labor migration and subsequent disintegration of family units, as well as the Arab slave trade, have all been suggested by early research.[2,3] The French physician and anthropologist Anne Retel-Laurentin published accounts in the early 1970s about the medical and social dimensions of the problem and urged it be addressed as part of a truly comprehensive population policy.[4,5] Between 1979 and 1984, the WHO instituted a task force to investigate the scope of infertility in developing countries and ran a multinational study surveying patients affected by involuntary childlessness in selected African hospitals.[6] During the 1990s, more analyses using population-based survey data showed that infertility patterns in Africa are distinctive. The "central African infertility belt," as it was called in the 1960s,[7] actually expanded into southern and western Africa.[8] Inhorn coined the term "fertility–infertility dialectic"[9] to describe the simultaneously high fertility and infertility rates in many developing countries, which occurred as a result of a cultural emphasis on procreation and the reality of widespread reproductive tract infections (RTIs).[10]

But apart from a few lone voices, mainly of anthropologists, the situation of infertile couples in developing countries was mostly ignored by both the medical and the social sciences for a long time. Policy makers in the population field were even less interested and used two main arguments, as crushing as they are cynical, against efforts to make infertility a significant topic on the global health agenda: (1) developing a medical infrastructure to diagnose and treat a nonfatal problem would be a waste of precious health resources, and (2) if anything, these regions should rather be concerned about "hyperfertility" and "overpopulation," not infertility.

CHAPTER 23

Infertility in Developing Countries: Scope, Psychosocial Burden, and the Need for Action

Anke Hemmerling, MD, MPH

Anke Hemmerling, MD, MPH, is affiliated with the the Department of Obstetrics, Gynecology, and Reproductive Sciences, for the University of California, San Francisco.

Ironically, it may be the HIV epidemic that is finally forcing policy makers to acknowledge infertility as a significant international health problem. Women feel pressured to start childbearing at a very early age, and the unfulfilled desire for a child leads many women and men to engage in unsafe and high-risk sexual practices.[9]

In the future, the new movement to reframe the neglect of women's health as a human rights issue should make it harder to maintain the course of silently overlooking involuntary childlessness in developing countries. In 1994, the UN International Conference on Population and Development (ICPD) in Cairo saw strong criticism of the top-down prioritization on family planning agendas that ignored other urgent issues in women's health. The discussions in Cairo resulted in a clear shift toward a more comprehensive approach to reproductive health.[9] As a first step, language requiring the "prevention and appropriate treatment of infertility where feasible" became part of the Cairo ICPD Programme of Action. Despite this, policies and infrastructure to fight infertility in developing countries are still extremely limited.

The Scope of Infertility in Developing Countries

There are several differing definitions and measurement methods for a couple's infertility. Although both partners may be the cause of childlessness, it is usually the woman's unsuccessful reproductive history that is used as the measurement stick.

Infertility is defined as a condition applying to women who fail to conceive after unprotected regular intercourse over a period of 1 or 2 years.[11,12] This definition may also be extended to women who fail to carry a pregnancy to term or those who fail to give birth to a living infant. *Primary infertility* describes women who have never conceived, while the term *secondary infertility* refers to women who remain without a live birth after having successfully conceived at least once.

Measuring infertility can be challenging. Small studies involving personal interviews with partici-

pants can better explore the details of reproductive history and more accurately access the duration and circumstances of involuntary childlessness. They can also exclude childless women currently using contraception or temporary abstinence and gain insight into possible male factors of infertility. Demographers often use larger population-based surveys, deriving their data on infertility from large preexisting datasets such as the Demographic and Health Surveys (DHS) or a national census. They usually count the number of women of fertile age who are in a marital union (assuming regular sexual intercourse), not using contraception, and remaining without a live birth for a defined timeframe of up to 7 years.[13,14] As can be imagined, the challenges of these methodological approaches are many and are described in detail elsewhere.[13,15]

Worldwide, about 8–12% of all couples, or 50 million to 80 million women, experience involuntary childlessness.[12,16,17] Infertility rates vary greatly among developing countries. Larsen and Raggers assessed the extent of primary infertility in sub-Saharan Africa with 3 million to 4 million women and of secondary infertility with more than 13 million women.[18] Other calculations for all developing countries combined (excluding China) concluded that as many as 186 million women aged 15–49 remain childless.[19]

The aforementioned WHO study showed that as many as 85% of infertility cases were caused by RTIs, a proportion twice as high as seen in Western countries.[6] Later studies by Larsen[7] and Erickson and Brunette[20] estimated that infertility in selected African countries affected about 19–26% of all women. National statistics often disguise remarkable regional fluctuations within countries.[20] In some regions as many as 30% of all couples experienced involuntary childlessness; mostly as secondary infertility after a previous pregnancy.[6,14,19]

Secondary infertility is mostly caused by RTIs, which are either sexually transmitted, as with chlamydiasis or gonorrhea, or acquired during septic delivery, unsafe abortion, or harmful traditional practices.[21] These infections often lead to pelvic inflammatory disease (PID) and damage to the ovarian tubes. Genital tuberculosis, schistosomiasis, filariasis, malaria, and micronutrient deficiencies as well as outdated treatment attempts such as dilatation and curettage[22] or cervical electrocauterization[23] also play a role.

Almost half of all infertility in developing countries is solely or partly due to male factors such as untreated varicocele and abnormal sperm counts caused by exposure to environmental toxins such as pesticides, arsenic, lead, or aflatoxins.[6,21,24,25]

Several authors have estimated that the burden on health systems of visits by desperate, childless couples is significant, accounting for 10–30% of all consultations.[10,22,26,27]

Data collected in interviews and focus groups conducted in various developing countries shows that more than 50% of couples affected by infertility reported seeking treatment. While some use the formal health sector,[22] many go to traditional healers first and foremost.[17,28,29]

Studies show that the widespread introduction of antibiotics for STI treatment, combined with a delayed age of sexual debut and behavior change, have facilitated a substantial decrease in infertility rates in some African regions since the 1950s.[3,14,30,31] But this development is not uniform throughout the continent. Some countries such as Mali or Cote d' Ivoire have seen no change in their infertility rates, while others, such as Ghana, Kenya, and Zimbabwe, have even experienced an increase.[18]

The Psychosocial Burden of Infertility in Developing Countries

Infertility research by social scientists emphasizes the distinction between infertility as a reproductive impairment and as a social and cultural construction. The cultural context and social conditions in which infertility occurs is of the utmost importance for how it is perceived and shapes the options for coping with this challenging life event.[9,32,33]

While in Western societies today the desire for a child is predominantly rooted in the attempt to gain personal happiness and fulfillment, additional needs and motives prevail in developing countries.

Children can provide economic security in old age. They increase the social status within society and often form the power base from which women negotiate and justify their existence. Fertility demonstrates the potency of the tribe,[34] and

children secure the continuation of the blood lineage. In many places, only a male offspring can continue the blood lineage and practice ancestor worship.[35,36] The worth of a new bride is primarily defined by her fertility, and the raising of children helps form a bond with the husband and the in-law family. Often, it is only the presence of children that can secure inheritance rights for a widow.

Modern Western concepts of fertility and sterility are often unknown or poorly understood in developing countries. In corners of the world as diverse as Cameroon,[34] Nigeria,[32] the Gambia,[22] Ghana,[37] Egypt,[10] Tanzania,[38] Malawi,[28] South Africa,[39] Mozambique,[40] Bangladesh,[36] India,[41] Vietnam,[42] and Pakistan[43], "barren" women face varying degrees of stigmatization. Many cultures believe foremost in supernatural causes for childlessness.[44] Infertile women are thought to be possessed by evil spirits that prevent the child's soul from implanting and growing in the womb.[32,36] Women in the grass fields of Cameroon lock their latrines at all times to prevent the evil spirits from entering their bodies.[34] Infertile women are sometimes believed to be witches who have their children in another world.[45] Infertility is often seen as God's punishment for "deviant" sexual behavior or disrespect toward ancestors. In Tanzania many people believe that the balance of health and fertility can be disturbed by the *mchango*, a force of physical and spiritual origin that inhabits a woman's body.[46,47] The more physiological models to explain infertility include weak "worms" (sperm), an "unclean" womb, a uterus bent backward after early teenage sex, or the failure of the couples' blood to "mix well."[36,46–49] In many places, the previous use of modern contraception is feared to lead to permanent infertility.[32,36,46,50–53] In short, biomedical explanations and traditional beliefs merge into what Kielmann has called the "the simultaneous logic of greedy spirits and faulty organs."[54] (p153)

Male infertility accounts for half of all cases in developing countries but is rarely acknowledged. It can be more easily hidden, while a woman's failure to become pregnant is very visible and so she is usually blamed for it. Greil wrote in 1997:

> The fact that gender roles are more important in conditioning the experience of infertility than the question of which partner

has the reproductive impairment is significant because it shows that what is essentially a social variable carries more weight than a medical factor.[33(p1694)]

In many cultures, if male infertility is suspected, clandestine arrangements are made within the blood family to impregnate the wife.[47,48,55] Although there is little research regarding male perspectives on infertility,[56] many women report that their partners refused to be tested because they fear public emasculation and the loss of social status.

Social repercussions of childlessness can be severe,[57, 58] as parenthood is mandated in many societies and the ideology of motherhood is internalized by women. Infertility in developing countries is therefore much more than a private misfortune: it poses a serious threat to gender identity and can be, in many cases, a life-threatening disaster.[22] As in the West, infertile women experience feelings of emptiness and guilt, grief and loss, anxiety and depression, and isolation and shame. But additionally, women are often publicly humiliated and ostracized by their families and communities. Some are even assaulted or pushed to suicide. They have no child to mourn for them after death and proper burial rights may be denied to childless women as it is believed that their remains may poison the fertility of the community land.[32] Graves may be marked to warn ancestors against reincarnation for the "unproductive." Childless women are barred from community functions as their presence is feared to endanger children[36,41] and negatively affect the fertility of other women.[40] They might even be held responsible for epidemics and droughts.[36] Women who suspect infertility in their partners may try to become pregnant with other men, and childless men may seek to assure their fertility elsewhere, dramatically increasing all partners' risk for STIs.[29,46,47,55] Domestic violence is common in such situations, and husbands may abandon their childless wives or take additional partners. The bride wealth has to be repaid in case of divorce,[47] and existing children stay with the father's family. Abandoned women often cannot return to their parents' homes because they have brought shame on their families. Out of desperation, some women experience hysterical pregnancies or they fake pregnancies to gain support and compassion from their communities for a pregnancy loss, in-stead of experiencing ostracism to punish them for their "barrenness."[34,36]

Strategies for Solutions

If involuntary childlessness continues to be solely viewed as a physical impairment only treatable using expensive and sophisticated medical technology and with moderate success, the options for improvement will arguably remain limited in many regions of the world for decades to come. If infertility is perceived as a marginal topic on a policy agenda that is aimed at limiting overall population growth, the need for action will remain unclear to many.

However, if infertility is approached as a preventable public health problem and human rights issue, the picture is brighter and strategies to fight infertility and its psychosocial consequences are many. Fourteen years after Cairo, it is time to challenge the continued skepticism of policy makers regarding the feasibility of fighting involuntary childlessness in developing countries. The strategies presented in the following sections should be pursued concurrently.

Prevention of Reproductive Tract Infections (RTIs)

The prevention of RTIs is undoubtedly the most promising, feasible, and cost-effective strategy to curb future infertility. Antibiotic treatment needs to be expanded beyond clinical symptomatic cases in order to catch the numerous incidences of asymptomatic chlamydia and gonorrhea infections that can damage fallopian tubes. Brady advocates using the emotionality of the topic and the visibility of childlessness to make a "triple protection" strategy attractive to women as a "safeguard of fertility." This three-pronged strategy includes: (1) condom use to prevent STIs, (2) safe deliveries to avoid postpartum infections, and (3) the use of family planning to decrease the number of septic abortions.[50] Promoting safe motherhood, legalizing abortions, and discouraging harmful practices would also significantly contribute to reducing the number of RTIs.[21]

Infertility Treatment

New reproductive technologies are still rarely available or are prohibitively expensive in many developing countries, and they are virtually nonexistent in sub-Saharan Africa.[59,60] Elite members of these societies travel to Egypt, the Gulf States, or South Africa, where infrastructures for infertility treatment have emerged in some cities during the last decade.[26,55] Most new reproductive technologies have been developed for a profit-oriented market in Western countries and are not easily transferable into settings with different needs and resources. However, cheap and efficient technologies such as the use of "old-fashioned" clomiphene for ovarian stimulation could be revived, and other less expensive technologies could be adapted.[48,55] Formal health sectors need to provide a minimum package of diagnostic services and treatment for infertility.[22] A tiered system could be implemented: simple local screening methods such as gynecological history taking, STI testing, explanation of menstrual cycles and fertile days and then, if needed, referral to better-equipped facilities for hormone and semen analysis and more advanced treatment options.[21,48,61] Today, childless couples in non-Western countries often turn first to traditional healers, religious leaders, or herbalists; they visit holy places or practice fertility rituals. The formal health sector is seen as a last resort because most people are either uninformed about medical causes of infertility, have low expectations, or have had unfavorable experiences with the health system.[41,62] We find the same dynamic with infertility as with voluntary counseling for HIV: if no treatment options are available, people will be much less inclined to seek diagnosis. To be culturally acceptable, any medical solution aiming to have an impact must seek to unite both medical and spiritual approaches to infertility treatment. Many traditional healers are aware of the importance of fertility treatment in their clients' lives. They are often already providing modern STI treatments and are sometimes eager to become a partner in the health network.[63,64]

Adoption

While socially acceptable in the West, adoption as a solution for involuntary childlessness is problematic in many developing countries. Adopting children from outside the family gene pool is often thought to weaken the bloodline.[10,42] Prospective parents fear that adopted children might not be accepted by the community, could be taken away later, or might refuse to provide financial security for their adopted, aging parents.[47] However, as the HIV epidemic continues to orphan millions of children, more advocacy for making adoption socially acceptable is of great importance, and childless couples may benefit from this change of cultural norms.

Education and Counseling

Education about infertility causes and prevention needs to be improved and intensified. Studies show that a better informed clientele receives more support within the family network and is more proactive in seeking treatment and practicing prevention.[36,41,43] Infertility, although mostly perceived as an issue affecting women, in reality involves both partners, and this fact needs to be accepted as such. Advocacy and educational efforts should seek to make the male's role in both fertility and infertility more visible. And, to do men justice, we need to take a closer look at men's roles beyond the unexamined assumption of hegemonic masculinity.[56,65] Counseling couples about their options to prevent, diagnose, and treat infertility as well as, in many cases, learning to cope with unresolved childlessness, needs to become a cornerstone of reproductive health education.

Only by moving people away from blaming the victim[66] and from viewing infertility as a supernatural curse can involuntary childlessness become socially acceptable. Such changes may seem to be a rather tall order, but cultural beliefs and explanations of sterility in some African countries today[44] are not dissimilar to the Freudian psychogenic theories[33,66,67] that dominated much of the 1900s. These theories posited infertility as rooted entirely in psychological problems and unconscious anxieties over motherhood—the "evil spirits" of Western civilization. Knowledge has the power to change our perceptions of the world—we should trust the potential of this universal paradigm.

Destigmatization and Empowerment

To address the psychosocial burden experienced by affected couples in developing countries, the importance of efforts to alleviate the social stigma of infertility cannot be overemphasized. The infertility debate was reframed as a human rights issue in Cairo, and it needs to be addressed as such in society at large. Cultural and social changes to decrease the pressures to procreate will not only help to improve the situation for childless women but also help women trying to space and limit their natural fertility by using family planning methods. Religious beliefs of any faith are an important source of hope. New church movements can help to strengthen women's roles in the community, as such movements often condemn polygyny, refuse ideology of lineage obligation, and socially reconstruct infertile bodies as valuable people.[32,39] An expansion of women's roles beyond motherhood is needed to give women the possibility to redefine their purpose and gain status and security even if they are unable to bear children. Formal education, economic empowerment, and the local enforcement of often already existing constitutional rights to land, inheritance, and child custody will all contribute to enabling women to claim their place in society.

Why Family Planning Policy Makers Should Pay Attention to Infertility

Little progress has been made fighting infertility in developing countries; the options for fertile women have not truly improved either.

The recent 2007 World Bank discussion paper "Population Issues in the 21st century"[68] details that in 35 surveyed countries, 31 of which are in Africa, no broad-based fertility decline has yet been achieved. Despite all efforts, in most of Africa total fertility rates remain high and contraceptive prevalence remains low, especially among the poorest quintile of the population. One valid reason is the lack of funds for population assistance, which fall short of required amounts as a great amount of resources has shifted during the last decade from family planning to HIV prevention and treatment.[69]

But lack of access to family planning services is not the only reason for the delayed African demographic transition. The demand for children remains high; in many places the prevailing cultural norms leave little room for voluntary subfertility

and virtually no room for voluntary or involuntary childlessness. Women need to prove their fertility in order to become accepted members of their husbands' families and within their communities, either immediately after marriage or already during the process of forming a marital union.[70] Consequently, many women will forgo contraception when it is available and strive to reach their desired family size as soon as they enter their reproductive years. Moreover, the literature shows that there is a deep and widespread fear that modern contraception could permanently forfeit the ability to bear children.[15,32,36,46,50-53,71-75]

Many of the researchers who have investigated infertility, such as Bergstrom,[76] Boerma and Mgalla,[15] Brady,[50] Larsen,[13] Retel-Laurentin,[4] Richards,[71] Sundby,[22] or Geelhoed,[37] have for years urged various stakeholders to rethink the position of infertility in global health policies and intervention research: "It is argued that childlessness represents a neglected aspect of family planning and that narrow-minded and goal-oriented population control is likely to be unsuccessful if it does not take into account all determinants of human reproductive failure."[76(p179)]

If family planning programs continue to downplay the role of cultural pressures on childbearing, ignoring the harsh implications of infertility for women's lives and choosing not to promote the fight against infertility as part of a broader family planning strategy addressing *all* of women's fertility needs, we will continue to see very little progress in many places. "(T)he young, less educated women especially are unlikely to use contraception as long as they feel susceptible to infertility, since their economic, social, and psychological status hinge on their ability to have children."[71(p91)]

Women's fears of remaining childless need to be taken seriously. Women need to be educated about their options and the relationships between infertility and early sexual debut, early childbirth, unprotected sex with multiple partners, unclean delivery, and unsafe abortion. Only then will a majority of women feel safe to postpone and space childbearing using modern contraception. Offering infertility diagnostic services and treatment, even if limited in scope, in addition to counseling and education, will build trust that reproductive health programs are designed to meet women's individual needs and will improve the acceptability of these services.[22]

Why Human Rights Advocates Should Pay Attention to Infertility

As health policy makers continue to focus on achieving the health-related Millennium Development Goals (MDG), attention to infertility may again fall short. At first glance, the goals of reducing child mortality (MDG 4) or improving maternal health and reducing maternal mortality (MDG 5) may not seem to include women whose most pressing problem is *not* to be mothers, and who do not directly contribute to the burden of maternal or child mortality nor to population growth. MDG 6, the third health-related goal, aims to combat major diseases and includes the prevention of sexually transmitted diseases, which in turn will curb infertility rates. Although MDG 3 strives to promote gender equality and to empower women, it focuses primarily on gender disparities in formal education systems. One could argue that the MDGs, which originally did not explicitly address reproductive or sexual health,[77] may not be the best available road map for addressing the totality of women's health.[78]

A human rights approach may indeed be more effective for addressing women's rights to comprehensive reproductive health care. Over the last 60 years, most countries have ratified major human rights treaties such as the Universal Declaration (UDHR), the Civil and Political Rights Covenant (ICCPR), the Economic, Social, and Cultural Rights Covenant (ICESCR), and the Convention on the Elimination of all Forms of Discrimination against Women (CEDAW). Additionally, declarations have been signed at various international conferences such as the Beijing Platform of Action at the Fourth World Conference on Women in 1995, as well as the ICPD in Cairo. The documents listed in Table 23-1 state a series of rights that address reproductive health and women's rights.[79]

Many of these human rights principles established by international treaties are now anchored in constitutions and the national body of law of many countries, and they could cover much ground for reproductive rights. The human rights framework supports a mandate for including infertility prevention, treatment, and destigmatization into national and global health policies.

TABLE 23-1

Rights Covered in International Documents	
Right	**Included in document**
The right to life, liberty, and security	UDHR, ICCPR, ICPD Cairo Programme of Action, Beijing Platform for Action
The right to health, reproductive health, and family planning	ICESCR, CEDAW, ICPD Cairo Programme of Action, Beijing Platform for Action
The right to decide the number and spacing of children	CEDAW, ICPD Cairo Programme of Action, Beijing Platform for Action
The right to consent to marriage and to equality in marriage	UDHR, ICESCR, CEDAW, ICPD Cairo Programme of Action, Beijing Platform for Action
The right to be free from discrimination on specific grounds	UDHR, ICCPR, ICESCR, CEDAW, ICPD Cairo Programme of Action, Beijing Platform for Action
The right to be free from practices that harm women and girls	CEDAW, ICPD Cairo Programme of Action, Beijing Platform for Action
The right not to be subjected to torture or other cruel, inhuman, or degrading treatment or punishment	UDHR, ICCPR, ICPD Cairo Programme of Action
The right to be free from sexual violence	CEDAW, ICPD Cairo Programme of Action
The right to enjoy scientific progress and to consent to experimentation	ICCPR, ICESCR, Beijing Platform for Action

At the ICPD in Cairo, infertility was reframed as a human rights issue and the "prevention and appropriate treatment of infertility where feasible" was explicitly included into the ICPD Programme of Action. Human rights advocates can help by reminding health policy makers that the major human rights treaties, as well as the goals set in Cairo and Beijing, commit us to helping all women achieve their chosen reproductive goals.

Conclusion

Infertility in developing countries is a serious and widespread problem with enormous psychosocial implications for affected couples. In the light of limited medical infrastructure to successfully treat involuntary childlessness once it has manifested itself, concerted efforts must be made to prevent reproductive tract infections that lead to infertility. We need to educate couples and demystify infertility in order to reduce stigma, and help women to expand their roles and status beyond motherhood. Women without a reproductive history must be enabled to pursue a productive future as respected members of their communities. The acceptability of family planning programs could benefit from the inclusion of infertility education and prevention into their service packages. From a human rights perspective, a continued silence on the topic is unacceptable.

DISCUSSION QUESTIONS

1. How can the knowledge about causes and prevention of infertility be disseminated effectively to reach the communities in developing countries?
2. How should the different levels of diagnosis and treatment for infertility be integrated into the existing health infrastructure, especially into family planning programs?
3. How can policy makers and human rights advocates help to foster a discussion within civil society in developing countries about women's social roles beyond motherhood?

REFERENCES

1. Leonard L. Problematizing fertility: "scientific" accounts and Chadian women's narratives. In: Inhorn M, van Balen F, eds. *Infertility Around the Globe*. Berkeley, CA: University of California Press; 2001:193-214.
2. Hunt N. STDs, suffering, and their derivatives in Congo-Zaire: notes towards an historical ethnography of disease. In: Becker C, ed. *Vivre et penser le sida en Afrique/ Experiencing and Understanding AIDS in Africa*. Paris, France: Codesria, IRD, Karthala; 1999:111-131.
3. Romaniuk A. Infertility in tropical Africa. In: Caldwell J, Okonjo C, eds. The population of Tropical Africa. Proceedings of the First African Population Conference sponsored by the University of Ibadan in cooperation with the Population Coun-

cil; January 3-6, 1966; University of Ibadan, Nigeria. London, UK: Longmans; 1968.

4. Retel-Laurentin A. Subfertility in black Africa—the case of the Nzakara in central African republic. In: Adadevoh B, ed. *Subfertility and Infertility in Africa*. Ibadan, Nigeria: Caxton Press; 1974:69-80.

5. Retellaurentin A, Benoit D. Infant-Mortality and Birth Intervals. *Popul Stud-J Demogr.* 1976;30(2):279-293.

6. Cates W, Farley T, Rowe P. Worldwide patterns of infertility: is Africa different? *Lancet.* 1985;2(8455):596-598.

7. Larsen U. Infertility in central Africa. *Trop Med Int Health.* 2003;8(4):354-367.

8. Larsen U. Sterility in sub-Saharan Africa. *Popul Stud* 1994;48:459-474.

9. Inhorn M, van Balen F. Introduction. Interpreting infertility: a view from the social sciences. In: Inhorn M, van Balen F, eds. *Infertility Around the Globe.* Berkeley, CA: University of California Press; 2002:3-32.

10. Inhorn M. Global infertility and the globalization of new reproductive technologies: illustrations from Egypt. *Soc Sci Med.* 2003;56(9):1837-1851.

11. Sciarra J. Infertility: an international health problem. *Int J Gynaecol Obstet.* 1994; 46(2):155-163.

12. Rowe P, Comhaire F, Hargreave T, et al. *WHO Manual for the Standard Investigation and Diagnosis of the Infertile Couple.* Cambridge, UK: Cambridge University Press; 1993.

13. Larsen U. Infertility in sub-Saharan Africa. In: *Reproductive Health in the Developed and Developing Countries: From Knowledge to Action* [Quetelet seminar]. Nov 17-20, 2004; Institute of Demography, University of Louvain at Louvain-Ia-Neuve. http://www.demo.ucl.ac.be/cq04/textes/Larsen.pdf. Accessed November 10, 2008 .

14. Larsen U. Primary and secondary infertility in sub-Saharan Africa. *Int J Epidemiol.* 2000;29(2):285-291.

15. Boerma J, Mgalla Z. Women and infertility in sub-Saharan Africa. *Reprod Health Matters.* 1999;7(13):183-188.

16. Fathalla MF. Reproductive health: a global overview. *Early Hum Dev.* 1992;29 (1-3):35-42.

17. Boivin J, Bunting L, Collins JA, et al. International estimates of infertility prevalence and treatment-seeking: potential need and demand for infertility medical care. *Hum Reprod.* 2007;22(6):1506-1512.

18. Larsen U, Raggers H. Levels and trends in infertility in sub-Saharan Africa. In: Boerma J, Mgalla Z, eds. *Women and Infertility in Sub-Saharan Africa: A Multi-Disciplinary Perspective.* Amsterdam, Netherlands: KIT Publishers; 2001:25-70.

19. Rutstein S, Shah I. *Infecundity, Infertility, and Childlessness in Developing Countries.* Calverton, MD. WHO, ORC Macro; 2004.

20. Ericksen K, Brunette T. Patterns and predictors of infertility among African women: a cross-national survey of twenty-seven nations. *Soc Sci Med.* 1996; 42(2):209-220.

21. Mayaud P. The role of reproductive tract infections. In: Boerma J, Mgalla Z, eds. *Women and Infertility in Sub-Saharan Africa: A Multi-Disciplinary Perspective.* Amsterdam, Netherlands: KIT Publishers; 2001:71-108.

22. Sundby J, Mboge R, Sonko S. Infertility in the Gambia: frequency and health care seeking. *Soc Sci Med.* 1998;46(7):891-899.

23. Inhorn M, Buss K. Ethnography, epidemiology and infertility in Egypt. *Soc Sci Med.* 1994;39(5):671-686.

24. Evers JL. Female subfertility. *Lancet.* 2002;360(9327):151-159.

25. Leke RJ, Oduma JA, Bassol-Mayagoitia S, et al. Regional and geographical variations in infertility: effects of environmental, cultural, and socioeconomic factors. *Environ Health Perspect.* 1993;101(Suppl 2):73-80.

26. Aboulghar M. The importance of fertility treatment in the developing world. *BJOG.* 2005;112(9):1174-1176.

27. Thomas C. Infertility—a challenge to South African health services. *Sex Reprod Health Bull.* 1995;1:7-8.

28. Barden-O'Fallon J. Associates of self-reported fertility status and infertility treatment-seeking in a rural district of Malawi. *Hum Reprod.* 2005;20(8):2229-2236.

29. Favot I, Ngalula J, Mgalla Z, et al. HIV infection and sexual behaviour among women with infertility in Tanzania: a hospital-based study. *Int J Epidemiol.* 1997;26(2):414-419.

30. WHO. *Infertility: A Tabulation of Available Data on Prevalence of Primary and Secondary Infertility.* Geneva, Switzerland: Programme on Maternal and Child Health and Family Planning, Division of Family Health; 1991.

31. White R, Zaba B, Boerma T, et al. Modelling the dramatic decline of primary infertility in sub-Saharan Africa. In: Boerma J, Mgalla Z, eds. *Women and Infertility in Sub-Saharan Africa: A Multi-Disciplinary Perspective.* Amsterdam, Netherlands: KIT Publishers; 2001:117-150.

32. Pearce TO. She will not be listened to in public: perceptions among the Yoruba of infertility and childlessness in women. *Reprod Health Matters.* 1999;7(13): 69-79.

33. Greil AL. Infertility and psychological distress: a critical review of the literature. *Soc Sci Med.* 1997;45(11):1679-1704.

34. Feldman-Savelsberg P. Plundered kitchens and empty wombs: fear of infertility in the Cameroonian grassfields. *Soc Sci Med.* 1994;39(4):463-474.

35. Pashigian M. Conceiving the happy family: infertility and marital politics in northern Vietnam. In: Inhorn M, van Balen F, eds. *Infertility Around the Globe.* Berkeley, CA: University of California Press; 2001:134-151.

36. Papreen N, Sharma A, Sabin K, et al. Living with infertility: experiences among Urban slum populations in Bangladesh. *Reprod Health Matters.* 2000;8(15):33-44.

37. Geelhoed DW, Nayembil D, Asare K, et al. Infertility in rural Ghana. *Int J Gynaecol Obstet.* 2002;79(2):137-142.

38. Larsen U, Masenga G, Mlay J. Infertility in northern Tanzania. *Int J Gynaecol Obstet.* 2005;90(1):80-81.

39. Dyer S, Abrahams N, Hoffman M, et al. Men leave me as I cannot have children. *Hum Reprod.* 2002;17(6):1663-1668.

40. Gerrits T. Social and cultural aspects of infertility in Mozambique. *Patient Educ Couns.* 1997;31(1):39-48.

41. Unisa S. Childlessness in Andhra Pradesh, India: treatment-seeking and consequences. *Reprod Health Matters.* 1999;7(13):54-64.

42. Wiersema N, Drukker A, Dung M, et al. Consequences of infertility in developing countries. *J Transl Med.* 2006;4:54.

43. Bhatti L, Fikree F, Khan A. The quest of infertile women in squatter settlements of Karachi, Pakistan: a qualitative study. *Soc Sci Med.* 1999;49(5):637-649.

44. Erny P. [Sterility and fertility rites in the African tradition]. *Afr Doc.* 1969(101): 47-61.

45. Orji E, Kuti O, Fasubaa O. Impact of infertility on marital life in Nigeria. *Int J Gynaecol Obstet.* 2002;79(1):61-62.

46. Roth Allen D. Mchango, menses and the quality of eggs: women's perceptions of fertility risks. In: Boerma J, Mgalla Z, editors. *Women and Infertility in Sub-Saharan*

Africa: A Multi-Disciplinary Perspective. Amsterdam, Netherlands: KIT Publishers; 2001;223-240.

47. Gijsels M, Mgalla Z, Wambura L. 'No child to send': context and consequences of female infertility in northwest Tanzania. In: Boerma J, Mgalla Z, eds. *Women and Infertility in Sub-Saharan Africa: A Multi-Disciplinary Perspective.* Amsterdam, Netherlands: KIT Publishers; 2001;202-222.

48. Sundby J, Jacobus A. Health and traditional care for infertility in the Gambia and Zimbabwe. In: Boerma J, Mgalla Z, eds. *Women and Infertility in Sub-Saharan Africa: A Multi-Disciplinary Perspective.* Amsterdam, Netherlands: KIT Publishers; 2001:247-259.

49. Boerma J, Mgalla Z. The discourse of infertility in Tanzania. In: Boerma J, Mgalla Z, eds. *Women and Infertility in Sub-Saharan Africa: A Multi-Disciplinary Perspective.* Amsterdam, Netherlands: KIT Publishers; 2001:189-202.

50. Brady M. Preventing sexually transmitted infections and unintended pregnancy, and safeguarding fertility. *Reprod Health Matters.* 2003;11(22):134-141.

51. Bogue D. Normative and psychic costs of contraception. In: Bulatao R, Lee R, eds. *Determinants of Fertility in Developing Countries.* New York, NY: Academic Press; 1983:151-192.

52. Caldwell J, Caldwell P. The cultural context of high fertility in sub-Saharan Africa. *Popul Devel Rev.* 1987;13:409-437.

53. Rutenberg N, Watkins SC. The buzz outside the clinics: conversations and contraception in Nyanza Province, Kenya. *Stud Fam Plann.* 1997;28(4):290-307.

54. Kielmann K. Barren ground: contesting identities of infertile women in Pemba, Tanzania. In: Lock M, Kaufert P, eds. *Pragmatic Women and Body Politics.* New York, NY: Cambridge University Press; 1997.

55. Pilcher H. IVF in Africa: fertility on a shoestring. *Nature.* 2006;442(7106):975-977.

56. Dyer S, Abrahams N, Mokoena N, et al. You are a man because you have children. *Hum Reprod.* 2004;19(4):960-967.

57. Donkor ES, Sandall J. The impact of perceived stigma and mediating social factors on infertility-related stress among women seeking infertility treatment in Southern Ghana. *Soc Sci Med.* 2007;65(8):1683-1694.

58. Dyer SJ. The value of children in African countries: insights from studies on infertility. *J Psychosom Obstet Gynaecol.* 2007;28(2):69-77.

59. Adamson GD, de Mouzon J, Lancaster P, et al. World collaborative report on in vitro fertilization, 2000. *Fertil Steril.* 2006;85(6):1586-1622.

60. Nachtigall RD. International disparities in access to infertility services. *Fertil Steril.* 2006;85(4):871-875.

61. Rowe P. Clinical aspects of infertility and the role of health services. *Reprod Health Matters.* 1999;7(13):103-111.

62. Sundby J. Infertility in the Gambia: traditional and modern health care. *Patient Educ Couns.* 1997;31(1):29-37.

63. Green EC, Makhubu L. Traditional healers in Swaziland: toward improved cooperation between the traditional and modern health sectors. *Soc Sci Med.* 1984;18(12):1071-1079.

64. Green EC. Sexually transmitted disease, ethnomedicine and health policy in Africa. *Soc Sci Med.* 1992;35(2):121-130.

65. Thompson C. Fertile grounds: feminists theorize infertility. In: Inhorn M, van Balen F, eds. *Infertility Around the Globe.* Berkeley, CA: University of California Press; 2002:52-78.

66. van Balen F. The psychologization of infertility. In: Inhorn M, van Balen F, eds. *Infertility Around the Globe.* Berkeley, CA: University of California Press; 2002:79-98.

67. Wischmann TH. Psychogenic infertility—myths and facts. *J Assist Reprod Genet.* 2003;20(12):485-494.
68. Lakshminarayanan R, May J, Bos E, et al. *Population Issues in the 21st Century.* Washington ,DC: World Bank; 2007.
69. Speidel JJ, Grossman RA. Family planning and access to safe and legal abortion are vital to safeguard the environment. *Contraception.* 2007;76(6):415-417.
70. Hattori MK, Larsen U. Motherhood status and union formation in Moshi, Tanzania 2002-2003. *Popul Stud (Camb).* 2007;61(2):185-199.
71. Richards SC. "Spoiling the womb": definitions, aetiologies and responses to infertility in north west province, Cameroon. *Afr J Reprod Health.* 2002;6(1):84-94.
72. Adinma JI, Okeke AO. The pill: perceptions and usage among Nigerian students. *Adv Contracept.* 1993;9(4):341-349.
73. Fakeye O, Babaniyi O. Reasons for non-use of family planning methods at Ilorin, Nigeria: male opposition and fear of methods. *Trop Doct.* 1989;19(3):114-117.
74. Castle S. Factors influencing young Malians' reluctance to use hormonal contraceptives. *Stud Fam Plann.* 2003;34(3):186-199.
75. Thapa S, Salgado M, Fortney JA, et al. Women's perceptions of the pill's potential health risks in Sri Lanka. *Asia Pac Popul J.* 1987;2(3):39-56.
76. Bergstrom S. Reproductive failure as a health priority in the Third World: a review. *East Afr Med J.* 1992;69(4):174-180.
77. Shaw D. Women's right to health and the Millennium Development Goals: promoting partnerships to improve access. *Int J Gynaecol Obstet.* 2006;94(3):207-215.
78. Human Rights Watch. Millennium Development Goals Ignore Fundamental Reproductive Rights Issues. In: *Women's Rights News.* 2005. http://hrw.org/women/newsletter/vol1_issue2.pdf. Accessed November10, 2008.
79. Reproductive rights are human rights. Center for Reproductive Rights Website. http://www.reproductiverights.org/pub_bo_rrhr.html. Accessed November 10, 2008.

CHAPTER 24

Vaccines and Women: Cultural and Structural Issues for Acceptability

INTRODUCTION

Seeking health can be conceptualized as a life-long process that includes both behaviors to cure or to seek relief from specific symptoms or illnesses, and behaviors to avoid symptoms and illnesses. Sociobehavioral research including both qualitative and quantitative methodologies can provide important information for understanding health practices and susceptibility to particular diseases with regard to gender, ethnicity, socioeconomic status, and political contexts.[1,2] Anthropologists and other social scientists have made significant contributions to understanding the perceived desirability, availability, and accessibility of sectors of healthcare systems including identifying critical influences in the acceptability and delivery of vaccine programs.[3-5] Sociobehavioral research on vaccines has included data on acceptability of existing vaccines[6] and hypothetical vaccines, such as HIV.[7] A number of variables that can be categorized as disease- or vaccine-related emerge as potentially salient to the decision-making process for vaccination. Such variables as perceived severity or characteristics of the disease[8] and personal vulnerability to the disease[9] have been recognized as contributing to acceptance and use of specific vaccines. Vaccine-related variables have included "comfort and confidence" in vaccines,[7] general positive attitudes toward immunization,[10] perceived benefits and risks of vaccination,[11] vaccine cost,[12] and characteristics and delivery of a vaccine, such as number of doses.[13]

Other vaccine-acceptance studies have relied more on a sociocultural and/or political-economic framework. In these studies, such variables as client–health worker communication, healthcare infrastructure, and media exposure regarding information about a particular vaccine are incorporated to understand acceptance and participation in vaccination programs.[14,15] In relation to vaccination acceptance, Nichter[4] has created two categories in reference to willingness to be vaccinated: "active demand" for vaccination in which an informed public perceives the benefits of vaccination and adheres to vaccination schedules, and "passive demand" in which individuals yield to recommendations and social pressures from health providers

Hala Azzam, PhD, MPH;
Linda M. Kaljee, PhD

Hala Azzam, PhD, MPH, is an Assistant Professor for the Department of Epidemiology of Preventive Medicine in the School of Medicine, University of Maryland, Baltimore, and the Emerging Pathogen Institute, College of Public Health, University of Florida.

Linda M. Kaljee, PhD, is an Associate Professor for the Wayne State University School of Medicine and for the Pediatric Prevention Research Center, Detroit, MI.

or community leaders. Streefland[16] has expanded on these definitions and concepts including three categories for "nonacceptance": (1) those willing to go but unable to attend for logistical reasons; (2) those who simply refuse to attend because of logistical or delivery issues; and, (3) those who question the need for vaccination.

In this chapter, we will explore how the social construction of gender and particularly the rights, roles, and responsibilities of women and girls affect vaccination utilization. A brief historical review in Europe and the United States suggests that women have been actively involved both in promotion and protest of government policies regarding vaccination since the introduction of smallpox inoculation. To date, there is little literature that explicitly addresses how gender affects vaccine use, though as we will discuss, women (or mothers) are most frequently the target of campaigns for childhood vaccines. In addition, we will consider how poverty can further exacerbate barriers for women in terms of receiving vaccines to prevent disease in themselves and their children. Within the last few years, the issue of women and vaccination has been a focus in relation to the recent availability of a human papillomavirus (HPV) vaccine for use with young adolescent girls both in the United States and internationally. We will discuss this literature on HPV and vaccination within the broader issues of gender and vaccines, as well as specific to the context of adolescent girls and sexuality in which the HPV vaccine has been cast. Finally, we will briefly review literature on participation in vaccine trials with a focus on implications with regard to gender differences in participation during clinical trials.

Smallpox, Religion, Liberty, and the Emergence of Vaccines

The earliest success with immunizing against disease in Western Europe occurred in 1721 with the introduction from Constantinople of variolation for smallpox using skin exudate from pox to produce a milder case of the disease than would be anticipated through natural exposure.[17,18] Prior to this introduction of inoculation to the West, however, evidence exists of the utilization and increasingly institutionalized use of inoculation for smallpox in China and in West Africa.[19,20]

In the 1700s during the introduction of smallpox inoculation in France, religion was at the forefront of arguments against utilization of inoculation. These arguments focused on disease as the will of God and punishment for sinners.[19] Religion also played a role in perceptions of inoculation in colonial America much along the same line of reasoning as across the Atlantic. In addition, inoculation as a general mechanism to avoid severe natural smallpox did not mesh with the medical and popular conception of the human body and disease control and treatment of the early 1700s. However, specific constructions of the disease course for smallpox related to a perceived need to encourage emergence of the pox in a controlled manner lead to increasing acceptance of the practice by mid-century. Regardless, acceptance of the practice varied across regions in the U.S. colonies.[18]

In the late 1700s, Edward Jenner's use of cowpox to immunize against smallpox gradually increased utilization of the method and affected policies and programs related to vaccination. However, until the mid to late 1800s, the primary method for vaccinating was arm to arm—and inherent in this practice was risk of contamination including recorded cases of syphilis, hepatitis, measles, streptococcal infections, and other bacterial infections, as well as smallpox.[21] With risks of contaminations and a decrease in immunity over time, the procedure elicited controversy. The antivaccination movement in England unfolded with the Compulsory Vaccination Act of 1853, which was linked to the unpopular Poor Law. For those individuals least able to afford any disruption to their income, the punishments for nonvaccination including imprisonment and fines could be devastating—yet parents still refused to have their children receive the smallpox vaccine. Within the discourse of the antivaccinators was a concern beyond fears of the vaccine, but regarding larger public health and social needs within their communities, such as clean water and living wages.[22] Compulsory vaccination laws were enacted throughout most of Western Europe by the late 1800s, as well as in the United States, though states in the Midwest and the South were slower to adopt these policies than in the North.[23]

Women's roles in promotion of vaccination can be traced to the Napoleonic era during which members of the Society for Maternal Charity instituted incentives to increase smallpox vaccination coverage of children under their care.[24] This reliance on women as volunteer labor for vaccination efforts remains evident in resource-poor countries. In the 1990s, Peru adopted a basic care health plan, and the implementation of components of the plan, including universal immunization for children, shifted responsibility from the state to the community and in particular to poor women.[25]

Outside of Europe and North America, vaccination campaigns were implemented throughout the colonized world in Africa and Asia, as well as within North America among Aboriginal groups.[20] These campaigns across the colonies were conducted by health and missionary organizations as well as through private companies, but were often also enforced through the colonizing power's military. Of particular interest, as we will discuss later in relation to the rejection of tetanus vaccination among girls in Cameroon in the late 1990s, these associations of vaccination with Western colonization and state control can reverberate through current public discourses regarding vaccination campaigns.[5]

The Expanded Programme for Immunization Experience

Even as public and political controversies continued regarding smallpox vaccination policies, in the late 1800s the development of Pasteur's rabies vaccine in 1885 and the diphtheria antitoxin in 1894 caught the population's imagination. Within a context of increasing mass media depictions of scientific discoveries, these developments were a part of the science that was recreating popular concepts of medicine.[26] Vaccines continued to be developed and marketed throughout the 1900s including those for pertussis, polio, measles, tetanus, tuberculosis (Bacille Calmette Guerin or BCG), and more recently *Haemophilis influenzae* type b (Hib) and hepatitis B virus (HBV).[27,28]

Despite rapid inclusion of new vaccines into immunization programs in the United States and Europe throughout the mid-1900s, relatively few children in low- and middle-income countries were receiving life-saving vaccines. In 1974, the Expanded Programme for Immunization (EPI) was implemented by WHO at which time immunization rates were less than 5% for children living in resource-poor countries. Today, through EPI, it is estimated that 80% of infants and children have received vaccines against several often fatal diseases, though coverage varies significantly across regions and within countries with warfare, civil unrest, and social and economic isolation, contributing to low coverage.[28] More recently through the establishment of the Global Alliance on Vaccines and Immunizations (GAVI). In 1999, coverage for these EPI vaccines has increased, and efforts are underway to further coverage for other vaccines including hepatitis B and Hib.[29]

EPI is designed to both deliver vaccines and to improve healthcare delivery systems within the public sector. Working through the public sector links the immunization programs to local and national governments. Streefland[30] notes that overall parents' acceptance of EPI is reflective of broader perceptions of the government, and country-specific EPI strategies range from promotion of vaccine uptake to coercive measures. Streefland further notes that in more repressive government environments both socioeconomic and gender inequality may contribute to increased participation in vaccination but not within a context of informed decision making. Questions that remain include how constructs of gender affect women's access and ability to utilize public health information and make informed decisions about EPI vaccines for their children and themselves, and how immunization decisions are made in cases when a woman is unable to carry out this responsibility in light of illness, death, or economic conditions in which she must work away from home.

A key component of EPI has been the mobilization of community-level health providers and utilization of health education to encourage participation in vaccination. Numerous studies have been conducted over the past 10 years that focus on these campaigns and participation and non-participation rates. These studies, as well as information, education, and communication (IEC) campaigns, primarily target the mothers of infants and young children who are perceived to provide the majority of health care and illness prevention. In studies in South Asia, mothers' general level of education or literacy level as well as specific knowledge of vaccination and EPI contribute to child immunization status. Research studies conducted in Dhaka, Bangladesh, indicate low socioeconomic status, mothers' education and employment status, and lack of knowledge of EPI-reduced rates of immunization among infants and children.[31,32] In addition, other factors affecting vaccination included the number of children in the household, distance to immunization sites and waiting times, numbers of home visits by health workers, costs associated with vaccination, fears of side effects, and loss of immunization cards.[32,33] Similar findings in relation to immunization coverage and mothers' levels of literacy have been documented in India and Ghana.[34-36] While mothers in Rajasthan, India, expressed overall positive attitudes toward immunization programs, lack of knowledge about vaccine diseases and schedules for doses negatively affected coverage. In this latter study, data also revealed that accessibility of services and family support were important factors for full participation in the immunization services.[35] In a separate study in Rajasthan, rural areas experienced lower rates of immunization coverage (45.1%) compared to urban areas (82.1%), and mothers' lack of information in regards to the need for immunization and busy schedules affected coverage rates. In addition, both health staff (56.4%) and family members (27%) were important sources of information regarding immunization.[37]

While the Rajasthan research did not find child gender differences in immunization coverage rates,[37] other research in India indicates differential vaccination coverage for girls compared to boys. In a study that utilized the 1992–1993 National Health Survey of the 17 largest states in India, gender inequality was evident in both urban and rural areas with fewer girls than boys being fully immunized. The greatest gender-based difference was in relation to children receiving no immunizations with 5% more girls than boys within this group irrespective of economic status. From analyses of these same data, evidence emerges that boys born after multiple daughters have the best outcomes in relation to nutritional and immunization status.[38,39] In a study of rural areas in 16 states in India, boys were immunized at higher rates than girls. However, across genders the literacy rate of mothers contributed significantly to overall higher rates of immunization as well as better nutritional status for all children. In this research, 67% of children of literate mothers were fully immunized, compared to 52% with literate fathers but illiterate mothers, and 42% of children in households with both parents illiterate.[40]

In Bangladesh, an analysis of both national-level and local district data also indicated that girls were less likely to be immunized than boys, with the differences increasing with numbers of doses for a particular vaccine. Overall, mother's education and father's job status increased rates of immunization, and lowest rates were in rural and ethnic minority groups.[41] In another study of 4075 children attending Dhaka Hospital between 1994 and 2003, 39% of girls compared to 61% of boys had received measles vaccination. In addition, those children not vaccinated were two times as likely to be stunted, underweighted, and/or wasted. Again, mother's literacy also affected coverage.[42]

Few studies have considered the impact of mothers' or other caregivers' health or day-to-day presence in the household in relation to immunization status. In particular, the effect of the HIV/AIDS epidemic on a household's utilization of immunization services has received slight attention. In areas with high rates of HIV/AIDS, the death or illness of one or both parents, particularly a child's mother, could significantly affect access to immunization programs. In one study in Zambia, DTP and polio coverage among HIV+ children found lower immunization rates for seropositive children with the mother's level of education contributing to rates.[43] Another study in Uganda found that a woman's positive HIV status increased likelihood of underutilization of immunization services for children.[44]

While the EPI is focused on childhood diseases and immunization of infants and young children, the immunization of women with the tetanus toxoid (TT) vaccine during pregnancy is another primary objective. High mortality rates are associated with tetanus infection among postpartum women and newborns. While increasing hygienic conditions during childbirth is one step toward decreasing the risk of tetanus, vaccination of women of childbearing age and pregnant women with the TT vaccine provides protection for both the woman and her infant. As of January 2008, maternal neonatal tetanus (MNT) remains a public health problem in 47 countries primarily in Africa and South and Southeast Asia. Maximum coverage requires six doses for those individuals immunized initially during childhood and five doses for those immunized during adolescence and adulthood. The vaccination schedule for pregnant women with an unknown history of tetanus coverage includes two doses during pregnancy.[45,46]

Research on coverage of women and adolescent girls in relation to the TT vaccine indicates similar issues as outlined for immunization of infants and children. In Karachi, a woman's knowledge about TT increased chances that she was immunized and that her children received EPI vaccines. Overall, 45% of the children had received full EPI coverage, and 57% of women had received two doses of TT during pregnancy.[47] In Indonesia, women's knowledge about tetanus disease and awareness of the TT vaccine increased vaccination. In addition, women who received antenatal care were 30 times more likely to have received the TT vaccine.[48] In Haryana, India, a survey of 11-year-old and 17-year-old girls revealed immunization rates for tetanus at 26.7% and 44.3%, respectively. Overall, girls in school (35%) were more likely to be vaccinated than out-of-school girls (13%).[49] While efforts to increase rates of immunization among girls and women for tetanus have shown success, there have been cases whereby local rumors and fears affected public health campaigns. An effort to vaccinate school-attending girls in Cameroon in the 1990s coincided both with political upheaval and implementation of policies to legalize contraceptive use and family planning. Public suspicions were raised among the adolescents, parents, and the Catholic Church, and warnings were issued out of concern that the vaccine would sterilize the girls. Mobile units that were utilized to carry out the vaccination campaign were linked to colonial efforts in Africa to implement smallpox vaccination, and the campaign process conjured fears of state power and control.[5]

Sexuality and Vaccination—The Introduction of the Human Papillomavirus (HPV) Vaccine

Genital HPV is the most common sexually transmitted disease, and estimates in the United States indicate that at least 50% of men and women contract HPV throughout their lifetime, while about 80% of women become infected by the age of 50 years.[50] More than 40 genital genotypes are known, and a majority of HPV infections are asymptomatic and resolve without intervention; however, specific genotypes can lead to genital warts, and 15 genotypes are classified as oncogenic. These latter genotypes (HPV 16, 18, 31, 33, 35, 39, 45, 51, 52, 56, 58, 59, and 66) are associated with 99% of all cervical cancers, though HPV infection alone is not sufficient to cause the cancer.[51,52] Of the 15 oncogenic genotypes, HPV 16 and 18 are the most highly carcinogenic and account for approximately 70% of cervical cancer worldwide.[53]

Cervical cancer is the second most common cancer in women worldwide. The development of the Papanicolaou (PAP) test to detect precancerous lesions has significantly decreased the risk of cervical cancer in higher-income Western countries.[54] The technology and moderately invasive procedures for PAP tests have limited availability and accessibility in many middle- and low-income countries. Thus, currently there are an estimated 500,000 new cases of cervical cancer and 275,000 deaths annually with 80% of these occurring in developing countries.[55,56]

Recently two HPV vaccines have been developed and are reaching the market including a quadrivalent vaccine (Gardasil, Merck & Company[57]) and a bivalent vaccine (Cervarix, Glaxo-Smith[58]). Both vaccines are based on the L1 core protein that can assemble into a viruslike particle and target HPV 16 and 18. In addition, the quadrivalent vaccine targets HPV 6 and 11, which cause more than 90% of genital warts.[59] Both vaccines have been shown to be 100% effective in preventing precancerous lesions resulting from HPV 16 and 18[60-66] as well as providing cross-protection against HPV 31[63]and 45.[63,64] Currently however, clinical trials are limited by the recent development of the vaccine, and protection data are only available through a five-year period.[63,65,66] Gardasil is approved in 80 countries, and in the United States it is licensed for women ages 9 to 26 years.[67] In Australia, the vaccine is also approved for boys 9 to 15 years.[68] Cervarix has been licensed in the European Union, Kenya, and Australia for women ages 10 to 45 years, and is awaiting approval in other countries including the United States.[68] Both vaccines require three doses, and immunization must be completed prior to sexual debut, as they are not effective after infection with HPV.

Several factors including issues regarding gender roles and sexuality can potentially affect acceptance and utilization of the HPV vaccine among young adolescent girls. As with other new vaccines, issues of safety, costs, delivery systems, and delivery logistics will be concerns in communities where the vaccine is introduced. The relative lack of information and knowledge in the general population regarding HPV could also affect acceptability of the vaccine. In addition, the utilization of the vaccine with young adolescent girls will raise concerns in reference to sociocultural ideals about virginity and promiscuity, and fears that the vaccine provides "license" for young women to engage in nonmarital sexual relations. The association of the vaccine with an STI could decrease acceptance. Alternatively, the corresponding association with prevention of a form of cancer might provide a positive balance in public opinion.

A recent systematic review on HPV vaccine acceptance research revealed 28 studies in the United States, 18 in the European Union, and only 3 in low- or middle-income countries.[69] Given the significantly higher risk for cervical cancer in developing regions of the world, we will focus in this chapter on four countries: Vietnam, Mexico, Turkey, and Hong Kong. Where possible, these findings will be contrasted and compared to findings in the United States, Europe, Australia, and Canada.

Vaccine safety and concerns about adverse events are generally one of the primary concerns among the public for both new and existing vaccines.[70] As of June 2008, 6697 cases of adverse events were reported by the Vaccine Adverse Event Reporting System (VAERS) after injection with Gardasil. A majority of conditions included nonserious side effects such as pain and swelling at the injection site, headache, fever, and vomiting. However, 103 life-threatening adverse events have been reported including syncope, seizures, and Guillian-Barre syndrome.[71] In a study in Mexico, 32% of respondents expressed fears that the vaccine could cause acquisition of HPV or development of cervical cancer.[72] In Hong Kong, both mothers and daughters expressed significant concerns regarding potential unknown side effects of the vaccine including impact of fertility and general health.[72,73]

Another general issue for vaccine acceptance particularly in relation to a new product is cost. Research on willingness to pay has indicated that individuals assess costs of a vaccine in relation to their knowledge and concerns about a particular disease.[75] The current market price for the Gardasil vaccine is $360 for the three-dose regimen. This cost is far above the ability to pay for a majority of residents in low- and middle-income countries, as well as lower-income families within the United States, Canada, Australia, and the European Union. Given the lack of knowledge and experience with HPV, and most likely cervical cancer, among potential vaccine recipients and parents, the cost of the vaccine may deter acceptance especially when compared to other vaccines or preventive measures for other endemic/epidemic diseases within any specific country.

Vaccine delivery for a three-dose regimen may also present challenges to providers and policy makers. In many countries adolescent girls are not in school, decreasing the effectiveness of a school-based delivery system.[76,77] Community-based approaches, including primary public healthcare facilities as well as the private sector, can be utilized, but there is the potential concern about stigmatization of girls attending clinics and receiving a vaccine for an STI. Also, in many settings, adolescent healthcare utilization is low and/or adolescent-friendly services are limited, and gender may affect access. In a review of data from national surveys in Burkina Faso, Ghana, Malawi, and Uganda, one in five adolescent girls versus one in three adolescent boys reported receiving health-related injections during the past year.[77] In relation to HPV vaccination, ongoing research is underway in Uganda, India, Peru, and Vietnam to increase understanding of vaccine acceptability, alternative vaccine schedules, potential cost-effective measures, and pilot testing for both school-based and community-based delivery.[78]

As noted, there is generally limited knowledge regarding HPV and the link between HPV and cervical cancer within the general population across countries.[69,79] In the United States, research indicates relatively high HPV vaccine acceptance despite low levels of knowledge and potential for increased acceptance with implementation of educational materials on vaccine benefits.[69] In Mexico, a study assessing 880 women's acceptance to participate in an HPV vaccine clinical trial found that only 2% of the women had knowledge of the link between HPV and cervical cancer. However, after education about the HPV vaccine and with the women's previous knowledge regarding usefulness of vaccines approximately 84% indicated they would be willing for themselves and/or their daughters to participate in a trial.[80] Similarly, in another pilot study in Mexico with mothers of adolescent children (ages 10 to 14) only 4% of respondents had good knowledge regarding HPV, but 83% and 63% were willing to use the HPV vaccine on themselves or their adolescent daughters respectively.[72] This situation is similar in Vietnam where vaccine acceptance was high among mothers of adolescent girls[81] (see Table 24-1).

A survey of 170 mothers with adolescent daughters and a series of focus groups with the same population in Hong Kong,[73,82] as well as focus groups with adolescent girls,[74] indicated a low level of knowledge and lack of information regarding HPV and cervical cancer. Further education efforts among both mothers and the young adolescent girls increased acceptance from 32% to 52% and from 51% to 69% respectively.[74,82] Finally, a recent study in Turkey showed a surprisingly high (95%) acceptability of HPV vaccine following some educational material regarding the benefit of the HPV vaccine.[83]

In trying to assess the HPV vaccine's acceptability, stigmatization regarding sexually transmitted infections and the role of sociocultural gender constructs and attitudes regarding sexuality are primary factors. The HPV vaccine is mainly marketed to adolescent women who stand to gain the most from it through its potential to prevent death from cervical cancer. However, vaccination of women alone raises questions regarding stigmatization of STIs and vaccinated women as promiscuous. In addition, parents may worry that vaccination be interpreted by their adolescent daughters as condoning early sexual behavior, especially in cultures where sexual debut is linked to marriage and adulthood.

While recognition of HPV as an STI is relatively low worldwide,[69] in the Hong Kong studies women discuss a connection between cervical cancer and its association with promiscuity and multiple partners.[74,82] In addition, women participating in focus group studies in Hong Kong revealed fear of stigmatization and concern over accusations of infidelity and partner loss if HPV

were generally known to be sexually transmitted and associated with cervical cancer.[74]

Adolescent girls in Hong Kong worried their parents might perceive them as promiscuous should they get vaccinated at an early age;[74] however, this was not reflected in data from mothers in Hong Kong, in which only 2–10% were concerned that the vaccine would increase sexual behaviors among their daughters.[73,74] Alternatively, in Mexico 25% of mothers were not willing to vaccinate their daughters and cited lack of sexual activity by their daughters as the main reason.[72] Several studies have shown however that parents are unaware of the age of their daughter's sexual debut.[72,84] In addition, in the study in Mexico 38% of respondents stated that the Catholic Church would not approve use of the vaccine for adolescent girls, and 34% of respondents stated they would support the church's decision.

Finally, it is important to note that traditional and alternative conceptualization of disease treatment and prevention may affect vaccine acceptance. In some belief systems, "God's will" is associated with contracting disease, and cervical cancer is not an exception.[82] And in this century, like 18th-century reactions to the smallpox vaccine, members of some religious groups perceive vaccines as unacceptable in relation to their religious beliefs including benevolence of God and rejection of intake of chemical substances.[85]

Also with between 50–80% of the world population practicing some form of traditional or alternative medicine, conflicting beliefs and attitudes will exist with biomedical models.[86] For example, in regards to the HPV vaccine, in focus groups with late adolescent girls in Vietnam concern was raised regarding the need for three doses in relation to perceptions of Western medicines as "hot." These respondents discussed parallel concerns about the rabies five-dose postexposure vaccine as dangerous for children and adolescents because too much "hot" Western medicine inhibits physical and mental development (unpublished data).

Gender and Participation in Clinical Trials

Vaccine clinical trials are designed to assess the safety, efficacy, and effectiveness of vaccine candidates through a rigorous multiphased methodology.

TABLE 24-1

Summary of Studies Assessing HPV Knowledge and Acceptability

Author	Country/ location	Study design	N	Age (years)	Gender	HPV link to cervical cancer	HPV vaccine acceptability
Lazcano-Ponce, 2001[80]	Mexico, urban	Survey	880	15 to 49	F	2%	84% daughter
Moraros, 2006[72]	Mexico, urban	Survey	60	24 to 52	F	4%	83% self, 63% daughter
Lee, 2007[82]	Hong Kong, urban	Survey, pre- and posteducation	170	NA	F	14%	Pre: 32% daughter Post: 52% daughter
Chan, 2007[73]	Hong Kong, urban	Focus group Pre- and posteducation	49	18 to 58	F	Practically none	Majority
Kwan, 2008[74]	Hong Kong, urban	Focus group Pre- and posteducation	64	13 to 20	F	Practically none	Pre: 51% self, Post: 69% self
Dinh, 2007[81]	Vietnam, urban	Survey	181	26 to 60	F	NA	68–91% daughter
Baykal, 2008[83]	Turkey, urban	Survey	143	17– >35	F	17%– >35%	95% self, 98% daughter, 95% sons
Brewer, 2007[69]	United States, results of several studies	Surveys and focus groups	Not available	Adolescents and adults	F/M	1–89% (mean 44%)	55–100% daughter

While vaccine research and development has been ongoing since the 1700s, the methodologies incorporated within clinical trials for assessing efficacy and toxicity of vaccines are relatively recent. The first blinded, randomized-control medical trial was conducted in 1948 for use of streptomycin for pulmonary tuberculosis, and the first large-scaled vaccine trial was in 1954 with the Salk poliomyelitis injectable vaccine. This trial included 650,000 children and 150,000 adult volunteers across the United States.[86,87]

To date, there have been significantly fewer studies examining vaccine trial participation compared to research on participation in immunization public health campaigns with a majority of studies on clinical trial participation conducted in the United States and other Western countries.[88] In a trial of the typhoid fever polysaccharide Vi vaccine with children 6–18 years in Hue, Vietnam, sociobehavioral pre- and postvaccination data indicated several factors that contributed to participation including knowledge about typhoid fever, adherence to traditional perceptions of disease causality, and past healthcare utilization practices. Positive perceptions of the campaign information and the consenting procedures were also associated with participation.[89] In another trial of this same vaccine in Kolkata, India, individual factors associated with trial participation included religion (Muslim and Hindu) and education. However, other significant differences related to trial participation included community sources of information about the trial and decision-making practices within households. In terms of the latter, the role of male and female adults within the household affected the percentage of household members vaccinated during the trial. Lowest levels of participation were among households where female respondents stated they independently made the decision about household member participation, and highest rates were among households where both the survey respondent and his or her spouse made the decision regarding trial participation.[90]

In HIV vaccine trials, gender has been a significant issue in relation to women's access and willingness to participate. In countries in which women have limited mobility, they may not be able meet trial requirements including clinic visits. In these trials, women are required to utilize contraception during the trial period, and they may not have control over choice of contraceptive use within their relationships. In HIV trials in India, high dropout rates resulted as women feared testing and needed partner permission to participate. Privacy and child care were also concerns for these women. In Thailand, during the vaccine trial women were provided with easy access to the site, a range of educational materials, and were provided free contraceptives.[91]

Women's ability to choose to enroll and participate in vaccine trials is of importance in relation to biological differences between men and women in antibody responses to various vaccines.[91,92] Sufficient numbers of men and women need to enroll in trials to ensure sufficient power to differentiate potential gender differences in response to the vaccine. In addition, for diseases like HIV to which women are particularly vulnerable both socially and biologically, their involvement in trials is essential to producing a vaccine that is equally efficient and protective regardless of gender.[91]

Conclusion

A model for vaccine acceptance within any population group must incorporate multiple levels of sociocultural and political-economic factors with individual determinants for utilization[93,94] (see Figure 24-1). Within this framework, issues related to the social construction of gender and the day-to-day reproduction of these constructs can be explicated for specific diseases and vaccines as well as a more generic contextual understanding of vaccination.

At the sociocultural and political-economic level, poverty can affect vaccine utilization even if vaccines are free of charge. A recent review of immunization coverage worldwide found that economic inequalities play a significant role and may be more important than gender inequalities with the exception of South Asia.[95] Thus, for some women, immunization of their children through EPI is inhibited by competing needs of other day-to-day responsibilities. For many women, there is insufficient time to provide for household needs. Poverty also affects education, and many women do not attend school or they must leave school at an early age. Literacy levels of mothers of infants and children significantly affect vaccination and

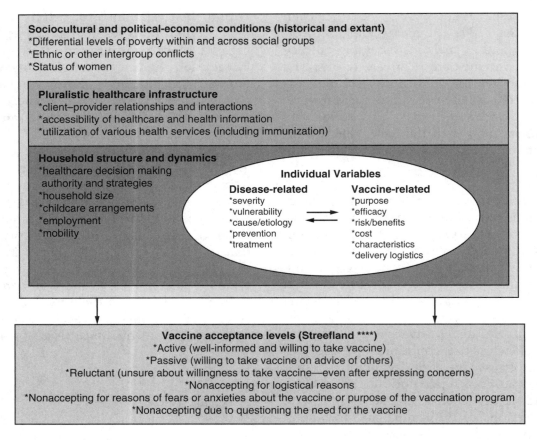

FIGURE 24-1 Vaccine acceptance model

From Kaljee, L. Sociobehavioral research methods for the introduction of vaccines in the diseases of most impoverished programme. *JHPN.* September, 2004.

increase the risks for these women and children of many preventable diseases. Stigmatization of women in relation to their sexuality and the values placed on a woman's virginity clearly can affect her ability to access the HPV vaccine. Likewise, in many cultures parents fear their adolescent daughters' use of the HPV vaccine and resulting stigma or actual premarital sexual debut, which can affect the girls' ability to be married and their access to economic resources.[5]

Sociocultural values of children, and particularly girls, can have a profound effect on utilization of vaccination services. In patrilineal societies, male children are highly valued, and limited household resources may be used to ensure their survival. Again, even in instances when vaccines are free, the time and resources needed to access these programs may favor boys. In cases such as HPV, the cost of a vaccine for girls for a

disease that is relatively unknown could significantly decrease participation in public campaigns to promote the vaccine.

At a political-economic level, governments may use a range of promotion methods for vaccination, some of which may be coercive in nature. While these methods may increase rates of participation, they do not create an informed public and may benefit from attention to social, economic, and gender inequalities. Within some government systems, public involvement may also create resistance to vaccination as clearly illustrated in 19th-century efforts to mandate smallpox inoculation in the United States, the United Kingdom, and within Western colonies in Africa and Asia. More recently, association of vaccines and biomedicine with colonization and with repressive political tactics can create an atmosphere of resistance as evident in Cameroon.

The public healthcare system can be closely associated with local and/or national government. The relationship between these systems and the public, however, are also dependent on day-to-day contact through various health services. Economic conditions often minimize availability of services including those specific for women such as cervical cancer screening (PAP) and adequate antenatal and childbirth facilities. These services not only put women at risk of disease and complications from pregnancy and childbirth but may also decrease regular contact with health providers. As indicated in research in Indonesia, visits to antenatal clinics significantly increased participation in TT vaccination among pregnant women.[48] In addition, women both formally and informally provide health care and education to other women in the communities. Often public health facilities are primarily staffed by women, and as noted in Peru, women are engaged in promoting immunization and other healthcare information within their neighborhoods. This role for women again reemphasizes the need for educational programs and services that target women and provide them with the information needed to make informed decisions regarding utilization of vaccines for their own health, the health of their children, and the well-being of other women in their families and communities. Finally, programs are needed to provide some form of continuing education for community healthcare providers to inform them about diseases and new treatments and prevention methods, such as vaccines. Highlighted in research in the United States, Thailand, and Mexico was the need to educate healthcare providers about HPV and cervical cancer prevention.[79,96,97] This is particularly important as physician and other healthcare provider recommendations were cited by women as playing an important role in acceptance of the HPV vaccine.

At the household level, woman in a majority of societies are the primary providers for children including prevention and treatment of disease. Alternatively, many women lack the authority within their households both in relation to economic resources and decision making. In some conservative societies, women may also experience limited mobility outside of the household decreasing opportunities for her to access health services including the EPI and national immunization days. A lack of access to family planning can also increase number of children, decrease a woman's time and resources, and further lead to gender discrimination for vaccination. Adolescent girls' roles in the household will also affect their access to the HPV vaccine. Household resources may force daughters to withdraw from school or may limit a young woman's contact with community-based health services. In some cultures, girls represent a resource for the household at time of marriage, and risks of stigma associated with the HPV vaccine could be perceived as decreasing a daughter's value. Alternatively, adolescents' roles in their own utilization of the HPV vaccine cannot be necessarily negated. In a trial of the polysaccharide typhoid fever vaccine in Vietnam, parents noted their decision to not participate also reflected the desires of their adolescent children.[89] In the research in Hong Kong, while many adolescents accepted the vaccine in a broader sense, they did not necessarily see the immediate urgency for vaccination citing concerns both about the vaccine (safety, efficacy) and about social consequences, parental disapproval, and social perceptions of sexual impropriety.[74]

These research findings suggest the need for targeted health education programs regarding vaccinations and associated diseases for adolescent girls for themselves and as they assume responsibility for the health care of their children.

For EPI vaccines, within low- and middle-income countries the severity and potential vulnerability of young children and women to diseases including tetanus, measles, diphtheria, polio, and tuberculosis are current or within recent memory. Limited access to treatment because of economic conditions or inaccessibility of facilities compounds the threat of these diseases. However, women may not have sufficient information regarding how vaccines can prevent familiar diseases and may not be fully informed of the benefits of immunization. While the general public has limited information about HPV, and the information they have has only become available very recently, cancer as a generic disorder is recognized and often perceived in the public eye as terminal. The branding of the HPV as the "cervical cancer vaccine" distances the vaccine from sexuality and gender and situates it as preventive of a much dreaded and less stigmatized condition.[98,99] Alternatively, the association between HPV and cervical cancer may prove to stigmatize women diagnosed with the cancer.

Vaccine-related knowledge and attitudes relate to real and perceived adverse events, efficacy, cost, and characteristics and delivery. In addition, in a majority of countries, vaccines are a part of a pluralistic medical system that includes both traditional/alternative medicine and biomedicine. In the United States, the nature of HPV as a sexually transmitted disease has been less of a factor on vaccine acceptance than vaccine efficacy and safety.[100] This is in alignment with vaccine safety concerns in the United States and other Western countries in recent years through association of vaccination with conditions such as autism as well as lack of experience or exposure among these parents in the previous decades with the targeted diseases.[101,102]

In low- and middle-income countries concerns of safety are also paramount in relation to vaccine acceptance. Such concerns are also often integrated within nonbiomedical belief systems. There is a need to incorporate the beliefs associated within multiple health systems to better inform individuals about vaccine safety as well as to develop and provide materials that can explain concepts of protection and vaccine efficacy. These needs are challenged by levels of illiteracy, particularly among women who may be the target population for such messages.

Indirect costs of vaccines are an issue and can relate to travel, time, and lost work opportunities. Women may be least able to afford such losses of time and income, yet may be the primary providers for childcare within their households.

Finally, recruitment and retention efforts for vaccine trials need to recognize the specific needs of women within the sociocultural contexts of the trials. Women's participation in these trials is essential to the development of highly efficacious and protective vaccines. Pretrial assessments must identify the needs of potential participants and be cognizant of gender issues, and pretrial information campaigns may often need to differentiate needs and concerns of women.

Vaccines are one part of public health efforts to decrease disease burden worldwide. Increasing efforts to develop and implement new vaccines as well as expand utilization of existing vaccines has become a focus of public and private funds in the last 10 years.[103] While biological and clinical research efforts are clearly recognized as essential toward reaching goals for immunization coverage and disease control and eradication, sociocultural research on the contexts for vaccine introduction and delivery, particularly in relation to economic conditions and gender constructs, must be integrated within the methodologies and models for clinical vaccine trials and public health campaigns.

DISCUSSION QUESTIONS

1. What are some of the barriers for vaccine implementation in developing nations versus the developed world? What are some potential solutions?

2. Is the HPV vaccine the only vaccine for STIs? Can you think of another existing vaccine? Are the barriers for the HPV vaccine implementation similar to that other vaccine? What are some of the differences?

REFERENCES

1. Kleinman A. *Patients and Healers in the Context of Culture: An Exploration of the Borderland between Anthropology, Medicine, and Psychiatry*. Berkeley, CA: University of California; 1980.
2. Baer H, Singer M, Susser I. *Medical Anthropology and the World System: A Critical Perspective*. Westport, CN: Bergin & Garvey; 1997.

3. Nichter M. Use of social science research in improving epidemiologic studies and interventions for diarrhea and dysentery. *Rev Infect Dis.* 1991;13(4):S265-S271.

4. Nichter M. Vaccinations in the Third World: A consideration of community demand. In: Nichter M, Nichter M, eds. *Anthropology and International Health: Asian Case Studies.* Australia: Gordon and Breach; 1996:329-366.

5. Feldman-Savelsberg P, Ndonko FT, Schmidt-Ehry B. Sterilizing vaccines or the politics of the womb: a retrospective study of a rumor in Cameroon. *Med Anthropol Q.* 2000;14(2):159-179.

6. Rhodes SD, Hergenrather KC. Using an integrated approach to understand vaccination behavior among men who have sex with men: stages of change, the health belief model, and self-efficacy. *J Community Health.* 2003;28:347-362.

7. Van de Van P, Artholow B, Rawstorne P, et al. Scaling HIV vaccine attitudes among gay men in Sydney, Australia. *AIDS Res Hum Retroviruses.* 2002;18:1333-1337.

8. Mays RM, Sturm LA, Zimet GD. Parental perspectives on vaccinating children against sexually transmitted infections. *Soc Sci Med.* 2004;58(7):1405-413.

9. Zimet GD, Liau A, Fortenberry VD. Health beliefs and intention to get immunized for HIV. *J Adolesc Health.* 1997;20:354-359.

10. Impicciatore P, Cosetti C, Schiavio S, et al. Mothers as active partners in the prevention of childhood diseases: maternal factors related to immunization status of preschool children in Italy. *Prev Med.* 2000;31:49-55.

11. Ramsay ME, Yarwood J, Lewis D, et al. Parental confidence in measles, mumps, and rubella vaccine: evidence from vaccine coverage and attitudinal surveys. *Brit J Gen Pract.* 2002;52:912-916.

12. Sansom S, Barker L, Corso PS, et al. Rotavirus vaccine and intussusception: how much risk will parents in the United States accept to obtain vaccine benefits? *Am J Epidemiol.* 2001;154:1077-1085.

13. Liau A, Zimet GD. The acceptability of HIV immunization: examining vaccine characteristics as determining factors. *AIDS Care.* 2001;13:643-650.

14. Smailbegovic MS, Laing GL, Bedford H. Why do parents decide against immunization? The effect of health beliefs and health professionals. *Child: Care Health Dev.* 2003;29:303-311.

15. Evans M, Stoddart H, Condon L, Freeman E, Grizzell M, Mullen R. Parents' perspectives on the MMR immunization: a focus group study. *Br J Gen Pract.* 2001;51:904-910.

16. Streefland P, Chowdhury AM, Ramos-Jimenez R. Patterns of vaccination acceptance. *Soc Sci Med.* 1999;49:1706-1716.

17. Theves G. Smallpox: an historical overview (English abstract). *Bull Soc Sci Med (Luxembourg).* 1997;134(1).

18. Gronim SS. Imagining inoculation: smallpox, the body, and social relations of healing in the eighteenth century. *Bull Hist Med.* 2006;80:247-268.

19. Heinrich L. How China became the "cradle of smallpox": transformations in discourse, 1726-2002. *Positions.* 2007;15:7-34.

20. Hackett P. Averting disaster: the Hudson's Bay Company and smallpox in Western Canada during the late eighteenth and early nineteenth centuries. *Bull Hist Med.* 2004;78:575-609.

21. Huygelen C. Jenner's cowpox vaccine in light of current vaccinology (English abstract). *Verh K Acad Geneeskd Belg.* 1996;58(5):479-536.

22. Durbach N. *Bodily Matters: The Anti-Vaccination Movement in England, 1853-1907.* Durham, NC: Duke University; 2005

23. Anderson W. Immunization and hygiene in the colonial Philippines. *J Hist Med Allied Sci.* 2006;62(1):1-21.

24. Adams C. Maternal societies in France: private charity before the welfare state. *J Women's Hist*. 2005;17(1):87-111.

25. Ewig C. Global processes, local consequences: gender equity and health sector reform in Peru. *Soc Polit*. 2006;13(3):427-455.

26. Hansen B. New images of a new medicine: visual evidence for the widespread popularity of therapeutic discoveries in America after 1885. *Bull Hist Med*. 1999;73(4):629-678.

27. Vaccine Information. National Network for Immunization Information. http://www.immunizationinfo.org/vaccineinfo/vaccine_detail.cfv?id=21. Accessed June 17, 2008.

28. World Health Organization. Diseases and vaccines: the history of vaccination. http://www.childrensvaccine.org/files/WHO-Vaccine-History.pdf. Accessed June 17, 2008.

29. GAVI Alliance. http://www.gavialliance.org. Accessed June 17, 2008.

30. Streefland P. Public doubts about vaccination safety and resistance against vaccination. *Health Policy*. 2001;55:159-172.

31. Rahman M, Islam MA, Mahalanabis D. Mothers' knowledge about vaccine preventable diseases and immunization coverage in a population with a high rate of illiteracy. *J Trop Pediatr*. 1995;6:376-378.

32. Perry H, Weierbach R, Hossain I, Islam R. Childhood immunization coverage in zone 3 of Dhaka City: the challenge to reaching impoverished households in urban Bangladesh. *Bull WHO*. 1998;76(6):565-573.

33. ICDDR, B. *Barriers to Immunization Among Women and Children Living in Slums of Zone 3 of Dhaka City*. Dhaka: ICDDR, B; 2002.

34. Singh P, Yadar R. Immunization status of children in BIMARU states. *Indian J Pediatr*. 2001;68(6):495-500.

35. Manjunath U, Pareek RP. Maternal knowledge and perceptions about the routine immunization programme: a study in semi-urban areas in Rajasthan. *Indian J Med Sci*. 2003;57(4):158-163.

36. Browne EN, Bonney AA, Agyapong FA, Essegbey I. Factors influencing participation in national immunization days in Kumasi, Ghana. *Annu Trop Med Parasitol*. 2002;96(1):93-104.

37. Gupta RS, Gupta A, Gupta HO, Venkatesh S, Lal S. Mother and child service coverage: reproductive and child health programme in Alwar district, Rajasthan State. *J Commun Dis*. 2006;38(1):79-87.

38. Pande R. Selective gender differences in childhood nutrition and immunization in rural India: the role of siblings. *Demography*. 2003;40(3):395-418.

39. Pande R, Yazbeck AS. What's in a country average? Wealth, gender, and regional inequalities in immunization in India. In: Gwatkin DR, Deveshwar-Bahl G, eds. *Overview of Socio-economic and Gender Differentials in Developing Countries*. http://poverty2.forumone.com/files/8970_Imm._Paper_Text_(Final)_gwatkin.pdf. Accessed June 17, 2008.

40. Boorah VK. Gender bias among children in India in their diet and immunization against disease. *Soc Sci Med*. 2004;58:1719-1731.

41. Chowdhury AM, Bhuiya A, Mahmud S, Abdus Salam AK, Karim F. Immunization divide: who do get vaccinated in Bangladesh. *J Health Popul Nutr*. 2003;21(3):193-204.

42. Chowdhury F, Khan A, Hossain MI, et al. Young children non-immunized against measles: characteristics and programmatic implications. *Acta Paediatrician*. 2006;95(1):44-49.

43. Setse RW, Cutts F, Monze M, et al. HIV-1 infection as a risk factor for incomplete childhood immunization in Zambia. *J Trop Pediatr.* 2006;52(5):324-328.

44. Mast TC, Kigozi G, Wabwire-Mangen F, et al. Immunization coverage among children born to HIV-infected women in Rakai district, Uganda: effect of voluntary testing and counseling (VCT). *AIDS Care.* 2006;18(7):755-763.

45. World Health Organization. Tetanus Vaccine: WHO Position Paper, Weekly Epidemiological Report (May 19 2006). http://www.who.int/immunization /wer8120tetanus_May06_position_paper.pdf. Accessed June 9, 2008.

46. World Health Organization. Maternal Neonatal Tetanus Elimination. http://www.who.int/immunization_monitoring/diseases/MNTE_initiative/en/. Accessed June 9, 2008.

47. Siddiqi N, Khan A, Nisar N, Siddiqi AF. Assessment of EPI (expanded program of immunization) vaccine coverage in a peri-urban slum. *J Pakistani Med Assoc.* 2007;57(8):391-395.

48. Roosihermiatie B, Nishyama M, Nakae K. Factors associated with TT (tetanus toxoid) immunization among pregnant women, in Saparua, Maluku, Indonesia. *Southeast Asian J Trop Med Public Health.* 2000;31(1):91-95.

49. Singh A, Arora AK. Tetanus immunization among adolescent girls in rural Hryana. *Indian J Pediatr.* 2000;67(4):255-258.

50. Center for Disease Control and Prevention. Genital HPV Infection CDC Fact Sheet. 2004. http://www.cdc.gov/std/HPV/STDFact-HPV.htm. Accessed June 19, 2008.

51. IARC. *Human Papillomaviruses* [monographs on the Evaluation of Carcinogenic Risks to Humans]. Vol. 90. Lyon, France: IARC; 2005.

52. Walboomers JM, Jacobs MV, Manos MM, et al. Human papillomavirus is a necessary cause of invasive cervical cancer worldwide. *J Pathol.* 1999;189(1):9-12.

53. Clifford GM, Smith JS, Plummer M, et al. Human papillomavirus types in invasive cervical cancer worldwide: a meta-analysis. *Br J Cancer.* 2003;88(1):63-73.

54. Center for Disease Control and Prevention. Quadrivalent human papillomavirus vaccine recommendations of the Advisory Committee on Immunization Practices (ACIP). *MMWR.* 2007;56(No. RR-2):1-26.

55. Ferley J, Bray F, Pisani P, Parkin DM. GLOBOCAN 2002 cancer incidence. Mortality and prevalence worldwide. *IARC Cancer Base.* 2004;5(version 2.0). Lyon, France: IARC.

56. Denny L, Quinn M, Sankaranarayanan R. Screening for cervical cancer in developing countries. *Vaccine.* 2006;24(Suppl. 3):S71-S77.

57. Gardasil product information. Merck & Company. http://www.gardasil .com/downloads/gardasil_pi.pdf. Accessed June 17, 2008.

58. Cervarix Product Information, GlaxoSmith. http://www.gsk.com/media /press-kits/cervarix-clinical-trials.pdf. Accessed June 17, 2008.

59. Garland SM, Hernandez-Avila M, Wheeler CM. Quadrivalent vaccine against human papillomavirus to prevent anogenital diseases. *N Engl J Med.* 2007;356:1928-1943.

60. Koufsky LA, Harper DM. Current findings from prophylactic HPV vaccine trials. *Vaccine.* 2006;24(Suppl 3):114-121.

61. Villa LL. Overview of the clinical development and results of a quadrivalent HPV (types 6, 11, 16, 18) vaccine. *Int J Infect Dis.* 2007;11(Suppl 2):S17-S25.

62. Future II Study Group. Quadrivalent vaccine against human papillomavirus to prevent high grade cervical lesions. *N Engl J Med.* 2007;356:1915-1927.

63. Harper DM, Franco EL, Wheeler CM et al. Sustained efficacy up to 4.5 years of a bivalent L1 virus-like particle vaccine against human papillomavirus types 16

and 18: follow-up from a randomized control trial. *Lancet.* 2006.367(9518): 1247-1255.

64. Smith JF, Brownlow M, Brown M, et al. Antibodies from women immunized with Gardasil cross-neutralize HPV 45 pseudovirions. *Hum Vaccin.* 2007; 3(4):109-115.

65. Villa LL, Costa RL, Petta CA, et al. High sustained efficacy of a prophylactic quadrivalent human papillomavirus types 6/11/1618 L1 virus-like particle vaccine through 5 years of follow-up. *Br J Canc.* 2006;95:1450-1466.

66. La Torre G, de Waure C, Chiaradia G, et al. HPV vaccine efficacy in preventing persistent cervical HPV infection: a systematic review and meta-analysis. *Vaccine.* 2007;25:8352-8358.

67. Centers for Disease Control and Prevention. Quadrivalent human papillomavirus vaccine: recommendations of the Advisory Committee on Immunization Practices (ACIP). *MMWR.* 2007;56(RR-2):1-26.

68. Path HPV vaccine adoption in developing countries: cost and financing issues. http://www.iavi.org/file.cfm?fid=47496. Accessed June 12, 2008.

69. Brewer NT, Fazekas KI. Predictors of HPV vaccine acceptability: a theory-informed, systematic review. *Prev Med.* 2007;45(2/3):107-114.

70. Jheeta M, Newall J. Childhood vaccination in Africa and Asia: the effects of parents' knowledge and attitudes. *Bull WHO.* 2008;86(6):419.

71. VAERS. http://www.nvic.org/Diseases/HPV/HPVrpt.htm. Accessed June 19, 2008.

72. Moraros J, Bird Y, Barney DD, et al. A pilot study: HPV infection knowledge and HPV vaccine acceptance among women residing in Ciudad Juárez, México. *Calif J Health Prom.* 2006;4(3):177-186.

73. Chan SS, Cheung TH, Lo W, Chung T. Women's attitudes on human papillomavirus vaccination to their daughters. *J Adolesc Health.* 2007;41(2):204-207.

74. Kwan TTC, Chan KKL, Yip AMW, et al. Barriers and facilitators to human papillomavirus vaccination among Chinese adolescent girls in Hong Kong: a qualitative-quantitative study. *Sex Transm Infect.* 2008;84(3):227-232.

75. Kim D, Canh DG, Poulos C, et al. Private demand for cholera vaccines in Hue, Vietnam. *Value Health.* 2008;12(1):119-128.

76. Jacob M, Bradley J, Barone MA. Human papillomavirus vaccines: what does the future hold for preventing cervical cancer in resource-poor settings through immunization programs? *Sex Transm Dis.* 2005;32(10):635-640.

77. Biddlecom A, Bankole A, and Patterson K. Vaccine for cervical cancer: reaching adolescents in sub-Saharan Africa. *Lancet.* 2006;367(9519):1299-300.

78. Path. *Vaccine Project Fact Sheet.* http://www.rho.org/files/PATH_CC_vaccine _project_fact_sheet_update_Dec_07.pdf. Accessed June 20, 2008.

79. Zimet GD, Liddon N, Rosenthal SL, et al. Psychosocial aspects of vaccine acceptability. *Vaccine.* 2006;24(Suppl 3):201-209.

80. Lazcano-Ponce E, Rivera L, Arillo-Santillan E, Salmeron J, Hernandez-Avila M, Munoz N. Acceptability of a human papillomavirus (HPV) trial vaccine among mothers of adolescents in Cuernavaca, Mexico. *Arch Med Res.* 2001;32(3):243-247.

81. Dinh TA, Rosenthal ST, Doan ED, et al. Attitudes of mothers in Da Nang, Vietnam, toward a human papillomavirus vaccine. *J Adolesc Health.* 2007;40: 559-563.

82. Lee PW, Kwan TT, Tan KF, et al. Beliefs about cervical cancer and human papillomavirus (HPV) and acceptability of HPV vaccination among Chinese women in Hong Kong. *Prev Med.* 2007;45(2-3):130-134.

83. Baykal CA, Al A, Ugur MG, et al. Knowledge and interest of Turkish women

about cervical cancer and HPV vaccine. *Eur J Gynaecol Oncol.* 2008;29(1): 76-79.

84. Wong WC, Lee A, Tsang KK. Correlates of sexual behaviors with health status and health perception in Chinese adolescents: a cross-sectional survey in schools. *AIDS Patient Care STDS.* 2004;18:470-480.

85. Boodman SG. Faith lets some kids skip shot. *The Washington Post.* June 10, 2008; HE01.

86. Matthews JR. *Quantification and the Quest for Medical Certainty.* New Jersey: Princeton; 1995.

87. Lambert SM, Markel H. Thomas Francis Jr., M.D. and the 1954 Salk Poliomyelitis vaccine field trial. *Arch Pediatr Adolesc Med.* 2000;154(5):512-517.

88. Ross S, Grant A, Counsell C, Gillespie W, Russell I, Prescott R. Barriers to participation in randomized controlled trials. *J Clin Epidemiol.* 1999:52(12): 1143-1156.

89. Kaljee L, Pham V, Son ND, et al. Trial participation and vaccine desirability for Vi polysaccharide typhoid fever vaccine in Hue City, Vietnam. *Trop Med Int Health.* 2007;12(1):25-36.

90. Sur D, Manna B, Chakrabarty N, et al. Vaccine desirability during an effectiveness trial of the typhoid fever polysaccharide Vi vaccine, Kolkata, India (manuscript submitted).

91. WHO-UNAIDS Expert Group. Gender, age, and ethnicity in HIV vaccine related trials. Report from a WHO-UNAIDS consultation, August 26-28, 2004; Lausanne; Switzerland. *AIDS* 2005;19(17):7-28.

92. Cook IF. Sexual dimorphism of humoral immunity with human vaccines. *Vaccines.* 2008; doi: 10.1016/j.vaccine.2008.04.054.

93. Sia D, Kobiane JF, Sondo BK, Fournier P. Individual and environmental characteristics associated with immunization of children in rural areas in Burkina Faso: a multi-level analysis. (English Abstract). *Sante.* 2007;17(4):201-206.

94. Kaljee L, Genberg B, von Seidlein VD, et al. Issues of acceptability and accessibility of a shigellosis vaccine, Nha Trang, Vietnam. *J Health Popul Nutr.* 2004;22:150-158.

95. Gwatkin DR, Deveshwar-Bahl G. Immunization coverage inequalities: an overview of socio-economic and gender differentials in developing countries. World Bank. http://siteresources.worldbank.org/INTPAH/Resources/Publications/Recent-Papers/8970_Imm._Paper_-_Text_(Final)_gwatkin.pdf. Accessed June 19, 2008.

96. Nganwai P, Truadpon P, Inpa C, et al. Knowledge, attitudes and practices vis-a-vis cervical cancer among registered nurses at the faculty of medicine, Khon Kaen University, Thailand. *Asian Pac J Cancer Prev.* 2008;9(1):15-18.

97. Aldrich T, Becker D, Garcia SG, et al. Mexican physicians' knowledge and attitudes about the human papillomavirus and cervical cancer: a national survey. *Sex Transm Infect.* 2005;1(2):135-141.

98. Hawkes N. *The Times.* GlaxoSmithKline wins NHS contract to supply cervical cancer vaccine. http://www.timesonline.co.uk/tol/life_and_style/health/article4166423.ece. Accessed June 20, 2008.

99. Stein R. Cervical cancer vaccine gets injected with a social issue. *The Washington Post.* October 31, 2005; A03.

100. Zimet GD. Improving adolescent health: focus on HPV vaccine acceptance. *J Adolesc Health.* 2005;37(6S):S17.

101. Bardenheier B, Ysuf H, Schwartz B, et al. Are parental vaccine safety concerns

associated with receipt of measles-mumps-rubella, diphtheria and tetanus toxoids with acellular pertussis, or hepatitis B vaccines by children? *Arch Pediatr Adolesc Med.* 2004;158(6):569-575.

102. Allred NJ, Shaw KM, Santibanez TA, et al. Parental vaccine safety concerns: results from the National Immunization Survey, 2001-2002. *Am J Prev Med.* 2005;28(2):221-224.

103. Plotkin SA. Vaccines, vaccination, and vaccinology. *J Infect Dis.* 2003;187: 1349-1359.

CHAPTER 25

Infectious Diseases and Women's Human Rights

Natasha Anandaraja, MD;
Nils Henning, MD, PhD

Natasha Anandaraja, MD, is an Assistant Professor in the Department of Medical Education in Mt. Sinai School of Medicine, New York, NY.

Nils Henning, MD, PhD, is an Assistant Professor of Community and Preventive Medicine in the Department of Pediatric Infectious Diseases at the Mount Sinai School of Medicine, New York, NY.

Gender Equity

In the arena of infectious disease, the rights of women are best examined through the study of gender equity. The term *gender* encompasses those aspects of being male or female that are determined by society, rather than biology, and that translate into the "experience" of being male or female with its attendant roles and expectations. An individual's experience of gender will therefore vary according to cultural context and at different stages along the life continuum.

When looking at health from a human rights perspective, *equity* is the standard by which we assess justice in the allocation of health resources and in health outcomes.

Gender equity in health refers not only to fairness in the allocation of resources between men and women but to recognition of the different attributes and vulnerabilities of male and female gender and the appropriate design of health interventions to ensure equity of healthcare access and health outcomes.[1]

Gender Analysis in Infectious Disease

The importance of the "gender agenda" in the control of infectious disease has been increasingly recognized in the fields of tropical medicine, communicable disease, and global public health. There has been a call for the integration of gender-sensitive programming at all levels of health and development programming.[2-5] So-called mainstreaming of gender equity in health is described as involving two core approaches: "(1) integrating gender and equity into ongoing monitoring and evaluation strategies and related research, and (2) training and resources to develop, implement, and evaluate ways to promote resilience to communicable disease and the ability to access quality preventive and curative care for different groups of men and women."[2] The extent to which stated commitments to mainstreaming of gender actually translate into policy or programmatic change is variable.[6] However, gender issues are increasingly represented in health literature, research, and policy. The

World Health Organization (WHO) and the Special Programme for Research and Training in Tropical Diseases have developed conceptual frameworks for "gender analysis" of communicable disease.[5,7] Gender analysis attempts to shift our focus from biological differences in vulnerability and response to disease toward differences in gender-related experiences of health and healthcare. This involves asking questions about the effect of gender on exposure and vulnerability to disease, perception of illness and health-seeking behavior, diagnosis, access to and utilization of healthcare, experience of stigma, and health outcomes. Gender analysis ultimately attempts to identify points along the illness and health-seeking continuum that are marked by gender disparities and are therefore potential targets for intervention.

Gender, Infectious Disease, and Poverty

Gender inequity in health is driven by a long history of social inequality and structural violence against women. Women's lack of social capital often translates into economic disadvantage, thus the interaction between poverty and infectious disease becomes an important consideration. As of 2001, 1.2 billion people were living in extreme poverty,[8] and the majority of these were women.[9] Despite the existence of effective prevention and treatment strategies, 5 of the 10 leading causes of death in low- and middle-income countries are infectious diseases, including lower respiratory infections, HIV/AIDS, diarrheal diseases, tuberculosis, and malaria.[10] This is not surprising given the links between infectious disease and overcrowding, malnutrition, and poor sanitation. Although poverty is not unique to women, social inequality renders women who are living in poverty more vulnerable to its disadvantages. The 1979 Convention on the Elimination of All Forms of Discrimination Against Women (CEDAW) states: "In situations of poverty, women have the least access to food, health, education, training, and opportunities for employment and other needs."[11]

The costs that female morbidity and premature mortality inflict on society should not be underestimated. In addition to the loss of economic productivity (women are responsible for up to 80% of food production and 60% of household income globally[12]), there is substantial cost in loss of care for children and sick household members. Studies in Columbia showed that although women's disease burden from malaria was lower than that of men in the same community, their additional work burden, the amount of time lost to sick episodes, and therefore the additional indirect economic burden of the disease on the individual and community was greater for women.[13] Given the correlation between maternal death and early childhood mortality, female mortality from infectious disease has a double impact on family well-being. These indirect costs of female ill-health are difficult to estimate and are not fully reflected in mortality statistics or lost disability-adjusted life years (DALYs), but must be considered in estimations of the global impact of women's infectious disease.

Gender disparities in infectious disease are difficult to quantify owing to a general lack of sex-disaggregated data, especially from those countries with the highest burden of communicable disease.[3] Qualitative data on the influence of gender is even rarer. In this chapter we explore the effect of female gender on the experience of infectious disease using existing data on five tropical communicable conditions. Tuberculosis, perhaps the most extensively studied of the five, is reviewed through the lens of the gender analysis framework. An overview of gender-related issues is also provided for malaria, leprosy, filariasis, and leishmaniasis. We discuss potential gender-based interventions for infectious disease control and future research directions. Our discussion is focused on data from resource-poor countries as the burden of morbidity and mortality for these largely "neglected" diseases is observed predominantly in these settings.

Tuberculosis

Tuberculosis is a disease of poverty; among the poor and under-privileged, poor women are at greatest risk, and they face the greatest obstacles to seeking complete cure.

—Dinesh M. Nair[14]

Tuberculosis is a bacterial infection caused by *Mycobacterium tuberculosis* (MTB). MTB is spread through inhalation of infectious droplets, and therefore transmission is related to crowding and proximity to infectious or sputum-positive cases. Infection results in primary disease that triggers a host immune response resulting in suppression of the infection to a latent state within the body. Progression to active disease is most common in the two years immediately following infection and is often precipitated by changes in immune function, most notable being that of acquisition of the AIDS virus. An infected individual's lifetime risk of progression to active TB ranges from 5–20%, compared to a 10% *annual* risk in HIV-positive individuals.[15] Active infection most commonly affects the lungs (pulmonary TB or PTB) but can also manifest in extrapulmonary sites, such as bone, genital, and lymphatic disease. The gold standard for MTB diagnosis is sputum culture, but in resource-poor and endemic settings diagnosis is made on clinical assessment, by chest radiography or identification of MTB bacteria on smear microscopy. Treatment of uncomplicated disease involves six months of therapy with a combination of antituberculosis medications. The WHO standard for therapy is directly observed therapy short-course (DOTS) based on voluntary presentation of patients to public health services, diagnosis by smear microscopy, and six months of daily or thrice weekly medication administered by healthcare workers to ensure compliance. On a population level, the DOTS strategy has been deemed effective and cost-effective,[16] with global cure rates of 84% in 2005, but case detection rates lower than projected at only 60%.[17] However, despite its success as a public health measure, the DOTS strategy does not necessarily deliver equitable care for those most at risk of marginalization, among whom women must be considered predominant.

TB Epidemiology

It is estimated that one-third of the world's population is infected with tuberculosis. In 2005, 1.6 million people died of TB. The link between TB and poverty is strong; about 90% of the burden of TB morbidity and mortality occurs in developing countries,[18] with 7.4 million of an estimated 8.8 million new TB cases in 2005 occurring in Asia and sub-Saharan Africa.[17] Globally, TB is the second leading cause of death due to infectious disease,[19] and it is the leading cause of death due to infectious disease in women; half a million women die every year from TB. In 2002, TB accounted for 2.0% of all deaths in women, ahead of maternal conditions (1.9%) and breast cancer (1.8%).[18] In 2001, TB was responsible for the loss of 35.87 million DALYs, representing 2.6% of the total global DALY burden.[10] Although TB accounts for a significant proportion of the global burden of lost DALYs, this measurement fails to recognize the broader detrimental effects that a woman's TB has on her family and community. This is especially significant as the greatest burden of TB mortality occurs in women aged 15–44 years, those at their most productive age, economically and reproductively.[20]

Gender Differentials in TB

Prevalence Globally, tuberculosis prevalence is lower in women than in men. The global ratio of male to female cases in 2007 was 1.8:1.0, with a greater discrepancy in Asian than African regions (see Table 25-1).[17] However, whether this represents an *actual* difference in prevalence based on greater biological risk and exposure in males or an *apparent* difference related to underreporting of female cases is still debated. Multiple studies from industrialized countries with well-developed reporting systems in the mid-1900s demonstrated equivalent passive notification rates in males and females until adolescence, with rates 10–35% higher in females in their mid-twenties to early thirties. However, recent studies of TB infection in developing countries with overall notification rates similar to the industrialized countries in the mid-1900s show equivalent rates of TB in males and females prior to 14 years of age giving way to higher rates in males from that age onward.[21] The discrepancy between historical and current data raises concerns regarding underreporting of female cases. Although the consistency of male dominance in TB notification data across global regions and socio-economic settings makes it less likely that underreporting is solely responsible for the male:female prevalence differential, the indication that female TB cases are going undetected cannot be ignored.

TABLE 25-1

Male-Female Ratio in Smear-Positive Case Notification by WHO Region, 2005	
WHO World Region	**Male:Female Ratio**
Africa	1.3
The Americas	1.6
Eastern Mediterranean	1.2
Europe	2.1
Southeast Asia	2.0
Western Pacific	2.2
Global	1.8

Source: WHO, 2007. Geneva, Switzerland: World Health Organization.[17]

TB Exposure Gender disparity in rates of TB infection and disease first appear in adolescence.[21] This disparity has been related to culturally based differentiation of gender roles at the onset of adulthood, resulting in changes to male and female patterns of exposure to TB and to changes in health-seeking behavior. In their teenage years girls in many cultures become socially restricted to the home and household activities, while men take on work and responsibilities outside of the immediate household. It has been proposed that this wider social exposure approximates to a greater risk of exposure to TB in men. There is some support for this theory in a study demonstrating that Indian women who work outside the home have TB rates approaching those of men in the same community.[6] However, gender roles often assign women the task of looking after the sick, so in regions of high TB prevalence a woman's risk of daily close contact with active TB cannot be underestimated.[22] The drop-off in female incidence in adolescence corresponds with entrance into marriageable age; fears that detection of TB will decrease marriage prospects may also lead to decreased health-seeking behavior and diagnosis.

TB Health Seeking Delays in presentation to healthcare significantly affect the course and outcome of TB. Women with symptoms of TB take longer to present to healthcare services than men.

Women may perceive TB symptoms or TB disease as less significant or curable in themselves compared to men. In Vietnam, women's TB was believed to have a genetic or mental health component, and therefore regarded as less curable and less serious than TB disease in men.[23]

Limited access to health education also contributes to delayed recognition of symptoms and late presentation to health care. Because of their work burden, women in rural India were less likely than men to be reached by mass media public health announcements, or to cite health facilities as sources of information. Women were also less optimistic about treatment outcomes, and less likely to seek appropriate levels of care for TB symptoms.[24] A study in Pakistan revealed low levels of knowledge about TB symptoms among rural females, and significantly less knowledge about the importance of completing treatment among women compared to men.[25] Studies in Pakistan also reveal that access to healthcare facilities is restricted by women's reliance on male family members for mobility.[26] Dependence on men for permission to seek care or start treatment is a real consideration in the many developing countries where men are the sole decision makers for family health issues (see Figure 25-1).[12]

Studies from multiple countries demonstrate that women are less likely to access public health facilities than men. Women often present first, and sometimes solely, to private or traditional healers, or use pharmacies rather than medical clinics for medical advice and medication. Reasons for this include discomfort with male physicians, discomfort with attitudes of public healthcare workers in general, unacceptable levels of privacy at public facilities, and poor access to these facilities due to distance, timing of opening hours, or costs.[7,24,27-34] Delay in reaching public facilities because of initial interactions with private services has been shown to lead to delay in diagnosis and treatment of TB.[34,35] Reliance on private services, unregulated by governmental standards and often not DOTS-based, can result in suboptimal care. Private facilities often rely on diagnosis by chest radiograph rather than sputum microscopy and may not prescribe an effective regimen of medications. Costs of medication within the private sector may also prohibit completion of a full course of treatment. Moreover, the majority of cases that are treated in the private sector are presumably not reported to

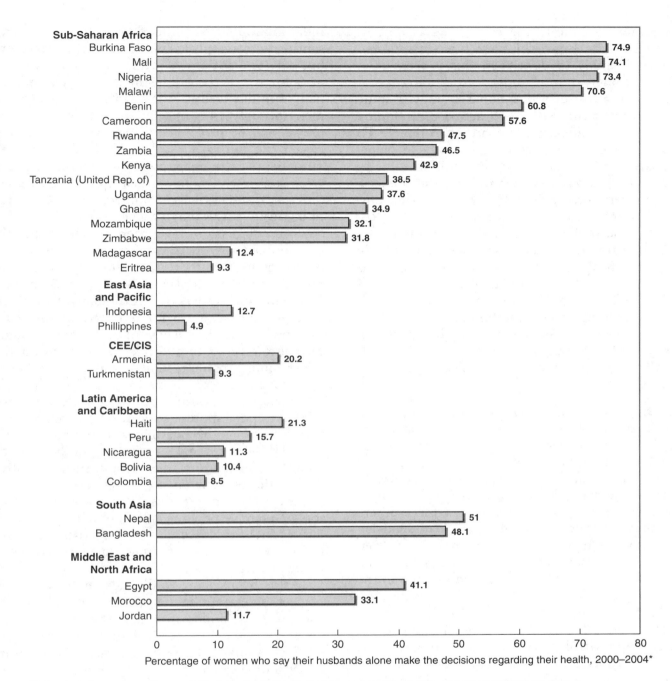

Sub-Saharan Africa

Country	Value
Burkina Faso	74.9
Mali	74.1
Nigeria	73.4
Malawi	70.6
Benin	60.8
Cameroon	57.6
Rwanda	47.5
Zambia	46.5
Kenya	42.9
Tanzania (United Rep. of)	38.5
Uganda	37.6
Ghana	34.9
Mozambique	32.1
Zimbabwe	31.8
Madagascar	12.4
Eritrea	9.3

East Asia and Pacific

Country	Value
Indonesia	12.7
Phillippines	4.9

CEE/CIS

Country	Value
Armenia	20.2
Turkmenistan	9.3

Latin America and Caribbean

Country	Value
Haiti	21.3
Peru	15.7
Nicaragua	11.3
Bolivia	10.4
Colombia	8.5

South Asia

Country	Value
Nepal	51
Bangladesh	48.1

Middle East and North Africa

Country	Value
Egypt	41.1
Morocco	33.1
Jordan	11.7

Percentage of women who say their husbands alone make the decisions regarding their health, 2000–2004*

*Data refer to the most recent year available during the period specified. All countries with available data are presented in the chart.

FIGURE 25-1   Many husbands are making decisions alone on their wife's health.
From The State of the World's Children 2007: Women and children—The double dividend of gender equality. UNICEF, 2006.

local governmental health authorities, and women attending these services are therefore unrepresented in national TB notification data.

Passive case finding, dependent on a patient's recognition of his or her symptoms and health-seeking behavior, is the basis of the global TB con-trol strategy. Data from passive case finding reflects TB "notification" rates, rather than true incidence. One should approximate the other where there are negligible barriers to accessing diagnostic services and where physician care is equitable and diagnostic services are of good quality. However this is not necessarily the case in environments where TB is most prevalent, and women are often more vulnerable to deficits in this process than men. Although routine active case finding is not regarded as a cost-effective global strategy,[36] some studies comparing passive to active case finding have found significant discrepancies in female TB rates using the two methods. A study in Nepal compared active case finding by mobile teams to case finding through self-referral to local services. Of self-referred cases only 28% were female, compared to 46% among the active case finding cohort.[37] A second study in rural Nepal found that the proportion of female cases rose from 35% in clinics and health posts to 53% in microscopy outreach camps.[38] Development of regional models of TB epidemiology based on current trends suggest that adding active case finding to the DOTS strategy could decrease TB mortality by up to one-third overall.[36] It can be extrapolated that a significant proportion of these averted deaths would be female.

TB Diagnosis   Once women present to health care, they can expect a higher rate of diagnostic delay than men. Females in rural China experienced a health system delay six times that of males.[35] In Vietnam, healthcare provider delay to diagnosis was longer for women despite similar health-seeking behavior; 5.4 weeks for women, 3.8 weeks for men.[39] In Malaysia, patient delay was also found to be more common in women than men, although there was no recognized social status difference between men and women in the community under study.[40]

Many reasons have been cited for gender discrepancy in TB diagnostic delay. Acceptance of male symptomatology as a normative presentation for TB may lead to female cases going unrecognized. Women with sputum-positive TB are less likely to present with the "typical" symptoms of cough, hemoptysis, and sputum production.[34] In Vietnam, absence of cough and sputum expectoration in women was directly linked to increased doctor delays.[41]

Reliance on sputum positivity to detect TB also underestimates female disease incidence. Numerous studies have found that women have a lower sputum submission rate and lower sputum positivity rate than males. A review of management of over 2000 patients at a nongovernmental clinic in

India found that two out of every three men presenting with symptoms was given a sputum exam, but only one out of every three women with similar symptoms received testing.[7] Similarly, in Vietnam, sputum testing was carried out in 36% of men and only 14% of women in a setting where prevalence of prolonged cough was similar between the two groups.[28] In Bangladesh, among outpatients with respiratory symptoms, women were less likely to have their sputum examined (OR 0.72), and if it was examined, it was less likely to be positive (OR 0.64).[33] Discrepancy in rates of sputum submission have been related to healthcare worker bias, social constraints on women expectorating in public, inability of females to provide sputum samples without permission from male family members, lack of independent transport preventing return for repeated sputum submission, lower frequency of productive cough, refusal to give sputum due to social stigma, and a belief among patients that chest x-ray is better than sputum for diagnosis of TB.[7,34,42] The gender disparity in sputum positivity rates has been related to poor sputum expectoration technique in females and to the possibility of sex-related biological differences in TB pathology, both of which could render sputum microscopy a less sensitive diagnostic test in women.

Difficulties in relationships between male doctors and female patients and a propensity to spend limited household funds on diagnostic tests for males were also found to hinder diagnosis of TB in female patients.[42]

Aside from failure to diagnose pulmonary TB, neglect of extrapulmonary forms of the disease leads to gross underestimation of overall TB incidence in women. Of particular importance is genital TB, estimated to be the causative factor in up to 19% of cases of female infertility in the developing world.[43] Genital TB often goes undiagnosed because of chronic nonspecific presenting symptoms and lack of simple diagnostic techniques.

TB Treatment and Adherence   Once women begin treatment they have better rates of adherence than men.[34] Reasons for treatment default among women often relate to household pressures or social stigma. In Bombay, India, men dropped out because of pressures to return to work or because of alcohol or drug addiction, whereas women dropped out because of the strain of keeping their diagnosis secret from family members.[14] Concerns regarding taking medications during pregnancy and lactation also affect women's adherence to treatment. One study from the Philippines tracked a high default rate among pregnant and lactating women to a fear of milk "drying up" or harm to the unborn infant.[44]

The DOTS program is the foundation of the WHO Stop TB Strategy, and as of 2005 was being applied in 187 countries.[17] However, it is not necessarily an appropriate model of service delivery for women, necessitating frequent travel to clinics and exposing women to stigma incurred by the frequent visits of health workers to their homes. In South India, social stigma was cited as a reason for not receiving DOTS more commonly among women than men, and was associated with treatment failure.[45] In Maharastra, a majority of women (85%) reported that the DOTS program was inconvenient for them because of responsibilities for young children, travel expenses, transport problems, difficulty in walking to the clinic, or weakness. Swallowing medications in front of male staff was also unacceptable.[31] Similarly in Pakistan, women cited cost and duration of travel, as well as social constraints on traveling alone as reasons for treatment default.[26] It is notable that despite evidence of the impact of gender on access to TB care, gender-specific barriers and their implications for effective TB control are not addressed in the DOTS strategy and receive no mention as of 2007 in the annual WHO report on global tuberculosis control. [17]

TB Stigma and Social Consequences

In many cultures the social consequences associated with the diagnosis of TB fall most heavily upon women. Difficulties in finding a marriage partner, or divorce or abandonment among those already married were significant consequences for women in Pakistan, Vietnam, India, and the Gambia.[14,20,24,27,30,46] Fear of social consequences can translate into delayed or absent health-seeking behavior: in Vietnam fear of social isolation was cited as the main reason for delaying seeking of treatment among women,[27] whereas for males delay was related more strongly to the economic consequences of treatment. A similar pattern was reported in rural India.[24] Unmarried urban Indian women, less likely than men to be self-employed, feared loss of employment in addition to loss of

marriage opportunities.[14] In India there was greater perceived support for married men and single women than married women or single men. Men expected and received care from their wives, but married women were often abandoned by the family that they had married into.[20,24] In the Gambia, women perceived more stigmatization than men and therefore put greater value on anonymity during medical interactions.[30] A WHO multicountry study reported increased potential for stigmatization among TB patients in Malawi due to the growing association of TB with HIV.[34] This added burden of social stigma can be expected by TB patients throughout the developing world as rates of HIV, especially among young women, increase. HIV infection is now considered a major factor responsible for increasing rates of TB disease in women of reproductive age both in developing countries and in industrialized nations such as the United States.[47]

TB Outcomes

In general, women who receive antituberculosis therapy have better outcomes in terms of treatment completion and cure then men.[48] However, women of reproductive age are at increased risk of progression from latent TB infection to active disease compared with men in the same age group. A study from Bangalore in the 1970s actively screened participants with TB infections for progression to active disease. The study demonstrated 130% greater risk of progression from latent to active disease in women between the ages of 10 and 44 years compared to men.[21] The reasons for this discrepancy remain unclear. It is possible that higher rates of reporting occur in a woman's reproductive years because of her increased interaction with the health system during pregnancy, childbirth, and child health visits. However, this would not have been an influence in the Bangalore study, which carried out active case finding. The increase in progression may be related to changes in immune status during pregnancy, but a clear link between pregnancy and increased incidence of TB has not been found.[21,49] Higher mortality and higher case fatality has also been reported in women of reproductive age. The aforementioned Bangalore study reported case fatality rates 27–41% higher in untreated women and girls between 5 and 24 years of age compared to men.[21] Again, the reason for this discrepancy in unknown, but may be related to diagnostic delay,

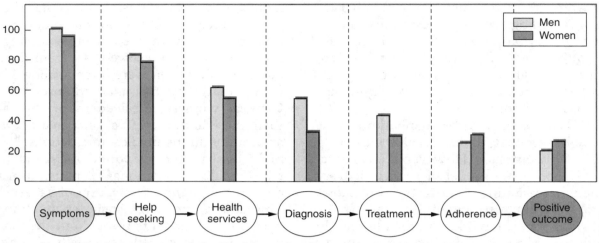

Stepwise barriers and tentative indication of the number of men and women reaching each step in the recognition, treatment, and cure of TB.

FIGURE 25-2   Stepwise model of attrition in the course of TB control.
From Uplekar, M. W., S. Rangan, et al. Attention to gender issues in tuberculosis control. *Int J Tuberc Lung Dis.* 2001;5(3): 220–224.

late presentation, or poor nutritional status. In pregnancy, TB that is treated early and adequately has outcomes equivalent to those in nonpregnant women. However, studies have reported a four-fold increase in obstetric mortality with increased incidence of spontaneous abortion and preeclampsia, and a nine-fold increase in preterm labor in cases where TB was diagnosed late.[50] Adverse perinatal outcomes for infants born to mothers with inadequately treated or advanced active TB have also been reported with significantly increased rates of prematurity, low birth weight, small for gestational age, and perinatal death.[51,52]

Summary

Gender analysis identifies several points along the continuum of tuberculosis diagnosis and care at which women are lost because of gender-specific obstacles. Figure 25-2 provides a graphic representation of this process of attrition.

Malaria

Women have the greatest responsibility for caring for those who fall ill from malaria,

yet in most endemic countries these same women have the least access to information, decision making power, and financial resources that would allow for effective disease prevention and treatment at the community level.

—Dr. Awa Marie Coll-Seck, Executive
Secretary of the Roll Back Malaria
Partnership[53]

Malaria is a communicable disease caused by four species of the *Plasmodium* parasite: *P. malariae*, *P. falciparum*, *P. vivax*, and *P. ovale*. Humans serve as the reservoir for malarial disease. The parasite is transmitted between humans by the female *Anopheles* mosquito, and once inside the human host it undergoes a series of changes as part of its complex life cycle. Its various stages allow the parasite to evade the human immune system, infect the liver and red blood cells, and infect a mosquito again when it bites an infected person. Malaria symptoms appear 9 to 21 days after the infection. Malaria produces fever, headache, vomiting, and flulike symptoms. The infection can progress rapidly and become life threatening, especially when caused by *P. falciparum*. Malaria usually kills by infecting and destroying red blood cells (anemia) and by clogging the capillaries that carry blood to the brain (cerebral malaria).[53]

Malaria Epidemiology

Malaria is present in over 100 countries around the world and threatens half the world's population, mainly in tropical Asia, Africa, and Latin America. Malaria was a serious threat in much of Europe and North Africa until recent decades. Although a worldwide program to eradicate malaria was launched in 1955, more people are dying of malaria now than in the 1950s. Every year, 350 to 500 million cases of malaria occur worldwide, more than 90% of them in tropical Africa.[54] Malaria causes an estimated 700,000 to 2.7 million deaths each year, mainly (greater than 75%) among African children.[55] The child death rate from malaria doubled between 1990 and 2002.[56] Today, malaria remains the single largest cause of death for children under 5 years in Africa, where it kills one child every 30 seconds—this translates to the deaths of approximately 3000 children every day. The World Bank ranks the disease as the leading cause of lost DALYs in Africa.[57]

Today, Roll Back Malaria (RBM), a priority project established by the cabinet of the WHO in 1998, has the more modest goal of malaria control. The objectives of RBM are a 50% reduction in malaria-associated mortality by 2010 and another 50% reduction by 2015.[58] The RBM strategy calls for the following:

1. Disease management through prompt and affordable access to effective treatment, including artemisinin-based combination therapy (ACT)

2. Disease prevention through personal and community protective measures, primarily increased access to insecticide-treated bed nets (ITN)

3. Targeted disease control and prevention for pregnant women with intermittent preventive treatment (IPT)

4. Epidemic control through early detection and response[58]

There are a number of reasons why the achievement of these objectives is highly unlikely, including lack of political will, lack of funding, war, and local differences in parasites, vectors, epidemiologic situation, national capacity and interest, and community participation. The prevalence and geographical range of malaria have actually increased in recent years, facilitated in part by tourism, migrant workers, refugees from conflict areas, and other travel. There has been resurgence of the disease in countries in temperate zones where it has previously been controlled, such as Azerbaijan, Turkey, Tajikistan, and Iraq.[59] Other factors responsible for the spread of malaria are environmental; they include changes in land use and global climate.[60] Antimalarial vaccines are currently not available (although considered an achievable goal),[61] and widescale chemoprophylaxis is not recommended because of the development of drug resistance, cost, and sustainability.[58] IPT, in which pregnant women, infants and children are presumptively treated with antimalarial drugs at specific intervals, has shown success and is gaining acceptance. ITNs have proven in numerous studies to be highly effective in reducing childhood mortality and morbidity from malaria. Challenges for the future include guaranteeing access for affordable ACT treatment and developing a scheme to subsidize treatments and prevention for those who can't afford it. Recently the Bill and Melinda Gates Foundation brought a campaign for malaria eradication back to the table.

Gender Differentials in Malaria

The risk of acquiring malaria infection and developing the disease depends on a number of factors. In highly endemic areas limited immunity develops in adults due to constant reinfection. Those at highest risk of severe disease are infants and children aged six months to five years who have not yet developed immunity, pregnant women who have depressed immune function, populations in unstable malarial areas, and individuals from non-malarial areas who enter malaria endemic areas (migrant workers, displaced persons, travelers).[62] The decreased immunity of pregnant women more than doubles their chances of contracting and dying of malaria.[63] Pregnant women who contract malaria have an increased risk for severe maternal anemia and the consequent impaired fetal growth contributes to low birth weight in newborns. Malaria during pregnancy causes 10,000 maternal deaths each year, 8–14% of all low birth weight babies, and 3–8% of all infant deaths in certain parts of Africa.[63] Pregnant women are more "attractive" to mosquitoes, possibly due to a 21% increase in exhaled air and 0.7°C increase in body heat that make them easier to detect by mosquitoes. Pregnant women are therefore more likely to be bitten, increasing their exposure to malaria.[64,65]

Gender roles play a major part in determining exposure to mosquitoes. Women's household responsibilities such as cooking the evening meal outside, or waking up for household tasks before sunrise, put them at risk of malaria infection.[66,67] Use of insecticide-treated nets (ITN) is strongly linked to culturally accepted sleeping patterns. If a household has only one net, priority is often given to the male head of household, therefore putting women and children at higher risk.[53] In some cultures, wives leave the matrimonial bed midway through pregnancy to sleep on the floor, leaving them unprotected against mosquito bites when they are most vulnerable.[53]

Proven methods for reducing death and disease due to malaria in pregnant women do exist. A study in Kenya has shown that women protected by ITNs every night during their first four pregnancies have 25% less underweight or premature babies.[53] A study in Malawi evaluating IPT showed a decrease in placental malaria infection from 32% to 23% and a decline of low birth weight babies from 23% to 10%.[53,68] When offered, 75% of all pregnant women took IPT.[68]

Malaria and HIV/AIDS coinfection is a health problem that is only recently gaining recognition. Both diseases take their greatest toll among poor populations living in developing countries. Women make up a relatively larger proportion of poor populations than men, and are also overrepresented in the malaria and HIV/AIDS coinfection group.[53] People living with HIV/AIDS have twice the risk of developing malaria compared with HIV-negative individuals.[53] HIV/AIDS also decreases the response to standard malaria treatment and IPT. As a cause of anemia, malaria frequently leads to blood transfusion, which is in itself a risk factor for HIV infection. Malaria also leads to a higher HIV viral load, increasing the rate of mother-to-child transmission of HIV during pregnancy and breast feeding.[53] HIV/AIDS impairs treatment of malaria during pregnancy, increasing the risk of anemia in the mother, premature birth, intrauterine growth retardation, and low birth weight infants. Studies have demonstrated that the highest

negative synergy between malaria and HIV infections occurs among adolescent girls.[69]

Gender roles and relations within the household are of crucial importance to the management and prevention of malaria. Women's access to resources and their bargaining power within the household have a significant influence on their treatment-seeking behavior for themselves and for their children with malaria. A study in the Volta region in Ghana found that behavioral responses to malaria in children were influenced at the household level by the social and economic power of women and men at different levels of seniority.[62] Women who lacked short-term or long-term economic support from relatives, or who disagreed with their husbands or family elders, faced difficulties in accessing appropriate treatment for children with malaria. A study in Ethiopia showed that married women were willing to pay more to prevent malaria in their household than married men.[70] Elderly women who have greater decision-making powers and can mobilize younger women in the community have shown to be helpful in promoting the use of ITNs.[71]

Summary

In 2005 a gender and malaria statement at the RBM Partners' Forum acknowledged that the gender perspective in malaria research and malaria control has been neglected in the current global response to the disease.[72] It was concluded that both social and biological factors contribute to the different impact malaria has on women and men, both as patients and as caregivers, with women in Africa proving especially vulnerable. "A gender perspective is essential for substantial reduction and elimination of malaria. Malaria is not only a health and poverty issue—it is also a gender equality priority."[72]

Leprosy

Leprosy is a chronic infectious disease caused by *Mycobacteria leprae*. The leprae bacillus multiplies very slowly and the incubation period of the disease is approximately 5 years, with symptoms taking as long as 20 years to appear.[58] Leprosy can be transmitted via inhalation of infected droplets or through skin-to-skin contact; however, it is not a highly contagious disease and actual disease transmission requires close and frequent contacts with untreated cases.[73] If untreated, leprosy can be progressive, causing permanent damage to the skin, nerves, limbs, and eyes. The diagnosis of leprosy is made clinically and by histopathologic examination of tissue biopsy material.[58] Infected individuals require treatment for a long time after they feel well, complicating adherence. Past attempts to control leprosy with prolonged dapsone therapy failed, partly due to the development of resistance and the difficulty of ensuring multiple-year patient compliance. Multidrug treatment with two or three antimicrobial agents has lead to shorter treatment regimes, higher compliance, and success in fighting leprosy in the last 20 years. Still, the long incubation period, the possibility of transmission before becoming symptomatic, the cost of multidrug therapy, reduced international funding in fighting leprosy, and an apathy regarding the social conditions that breed the disease, make it likely for leprosy to continue to be a health threat for neglected populations in affected countries.

Leprosy causes enormous stigmatization, largely due to the disfigurement that it can produce and the belief in many cultures that it represents some form of divine punishment.[58] Therefore, psychological and social suffering are often as problematic as the physical aspects of the disease.

Leprosy Epidemiology

Leprosy was recognized in the ancient civilizations of China, Egypt, and India, and written mention of the disease dates back to 600 BCE. Leprosy was endemic in Europe during the Middle Ages, but had virtually disappeared by the 1700s. One theory is that the rise of TB in Europe, lead to cross-immunity to leprosy. This is supported by the observation that Bacille Calmette-Guerin (BCG), the vaccine intended to prevent the worst cases of TB in children, is effective in preventing leprosy.[58]

At the beginning of the new millennium, leprosy is still endemic in many low- and middle-income countries, particularly affecting the poorest segments of these societies. Overall, the global disease burden has dropped dramatically in recent years. While the WHO reported 5.2 million cases in 1985, approximately 410,000 new cases were detected during 2004, and 290,000 cases were undergoing treatment at the beginning of 2005.[74] Nine countries in Asia, Africa, and Latin America account for 75% of the global disease burden. India alone accounts for 55% of the burden, making it the country with the largest number of leprosy cases.[75,76] Other countries not meeting the leprosy elimination target set by the World Health Assembly (a prevalence rate of less than one case per 10,000 persons) are Brazil, Madagascar, Mozambique, and Nepal.[74]

Gender Differential in Leprosy

Although some countries such as Burkina Faso, Kenya, Uganda, and Malawi record a higher prevalence of leprosy in women, in the great majority of affected countries the incidence and case detection rates of leprosy in men are about twice that in women.[77-80] Recent studies indicate that female cases might be underreported. For example in Brazil, case detection of leprosy in females has been increasing since women started working outside the home, and the male to female ratio is now 1:1.[4] A study in Bangladesh showed a decrease in the male-to-female ratio, from 2.3 to 1.6, with the introduction of active case finding.[81] Interestingly this trend in case detection was not reflected in the 15–30 year age group. This is because of a combination of gender-related factors: reduced exposure to leprosy of women in this age group due to cultural restrictions in social activities, a fear of presenting for diagnosis because of the possibility of jeopardizing marriage prospects or of separation from husbands and children, and reluctance to present and be examined by male health workers.[81] In general, women present for treatment of leprosy later and consequently suffer more severe symptoms than men.[4] In Nigeria the period between first signs or symptoms and presentation for diagnosis in female leprosy patients was twice that of males.[82] As a result, they suffered a higher proportion of disabilities.[82] However, research also shows that nonpregnant women develop stronger and more effective immune reactions to subclinical disease than men.[77,83] Some data suggest higher rates of subclinical than overt infection in women, and that lower incidence and less severe clinical forms of the disease are associated with the presence of estrogen and other female hormones.[84] However, pregnancy weakens the immune system. A study in Ethiopia showed that combined effects of puberty and first pregnancy resulted in relapse in female participants.[85] Nerve damage was accelerated in pregnant and lactating women.[86] Congenital transmission is possible but rare.[87] Other studies show seemingly contrary results regarding differences in frequency and type of deformities seen in leprosy according to sex.[4] Males experience twice as many Grade I and Grade II deformities as women, while paradoxical immune reactions are more common among women.[77,87-89] These findings underline the need for further clinical and social research.

Summary

The experience of living with leprosy shows clear gender differences and has a greater negative impact on women. The proportion of illiterate and unemployed female leprosy patients is considerably higher than the proportion of illiterate and unemployed males.[90] While both men and women are negatively affected in terms of their family and marital lives, women suffer more isolation and rejection.[87] Psychologically, women are more vulnerable because they are deprived of personal contact with others in the domestic environment where they are accustomed to receiving their greatest emotional support.[87,91] Women report that indifference to them by other family members, or seeming negation of their presence, cause them the greatest suffering.[87] Support is critical for women, who often lack access to the variety of outside advice and assistance available to men.

Filariasis

The threadlike, parasitic filarial worms *Wuchereria bancrofti* and *Brugia malayi* that cause lymphatic filariasis live almost exclusively in humans. These worms lodge in the lymphatic system, where they live for four to six years, producing millions of immature microfilariae that circulate in the blood. Mosquitoes functioning as vectors bite infected humans and pick up the microfilariae, which develop, inside the mosquito, into the infective stage in a process that usually takes 7–21 days. The larvae then migrate to the mosquitoes' biting mouthparts, ready to enter the punctured skin of another human reservoir, thus completing the cycle.[92] Although the infection is generally acquired early in childhood, the disease may take years to manifest. In its most obvious manifestations, lymphatic filariasis, also known as elephantiasis, causes chronic lymphedema and enlargement of the entire leg or arm, the genitals, vulva, and breasts. Acute episodes of local inflammation involving skin, lymph nodes, and lymphatic vessels often accompany the chronic process. Inflammation is due in part to the body's immune response to the parasite, but is largely the result of bacterial infection of skin where normal defenses have been partially lost due to underlying lymphatic damage. The psychological and social stigmas associated with the disease are immense.

In endemic areas, chronic and acute manifestations of filariasis tend to develop sooner and more frequently in refugees or newcomers than in local populations that are continually exposed to infection. Lymphedema may develop within six months and elephantiasis as quickly as a year after arrival.[92] The disease also causes hidden, internal damage to the kidneys and the lymphatic system.[58] The psychological and social stigmas associated with the disease are immense.

Until recently, diagnosing lymphatic filariasis had been extremely difficult, since parasites had to be detected microscopically in the blood, and nocturnal periodicity restricts their appearance in the blood to the hours around midnight. However, the development of an antigen test using finger-prick blood droplets taken any time of the day, and which does not require laboratory facilities, has transformed the approach to diagnosis.[92]

The primary goal of treating affected communities is to eliminate microfilariae from the blood of infected individuals so that transmission of the infection by the mosquito can be interrupted. The use of single doses of two drugs administered concurrently (optimally albendazole with diethylcarbamazine or ivermectin) is 99% effective in removing microfilariae from the blood for a full year after treatment.[92] For individual treatment, both albendazole and DEC have been shown to be effective. It is clear that antiparasitic treatment can result in improvement of patients' elephantiasis and hydrocele especially in the early stages of disease, but the most significant advancement in treatment of those with elephantiasis arose from the recognition that much of the progression in pathology results from bacterial and fungal "super-infection" of tissues with compromised lymphatic function. Rigorous hygiene of the affected limbs, with accompanying adjunctive measures to minimize infection and promote lymph flow, has shown the best results in reducing the frequency of acute episodes of inflammation ("filarial fevers") and in improving the elephantiasis itself.[92] The strategy of the Global Program to Eliminate Lymphatic Filariasis by the WHO has two components: to stop the spread of infection (i.e., interrupt transmission), and to alleviate the suffering of affected individuals (i.e., morbidity control).[92]

Filariasis Epidemiology

More than a billion people in more than 80 countries are at risk of acquiring filariasis. Over 120 million have already been affected, and over 40 million of them are seriously incapacitated and disfigured by the disease. One-third of the people infected with the disease live in India, one-third live in Africa, and most of the remainder in South Asia, the Pacific, and the Americas.[58,92] In tropical and subtropical areas the prevalence of the infection continues to increase. A primary cause of this increase is the rapid and unplanned growth of cities, which creates numerous breeding sites for the *Culex* and *Anopheline* mosquitoes that transmit the disease.[92]

Gender Differential in Filariasis

The ratio of male-to-female cases of filariasis varies by geographical area and parasite, and is due to a combination of gender bias in case detection and gender-based difference in patterns of exposure. In India, men and women are found to be equally susceptible to Bancroftian filariasis, but prevalence of the chronic disease is reported to be higher in males.[93–96] In southern Ghana, where women are

working in the mangrove swamps and are exposed to the filariasis mosquito, prevalence of lymphedema is higher in women than in men.[97] Some studies show that lymphedema affects women more frequently than men in Bancroftian filiriasis.[98,99] As these differences in susceptibility are only apparent in the reproductive years, some researchers have suggested a pregnancy-associated immune response.[100] In areas endemic for Brugian filariasis, infection and lymphedema cases are more prevalent in men.[98] Lymphedema of the leg seems to be 10 times more likely in women than men according to a study in Haiti.[99] The prevalence of lymphedema of the vulva and other urogenital symptoms in women are often underreported due to the reluctance of women and health providers to examine the genitals of female patients. In a survey in Tanzania for example the physical examination of males included the genitals, arms, and legs, while the examination of women was restricted to the arms and legs.[101]

Quality-of-life studies of affected women describe a spectrum of consequences associated with their lymphedema.[4] In general, women affected by lymphedema are often considered undesirable, and when their lower limbs and genital parts are enlarged they can be severely stigmatized.[102] Marriage, in many situations an essential source of security, is often impossible. Embarrassment, shame, cultural constraints, and social taboos often prevent women from seeking healthcare.[103] Women's lives are substantially burdened both socially and economically by the physical impairment of elephantiasis, most notably in the loss of income due to restrictions on mobility. Interestingly, physical, functional, and psychological limitations were not always associated with severity of lymphedema.[102]

Leishmaniasis

Leishmaniasis is caused by parasitic protozoa of the genus *Leishmania*. The disease can be traced back many hundreds of years, and representations of skin lesions and facial deformities have been found on pre-Inca potteries from Ecuador and Peru dating back to the first century CE.[104] Humans are usually infected via the bite of phlebotomine sand flies, which breed in forest areas, caves, or the burrows of small rodents. There are three main types of the disease:

- In cutaneous forms (CL), skin ulcers usually form on exposed areas, such as the face, arms, and legs. These usually heal within a few months, leaving scars. Diffuse cutaneous leishmaniasis, a subform of CL, produces disseminated and chronic skin lesions resembling those of lepromatous leprosy. Diffuse cutaneous leishmaniasis is difficult to treat.

- In mucocutaneous forms, the lesions can partially or totally destroy the mucous membranes of the nose, mouth, throat, and surrounding tissues.

- Visceral leishmaniasis (VL), also known as kala azar (black sickness) in India, is characterized by high fever, substantial weight loss, swelling of the spleen and liver, and anemia. If left untreated, the disease has a fatality rate of approximately 90% within two years.[104]

Chemotherapy remains the most important element in the control of VL, with antimonials used as the primary first line of treatment in most parts of the world, except in India which has high levels of drug resistance. The number of treatments available for VL has significantly grown over the past decade, with both new drugs and new formulations of old drugs either recently approved or in clinical development (amphotericin B liposome, miltefosine, and aminosidine). All these drugs have significant drawbacks: route of administration, length of treatment (21 to 28 days), toxicity, and cost, which limit their utilization in disease-endemic areas.

Leishmaniasis and HIV infection coexist in a deadly synergy. The spread of HIV infection is bringing severe VL to new geographical areas. In persons infected with HIV, leishmaniasis accelerates the onset of AIDS by cumulative immunosuppression and by stimulating replication of the virus.[104] The epidemiological significance of asymptomatic carriers of the parasite has also been amplified by the advent of HIV, as coinfection activates disease in parasite carriers. Treatment of leishmaniasis is much more difficult in patients with HIV.

Leishmaniasis Epidemiology

The spread of leishmaniases are related to environmental changes such as deforestation, building of dams, new irrigation schemes, urbanization, and migration of nonimmune people to endemic areas. Epidemics have significantly delayed the implementation of numerous development programs. This is particularly true in the Amazon basin, the tropical regions of the Andean countries, Morocco, and Saudi Arabia.[104] For many years, the public health impact of leishmaniasis has been grossly underestimated, mainly due to lack of awareness of its serious impact on health. Over the last 10 years, endemic regions have been spreading further, and there has been a sharp increase in the number of recorded cases of the disease.[104] As notification is compulsory in only 32 of the 88 countries affected by leishmaniasis, a substantial number of cases are never recorded. In fact, 2 million new cases (1.5 million for CL and 500,000 for VL) are considered to occur annually, with an estimated 12 million people presently infected worldwide. The great majority of cases can be distributed to less than a dozen countries[104]:

- 90% of all VL cases occur in Bangladesh, Brazil, India, Nepal, and Sudan.
- 90% of mucocutaneous leishmaniasis occurs in Bolivia, Brazil, and Peru.
- 90% of CL cases occur in Afghanistan, Brazil, Iran, Peru, Saudi Arabia, and Syria.

Gender Differentials in Leishmaniasis

The risk of leishmaniasis infection among males and females seems to be equal in childhood, but more male cases are reported from around seven years of age.[105-107] The higher prevalence in adolescent and adult males is often explained by higher risk of exposure. Leishmaniasis is recognized as an occupational disease, common in male-dominated employment such as building of roads and railroads, oil and gold extraction, deforestation, hunting, and military service.[108,109] In India, a five-fold higher rate of leishmaniasis in males compared with females by hospital reporting likely reflects the greater likelihood of treatment for males.[107] Community surveys reveal much higher rates among women than is evident from hospital records.[107] Sociocultural and economic circumstances hinder women's presentation in hospitals and lead to underreporting. In Brazil, where gender discrimination is less common than in Southeast Asia, there is no significant difference in prevalence between men and women.[105,110] A study of the prevalence of Chagas' disease and VL in Columbia also reported similar rates in men and women.[111]

In terms of social and economic consequences, cutaneous and mucosal leishmaniasis are especially damaging for women and girls owing to the cosmetic impact of lesions. The author has seen several cases of severe stigmatization in Afghanistan, making marriage, in many situations an essential source of security, impossible.

Interventions for Gender Equity in Infectious Disease

Attention to Health Education

The beneficial effect of maternal education on a broad spectrum of maternal and child health parameters is well documented.[112] In South Africa, maternal literacy was associated with improved treatment-seeking and better case notification rates among children with TB.[113] In Yemen, illiterate patients had a longer delay to TB diagnosis than literate patients, and in India significantly less women accessed the media for healthcare information than men.[24,114] As female literacy rates continue to lag behind males in most developing countries,[12] the development of educational materials that are sensitive to illiteracy, which counter negative gender stereotypes and are effectively targeted to women, are of great importance.

Improving Access to Health Care

Limitations on a woman's time, mobility, and finances make visits to healthcare facilities a formidable barrier. The stigma attached to many communicable diseases, such as leprosy and TB, also prevents health-seeking behavior. Interventions to improve accessibility to healthcare while preserv-

ing patient privacy are therefore essential in promoting gender-equitable access to health services.

Improving physical accessibility by increasing numbers and strategic placement of community clinics, extending opening hours, and reducing costs of treatment are basic interventions with great potential for positive impact. Integration of infectious disease programming into existing community-based care initiatives (such as antenatal health or childhood primary care services) would further increase accessibility by both consolidating time spent on family healthcare and providing anonymity to patients requiring infectious disease services. Considering women's preference for seeking healthcare outside the public sector, integration of traditional healers, pharmacies, and private practitioners into infectious disease programming is an important consideration. Public-private partnerships have already demonstrated success in the field of TB control,[115] and innovative partnerships between national control programs and workplace programs can successfully provide on-site education, testing, and treatment.[116]

Improving Diagnostic Methods

As gender analysis of tuberculosis suggests, basing screening protocols and diagnostic criteria on male symptomatology can lead to underestimation of female disease, delay in diagnosis, and poor outcome. These techniques must be revised to increase sensitivity for female disease. Female genital manifestations of infectious diseases such as TB and filariasis are often neglected due to lack of facilities for evaluation in the community setting. Equipping and training community health providers, modifying screening procedures, and developing diagnostic protocols and rapid diagnostic tests for use at the community level are essential steps toward increasing case detection among women.

Modifying the Healthcare Workforce

Cultural restrictions on female social interactions and discomfort with male healthcare providers is a cause of delay in health-seeking behavior particularly evident in the examples of tuberculosis and leprosy.[7,31,42,82] Increasing the numbers of female healthcare providers is an integral step in providing appropriate and accessible care in these situations. Ongoing monitoring of gender disparities in infectious disease programming is essential so that issues of provider bias and missed opportunities for diagnosis of female disease can be identified and addressed.

Minimizing Financial Loss

Cost of care and lost income due to infectious disease are catastrophic for families living in poverty. Studies on TB in India reflect global trends, with an average loss of three to four months of work time and 20–30% of annual household income.[117] Women are often the last members of the family to have resources allocated to their well-being. Healthcare programs that integrate income generation or income-support strategies, financial incentives for completion of treatment, support for costs of travel, and free diagnostics and medications will therefore increase the likelihood that women in resource-poor settings will ultimately receive care.

Reducing Stigma and Increasing Community Support

Fear of social isolation owing to the stigma of infectious disease is known to be a significant deterrent to health-seeking behavior in women. Interventions that foster acceptance and support of those with communicable diseases therefore address a significant barrier to care. In Bangladesh, community health volunteers with the Bangladesh Rural Advancement Committee reported that stigma around TB had decreased with the growing awareness of potential for cure.[7] Peer support for TB patients has been shown successful in North Ethiopia where participation in TB "clubs" improved knowledge about tuberculosis, reduced social isolation, and improved rates of treatment completion.[118]

Empowering Women

The empowerment of women through education, policy, and social structural change is an essential process without which all other gender-related interventions will ultimately prove superficial and short lived. In the field of health, women's empowerment has significant impact; ensuring that women have decision-making and financial power is a direct way to counter gender inequity and to improve the health of women and their families. In Benin, women's involvement in community income generation activities and local credit groups was significantly associated with use of ITNs. Women were also found to be more likely to spend household money on health items (including ITNs)[119] and malaria treatment for family members,[70] than men. Empowering women to provide healthcare, not just for themselves and their families, but for their entire community has proven successful in many low-income settings where community healthcare workers (CHWs) are first-line primary care providers.[120,121] In the field of infectious disease, onchocerciasis control programs have demonstrated that using female community health workers and involving women in leadership roles in community initiatives improved female participation and outcomes.[122] Likewise in Central Sudan female health workers played an important role in malaria control through community organization, vector control, and health education.[123] However, female participation must be carefully planned to avoid overburdening women with additional work or alienating male community members.[123,124]

Including Men

Given the gender-associated power dynamics within families and communities, the importance of educating and enlisting men in infectious disease programming cannot be ignored. In vector control especially, gender roles often necessitate involvement of men in water control and insecticide-spraying initiatives. However, from the most basic standpoint, eradication of disease from the female population cannot be attained while males still serve as a disease reservoir. This is particularly relevant for diseases such as TB where men have been shown to have higher treatment default rates than women. Control programs must therefore ensure that barriers to care that may be specific to males are also investigated and addressed.

Prioritizing Gender-Sensitive Research

Collection of high quality sex- and age-disaggregated mortality and morbidity data is the first step toward tracking the effect of gender on infectious disease. This must include investigation into the burden of female disease that exists within the private sector and which is therefore unrepresented in national data. Efforts to identify and understand gender differences in rates of disease will ultimately require combined epidemiological and social science research.

Fair representation of women in clinical and biomedical trials is essential to elucidate potential differences in female responses to treatment regimens and differing sensitivity of diagnostic tools in females versus males. Special attention must be focused on evidence of changes in immune responses during female reproductive years and on safety and efficacy of standard treatment regimens during pregnancy and lactation.

Many risk factors for infectious disease disproportionately effect women. These include malnutrition, poverty, and exposure to indoor air pollution. Research to elucidate the effects of these factors on vulnerability to disease and treatment outcomes can provide new and effective intervention strategies.

Many existing infectious disease control strategies fail to address the specific needs of women. Carefully targeted operational research is needed to clarify the influence of healthcare-provider gender, passive versus active case-finding strategies, and models of integrated community-based care on the diagnosis and treatment of female patients. In addition to investment in high-quality outcomes research, the integration of gender-sensitive indicators into program monitoring strategies is an essential step toward ensuring gender equity.

Conclusion

The gender-based review of infectious disease reveals that women are disproportionately affected on several levels:

1. As individuals who face significant disadvantages in accessing healthcare

2. As community members who suffer damaging social and economic consequences from illness

3. As primary caregivers whose work burden is increased by illness in family members

Ultimately, gender disparities in health reflect inequity in the distribution of social capital, power, and money. As such, the fight for gender equity reflects a larger global struggle. In this context, failure to address women's poverty, lack of education, and lack of social capital will lead to failure in disease control. Therefore, the gender approach must extend beyond infectious disease programming into social, economic, and political development strategies. Whether it is regarded as a human right, as an isolated component of effective health programming, or as a necessity for global well-being, the need to promote gender equity in approaching infectious disease is clear and immediate.

Tuberculosis, malaria, leprosy, filariasis, and leishmaniasis are regarded as "neglected diseases," disproportionately affecting those living in poverty. Women are overrepresented in this group. All of these diseases are seriously disabling or life threatening, affect large populations, lack adequate treatment options, and require therapeutics that have insufficient market potential to attract a private-sector response. Current trends in research and development do not address the health needs of the populations that suffer from these diseases. Only 1% of the drugs that have come to the market in the last 30 years were developed for tropical diseases or TB, and the existing medications for these diseases are limited by toxicity and increasing microbial resis-tance.[125] Thus, current systems of health research and health delivery are failing the majority of the world's population, reinforcing the increasing gap between the haves and the have-nots. Failed redistribution, failed accountability, and the cycles of exclusion, denial of rights, and aggression continue to escalate globally. What is needed is a paradigm shift to address the interests of neglected populations worldwide, and gender-specific research and interventions must be part of the solution. Several initiatives have been formed in the last few years to raise awareness and address this gap, including the Drugs for Neglected Disease Initiative, UNDP/World Bank/WHO's Special Program for Research and Training in Tropical Diseases, and the Bill and Melinda Gates Foundation. However, to make a tangible and lasting change what is needed is not merely charity and awareness, but the implementation of structural change.

DISCUSSION QUESTIONS

1. Discuss research strategies to elucidate whether the marked differential in male and female TB incidence is due to underreporting of female cases or true sex-based differences in disease incidence.

2. Discuss the advantages and disadvantages of community-based programs for the control of communicable disease with a focus on women's access to services.

3. "Preferential resource allocation for diagnosis and treatment of infectious disease in males is justified given their primary role as economic providers in most cultural contexts." Please discuss.

4. Explain and discuss the higher prevalence of leishmaniasis, filariasis, and leprosy in passive case reporting versus active case reporting.

5. Discuss the consequences of coinfection of tuberculosis, malaria, and leishmaniasis with HIV/AIDS.

6. What is the current state of research and development on the safety of new antimalarial drugs for pregnant women? What are your recommendations for research priorities in the treatment of malaria?

REFERENCES

1. Gwatkin DR, Guillot M, Heuveline P. The burden of disease among the global poor. *Lancet.* 1999;354:586-589.

2. Theobald SR, Tolhurst R, Squire SB. Gender equity: new approaches for effective management of communicable diseases. *Trans Royal Soc Trop Med Hyg.* 2006;100:299-304.

3. United Nations Department of Economic and Social Affairs—Statistics Division. *The World's Women 2005: Progress in Statistics.* New York, NY: United Nations Publications; 2006. http://unstats.un.org/unsd/demographic/products/indwm/ww2005_pub/ww2005_complete_report.pdf. Accessed July 29, 2008.

4. Allotey P, Gyapong M. The gender agenda in the control of tropical diseases: a review of current evidence. Geneva, Switzerland: Special Programme for Research and Training in Tropical Diseases, World Health Organization; 2005. Special Topics No. 4. http://www.who.int/tdr/publications/publications/pdf/seb_topic4.pdf. Accessed February 25, 2008.

5. Periago MR, Fescina R, Ramon-Pardo P. Steps for preventing infectious diseases in women. *Emerg Infect Dis.* 2004;10(11):1968-1973

6. World Health Organization. Gender in tuberculosis research. *Gender and Health Research Series* [serial online]. 2004. http://www.who.int/gender/documents/TBlast2.pdf. Accessed July 29, 2008.

7. Uplekar M, Rangan S, Ogden J. *Gender and Tuberculosis Control: Towards a Strategy for Research and Action.* Geneva, Switzerland: World Health Organization; 1999. WHO/CDS/TB/2000.280.

8. World Bank. *World Development Report 2000/2001: Attacking Poverty.* New York, NY: Oxford University Press; 2001.

9. Beijing Declaration and Platform for Action. Official Report of the Fourth World Conference on Women, Beijing. September 1995. http://www.un.org/esa/gopher-data/conf/fwcw/off/a—20.en . Accessed February 4, 2008.

10. Lopez AD, Mathers CD, Ezzati M, Jamison DT, Murray CJL. Global and regional burden of disease and risk factors, 2001: systematic analysis of population health data. *Lancet.* 2006;367(9524):1747-1757.

11. The Convention on the Elimination of All Forms of Discrimination Against Women (CEDAW). The Division for the Advancement of Women Web site. http://www.un.org/womenwatch/daw/cedaw/. Accessed February 8, 2008.

12. UNICEF. The State of the World's Children 2007: *Women and Children—The Double Dividend of Gender Equality.* 2006. http://www.unicef.org/publications/index_36587.html. Accessed February 7, 2008.

13. Bonilla E, Rodriguez A. Determining malaria effects in rural Columbia. *Social Science and Med.* 1993:37(9):1109-1114.

14. Nair DM, George A, Chacko KT. Tuberculosis in Bombay: new insights from poor urban patients. *Health Policy Plann.*1997;12(1):77-85.

15. Corbett EL, Watt CJ, Walker N, et al. The growing burden of tuberculosis: global trends and interactions with the HIV epidemic. *Arch Intern Med.* 2003;163:1009-1021.

16. Murray CJ, Saloman JA. Modeling the impact of global tuberculosis control strategies. *Proc Natl Acad Sci* 1998;95:13881-13886

17. World Health Organization. Global tuberculosis control: surveillance, planning, financing: WHO Report 2007. http://www.who.int/tb/publications/global_report/2007/en/. Accessed July 29, 2008.

18. World Health Organization. *The World Health Report 2003: Shaping the Future.* Geneva, Switzerland: WHO; 2003. http://www.who.int/whr/2003/en/whr03_en.pdf. Accessed July 29, 2008.

19. Frieden TR, Sterling TR, Munsiff SS, Watt CJ, Dye C. Tuberculosis. *Lancet.* 2003;362:887-899.

20. Hudelson P. Gender differentials in tuberculosis: the role of socioeconomic and cultural factors. *Tubercle Lung Dis.* 1999;77:391-400.

21. Holmes CB, Hausler H, Nunn P. A review of sex differences in the epidemiology of tuberculosis. *Int J Tuberc Lung Dis.* 1998;2(2):96-104.

22. Diwan VK, Thorson A. Sex, gender, and tuberculosis. *Lancet.* 1999;353:1000-1001.

23. Long NH, Johansson E, Diwan VK, Winkvist A. Different tuberculosis in men and women: beliefs from focus groups in Vietnam. *Soc Sci Med.* 1999;49:815-822.

24. Atre SR, Kudale AM, Morankar SN, Rangan SG, Weiss MG. Cultural concepts of tuberculosis and gender among the general population without tuberculosis in rural Maharashtra, India. *Trop Med Int Health.* 2004;9(11):1228-1238.

25. Agboatwalla M, Kazi GN, Shah SK, Tariq M. Gender perspectives on knowledge and practices regarding tuberculosis in urban and rural areas in Pakistan. *East Mediterr Health J.* 2003;9(4):732-740.

26. Khan A, Walley J, Newell J, Imdad N. Tuberculosis in Pakistan: socio-cultural constraints and opportunities in treatment. *Soc Sci Med.* 2000;50:247-254.

27. Johansson E, Long NH, Diwan VK, Winkvist A. Gender and tuberculosis control. Perspectives on health seeking behaviour among men and women in Vietnam. *Health Policy.* 2000;52:33-51.

28. Thorson A, Hoa NP, Long NH. Health-seeking behaviour of individuals with a cough of more than 3 weeks. *Lancet.* 2000;356(9244):1823-1824.

29. Yamasaki-Nakagawa M, Ozasa K, Yamada N, et al. Gender difference in delays to diagnosis and healthcare seeking behaviour in a rural area of Nepal. *Int J Tuberc Lung Dis*. 2001;5(1):24-31.

30. Eastwood SV, Hill PC. A gender-focused qualitative study of barriers to accessing tuberculosis treatment in The Gambia, West Africa. *Int J Tuberc Lung Dis*. 2004;8(1):70-75.

31. Morankar S, Weiss MG. Impact of gender on illness experience and behaviour: implications for tuberculosis control in rural Maharastra. *Health Admin*. 2003;15(1-2):149-155.

32. Xu B, Fochsen G, Xiu Y, Thorson A, Kemp JR, Jiang CW. Perceptions and experiences of health care seeking and access to TB care: a qualitative study in rural Jiangsu Province, China. *Health Policy*. 2004;69(2):139-149.

33. Begum V, de Colombani P, Das Gupta S. Tuberculosis and patient gender in Bangladesh: sex differences in diagnosis and treatment outcome. *Int J Tuberc Lung Dis*. 2001;5(7):604-610.

34. Weiss MG, Auer C, Somma DB, et al. Gender and tuberculosis: cross-site analysis and implications of a multi-country study in Bangladesh, India, Malawi, and Columbia. Geneva, Switzerland: World Health Organization, Special Programme for Research & Training in Tropical Diseases; 2001.

35. Cheng G, Tolhurst R, Li RZ, Menga QY, Tang S. Factors affecting delays in tuberculosis diagnosis in rural China: a case study in four counties in Shandong Province. *Trans Royal Soc Trop Med Hyg*. 2005;99:355-362.

36. Murray CJL, Salomon JA. Expanding the WHO tuberculosis control strategy: rethinking the role of active case-finding. *Int J Tuberc Lung Dis*. 1998;2(9):S9-S15.

37. Cassels A, Heineman E, LeClerq S, Gurung PK, Rahut CB. Tuberculosis case-finding in Eastern Nepal. *Tubercle*. 1982;63:175-185.

38. Harper I, Fryatt R, White A. Tuberculosis case finding in remote mountainous areas—are microscopy camps of any value? Experience from Nepal. *Tubercle Lung Dis*. 1996;77:384-388.

39. Long NH, Johansson E, Lönnroth K, et al. Longer delays in tuberculosis diagnosis among women in Vietnam. *Int J Tuberc Lung Dis*. 1999;3(5):388-393.

40. Chang CT, Esterman A. Diagnostic delay among pulmonary tuberculosis patients in Sarawak, Malaysia: a cross-sectional study. *Rural Remote Health*. 2007;7:667-675.

41. Long NH, Diwan VK, Winkvist A. Difference in symptoms suggesting pulmonary tuberculosis among men and women. *J Clin Epidemiol*. 2002;55: 115-120.

42. Thorson A, Johansson E. Equality or equity in health care access: a qualitative study of doctors' explanations to a longer doctor's delay among female TB patients in Vietnam. *Health Policy*. 2004;68:37-46.

43. Chowdhury NN. Overview of tuberculosis of the female genital tract. *J Indian Med Assoc*. 1996;94(9):345-456, 361.

44. Nichter M. Illness semantics and international health: the weal lungs/TB complex in the Philippines. *Soc. Sci. Med*. 1994;38(5):649-663.

45. Balasubramanian VN, Oommen K, Samuel R. DOT or not? Direct observation of anti-tuberculosis treatment and patient outcomes, Kerala State, India. *Int J Tuberc Lung Dis*. 2000;4(5):409-413.

46. Harper M, Ahmadu FA, Ogden JA, McAdam KP, Lienhardt C. Identifying the determinants of tuberculosis control in resource-poor countries: insights from a qualitative study in The Gambia. *Trans Royal Soc Trop Med Hyg*. 2003;97: 506-510.

47. Thillagavathie P. Current issues in maternal and perinatal tuberculosis: impact of the HIV-1 epidemic. *Semin Neonatol.* 2000;5:189-196.

48. Borgdorff MW, Nagelkerke NJ, Dye C, Nunn P. Gender and tuberculosis: a comparison of prevalence surveys with notification data to explore sex differences in case detection. *Int J Tuberc Lung Dis.* 2000;4(2):123-132.

49. Crampin AC, Glynn JR, Floyd S, et al. Tuberculosis and gender: exploring the patterns in a case control study in Malawi. *Int J Tuberc Lung Dis.* 2004;8(2):194-203.

50. Ormerod P. Tuberculosis in pregnancy and the puerperium. *Thorax.* 2001;56:494-499.

51. Jana N, Vasishta K, Jindalb SK, Khunnu B, Ghosh K. Perinatal outcome in pregnancies complicated by pulmonary tuberculosis. *Int J Gynecol Obstet.* 1994;44:119-124.

52. Figueroa-Damián R, Arredondo-García JL. Neonatal outcome of children born to women with tuberculosis. *Arch Med Res.* 2001;32:66-69.

53. Roll Back Malaria. *A Guide to Gender and Malaria Resources.* Stockholm, Sweden: Kvinnoforum; 2006.

54. World Health Organization. World malaria situation in 1994. Part 1. Population at risk. *Weekly Epidemiological Record.* 1997;72:269-274.

55. Breman JG. The ears of the hippopotamus: manifestations, determinants, and estimates of the malaria burden. *American J Trop Med Hyg.* 2001;64(1-2 Suppl):1-11.

56. Drugs for Neglected Diseases Initiative. Neglected diseases. http://www.dndi.org/cms/public_html/insidecategoryListing.asp?CategoryId=89. Accessed February 14, 2008.

57. World Bank. *Investing in Health: World Development Report.* New York, NY; Oxford University Press; 1993.

58. Merson M, Black R, Mills A. *International Public Health.* 2nd ed. Sudbury, MA: Jones and Bartlett; 2006.

59. World Health Organization. Malaria fact sheet: Fact sheet No. 94. May 2007. http://www.who.int/mediacentre/factsheets/fs094/en/index.html. Accessed July 29, 2008.

60. Nchinda T. Malaria: a re-emerging disease in Africa. *Emerg Infect Dis.* 1998;4:398-403.

61. Moorthy VS, Good MF, Hill AV. Malaria vaccine developments. *Lancet;* 2004;363(9403):150-156.

62. Tanner M, Vlassoff C. Treatment seeking behaviour for malaria: a typology based on endemicity and gender. *Soc Sci Med.* 1998;46:523-532.

63. Geberding JL. Women and infectious diseases. *Emerg Infect Dis.* 2004;10:1965-1967.

64. Dobson R. Mosquitoes prefer pregnant women. *BMJ.* 2000;320:1558.

65. Lindsay S, Ansell J, Selman C, et al. Effect of pregnancy on exposure to malaria mosquitoes. *Lancet.* 2000;355:1972.

66. Tolhurst R, Nyonator FK. Looking within the household: gender roles and responses to malaria in Ghana. *Trans R Soc Trop Med Hyg.* 2006;100(4):321-326.

67. Vlassoff C, Manderson L. Incorporating gender in the anthropology of infectious diseases. *Trop Med Int Health.* 1998;3:1011-1019.

68. Roll Back Malaria. Malaria in pregnancy: RBM InfoSheet. http://www.rbm.who.int/cmc_upload/0/000/015/369/RBMInfosheet_4.htm. Accessed July 29, 2008.

69. Brabin L, Brabin BJ. HIV, malaria and beyond: reducing the disease burden of female adolescents. *Malaria J.* 2005;4:2;1475-2875.

70. Lampietti JA, Poulos C, Cropper ML, Mitiku H, Whittington D. Gender and preferences for malaria prevention in Tigray, Ethiopia. Policy Research Report on Gender and Development, Working Paper Series, No. 3. North Carolina; World Bank; 1999.

71. Minja H, Schellenberg JA, Munkasa O, et al, Introducing insecticide-treated nets in the Kilombero Valley, Tanzania: the relevance of local knowledge and practice for an Information, Education and Communication (IEC) campaign. *Trop Med Int Health.* 2000;6(8):614-623.

72. Roll Back Malaria. Gender and malaria statement. Presented at United Against Malaria Forum V; November 18-19, 2005; Yaoundé, Cameroon.

73. Noordeen SK. Epidemiology and control of leprosy—a review of progress over the last 30 years. *Trans Royal Soc Trop Med Hyg.* 1993;87:515-517.

74. World Health Organization. Leprosy Forum Report; May 26, 2006; Geneva, Switzerland.

75. Visschedijk J, Broek J, Henk E, Lever P, Beers S, Klatser P. *Mycobacterium leprae*-millennium resistant! Leprosy control on the threshold of a new era. *Trop Med Int Health.* 2000;5:388-399.

76. Zodpey SP, Tiwari RR, Salodkar AD. Gender differentials in the social and family life of leprosy patients. *Leprosy Rev.* 2000;71:505-510.

77. Tiendrebeogo A, Toure I, Zerbo P. A survey of leprosy impairments and disabilities among patients treated by MDT in Burkina Faso. *Int J Leprosy Other Mycobacter Dis.* 1996;64:15-25.

78. Ulrich M, Zulueta AM, Caceres-Ditmar G, et al. Leprosy in women—characteristics and repercussions. *Soc Sci Med.* 1993;37:445-456.

79. Kaur H, Ramesh V. Social problems of women leprosy patients—a study conducted at two urban leprosy centres in Delhi. *Leprosy Rev.* 1994;65:261-271.

80. Le Grand A. Women and leprosy: a review. *Leprosy Rev.* 1997;68:203-211.

81. Richardus JH, Meima A, Croft RP, Habbema JDF. Case detection, gender and disability in leprosy in Bangladesh: a trend analysis. *Leprosy Rev.* 1999;70: 160-173.

82. Peters ES, Eshiet AL. Male-female (sex) differences in leprosy patients in south eastern Nigeria: females present late for diagnosis and treatment and have higher rates of deformity. *Leprosy Rev.* 2002;73(3):262-267.

83. Rao S, Subramanian M, Subramanian G. Deformity incidence in leprosy patients treated with multi drug therapy. *Int J Leprosy.* 1994;66:449-454.

84. Ulrich M, Smith P, Sampson C, et al. IgM antibodies to native phenolic glycolipid I in contacts of leprosy patients in Venezuela: epidemiological observations and a prospective study of the risk of leprosy. *Int J Leprosy Other Mycobacter Dis.* 1991;59:405-415.

85. Noordeen S. The epidemiology of leprosy. In: Hastings R, ed. *Leprosy.* Edinburgh, Scotland: Churchill Livingstone; 1985.

86. Duncan ME, Pearson JM. Neuritis in pregnancy and lactation. *Int J Leprosy.* 1982;50:31-38.

87. Vlassoff C, Khot S, Rao S. Double jeopardy: women and leprosy in India. *World Health Stats Q.* 1996;49:120-126.

88. Tiendrebeogo A, Toure I, Zerbo PJ. A survey of leprosy impairments and disabilities among patients treated by MDT in Burkina Faso. *Int J Leprosy Other Mycobacter Dis.* 1996;64:15-25.

89. Scollard DM, Smith T, Bhoopat L, et al. Epidemiologic characteristics of leprosy reactions. *Int J Leprosy Other Mycobacter Dis.* 1994;62:559-567.

90. Rao S, Garole V, Walawalker S, Khot S, Karandikar N. Gender differentials in the social impact of leprosy. *Leprosy Rev.* 1996;67:190-199.

91. Behere PB. Psychological reactions to leprosy. *Lepr India.* 1981;53:266-272.

92. World Health Organization. Lymphatic filariasis fact sheet, Fact sheet No 102. Revised September 2000. Geneva, Switzerland: WHO.

93. Sahoo PK, Babu Geddam JJ, Satapathy AK, Mohanty MC, Ravindran B. Bancroftian filariasis: prevalence of antigenaemia and endemic normals in Orissa, India. *Trans Royal Soc Trop Med Hyg.* 2000;94:515-517.

94. Gyapong JO, Gyapong M, Adjei S. The epidemiology of acute adenolymphangitis due to lymphatic filariasis in northern Ghana. *Am J Trop Med Hyg.* 1996;54:591-595.

95. Kazura JW. Filariasis and onchocerciasis. *Curr Opinion Infect Dis.* 1997;10:341-344.

96. Pani SP, Srividya A, Krishnamoorthy K, et al. Rapid assessment procedures (RAP) for lymphatic filariasis. *Natl Med J India.* 1997;10:19-22.

97. Gyapong JO. Lymphatic filariasis in Ghana: from research to control. *Trans Royal Soc Trop Med Hyg.* 2000;94:599-601.

98. Michael E, Bundy DA, Grenfell BT. Re-assessing the global prevalence and distribution of lymphatic filariasis. *Parasitology.* 1996;112:409-428.

99. Coreil J, Mayard G, Louischarles J, Addiss D. Filarial elephantiasis among Haitian women—social context and behavioural factors in treatment. *Trop Med Int Health.* 1998;3:467-473.

100. de Almeida AB, Freedman DO. Epidemiology and immunopathology of Bancroftian filariasis. *Microbes Infect.* 1999;1:1015-1022.

101. Simonsen PE, Meyrowitsch DW, Makunde WH, Magnussen, P. Bancroftian filariasis—the pattern of microfilaraemia and clinical manifestations in three endemic communities of northeastern Tanzania. *Acta Tropica.* 1995;60:179-187.

102. Person B, Addiss D, Bartholomew LK, et al. A qualitative study of the psychosocial and health consequences associated with lymphedema among women in the Dominican Republic.2007;103(2):90-97

103. Bandyopadhyay L. Lymphatic filariasis and the women of India. *Soc Sci Med.* 1996;42(10):1401-1410.

104. World Health Organization. Leishmaniasis: burden of disease. http://www.who.int/leishmaniasis/burden/en/. Accessed July 29, 2008.

105. Vélez ID, Hendrickx E, Roman O, Agudelo S. *Gender and Leishmaniasis in Colombia: A Redefinition of Existing Concepts.* Geneva, Switzerland: UNDP/World Bank/WHO Special Programme for Research and Training in Tropical Diseases; 1997. WHO/TDR/GTD/RP/97. http://whqlibdoc.who.int/hq/1997/WHO_TDR_GTD_RP_97.1.pdf. Accessed July 29, 2008.

106. Thakur CP. Socio-economics of visceral leishmaniasis in Bihar (India). *Trans Royal Soc Trop Med Hyg.* 2000;94:156-157.

107. Bora D. Epidemiology of visceral leishmaniasis in India. *Natl Med J India.* 1999;12:62-68.

108. Klaus SN, Frankenburg S, Ingber A. Epidemiology of cutaneous leishmaniasis. *Clin Dermatol.* 1999;17:257-260.

109. Wijeyaratne PM, Jones Arsenault LK, Murphy CJ. Endemic disease and development: the leishmaniasis. *Acta Tropica.* 1994;56:349-364.

110. Brandao-Filho SP, Campbell-Lendrum DH, Brito MEF, Shaw JJ, Davies CR. Epidemiological surveys confirm an increasing burden of cutaneous leishmaniasis in north-east Brazil. *Trans Royal Soc Trop Med Hyg.* 1999;93:488-494.

111. Corredor Arjona A, Alvarez Moreno CA, Agudelo CA, et al. Prevalence of *Trypanosoma cruzi* and *Leishmania chagasi* infection and risk factors in a Colombian indigenous population. *Revista Instit Med Trop Sao Paulo.* 1999;41:229-234.

112. Grown C, Rao Gupta G, Pande R. Taking action to improve women's health through gender equality and women's empowerment. *Lancet.* 2005;365: 541-543.

113. van Rie A, Beyers N, Gie RP, Kunneke M, Zietsman L, Donald PR. Childhood tuberculosis in an urban population in South Africa: burden and risk factor. *Arch. Dis. Child.* 1999;80:433-437.

114. Date J, Okita K. Gender and literacy: factors related to diagnostic delay and unsuccessful treatment of tuberculosis in the mountainous area of Yemen. *Int J Tuberc Lung Dis.* 2005;9(6):680-685.

115. Dewan PK, Lal SS, Lonnroth K, et al. Improving tuberculosis control through public-private collaboration in India: literature review. *BMJ.* 2006;332:574-578.

116. World Health Organization, International Labour Organization. *Guidelines for workplace TB control activities: the contribution of workplace TB activities to TB control in the community.* Geneva, Switzerland: WHO; 2003. WHO/CDS/TB/2003.323. http://whqlibdoc.who.int/publications/2003/9241546042.pdf. Accessed July 29, 2008.

117. World Health Organization. *Stop TB Guidelines for Social Mobilization: A Human Rights Approach to Tuberculosis.* Geneva, Switzerland: WHO; 2001. WHO/CDS/STB/2001.9.http://www.stoptb.org/events/world_tb_day/2001 /H.RightsReport2001.pdf. Accessed July 29, 2008.

118. Demissie M, Getahun H, Lindt B. Community tuberculosis care through "TB clubs" in rural North Ethiopia. *Soc Sci Med.* 2003;56:2009-2018.

119. Rashed S, Johnson H, Dongier P, et al. Determinants of the permethrin-impregnated bednets (PIB) in the Republic of Benin: the role of women in the acquisition and utilization of PIBs. *Soc Sci Med.* 1999;49:993-1005.

120. Barzgar MA, Sheikh MR, Bile MK. Female health workers boost primary care. *World Health Forum.* 1997;18(2):202-210.

121. Haines A, Sanders D, Lehmann U, et al. Achieving child survival goals: potential contribution of community health workers. *Lancet.* 2007;369:2121-2131.

122. Katabarwa MN, Habomugisha P, Agunyo S. Involvement and performance of women in community-directed treatment with ivermectin for onchocerciasis control in Rukungiri District, Uganda. *Health Soc Care Community.* 2002;10(5): 382-393.

123. A/Rahman SHA, Mahamedani AA, Mirgani EM, Ibrahim AM. Gender aspects and women's participation in the control and management of malaria in Central Sudan. *Soc Sci Med* 1996;42(10):1433-1446, 1995

124. Manderson L, Mark T, Woelz N. Women's participation in health and development projects. Geneva, Switzerland: WHO; 1996. http://www.who.int/tdr /publications/publications/pdf/WHO_TDR_GTD_RP_96.1.pdf. Accessed July 29, 2008.

125. Trouiller P, Olliaro P, Torreele E, Orbinski J, Laing R, Ford N. Drug development for neglected diseases: a deficient market and a public-health policy failure. *Lancet.* 2002;359:2188-2194.

CHAPTER 26

Women and Disability

Tom Fryers, MB, ChB, DRCOG,
DPH, MD, PhD, FFPH

Tom Fryers, MB, ChB, DRCOG, DPH, MD, PhD, FFPH, is a Professor of Public Mental Health, University of Leicester, UK.

INTRODUCTION

Although women are often disabled, and necessarily face some specific issues, those issues have been little addressed until recently. Women's rights have achieved a high profile for the relative oppression of women in most cultures, but disabled women and their specific concerns are still largely ignored.[1–5] Community-based rehabilitation (CBR) projects have proliferated in developing countries for about 30 years, with accompanying literature, but have seldom addressed the specific concerns of disabled women.[1,2,4,6,7,8]

This double jeopardy is compounded in many societies by poverty, which affects women disproportionately,[1,5,6,8,9] and by caste or class,[10,11] but there is a dearth of research that provides hard facts; most published material, including official reports, is based largely upon anecdotes, personal experience, and material from earlier, similarly nonscientific papers.[12] However, there can be no doubt that disabled women face many different problems than do disabled men; some are intrinsic to being a woman, but many arise from cultural assumptions about women's roles, expectations, and cultural stereotypes about disabilities, thus varying a great deal from country to country and culture to culture.[3,6,11,13] Disabled women do not form a homogeneous group; their situations and their problems are immensely varied and cannot be understood or addressed outside their culture.[3,6,8] Nevertheless, there are many common concerns that represent universal issues relating to care received as a child, education, fulfilling satisfactory roles in society, marriage, childbearing and child rearing, family relationships, and a place in society with increasing age.

The emphasis of this chapter is on developing countries, where most of the problems are and where the issues arise most dramatically. But, because there is little hard data or scientific literature it is inevitably unbalanced; examples from the literature come predominantly from the Middle East and South Asia. Hence, personal experience is geographically wider, but necessarily without the depth of cultural understanding. This cannot be a comprehensive review, but may, perhaps, arouse interest in a neglected field, and point readers in a profitable direction.

Numbers and Types of Disability

In all countries, collecting statistics on disability is a huge challenge. Definitions are notoriously inconsistent and contentious; the relationship between physical or mental incapacity, functional disablement, and social disadvantage are subtle and complex, encompassing physiological, personal, social, and cultural factors. Arguments about "medical" and "social" models seem fruitless, as both are important, and both will need to be accommodated in any rehabilitation program.

The headline figure for children of "One in Ten" promoted for many years by international agencies is not useful; the proportion of children considered "disabled" depends on the definition used and the methods of measurement. In general, 2–3% of children in most communities have a disability that significantly affects their lives, but some communities will have a greater number for specific reasons such as war, endemic disease, epidemics, or a hostile environment.[14] In the UK, in 1989, 3.7% of boys and 2.6% of girls were considered disabled in the National Survey of Childhood Disability.[15] Up to 14% were obtained in the first adult survey, depending on severity; but this included the elderly population, which has increasing disability with age.[16] Most developing countries have only small populations of elderly people. Thus, disability affects many people and their families; it is not merely an issue for a small minority.

There are very many causes of disability, but cerebral palsy (CP) syndromes are prevalent in all communities, more in males than females.[17] Polio has been a major cause of disability for boys and girls, but there have been few cases since 2002, though some still arise, especially in India and Nigeria.[18] For both CP and polio, neglect of active habilitation in early childhood is a major contributor to later disability. Congenital abnormalities vary, but high rates of consanguineous marriage, characteristic of many cultures, increase them significantly.[14] Injuries are important, but very variable; accidents may be more common in men, but

injuries from personal violence are more common in women.

> Domestic violence is the biggest cause of injury and death to women worldwide. Gender-based violence causes more deaths and disability among women aged 15 to 44 than cancer, malaria, traffic accidents, and war.[3]

Severe mental retardation also has many causes and affects males and females roughly equally. Reliable studies suggest prevalence rates of 1–5 per 1000, but the rate in any one community depends upon the balance of causes and survival. For example, in iodine-deficient environments, congenital hypothyroidism (cretinism) can boost the rate to much higher figures.[14] Depressive illness, both major and minor, varies between countries, but generally is twice as common in women as men. Schizophrenia, with a lifetime risk of about 1%, shows no consistent gender differences except age of incidence, which is a few years later for women than men.[19]

Other estimated statistics also help to set the scene: the majority of the world's poor are women: around 70% of the 1.3 billion people who live in extreme poverty (on less than US $1 a day) are women and girls. Two-thirds of children denied primary education are girls, and 75% of the world's 876 million illiterate adults are women.[9]

Visibility and Audibility

Many writers on gender and disability emphasize the lack of interest in disabled women shown by women's organizations, and in women's special needs by disabled organizations. Sands[1] writes "The interconnection between disability and gender identity is largely invisible within women's rights, disability rights, and development agendas." Similarly in a World Bank Report of 2004[6]: "Those committed to gender equity, by failing to consider disability, and those committed to disability equity, by failing to consider gender, have unwittingly rendered girls with disabilities invisible." Abu-Habib[3] wrote: "In the Middle East and India, disabled women have not been fully integrated in either the disability movement or the women's movement."

She quoted Sherr, Canadian feminist filmmaker, in 1992: "There is clearly a conflict between feminism's rhetoric of inclusion and failure to include disability." And Oliver[4] quoted Deegan & Brooks in 1985[20]: "The disability movement has often directed its energies toward primarily male experiences. Male concerns and employment issues, for example, have received more attention than child-bearing problems."

The literature also largely ignores disabled women. Even in the UK, Lonsdale in 1990 could write[7]: "Women with disabilities are almost invisible in the literature on disability, and to some extent in society." The African Union Protocol on the Rights of Women in Africa (2004) makes only one incidental mention of disability.[21] The current Gender Equality Guides from Oxfam make no mention. The important section on women in poverty in the UK Open University Text, "Third World Lives of Struggle,"[22] does not address disability. A recent book on CBR in community development makes only occasional brief mention of girls or women as facing particular issues.[23]

However, in that book, Coleridge testifies to a recent dramatic change on the part of the World Bank: "The *Poverty Reduction Source Book*[24] places disabled people, along with children, old people, and the chronically sick in the basket marked 'not able to be economically active, in need of special care and welfare'." But since the inception of President James Wolferson, "The Bank has now adopted a policy of mainstreaming disability in all its programmes." The results include an excellent and important 2004 report: *Education for All: A Gender and Disability Perspective.*[6] In 2003, the UN Economic and Social Commission for Asia and the Pacific[5] reported specifically on women's issues and their previous neglect. In 2006, the UN Committee on the International Convention on the Rights and Dignity of Persons with Disabilities adopted a draft convention specifically encompassing women's needs and gender issues.[25]

In spite of these, documentation generally mirrors the reality for most women in their various communities. If Lonsdale[7] considers disabled women almost invisible in the UK, women in most developing countries are infinitely worse off. In some cultures, all women are almost invisible— what can integration mean for disabled women in Afghanistan and those other Asian countries where most women are kept separate and private?[13,26,27] In other countries, disabled girls and women may be restricted to the house because of stigma or overprotectiveness of the family.

Women have been poorly represented in many local disabled person's groups or organizations. Leadership roles may not be readily available to women in some cultures, but disabled women have also been poorly represented in women's groups and organizations, though there are exceptions; for example in southern Andhra Pradesh, India, women are active and prominent in local and district leadership. The tendency for girls, especially if disabled, to be given less priority in education and training, and their lack of information about disability and rehabilitation, also minimizes their capacity to be heard in the community.

Women have also often been invisible and unheard by rehabilitation services. Services often arise after armed conflict, predominantly for injured men. They are neither designed for women nor suitable for women. Where both men and women are injured, men might be heroes, while women are ignored (such as in the Palestinian Intifada[2]). Even in CBR programs, women may be less visible and fail to have their voices heard.[8] Disabled women of low caste, low social class, or from poor areas or rural communities may suffer multiple disadvantages.

The Importance of Culture

It cannot be overemphasised that the situation and experience of women with disabilities depends upon the culture of the population that gives them identity. In Western countries we have grown accustomed to societies that combine many cultures, where cultures change, fluctuate, merge, and decline, becoming ill-defined for many individuals. This may be appropriate for societies where individual autonomy and self-fulfillment are primary goals. But in most developing countries, a large proportion of the population still enjoy a fairly stable, traditional culture in which beliefs, values, and expectations are widely shared, even unquestioned.

Many of these features of traditional societies are perceived as under threat from alien Western values, by armed imposition, trade imbalance, media exposure, or aid programmes. Cultural values, such as those regarding the status and roles of women, may be so fundamentally different that communication about them is very difficult. But if abuse and oppression of women, especially of disabled women, are to be addressed, then the traditional values that the women themselves share must be understood, accepted, and honoured. To attempt to override or subvert deep cultural values only arouses conflict and precludes successful outcomes in any programme.

In many communities, especially in South Asia, disability is viewed in terms of karma, fate, or God's will; this can encourage acceptance, but it can also inhibit initiatives toward change. However, Dalal,[28] in an interesting discussion, perceives that most people are in practice quite pragmatic, and when there is evidence of some technique or service that does improve their situation, they will readily accept it, but it needs to be demonstrated.

It is clear that you cannot generalize about cultures, about the situation of women or disabled women. Any aid programme, especially those such as CBR, that must be embedded in the community must first understand the local culture in-depth and take account of cultural issues in all aspects of programme design and application.[8,13,28]

There is, however, a dilemma for those promoting rehabilitation in traditional societies. An essential part of the work is to change negative attitudes toward disabled people, to inform and educate the community about disability prevention (such as consanguineous marriage), to encourage and stimulate new ideas about employment and income generation for disabled people, and to assist the poor and disadvantaged whose voice is not heard.

Such aims and activities can indeed be a threat to traditional values. It is important, therefore, that change is promoted from within the culture by those who share the values but can see opportunities for development and understand how change can be wrought. At the very minimum, development agencies must "devise effective strategies for dealing with culturally sensitive issues, such as forging partnerships with indigenous social movements."[29] A study of disabled women in rural Haryana, India, concluded that state policies will fail "unless informed by microlevel realities and greater sensitivity to cultural nuances."[30] At best, local people are recruited and trained and run the programme within their understanding of the culture.

Attitudes to women are likely to expose the most fundamental cultural conflicts. For example, throughout the Middle East and South Asia, families and communities are very male dominated with all decisions being made by the father.[3] Both Hindu and Islamic historic texts emphasize the subservience of women to father, husband, or son.[8] In some cases, all women are kept hidden and separate.[13] Disabled person's organizations and rehabilitation personnel also tend to be dominated by men, which can lead to further neglect of women's interests.[31] Women and disabled people may be considered in the same light—as passive, necessarily dependent, and of low intrinsic value to the community.[4] On basic human rights grounds, such attitudes must be challenged by development and rehabilitation programmes, but to be successful, it must be from within the culture.

Fortunately, cultures are not completely static, all are subject to change, though some are more resistant than others.[27] Some individuals transcend their culture to be strong role models for change, though they may be predominantly from wealthier and more educated families.[3,6,32] Some men fulfill their cultural expectations with humanity, deep personal affection, and compassion.[3] Many groups of women and disabled people have successfully challenged cultural stereotypes that previously kept them powerless.[3,8,33] Some CBR programmes have created new social situations where changed attitudes allow disabled women to emerge, to thrive, and to lead their communities.[23]

Women and people with disabilities can become influential enough even to change government policy against cultural traditions—Uganda's new constitution of 1995 included the remarkable Article 32.1: "Notwithstanding anything in this Constitution, the State shall take affirmative action in favour of groups marginalised on the basis of gender, age, disability or any other reasons created by history, tradition or custom, for the purpose of redressing imbalances which exist against them".[32] This resulted, among other things, in positive discrimination for disabled children in Ugandan schools.[34]

To be successful for disabled women, development programmes need to foster, encourage, and build on these intrinsic, indigenous resources. However, economics also plays a large part, and poverty tends to sustain tradition. In well-off societies, most disabled women will obtain at least a large part of what they need and live relatively "normal" lives.[7] This is not so for women in poor communities, though it may be true for well-off women in those same societies.[3,6]

Personal Situations of Disabled Girls and Women

Both individual needs and social situations are widely varied, but generalizations have to be made. Commonly, girls are not valued as much as boys, in some societies to the point of infanticide. Any disabled child may be kept hidden because of shame and stigma[35] (even in Western countries until relatively recently). Disabled girls may be neglected in favour of boys and die early. They may be cared for physically but not emotionally and overprotected by near-imprisonment at home. They are commonly excluded from education: UNESCO estimated that only 2% of disabled children are in school, with far fewer girls than boys.[6]

These all leave disabled women at a huge disadvantage. Such general discrimination can be tackled in several ways.[36] Educating the community requires the recruitment of local leaders to the campaign. Role models of successful women with disabilities can be invaluable if they can be found; they can be created by selection of disabled women for training as rehabilitation or development workers in their own communities.[13,36] Disabled self-help groups, so potent in many communities, can ensure that women, and parents of disabled girls as well as boys, are fully involved, and women's groups can incorporate disabled women and their special interests.

Negative attitudes, assumptions, and stereotypes are common in most communities, even shared by the family. Girls and women with obvious disabilities, of whatever type, may be assumed to be totally incapable of anything and utterly useless.[8] This needs challenging at an individual level, by demonstrating the positive gifts of girls, their capacity to learn self-care, and the benefits to the family in doing so. They are often excluded from information normally available to girls and may, for example, find it very difficult to cope with menstrual hygiene.

In many societies it is assumed that girls with disabilities are virtually sexless, could certainly not be married, and would be unable to have children or care for them if they did.[2,3,7,11,33,37] For most disabled girls none of these is true, but collectively they represent a huge barrier to be overcome in societies where a girl's main value lies in her marriage prospects, and where marriage is the only acceptable status for a woman.[6] In many cultures there is an assumption that a woman's first responsibility is to look beautiful, something that still lingers in Western stereotypes.[7] For women with disabilities, this is assumed to be impossible; and they may not, therefore, be considered for marriage.

In some communities where not to be married is a disaster, few disabled women are married.[3] Additionally, they may be married to someone quite unsuitable. Divorce is much more common for disabled women than others.[3,8] As marriage is more difficult to arrange, families may feel forced to select a very close relative, though this is often the norm for all women. Occasionally, a disabled woman may be married as a second wife; the only example known to the author was a compassionate act by the sister and brother-in-law of a young deaf women with no speech, and it appeared to work extremely well.

A close link between disability and poverty has appeared self-evident to many commentators, especially for women, but most reports are not evidence-based. A recent rigorous literature review[12] found very little scientific evidence, most literature being anecdotal, relying on personal experience and previous authors, and equally nonevidence-based. Even major reports from bodies such as the World Bank used mostly nonscientific sources in the same way. The review was limited to methodologically reliable studies, but most of these were small scale and local, so general disability across cultures is far from certain. The review also had to limit analysis to those studies that used reasonably consistent definitions of both disability and poverty.

They concluded that whether disability leads to poverty or not is related to local culture, especially to social values. Stigma commonly accompanies disability, often leading to exclusion, rendering the disabled person at greater risk of poverty. So disability can lead to poverty, but only where there is discrimination and social exclusion. (This is probably true also in developed countries.)

Poverty can also lead indirectly to disability, through poor nutrition, disease, delayed medical consultation, and poor access to treatment, the effects of which may increase the risk of further poverty. The authors believe that solutions lie in community education and action—reducing stigma and discriminatory practices and empowering disabled people—a human rights approach.[12]

Any human rights approach would need to overtly address the discrimination of women, and specifically of disabled women, because poverty seems to affect women disproportionately. Empowering disabled people, especially women, should surely include microfinancing—the small-loan systems that have become so widespread, particularly in the Indian subcontinent, and which can have a powerful effect in raising women out of poverty, giving them a degree of economic independence and hope of a perpetual source of income. From personal experience in rural Andhra Pradesh, India, microloans are one of the key features of any rehabilitation programme, with long-term benefits for women and whole families.

Abuse and Violence

There is a great deal of evidence, though mostly anecdotal, that disabled girls and women are especially subject to physical, mental, and sexual abuse. This may be true in all countries.[2,5,6,8,31] Sands, in 2005, summed up her experience in Australia and the Pacific Region[1]: "Women with disability have compiled the most comprehensive information about themselves. This information provides a global picture of exclusion, discrimination, poverty, violence, and human rights abuse."

Such women are often less able to stand up for themselves physically, or to escape unwanted attention, which renders them more vulnerable both inside and outside the home. They may also be less able to attract attention, cry, or run for help. They may be abused in the family home because they are considered worthless and a burden. They may be considered "less human" than able-bodied girls and therefore without feelings that matter; for example, Sands reported that in some Pacific Island communities, violence against a woman with a disability was not considered a crime.[1]

In Andhra Pradesh, many disabled women say that they were subject in adolescence to molesting and sexual exploitation by boys and men before the advent of the CBR programme. All accounts suggest that they are particularly susceptible to rape, including incest;[38] they may be less informed, either in a traditional or modern way, about sex or safe sex,[39] and are thus less able to resist sexual advances or negotiate safe sex, and are more exposed to unwanted pregnancy and sexually transmitted diseases including HIV/AIDS.[37,39,40]

Women considered unmarryable and excluded from normal expectations may seek or be forced into promiscuous relationships or prostitution.[37,39] It has been reported that they may be encouraged to have a child to look after them and reduce the burden on the family.[38] Child abuse is an issue in all countries and is not easily addressed in any, but the consequences are commonly serious and long lasting.[41] All of these issues are of great concern to those involved in CBR programmes. They need to be addressed with great sensitivity, and perhaps courage, but this can only be done by women workers who share the general culture of that community. In many places, recruiting and training such women is of the highest priority.

Rehabilitation

In many countries, rehabilitation was first seriously addressed as a response to war and injured soldiers. Its male orientation was appropriate, for example, in the UK after the First World War, but it is not appropriate after periods of armed conflict involving civilians. In Western countries, rehabilitation services have become technologically sophisticated and widely available, closely related to formal medical and social services. They are dominated by elderly people with disease-related disabilities increasing with age. Generally speaking, women have equal access, but Lonsdale (1990) thought there were still barriers to equal treatment.[7]

In most developing countries, rehabilitation was limited often to only orthopaedic workshops and a little surgery, until the advent of CBR around 1980. The primary concern of CBR was to address the basic needs of huge numbers of disabled people in rural communities throughout the world, who received no help whatsoever. There have been many programmes called CBR, often small and providing help in different ways, and misunderstandings have arisen. Perhaps the most common is to conceive it as merely community rehabilitation, that is, providing help within the village and home. Much can be done at this community level (Thomas says 70% of people can be helped[31]), but this is not enough; community-based rehabilitation is a rehabilitation programme *based* in the community but also encompassing higher levels of professional and specialist help to support and supplement what can be done locally.

A second common misunderstanding is that CBR is largely concerned with individual, medical, and physical interventions; some early manuals (e.g., WHO[42]) may have given this impression, but one of the earliest and longest-lasting CBR programmes, started by women activists in Bacolod, Philippines, using an early draft of the WHO manual, encompassed social, educational, employment, and economic aspects from the beginning.[43] A CBR programme should represent a comprehensive approach, or at least as comprehensive as local conditions and resources permit. It encompasses not only individual improvement of body function, but addresses issues of relationships (family and community); economic and social function (education, training, work, employment, and income generation); community attitudes and understanding (discrimination and stigma, inclusion and participation); and human rights.[44] It has close links with community development. CBR at its best applies both medical and social models of disability and rehabilitation.[31]

What can be done in the community, in the village, and the home, is most important and represents a new emphasis in rehabilitation. It recognizes that formal resources are scarce and have to be used carefully, so that simple interventions have priority, but also that the disabled person, family, and community have gifts and capacities that represent substantial resources if applied knowingly. The ideal is to recruit CBR workers from the local community, including disabled people wherever possible, and to involve the local disabled group and wider community fully in programme development. The most important work in CBR goes on at this level, but it needs to be supported by professionals, specialists, and re-

sources from outside the local community. This emphasis is also revolutionary—specialists and professionals support and facilitate the work in the community, not the other way round, through encouragement, training, consultation, and referral as necessary, and as available facilities permit. And all must be done in full recognition and understanding of the local culture.

The principles should, of course, apply equally to both sexes, but local cultural constraints often mean, as ever, that girls and women get less help, suffer discrimination, or are ignored even in CBR programmes. The point is that all programmes must accommodate the local culture to a large extent if they are to succeed. Programmes must be pragmatic if they are to serve disabled women's needs—what can *integration* mean for disabled women where all women are segregated?[13] In some communities, separate programmes for women are the only acceptable structure.[8,13,26] Nevertheless, frank discrimination against women needs to be challenged at all levels and wherever a voice might be heard. Even in the most segregated societies it is important to challenge attitudes that perceive women as of less value than men or that treat women as second-class citizens.[29,45]

However, there are less fundamental factors in discrimination against disabled women that provide potential for change. Women may receive little rehabilitation because men cannot serve them and few women are trained as rehabilitation workers. Cultural barriers to women taking up such work need to be addressed.[8] CBR managers need to work with existing disabled and women's groups to facilitate increasing participation of women. Rehabilitation techniques suited to women's needs should be developed, though if prescription is truly on an individual basis, this should arise as more women become involved.[7] Restoring or improving a woman's capacity to perform her allotted roles in a particular society is as important as rehabilitating men to theirs.

Common concern for disabled children and adults can permit a certain amount of flexibility in cultural behaviour. In Tunisia, in general, men worked with disabled older boys and men, and women worked with young children, older girls, and women. But of six home visitors in Sfax, who would visit homes with women present, two were men. The capacity for female staff to be vocal and fully participatory in meetings seemed to depend upon local relationships and personalities. This seemed to apply less to parents meetings, where men always dominated.

"Empowerment" is commonly used on behalf of women, disabled people, racial and low caste groups, and others to express their liberation from oppression in their society, but it can be a problematic term.[1,10,45,46] Thomas and Thomas[26] comment that "In many Asian countries, 'empowerment' of the individual, as understood in the Western context, is seen as a selfish and undesirable concept. Being altruistic for the sake of the family and for the larger society has a higher value." Similarly with unqualified independence or (even worse) autonomy, which in every society can only be relative, it is never achieved and is not even desirable.[47] The higher aim for a disabled person, man or women, is to achieve equitable mutual dependence in which one is able to make one's full contribution to the common good.

Of course, in many other cultures there are few formal or structural barriers to women receiving equitable attention within any programme. But constraints may lie in attitudes of acceptance, hopelessness, and depression of a disabled woman herself. A high degree of dependence as a disabled person, in receipt of privileges, may even be comfortable.[48] Commonly, the constraints lie in community attitudes, assumptions, and stereotypes that are susceptible to change if approached by those from within the culture who understand what they are doing. It is not always easy to find such people to run CBR programmes, but they are essential.

Poverty is common for disabled women who may not have independent access to money. Microfinancing schemes have become widespread in rural communities throughout the world, with remarkable success in raising families out of poverty. They may be available at various levels of community, and a CBR programme may first negotiate access for disabled people, especially women, not previously benefiting. But CBR self-help groups may create their own, either with outside capital or from regular small member subscriptions, as seen in India and Kenya, for example.

The loans may appear very small to outsiders, but in a subsistence economy may be substantial. They are commonly for one or two years; they are used to finance an income generation project (for example: a milk cow, lambs to raise, seed or seedlings, small machines, or a small shop); or for skills training. The loans are often managed by the group, so that there is common interest in regular payment of interest and repayment of the loan on time. In most cultures (but probably not all), the loans can specifically bring women, married or not, a degree of economic independence, and some regular income for the future. This adds also to self-esteem and community respect.

The SACRED (Social Action for Child Rehabilitation, Emancipation, and Development) CBR programme in southern Andhra Pradesh illustrates the huge potential that can be realized when the right people are involved. The programme now covers five districts and helps more than 3000 disabled people. The main vehicle for change is the village self-help group (Sangham)[11] for disabled people, modelled on the Sanghams for women, facilitated by trained rural development workers, backed up by the small staff of the organization, all from the same culture. The majority of workers are women, many of them disabled, who have very successfully created role models in the villages and wider community. Many leaders of disabled Sanghams are women, and they play a very active and vocal part.

Everything is done through and with the group, working also with women's groups and village leaders. The group identifies individual disabled person's needs with the family and involves health professionals and specialists as and when required, within the framework of general provision in the state. Unusually for CBR programmes, people with severe mental illness are fully included. Education is encouraged, training facilitated, employment and income-generation projects promoted, as much for girls and women as for boys and men. Microloan systems are firmly in place and widely used to lift men and women out of poverty. Because of group commitment, no disabled person has failed to repay their loan on time.

Community education is undertaken with wall paintings, street and school theatre, and direct contact with community leaders. What has been achieved has greatly enhanced the lives of disabled men, women, and children; their families; and the communities in which they live. These people with disabilities have achieved self-respect and an acknowledged status in the community, where negative attitudes are now much less common and positive support more frequent. The latest step, after 10 years of development in the earliest district, is for the disabled group to take responsibility for their own programme. The leaders of the women's groups are facilitating this.

Caregiver Issues

It is a commonplace to say that most informal home care of children, elderly people, and disabled people is by women, in the UK as elsewhere. This has been represented by feminists as oppressive to women,[49] though Keith[50] (a feminist writer, a disabled woman, and a caregiver), argued that feminist research and writing in proclaiming the unrecognized work of caregivers had ignored those who need care and reinforced negative public perceptions of disabled people as passive, helpless, and demanding. Nevertheless, she quoted Finch and Groves[51]: "In practice community care equals care by the family and care by the family equals care by women."[50]

It was therefore a surprise when the UK General Household Survey of 1985 showed almost as many men as women were informal caregivers.[49] This was confirmed in the first National Survey of Carers in 2000[52]: 18% of women and 14% of men. Care for disabled children and elderly parents was mostly provided by women, but caring for a disabled spouse was almost equally men. Of course, most are elderly couples and developing countries have, as yet, few of these.

Women, even in Western societies, are still perceived to be, in general, more natural caregivers than men, and taboos about men touching women's bodies are not equally reciprocated.[49] How oppressive caring is felt to be must vary with the relationship to the person cared for, the opportunities for alternate lifestyles, and the culture. Women caregivers in Australia followed the expectations of their Russian culture of origin, rather than their adopted Australian culture.[53] Oliver[4] argued that the assumed passivity of disabled people is entirely ideological[54] but did not argue the same for the assumed passivity of women in some cultures, which he discusses in relation to other authors, though this may have more face validity. Certainly

caregiving is often anything but passive; it is extremely demanding—physically and emotionally.[3]

Similarly in developing countries there needs to be a balance between the needs of the disabled person and the needs of the caregiver, though the caring role may be shared more in wider family groups. Abu-Habib[3] pointed out that women as caregivers are also forgotten in the Middle East, yet often carry a huge burden, not least as stigmatized, blamed mothers of disabled children. A recent study of mothers of children with cerebral palsy in Kerala, India, found that the most stressful factor was pessimism about the child's future capacity to care for him or herself.[55] (The present author recalls that mothers expressed similar concerns in Salford, UK, 40 years ago.) Abu-Habib also noted that the perception of the importance of women's caregiver roles in families was one reason for devaluing disabled women, on the assumption that they could not fulfill it.[2]

Women as caregivers should be involved in disabled persons' self-help groups where appropriate. Coleridge[11] noted what a difference the formation of Sanghams made. Similarly, in Palestine, a CBR programme for women who were principal caregivers provided "a way out of isolation, and the release of human resources within the community, especially for the care of disabled children."[56] As with Keith's experience in the UK, in the family the lives and emotions of caregiver and care-receiver were intertwined, because the relationship is important.

Conclusion

The literature on gender and disability has been small but is increasing. However, much of it is essentially anecdotal, feeding on previous similarly nonscientific reports, and not backed by serious research. It is hardly surprising that writers who do focus on this unpopular topic take the view that women and girls are generally discriminated against in most societies, especially where traditional cultures strictly separate men's and women's roles and give men domination of leadership and decision making. But other less segregated and rigid societies are also believed to ignore, neglect, devalue, and discriminate against disabled girls and women in education, health care, rehabilitation, marriage options, employment opportunities, and so on.

It would be possible to reject all these claims because they are not evidence-based in a scientific sense, but it would be wrong to do so. After all, there is some evidence to back them up, we have none to the contrary, and most of the claims have face validity and accord with the personal experience of many people. But we should, nevertheless, bear in mind the possibility that reports represent exaggerated and one-sided descriptions of a much more complex picture.

My own experience gives a different side of the picture, but is clearly biased. I have been involved with widely varied programmes for disabled children and adults in at least 15 developing countries encompassing a diversity of cultures, and I have seen girls and women apparently given the same degree of attention, opportunities, and resources as boys and men in all cases. But this is a distorted picture; I could not observe their experience before the programme, or others in communities with no such programme. However, it was clear that the various programmes, mostly CBR, were addressing the needs of girls and women with conscious determination and employing and training women in all the roles required.

This impression is backed up currently by my women colleagues on the SACRED CBR programme in southern Andhra Pradesh, India. They describe, from their own knowledge of the local culture and their own direct experience (many are also disabled) the various disadvantages, discriminations, and abuse suffered by girls and women in these communities before the advent of the CBR programme. They believe that the programme has changed things substantially by raising the profile of disabled women; by giving them a voice to speak out to the community at large and a new self respect; by helping them to access resources in education, health care, training, loans, and employment; and by involving other community groups and organizations, not least the powerful women's groups and the village leadership. They do not claim that no one is now abused, devalued or ne-glected, but the community in general is different, with different expectations and different standards of behaviour. Thus can culture change, but it takes time. And such change requires a cul-turally sensitive approach and a deliberate strategy from the beginning.[29,30]

There can be little doubt that, given those conditions, CBR is the approach most likely to improve the lot of disabled women and men in rural communities. There have been few attempts to do something similar in big towns, though the Philippines programme started in a very poor suburb of Bacolod City.[43] Big towns in most countries do have basic education and health facilities, but it remains unclear to me what the experience of disabled men or women is in towns of the developing world. There is a clear opportunity for investigation.

CBR is the only approach for poor communities that has stood the test of time; although there are many variants, it is widely understood to encompass social inclusion, human rights, and equal opportunities as well as improvement of bodily structure and function.[57] It is also an approach with a lot of history, with people experienced in starting and running programmes, and with documented evaluations. Because it comes with a strong ethical and human rights history, it should be a vehicle well suited to addressing discrimination against girls and women, as well as low-caste and low-class groups and the poor. As the SACRED programme has demonstrated, it is also possible to fully include people with serious mental illness.

The self-help group is a key to development in the village, providing mutual support, a common voice, and a public presence. It is small enough to encourage everyone to participate, and is as likely as any structure to give women a full voice and an opportunity for leadership. In some cultures, separate women's groups are necessary. Self-help groups in Maua, Kenya, were less formally structured into the CBR organization than in Andhra Pradesh but were effective in allowing everyone to participate in discussion of issues, forwarding complaints and requests, mediating in interpersonal conflicts, deciding means of helping people in particular need, managing the small loans scheme, and planning further developments.

Many disabled children, more girls even than boys, are assumed not to be capable of benefiting from education, or are kept out of school by practical problems such as transport. One of the tasks of CBR workers and local group leaders is to negotiate their access to school and to support the family and the school. Education is a way out of poverty and discrimination and is even more important for disabled children than others because of the reduced options they often have for work. This may be even more true for girls than boys because girls in many communities are restricted in access to jobs. Special education may be needed, such as blind children needing to learn Braille. It is the experience of some of the disabled women in the SACRED programme that education and a successful occupation create a new status and acceptance in the community.

It has been observed that in most cultures, where disabled and impoverished women might suffer great discrimination, those from a well-off family in the same community (depending on the degree and type of disability) often have all the opportunities they need for education, community participation, marriage, and family life. Such disabled women can act as role models, and make a difference, even in government,[32] but perhaps the more important lesson is that relief of poverty and the opportunity for a dependable income are likely to make a huge difference to other women. In many communities now, the principle strategy is not grants from aid budgets, but small, short-term loans through a microfinancing system. This needs capital, of course, and it is encouraging that the World Bank has been providing capital for such schemes for some years.

Another strategy with a proven record (at least by personal experience of many) is to recruit and train disabled women as rehabilitation workers at all levels. Since they often have diminished job opportunities, they bring great commitment, and their own experience as disabled women gives them an advantage in understanding others and being perceived as understanding others.

We end where we started: women's movements, organizations and groups, activists and writers must ignore their disabled sisters no longer. The advocacy of women for women in general has often been very powerful; it could surely be equally effective for women with disabilities. There are good programmes of CBR in many countries, which fully include disabled women and are liberating, but they are drops in the ocean; there remain millions of disabled women in the villages—and no doubt, the towns—of the third world, with little hope. They do much for themselves, but how much more could be achieved with the backing of women overall?

They also have something very special to offer the whole community: "Able-bodied women can learn from the disabled, who have had to learn this before they can truly cope; that the physical body is not as important as the person that lives inside."[58]

Case Studies

These brief life stories come from five disabled women from the same culture but with very different experiences. Three had polio as small children; two were born with severe bilateral talipes equinovarus (club foot) but received no treatment. They were all eventually recruited by SACRED of Anantapur, Andhra Pradesh, to work in the villages as rural development workers in the community-based rehabilitation programme previously mentioned in this chapter.

—Tom Fryers.

B. Chittemmer

One of the bitter experiences of my life is being born a disabled child to parents who were not bothered about my existence. They abandoned me, intending me to die. My grandmother rescued me, but the person whom I adore more than God is my grandfather. He is all in all to me because he acted the role of my parents; I remember him with every beat of my heart.

But for him I would not have survived the negative forces within my family who considered me a liability. He helped in my daily routines, including bathing, and I see in him both father and mother. I called him "Father" since I was seven, when he carried me to school every day. My grandmother, for reasons unknown, came to hate me and forced him to send me to a hostel in Dhone. But he couldn't bear the separation, and conditions in the hostel were not congenial to study, so I continued my education staying with my grandfather. He died after I completed my primary education. My grandmother repented and educated me by going for labouring work.

I experienced discrimination from an early age. Insults in the classroom and out made me conclude that disabled people are born to suffer, and society hardly cares for their existence. Continuous suffering strengthened my inner courage, and I had a strong determination to prove that I also could contribute toward the development of society, and I completed my tenth class. Then my grandmother forced me into marriage as she wanted to relinquish her commitment as my custodian. Though my husband was good, he had to listen to his parents who didn't cherish my presence in the family, so he abandoned me. I then trained in embroidery, and, after further training, became a teacher for children who had dropped out of school. Later, SACRED entered our village, noticed my miserable condition and tried to rehabilitate my collapsing life. My grandmother, with the help of SACRED staff, intervened and amicably settled the issue with my husband. He is not working, but now realizes that he should look after me nicely. He is trying to find a job, and we are at present living together happily. My parents provided everything for my older sister, two younger brothers, and one younger sister, but provided me with nothing.

Lingering feelings about this causes me a lot of pain and suffering, but I am determined to earn money independently because empowerment without improved finances is hardly possible. Disabled people have an equal right to live in society, and others should not exercise any say in their lives. My confidence has come from within; if disabled people are united they can achieve anything, nothing proves impossible. I am looking for a day when disabled people live with human dignity.

B. Chittemmer

M. Deepika

I am aged 24, and come from Raketla village in Uravakonda. I have one older sister and one younger brother, but I was the sole victim of polio when I was one year old. My parents, who were poor, took me to doctors who prescribed medicines and tonics, and advised them to use sand bags and some exercises. This contributed to my mobility, but my left leg remained weak.

My parents migrated to Anantapur in order to provide a good education for their children. I was admitted into Syfulla School, Navodaya colony, Anantapur. Both teachers and classmates were quite helpful, and I mingled and played with able-bodied children. Travelling to and from school was a little inconvenient as I grew bigger; my father was carrying me on his cycle. At home, people suggested that I should be admitted into a hostel, but my father didn't like their proposal. With great difficulty I completed my primary education, and went to a high school for girls in Anantapur. While in the seventh class my parents approached an orthopedic doctor who operated to release contractures. I lost much schooling, but my father used to provide reading materials and encouraged me to study.

I later went to college and completed both my intermediate and graduation (second class) in commerce. My parents arranged my sister's marriage, but my father encouraged me to join a computer course, in order to be independent. Other relatives always discouraged me because I am disabled, and I didn't go to any place other than my college, computer institute, and home. I learned desktop publishing and completed the postgraduate diploma in computer application. I applied for an NGO job, and was referred to SACRED who gave me an interview.

My parents doubted my abilities to do a job independently but I was determined, and they didn't object because of debts when my brother became ill. Joining SACRED was a turning point because I worked with so many disabled persons, gained experience in programs implemented by SACRED, and learned bank transactions. I procured articles necessary for my family and cleared all their debts, and saved one Lakh rupees and purchased 10 grams of gold. I contributed to my brother's education, and he is now a science graduate, and has become a school teacher. He is earning Rs.6000 per month and puts Rs.3000 into my bank account every month.

I am happy today because I can go to the SACRED office (with the help of a caliper) and use my computer skills. My family is highly cooperative, and I am able to forget my disability by moving with my kith and kin. There is good recognition because I became an earning member, contributing to the growth of my family. I now know that disabled people can be well recognized if they prove their hidden talents. I may not erase the negative feelings prevailing in present day society, but I can keep my thoughts positive.

M. Deepika

A. Umadavi

I am from Kakkulapalli village, Anantapur, and had polio at age three. My parents were poor agricultural labourers and borrowed money for my treatment. At six, I went to the local school; I could not go home for lunch because we lived far away, and I could only crawl. My parents were advised to get me wooden crutches made locally, which helped my mobility a lot, but my muscles were weak and I often used to fall.

After primary education, I went to the high school at Kalyandurg, completing the tenth class. My parents took me to a famous doctor in Tirupathi, who operated to release contractures, but mobility was not improved; they lost two months' wages and incurred debts. I could overcome all my suffering because of the concern showed by my parents and younger sister.

At the age of 18 my mother compelled me to marry her younger brother who was disinclined to accept me as his wife. I stayed with my parents, and my husband came every two months. I felt sad for marrying someone not interested in me. My parents worried about my future; they and my family were my only society; the outside world was unknown until an NGO started a self-help group in our village. Interaction with other disabled persons overcame my shyness and anxiety and improved my self-confidence and willpower. The group chose me as a volunteer for three villages, with an incentive of Rs.300 and travel expenses. Participation in meetings and training improved my communication skills, and I could forget my personal problems in the activities of the self-help groups. My mother tried to compel me to drop my work because others were commenting; I was still with my parents after marriage and my husband never even inquired of my welfare or whereabouts. At one time I decided to die because of the mental tensions.

The turning point was my appointment as animator with SACRED in June 2005. I then moved to my husband's place, but his family objected, and my husband scolded me. I told them that I was earning and they should accept me as a member of the family, but we were forced to leave, and took asylum in a new government house in the name of my husband. We were without food for two days, but my husband changed his attitude and accepted me as his wife. My parents had given me vessels, cloths, and provisions to set up a separate family.

I started work as an animator for eight villages, and my husband also started earning. We got our house electrified and got a gas connection; we purchased a colour television, a cell phone, and basic necessities. It created a lot of jealousy, and my husband's younger brother forced us to repay a Rs.3000 loan on the house. They locked us out until we paid, and were beaten up by him. I was going to lodge a police complaint, but the villagers settled the issue temporarily. My husband earns Rs.100 a day, and I earn Rs.2000 a month. I am now very happy to be living independently. I forget that I am disabled. My parents are happy that I am with my husband, but not that I have no children. I took homeopathy medicine, and I am glad to share that I am now pregnant. I now know that there will be satisfactory outcomes only when disabled people fight for their basic rights. Unless we raise our grievance against discriminations faced in our day-to-day life, we will hardly survive in the present day world.

A. Umadavi

B. Urukundamma

I was born at Pathikonda village, Kurnool, on July 19, 1979, and became disabled by polio at six months. I have three sisters and five brothers, all settled, and I am the only disabled person in the family. I studied from primary to intermediate level in my native village, overcoming both financial and mobility problems to do so, but I then had to discontinue my education due to financial problems. I got a small job as a teacher to supplement the family income, but I was sad about dropping my education. Since then, I decided to continue my education by working as a teacher, and applied to take a graduate course from the AMBEDKAR Open University (distance learning). I have successfully completed my first year course.

While I was pursuing my second year, I got an offer from SACRED to become one of their rural development workers. I am very happy with this because I can continue my education privately, and also contribute to my family's income. Moreover there is self-satisfaction because I am working for other disabled persons in our region. My message to other disabled persons is "Don't compromise with what you have achieved in life. Set up higher goals and work sincerely to reach them. Even if you fail in your attempt, don't get disappointed and frustrated. Learn from each experience and grow in life."

B. Urukundamma

R. Nagamani

I was born in a poor family; my parents had a consanguineous marriage and seven children died immediately after birth. I am the only living child to my parents, but unfortunately I was disabled. My father was always sick, and there were no others to extend any support to our family. There was lot of pressure on me to drop my education after the seventh class, but I was determined and worked hard, and completed the tenth class.

At the age of 14 years my parents performed my marriage. I was married to a man who was illiterate and not doing any job, and the maintenance of my family became very difficult. My parents and also my husband discouraged me from doing any work, because of my disability. I wanted to learn tailoring, but they didn't send me to a tailoring course. Even before I was 21 years of age I had three children, but I then got a family planning operation. I was working as an agriculture labourer, but also joined a tailoring course, and became a tailor in the village.

There was then a dispute with our relatives regarding a land issue. They abused me and used filthy language, and threatened that they would break my legs. I went to the police station to file a case against my relatives who created such a nuisance. The police warned them of the consequences of harassing a disabled person, and the issue was settled amicably, but I was in financial crisis.

At this time, SACRED entered our village. I was encouraged to join the organization, but I was fearful of moving out of the house independently. However, I took it as a challenge and joined the organization. I now have a different mindset with the help of which I am able to carry out my tasks with perfection. I have the inner strength to do my best for other disabled persons. I have realized that my society is much larger than what I was imagining, and I have the hope that I can achieve excellence in my job.

Acknowledgements

I would like to thank the many people, in many countries, with whom I have worked on disability projects, who have welcomed me and taught me much, especially colleagues on the SACRED programme in Andhra Pradesh, India, and particularly Lakshmi Prasana, who understands a great deal more than I about women with disability, and the five colleagues who have very willingly contributed their stories to add concrete and particular realities to my generalizations. I would also like to thank my wife Barbara and sister-in-law Margaret Hall for reading the first draft and making helpful suggestions. Mary Edmonds-Otter of the University of Leicester library was immensely helpful with literature searches.

DISCUSSION QUESTIONS

1. How would you define human rights for girls and women with disabilities in poor communities in developing countries?

2. How might you try to increase the interest and involvement of women and organizations active in women's rights in women with disabilities?

3. What human rights do you think should be considered so fundamental that they should transcend all cultures? What principles would you adopt to deal with situations where deep, long-standing cultures are in conflict with what you consider to be inalienable human rights for disabled women?

4. Within one culture of your choice, what do you consider to be the key issues to address to promote equality of opportunity for disabled girls and women?

5. To what extent do you think individuals and organizations from outside a community can work effectively to improve disabled girls' and women's access to education, economic activity, and family life? What strategies would you suggest?

REFERENCES

1. Sands T. A voice of our own: advocacy by women with disability in Australia and the Pacific. *Gender Dev.* 2005;13(3):51-62.

2. Abu-Habib L. 'Women and disability don't mix!': double discrimination and disabled women's rights. *Gender Dev.* 1995;3(2):49-53.

3. Abu-Habib L. *Gender and Disability—Women's Experiences in the Middle East.* Oxford, UK: Oxfam; 1997.

4. Oliver M. *The Politics of Disablement.* London, UK: Macmillan; 1990.

5. United Nations Economic and Social Commission for Asia and the Pacific. Consideration of regional framework for action towards an inclusive, barrier-free, and rights-based society for persons with disabilities in Asia and the Pacific. *Asia Pacific Disabil Rehab J.* 2003;Supplement.

6. Rousso H. *Education for All: A Gender and Disability Perspective.* Washington, DC: World Bank; 2004.

7. Lonsdale S. *Women and Disability.* London, UK: Macmillan; 1990.

8. Thomas M, Thomas MJ. Status of women with disabilities in South Asia. In: Thomas M, Thomas MJ, eds. Selected readings in community-based rehabilitation, series 2: disability and rehabilitation issues in south Asia. *Asia Pacific Disabil Rehab J.* 2002;27-34.

9. *Gender Equality: Further Guide to Gender Equality.* Oxford, UK: Oxfam; 2008.

10. Govinda R. The politics of the marginalised: Dalits and women's activism in India. *Gender Dev.* 2006;14(2):181-190.

11. Coleridge P. *Disability, Liberation and Development.* Oxford, UK: Oxfam; 1993.

12. van Kampen M, van Zijverden IM, Emmett T. Reflections on poverty and disability: a review of literature. *Asia Pacific Disabil Rehab J.* 2008;19(1):19-37.

13. Coleridge P. Disability and culture. In: Thomas M, Thomas MJ, eds. Selected readings in community-based rehabilitation, series 1: CBR in transition. *Asia Pacific Disabil Rehab J.* 2000;2-38.

14. Fryers T. Mental retardation. In: Tantam D, Appleby L, Duncan A. *Psychiatry for the Developing World.* London, UK: Gaskell; 1996:258-290.

15. Bone M, Meltzer H. *The Prevalence of Disability Among Children.* London, UK: HMSO; 1989.

16. Martin J, Meltzer H, Elliot D. *The Prevalence of Disability Among Adults.* London, UK: HMSO; 1988.

17. Stanley F, Alberman E. *The Epidemiology of the Cerebral Palsies.* Oxford, UK: Blackwell; 1984.

18. Global Polio Eradication Initiative: Wild Poliovirus Weekly Update, February 20, 2008. Geneva: WHO; 2008.

19. Piccinelli M, Homen FG. *Gender Differences in the Epidemiology of Affective Disorders and Schizophrenia.* Geneva, Switzerland; WHO:1997.

20. Deegan M, Brooks N, eds. *Women & Disability; the Double Handicap.* New Brunswick: Edison, NJ. Transaction Books; 1985:1.

21. Gawaya R, Mukasa RS. The African Women's Protocol: a new dimension for women's rights in Africa. *Gender Dev.* 2005;13(3):42-50.

22. Johnson H, Bernstein H. *Third World Lives of Struggle.* Oxford, UK: Heinemann/Open University; 1982.

23. Hartley S, ed. *CBR as Part of Community Development: A Poverty Reduction Strategy.* London, UK: University College Centre for International Child Health; 2006.

24. *Poverty Reduction Source Book.* Washington DC: World Bank; 1999.

25. United Nations Ad Hoc Committee on a Comprehensive and Integral International Convention on the Protection and Promotion of the Rights and Dignity of Persons with Disabilities. *Final Report of Eighth Session: Draft Convention on the Rights of Persons with Disabilities, and Draft Optional Protocol.* New York, NY: UN; 2006.

26. Thomas M, Thomas MJ. A discussion of some critical aspects in planning of community-based rehabilitation. *Asia Pacific Disabil Rehab J.* 2000;84-95.

27. Coleridge P. CBR in a complex emergency; study of Afghanistan. *Asia Pacific Disabil Rehab J.* 2002;35-49.

28. Dalal AK. Disability rehabilitation in a traditional Indian society. *Asia Pacific Disabil Rehab J.* 2002;17-26.

29. Sinha K. Citizenship degraded: Indian women in a modern state and a pre-modern society. *Gender Dev.* 2003;11(3):19-26.

30. Mehrotra N. Women and disability management in rural Haryana, India. *Asia Pacific Disabil Rehab J.* 2008;19(1)38-49.

31. Thomas M, Thomas MJ. Some Controversies in CBR. In Hartley S, ed. *CBR as a Participatory Strategy in Africa.* London: University College Centre for International Child Health; 2002:13-25.

32. Johnson D, Kabuchu H, Kayonga SV. Women in Ugandan local government: the impact of affirmative action. *Gender Dev.* 2003;11(3):8-18.

33. Nagata KK. Gender and disability in the Arab region: the challenges in the new millenium. *Asia Pacific Disabil Rehab J.* 2003;14(1):10-17.

34. Chavuta AHP, Kimuli E, Ogot O. CBR as part of inclusive education and development. In Hartley S, ed. *CBR as Part of Community Development: A Poverty Reduction Strategy.* London, UK: University College Centre for International Child Health; 2006: 64-73.

35. Try L. Gendered experiences: marriage and the stigma of leprosy. *Asia Pacific Disabil Rehab J.* 2007;17(2): 55-72.

36. Thomas M, Thomas MJ. Addressing needs of women with disabilities, in CBR. *Asia Pacific Disabil Rehab J.* 2003;26-33.

37. Groce NE. HIV/AIDS and individuals with disability. *Health Human Rights.* 2005;8(2):215-224.

38. Davidson L. HIV and AIDS, and Disability. In Hartley S, ed. *CBR as Part of Community Development: A Poverty Reduction Strategy.* London, UK: University College Centre for International Child Health; 2006:91-95.

39. Nganwa AB, Batesaki B, Balaba A, Serunkuma P, Yousafzai AK. HIV/AIDS and community based rehabilitation. In: Hartley S, ed. *CBR as a Participatory Strategy in Africa.* London, UK: University College Centre for International Child Health; 2002:185-196.

40. Glasier A, Gulmezoglu AM, Schmid GP, Moreno CG, Van Look PF. Sexual and reproductive health: a matter of life and death. *Lancet.* 2006;368:1595-1607.

41. Fryers T. *Childhood Determinants of Adult Mental Illness.* Helsinki, Finland: STAKES; 2007.

42. Helander E, Mendis G, Nelson G, Goert A. *Training in the Community for People with Disabilities.* Geneva, Switzerland: WHO; 1989.

43. Valdez JS. *Community-Based Rehabilitation Services: Provision in Poverty Stricken and Rural Areas.* Bacolod City, Philippines: Negro Occidental Rehabilitation Foundation; 1984.

44. Giacaman R. A community of citizens: disability rehabilitation in the Palestinian transition to statehood. *Disabil Rehab.* 2001;23(14):639-644.

45. Sweetman C. Women & citizenship [editorial]. *Gender Dev.* 2003;11(3):2-7.

46. Gill A, Rehman G. Empowerment through activism: responding to domestic violence in the South Asian Community in London. *Gender Dev.* 2004;12(1):75-82.

47. Gaylin W, Jennings B. *The Perversion of Autonomy.* New York, NY: The Free Press; 1996.

48. Coleridge P. Setting out the issues: an interview with B Venkatesh. In: Coleridge P, ed. *Disability, Liberation and Development.* Oxford, UK: Oxfam; 1993:13-26.

49. Julia Twigg J, ed. *Carers: Research and Practice.* London, UK: HMSO; 1992.

50. Keith L. Who cares wins? Women, caring and disability. *Disabil Soc.* 1992; 7(2):167-175.

51. Finch J, Groves D. Community care and the family; a case for equal opportunities. *J Soc Policy.* 1980;9:487-511.

52. Maher J. *Carers 2000.* London, UK: National Statistics; 2002.

53. Team V, Markovic M, Manderson L. Family care-givers: Russian-speaking Australian women's access to welfare support. *Health Soc Care Community.* 2007; 15(5):397-406.

54. Abberley P. The concept of oppression and the development of a social theory of disability. *Disabil Handicap Soc.* 1988;2(1):5-19.

55. Vijesh PV, Sukumaran PS. Stress among mothers of children with cerebral palsy attending special schools. *Asia Pacific Disabil Rehab J.* 2007;18(1):76-92.

56. Coleridge P. CBR as part of community development and poverty reduction. In: Hartley S, ed. *CBR as Part of Community Development: A Poverty Reduction Strategy.* London, UK: University College Centre for International Child Health; 2006:19-39.

57. Thomas M. Editor's Comment *Asia Pacific Disabil Rehab J.* 2007;18(1)1-2.

58. Duffy Y. *All Things Are Possible.* Michigan: AJ Garvin and Associates; 1981 (quoted in Coleridge P, ed. *Disability, Liberation and Development.* Oxford, UK: Oxfam; 1993:219).

CHAPTER 27

INTRODUCTION

On March 31, 2007, the UN General Assembly adopted by consensus a landmark treaty to promote and protect the rights of the world's 650 million disabled people. "We have now reached a global consensus: The disabled are entitled to the full range of civil rights that those without disabilities enjoy," said Haya Rashed Al Khalifa of Bahrain, the president of the 192-nation general assembly.[1]

Worldwide, the largest minority and arguably the least understood class of citizens are women with disabilities. These women are now being recognized as victims of a human rights dilemma. In the absence of an energized advocacy group or internationally recognized spokesperson, the disability rights movement has slowly gained credibility among the world's people. But women and particularly female children in many areas are still facing the greatest need in fulfilling the full range of civil rights that the nondisabled enjoy and as promised in the recently enacted UN treaty. As early as 1990 at the World Conference on Education for All, in Jomtien, Thailand, women's education was cited as a top priority for international development agencies. The Beijing Platform for Action, the outcome document of the 1995 United Nations Fourth World Conference on Women focused on 12 critical areas of concern. The education and training of women was one of the highlighted critical areas:

> Intensify efforts to ensure equal enjoyment of all human rights and fundamental freedoms for all women and girls who face multiple barriers to their empowerment and advancement because of such factors as their race, age, language, ethnicity, culture, religion, or disability, or because they are indigenous people.[2]

Among women with disabilities in the United States, the research suggests that legal changes that have increased women's access to education and in particular a bachelor's degree seems to be a key factor in determining parody between the disabled and nondisabled. Women with and

Women with Disabilities in Education: The United States and the Americans with Disabilities Act

Martin Patwell, EdD

Martin Patwell, EdD, is Director of the Office of Services for Students with Disabilities for West Chester University, West Chester, PA.

without disabilities are increasing their numbers significantly in postsecondary education, graduating and broadening their areas of interest. As a result of this advancement, it is these same women who are making inroads into employment areas that have previously been closed. Nevertheless, there is much that remains to be done in eliminating inequities and providing avenues for success.

Education

The value of women's education has received global recognition over the past two decades. The *Human Development Report 1995*,[3] produced by the UN's Development Program, and the UN's Millennium Development Goals (MDGs), with gender equality and women's empowerment as one of the goals, emphasizes the need to eliminate gender disparity at all levels of education.[4]

In the United States, emphasis on educational accommodations and social accessibility has been the key to the success of the Americans with Disabilities Act of 1990 (ADA) (42 U.S.C. 12102). The gradual inclusion into the social fabric of people with disabilities has been a transition from mendicants to entrepreneurs. In 1986, before the ADA, educational law had produced a generation of students with disabilities whose expectations were to graduate high school, but college was far down their list of attainable objectives. At that time the gap between disabled and nondisabled students with HS graduation was 24 percentage points (61% versus 85%).[5] By 2001 10 years after the ADA was implemented, students with disabilities had increased their rate of graduation by more than two-fold over the nondisabled, and the gap was reduced to 13 points (78% versus 91%).[6] Overall, women increased their participation in more college prep courses, and eliminated the gender gap by the beginning of the 1990s. Not only did women take harder courses in high school, but they had higher grade point averages (GPAs).[7]

Between 1990 and 2005 enrollment of women (age 25 and under) in higher education increased 45%, more than double the increase seen in males. As women have become the majority population on college campuses over the last decade they have also surpassed their male counterparts in important quality issues such as degree attainment and educational expectations.[8] From 1990 to 2000 women increased their level of degree attainment by 10%, and by 1994 were more likely than men to have attained a BA. Into the mid-1990s there was still a considerable gender difference among youth with disabilities. Girls were less likely to be employed, made less money than boys, and did not attend postsecondary education.[9]

Outside of school women with and without disabilities tend to be as engaged as males in work, training, or college, and most (75%) do a combination of work and training or college.[9] Women who entered postsecondary education by 1994 were more likely to graduate with a BA than men (50% versus 45%). Except for their preference in pursuing education and health careers, women persisted in choosing more academic majors.[10]

In addition to becoming the majority on campus, women's participation in higher education changed from mostly part time to mostly full time. Additionally, they made these gains against all odds. During this period, women continued to represent lower income, greater incidence of dependent children, and single parenthood. Likewise, over that time college admissions for students with disabilities had increased by some 49%.[11] Currently, a higher percentage of female undergraduates report a disability (11.4% versus 11.2%).[12] The conclusions are unmistakable: college works for students with disabilities, especially women. College has become more attainable for people with disabilities, and despite slow acceptance on college campuses, most colleges offer services for 80% of students with disabilities who need them.[13] The number of high school graduates with disabilities matriculating in postsecondary education has risen from 3% in 1978 to 19% in 1996.[12] More than 50% of students with disabilities enrolling in postsecondary education worked towards a degree or credential. And 67% of youth with disabilities who graduated with a bachelor of arts degree were working full time compared with 73% of people without disabilities holding the same degree.[13]

The degree makes all the difference for people with disabilities. While in all other economic aspects the disabled population lags significantly, persons with disabilities who attain a BA have an equal chance of securing a full-time job in their field.[14]

Some Problems Persist

Yet much needs to be done in preparing all youth with disabilities for life after high school. Twice as many persons with disabilities drop out of high school,[6] and they are much less likely to take the full curriculum of math, science, and foreign languages. Plus, despite the legal mandates for schools, youth with disabilities are not required to attend individual educational plan (IEP) meetings that discuss their disabilities, and thus they do not advocate for postschool transition plans nor prepare themselves for advocacy in college or work.[13] As we have seen, this is increasingly more of a problem for women who would take more advantage of participation in college preparation if it were offered.

Undermining academic success in college and the pursuit of a degree are the social dynamics inherent in transitioning to adult life. The social aspect of college life is critical to students with disabilities. Families who have a child with a disability are often not educated to convey the information about growing independently that their children need. We see this in "helicopter parenting" that continues beyond the mandatory participation in secondary educational planning into college and beyond. Like most families in the United States parents expect colleges to provide the transition to adulthood that is missing in our disintegrated social structure, with or without their direct help. Unfortunately, colleges are competing with media and losing. According to the Center on Institutional Research (CIRP) survey[15] of college freshman, overall they spent twice as much time watching TV and social networking on the Internet than face to face with groups, or reading. But female college students were different from men in some important ways. Women were more likely to use the net for socializing but also did a lot more reading than men. In fact they were better prepared for college than men and took the prospect of college more seriously. They took

more advanced placement classes, studied longer hours, volunteered more, did more research, and were less likely than men to party. As a result of all this preparation, women were more likely to feel overwhelmed and more open to counseling when they arrived at college. But more insidiously they were less apt than men to rate themselves highly on indicators for positive self-esteem, academic ability, competitiveness, emotional health, and self-confidence, both intellectual and social. To add to their stressors women were more interested in such extracurricular activities as joining a sorority, doing community service, participating in student clubs, or studying abroad.[15] They were also much more likely to anticipate working to pay for college. Yet despite their differences in approach and problems with self-esteem, women entering college today are almost identical to men in their expectations for financial success and recognition in their chosen field. In total numbers women are almost equal to men in science and math degrees, advancing in all other fields.[16]

Drawing out social differences between female colleges students with and without disabilities is difficult because of lack of research. However, beneath the data a lot of the noise that obscures the disability differences is all gender. For example, one area of disability that has been intensively studied is attention deficit hyperactivity disorder (ADHD). One of the leading researchers in the field, Russell A. Barkley, found that there were few differences between men and women with ADHD outside the usual differences between the sexes. For example, woman in general report higher rates of anxiety, and so do woman with disabilities.[17] Yet there are still reasons to suspect that women's difficulties in education and employment would be exacerbated by the effects of their disability. Consider a few of the findings from Barkley and colleagues from a gender equity perspective:

- Virtually all the ADHD adults in their Milwaukee study suffered from educational and occupational impairments, often the co-occurrence of learning disabilities or the effects of late diagnosed and untreated disabilities. Women with disabilities in his sample were less likely to be identified or referred for services at an early age. This is not disquieting until you realize that all of these women should have been referred since ADHD is a developmental disorder. Is the underrepresentation at earlier ages a sign of better coping or mere neglect, as many (mostly female) writers suggest?

- On the job women with ADHD were found to have more problems in client relations, he found. This too is a significant finding, if in fact it impairs occupational movement for women. And even more troubling, if it is paired with the fact that women were identified by others as being more aggressive than males with ADHD, it opens an entire area of potential gender disability and discrimination with regard to women.

- Women had different medical complaints associated with anxiety, depression, and somatization. When they were involved in criminal activity it was less social acting out and more social deprivation related, like forging checks. What does this say about the more desperate lives women with disabilities lead and the challenges they encounter?

- Women with ADHD were less likely to be married. Since ADHD people have poorer marriages it is not unrealistic to think that they are part of the increasing phenomenon of households led by women with disabilities. Estimates of ADHD among the offspring of ADHD adults range from 43% to 57% in some studies to 22% to 43% in the Milwaukee study. Thus the problems of women with ADHD who are single moms are going to be exacerbated by their genes.

Due to lack of emphasis on gender disparities and disability, research is lacking on the full range of problems of women with disabilities. We know that women with disabilities receive less financial support from the Office of Vocational Rehabilitation (OVR), one of the main suppliers of postsecondary service, and some suggest that women with disabilities are not encouraged to explore career opportunities offered to men.[18] Social Security Income (SSI), which is available for most students with disabilities, is restricted in its provisions for college savings and dependent on VR waivers to go beyond $2000 in a college fund.[13] Women with disabilities face additional obstacles in even attaining SSI.[18] Most students with disabilities have additional educational or medical expenses associated with the cost of attending postsecondary education, but few receive the full benefit of financial aid they are entitled to.[19] Most expenses, such as wheelchairs, hearing aids, and personal attendants, all very costly items that are not covered by insurances, can be added to the educational expenses under Pell grants, but this is rarely done, due to the disconnection between the federal loan program (FAFSA), which does not include such information in calculating students educational related costs, and the college financial aid offices information.[13] This is a tremendous burden on students who might have to choose between financial aid requirements for full-time status or being dropped from all health care.

Global trends reveal a growing representation of women in higher education in many regions—with the highest ratios in Europe, Latin America, and the Arab states and the lowest representations in sub-Saharan Africa and South Asia.[4] Despite improved ratios of access and participation over the past decades, there remains a definite pattern of gender tracking in most countries with women dominating certain courses or fields such as liberal arts, home economics, nursing, and teaching, while men dominate courses in law, agriculture, engineering, and natural sciences. Gender tracking, which channels women into careers that are basically extensions of their domestic responsibilities and allows men to acquire more marketable skills and enjoy greater earning power, only exacerbates the problem of unequal opportunities for women.[20] Women are now comparable to men in first degrees awarded in many of the Western countries (United States, UK, Italy, Canada, France, and Italy), and slightly less than half in Mexico, Japan, Korea, Turkey, and Germany.[16] If the evidence in the United States is any indication, however, there is a lot of work left to do to overcome years of discrimination once students graduate and enter the workforce.

Post-Postsecondary: What Happens After Graduation?

The status of woman with disabilities in the United States employment sector in the 1900s was largely determined by rehabilitation services. In the early part of the century, rehabilitation—physical, occupational, and other therapies—became true professions in the medical model of intervention. The average client of the rehabilitation system in the 1920s and 1930s was "white, male, and 31 years old."[21] The purpose of what came to be known as "vocational rehabilitation (VR)" in the 1920s focused on returning workers hurt on the job to productive employment; only 12,000 of the estimated 250,000 new persons with disabilities per year were actually "rehabilitated." The war years of the 1940s only increased the percentage of young males with disabilities. Rehabilitation was a government-funded insurance system for industry. The goal was to return the investment by concentrating on wage earners, not nonindustrial accidents or congenital disabilities. The guiding philosophy in the latter part of the 1900s was Menninger's "whole man theory": through rehabilitation the disabled could be made right again. But the template for rightness became stereotypical roles reinforced by the OVR system of "order of service." Men with mild disabilities were deemed more worthy of investment. Ironically, the modern rehabilitation system was founded by a woman, Mary Switzer, who became the Director of the OVR after WWII and helped pass legislation that became the Rehabilitation Act of 1954. Yet, Switzer remained opposed to what advocates called the "rights" argument of disability access to employment. This was not only in keeping with the American way of business but emphasized the OVR "creaming" approach to offering assistance.[21]

In that context it is worthwhile to consider the passage of social legislation that attempted to eliminate discrimination in hiring. By the 1980s a logical consequence of increased educational attainment for persons with disabilities was an upsurge in seeking employment. Added to the additional weight of the ADA as social legislation, we can actually distinguish two trends that are a direct consequence of the act. One of the chief arguments against the ADA as social legislation is the apparent lack of progress in employment for persons with disabilities.[11]

While there has been some progress made in the number of employed persons with disabilities living below the poverty line, it is still three times more likely for persons with disabilities to be making a poverty wage.[11]

The second fact to consider in employment trends is that only medium-sized and larger businesses were affected by the act. Businesses with fewer than 15 employees were exempt. So, we can compare the increase in employment between small and larger businesses to see the effect of the ADA in employment. Over the eight-year ADA initiation period, while employment actually declined overall, employment for persons with disabilities increased and narrowed the gap from 4.1% to 1.9%. In small industries, unaffected by the ADA, no such dramatic increase occurred, and the gap actually increased.[22]

Overall, since the passage of the ADA, the percentage of persons with disabilities who are able to work and are working has increased from 46% in 1986 to 56% in 2000.[23] But two-thirds of persons with disabilities who are unemployed in a time of relatively low unemployment would prefer to be working.[24]

Employment for women graduates continues to lag behind males despite the impressive gains in degree attainment. For BA recipients, more men were employed full time, they made more money, and even in fields where salaries were higher, women earned less. Nevertheless, as elsewhere, women's gains over the last decade surpassed men. There was no detectable difference, for the first time, in unemployment. And women's entries into fields that were male enclaves—science and engineering—increased as did their salaries. The gender gap in income in science, technology, engineering, and math [STEM] fields shrank from 71% to 84%.[16]

Young women with disabilities face the dual dilemma of their gender and their disability. Young men and women growing up with disabilities internalize the negative stereotypes about them and often quit before they can get started on a career. The vast majority are employed in menial jobs with no hope of advancement.[13] They also suffer from violence to a disproportionate degree.[25] And because they have less income, they lack access to the greatest leveler of all—assistive technology. While 47% of college graduates with disabilities have a computer, fewer than 13% of high school graduates have one, and among those with less than a high school diploma, only 2.4% have access to the Internet. What this means to a persons with disabilities who face obstacles to a quality education because of their disability is even further entrenchment as a second-class citizen. Isolated physically, sensorially, and educationally, without computer access these individuals are cut off from the services and support they desperately need.

Women with disabilities suffer even more job discrimination than men with lower rates of employment and lower incomes.[18] Currently unemployment in the United States among persons with disabilities is 68%,[26] a gap of 49% between the disabled and nondisabled. College graduation made a significant difference in unemployment, but women were still underpaid even for the same jobs. While unemployment increased for women overall, those with a BA were exempt from this downward trend. While a greater percentage of women earned higher salaries in 2001 compared to 1994, they still were making 83% of what men earned in the same professions.[12]

For women the burden is passed to their children. Families with a disabled member were much more likely to be living in poverty (12.8% versus 7.7%). According to U.S. Census data, families with a female head of household were more likely to report a member with a disability, and 43% of families with a female head of household who contained a person with disabilities were living in poverty.[27] The cost and impoverishment increases significantly with the number of members; families with two or more children with a disability are five times more likely to live in poverty.[27]

And yet, many government organizations and nongovernmental organizations (NGO'S) still believe that persons with disabilities prefer the meager SSI payments they receive. The stigma of services, medical rehabilitation, and special education among this population present the illusion of opportunity for a life that is as "good as it can be."[4] Despite the legal victories for persons with disabilities over the past three decades, the employment sector and general attitudes about disability have not substantially changed.[11] Neither has our youth-obsessed culture, which makes a cult of physical health and vitality. So the burden of change and adaptation is still squarely on the shoulders of the disabled.

Persons with disabilities continue to encounter discrimination in the workplace. According to the Center for an Accessible Society, 32% of employers thought their work could not be done by persons with disabilities; 60% provides no training to staff on accommodating persons with disabilities. Yet where persons with disabilities were employed employers said that 73% of them required no accommodation, and the majority (65%) state that accommodations were not costly.[28]

Since 1990 a number of employer surveys have addressed the issue of worker rights. In 2000, a Harris survey reported that 90% of employers favored the ADA's nondiscrimination policy. And a report on employer satisfaction found a "high willingness" to employ persons with disabilities.[21] In 2001, 36% of persons with disabilities continued to face discrimination on the job.[22] Four years later that number had decreased to 22%.[25] Although the overt discrimination of illegal hiring and firing may have ceased, the more subtle attitudinal shift takes much longer to take hold. Despite the gains made in the social environment, the gap in employment is still the best measure of the failure to meet the economic and social needs of persons with disabilities. According to the latest survey of life satisfaction, people with disabilities are less satisfied (34% versus 61%) than the nondisabled. Problems with accessible transportation (31% versus 13%), education, employment, and income top the list of complaints.[11]

Despite all the negative news, we can find hope in the prospects for any student with a disability who proceeds to gaining their BA. For women who have taken the dual advantage of the women's rights and disability rights movements to its natural conclusion, the news is quite bright indeed.[14]

Hopeful Trends in Education

One of the most promising vehicles for creating more receptive campuses is disability studies, a movement that has gained a great deal of energy and rhetoric from the women's rights and civil rights movements. Disability studies offer the opportunity to internally restructure the dialogue around society's relationship to persons with disabilities for the purpose of contributing to a change in perspective that ennobles the perceiver and normalizes the perceived. Historically, second-class status has been attributed to persons with disabilities based on perceived differences in appearance, sensory aptitude, mobility, or learning. Disability studies is "both a private and a public experience. . . . For some, disability represents a personal catastrophe to be avoided if at all possible. . . . For others, disability is a source of pride and empowerment."[29(p1)]

Just as with previous rights movements, there are various frames of reference in conceptualizing disability studies. The most often cited is contrasting the medical model of disability with a more progressive social model. Disability studies encompass a key aspect of the human experience, akin to gender, race, ethnicity, and sexual orientation. There is one key difference, however. All of us will experience disability in our lives (assuming we live long enough). Yet somehow disability, rather than being embraced and gaining in understanding over time, has become increasingly linked with ineptitude, personal catastrophe, and freakishness. It is the fragility of our life and health and the inevitability of disability that keeps us from embracing it as part of the natural cycle. We choose to live in a bubble surrounding ourselves with images of perfectionism. Disability studies could be an antidote to such sterility.

The study of disability as a social context for human experience has psychological, political, and economic import for our society as a whole. We experience disability in many ways, both as a regrettable fact of life and as a symbol of our modernity. We can reflect on a recent history of both unbelievable inhumanity and a dawning recognition of a common stake in a shared acceptance of difference.

One of the objects of disability studies is finding exceptions to the medical model that make the hope for a social model of disability more realistic. As an example, deafness is a hereditary trait, just as are blond hair and hemophilia. All occur with greater frequency the closer the bonds of a social group. In the colonial United States, the isolated community on Martha's Vineyard became such a haven. The original 28 families accounted for two-thirds of the population until the mid 1800s, and the incidence of deafness was four times the national average; in some towns it reached as high as 1 in 49. Naturally sign language was common, and as a device for communicating over distances and across the water it became as popular among the hearing as it was among the deaf. Newer emigrants complained that people gathered in community locations and spoke by sign in groups, only punctuating the silence with loud laughter when the joke reached its punch line. Eventually, schools that specialized in educating the deaf were started off the island, and the majority of deaf islanders spent up to 10 years at places like the American Asylum in Hartford. Thus, not only were the deaf islanders better educated than their contemporaries, they suffered none of the prejudices associated with disabilities elsewhere. Many experts in education and psychology were lampooning the idea of educating the deaf, comparing them to "savages of Patagonia." When the first college for deaf students opened in 1870, a leading authority was quoted as comparing the prospects of a deaf-mute as no higher than an orangutan.[30] Meanwhile, on Martha's Vineyard, deafness was not considered a disability, not because it was the right thing to do, but because the society worked better when people made a little effort. This could be a working definition of a social model.

Yet social models, unlike medical and legal models, are not something we can impose by fiat. Persons with disabilities in this century are still part of a "throw away" society in parts of the developing world. In the larger American society, disability access is still considered the province of medical and legal professionals. Many of the current prejudices that persons with disabilities face in the West were formed in the 1800s when our ideals about differences were that we would soon eradicate them; any opinions to the contrary were unscientific and often illegal: "If you couldn't cure it, make it illegal." The last of the "ugly laws," which made it a crime for persons with disabilities to appear in public, were on the books in many states until 1974.[29(pp39-41)] The first federal law eliminating discrimination based on disability was enacted in 1977, and the ADA was only passed in 1990. In between the era of legal segregation and the dawn of prohibition of discrimination there was no national renaissance of thinking. Activists simply made lawmakers uncomfortable. The reality is that until as a society we can admit that it is not biology nor demons that disables but our attitudes, society will not change.

Universal Design of Instruction

Students with disabilities in postsecondary education in the United States face a bewildering assortment of choices and decisions that their nondisabled peers do not. In an effort to create a nondiscriminatory environment and not lower academic standards, we require students to become knowledgeable and articulate about their disabilities and make the leap to an independent college environment that is, in the words of one such student overheard at one of our University's orientation sessions, "like a hotel run by kids."

Universal design for instruction (UDI) is a promising and growing movement within educational theory and disability studies. In brief, UDI asks faculty to design courses and approach their teaching with maximal flexibility in order to successfully teach more students—with or without disabilities. Under this approach, we should no longer be thinking of accommodations as defining how we will work with particular students with disabilities in the classroom, but rather, what can we do to make our work with students maximally accessible to all students, regardless of specific diagnoses. Just as UDI architectural design principles that resulted in curb cuts and automated sliding doors have been useful for all people, regardless of mobility issues, educators working to promote UDI maintain that these principles have radical potential to enhance the learning of every student in a given classroom.

UDI and disability studies encompass many facets of the values espoused for our students' education. Our hope is to incorporate these egalitarian approaches to education into the mainstream and eliminate the need for special treatment of persons with disabilities on our campus. However, without broad social support our attempts will not eliminate the inequities that exist in the employment sector, nor transform society into a more accepting and less judgmental environment.

Conclusion: Global Benefits to Society

Abroad, countries fear the US/UK model that has given rise to medical dependency, the "dole," while admiring the high-quality care affordable by the rich. The case of Christopher Reeves is a case in point. After his accident, "Superman" became a media darling by advocating rehabilitation and recovery. His news profiles featured him in state-of-the-art facilities, with round-the-clock care and experimenting with the latest discoveries. His foundation raised enormous funds for spinal cord

research, but critics in the United States and the UK found fault with the emphasis on recovery and faulted him for ignoring, in effect, the vast majority of spinal cord injured who could not afford the care he championed. Heather Mills, Paul McCartney's ex-wife, is likewise taken to task for having an expensive prosthesis and appearing on the British import TV show, "Dancing with the Stars." The problem is that since there are so few persons with disabilities on TV in roles other than victim that the exceptions need to be representative. If not, than even the back-handed compliments of "heroic," "inspirational," and so on, feel like ashes in the mouths of those who cannot afford the state-of-the-art treatment these celebrities enjoy.

As long as the medical model is dominant, the image of victimhood will forever be the fate of persons with disabilities. As long as there is one model of completeness, the emphasis will be on the ability of the person with disability to participate in or return to the same system that labels them as disabled in the first place. It is these systems that define how we as a society react to a person with a disability, help them as an act of charity, or ignore them in hopes that their courage will somehow surmount whatever obstacles we have placed in their way.

In the case of women the obstacles to "runway model" perfection lead to serious health and emotional complications among large numbers of girls. Among those with visible disabilities the obstacles to desirability, given the media's seeming obsession with physical perfection, can seem insurmountable. The new model of social change affords us all the opportunity to participate equally in recreating a society that is accepting of us now and as we shall become.

One rationale that justifies the changes in civil rights of women with disabilities is to look at the cost of treating them as second-class citizens, incapable of full expression of their rights to education and employment. The numbers of persons with disabilities are increasing in every country of the world.[1] Albrecht used the paradigm of the political economy to identify how in the United States, a "disability business" had grown up that has become a billion dollar enterprise consisting of medical, social welfare, rehabilitation, insurance, legal, pharmaceutical, medical supply, technology, and governmental organizations.[29] In his analysis, the market has created a vehicle for a two-prong approach that resides within our developed economy. People who rely on medical care are severely limited in their choices. Insurance companies demand that students, who would be continued under their parent's policy through graduation from postsecondary school, maintain full-time status. In addition to governmental policies in some developing countries that would link population control with sterilization of persons with disabilities, one of the countries that is a signatory to the UN treaty mentioned earlier is advocating selective sterilization for persons with disabilities.[31] Women with Disabilities Australia is fighting a proposal to authorize sterilization among minors with intellectual disabilities and blames the government for "blatantly disregarding the inherent principles of the Convention."[31] For a woman with disabilities whose history has been intertwined with sterilization practices the relationship with healthcare is even more complicated.

Since 1981, the year the UN declared the International Year of the Disabled Person, considerable efforts have been made to identify common constructs around basic issues of incidence, treatment, and needs of the disabled in various countries around the world. One of many issues is categorization of disabilities: What constitutes a disability and what degree of severity? What are the economic burdens? What social policies are in place, and what levels of protection from discrimination are available? In a 1995 UN document,[3] the prevalence of disabilities in 90 countries around the world ranged from 0.2% to 20% depending on definitions. Surveys of disability reveal the inherent conflicts in the area. Medical models such as those utilized in the WHO study were criticized by Keck,[32] among others, who contrasted the developing world's obsession with participation in employment and education with indigenous tribes in Papua, New Guinea, for whom any definition of personhood required a context that was not considered in the survey design. As my colleague Steve Brown of the University of Hawaii's disability studies program notes, local Hawaiian's notion of what we would consider disability would be a family member who cannot participate in the harvest of seaweed, similar to the Tswana folktale from Southern Africa that recognized the contributions of an albino child, who had been ostracized because of her deviant looks, only after her hard work was recognized.[32] In con-

trast are the studies by Weiss that found that 50% of the Israeli families who gave birth to "appearance impaired" children chose to leave them at the hospital rather than bring them home.[33] According to Ingstad and Whyte,[34] in many developing societies, the issue of disability and personhood is more a function of integration into the family economic structure than fitting into a social expectation of "normal." The question in developed societies becomes one of the relationships of people as a medical cost component of the families' financial burden.

As in the recent interest in land mine victims, not only are families affected by war, but the wounded are abandoned by governments who rely on foreign aid to meet their "short-term" approaches to medical care. This situation has been an ongoing one since missionaries began accompanying colonial powers. In times of war we honor the sacrifices of the men and women in battle, but behind the scenes, as we have seen recently in the United States, rehabilitation is often left to charitable organizations.[32] It is important in any consideration of program implementation to be highly sensitive to cultural conditions and perceptions of personhood before we speak about models of rehabilitation or educational reform for the disabled.

China is among the 80 countries that signed the UN declaration that was ratified in April 2007. An article in the *China Daily* from 2004 citing statistics from the Guangzhou Disabled Persons' Federation noted that one major city had 300,000 persons with disabilities and of that total 2000 were homeless.[35] As we move forward into the third decade of this "newest" civil rights movement we are all truly global partners in advancing the status of persons with disabilities. With record enrollment and graduation rates soaring (46% increase between 2004 and 2005) there are more challenges and more opportunities for China's colleges and universities. As more students with disabilities are being educated and specialized programs (including one college exclusively for the disabled) increase, more qualified students with disabilities will be applying to postsecondary education. In 2004, Guangzhou started a special education program with 38 students who were in a 4-year degree program. The program includes 800 hours of practical experience with persons with disabilities.

DISCUSSION QUESTIONS

1. What are the challenges faced by disabled women in the United States and other countries who try to improve their lifestyle?

2. What are some of the programs and policies in place to assist disabled women in the United States and in other countries?

3. How do policy makers, educational institutions, UN agencies, and local, state, and national governments work together to reduce the disparities disabled women experience worldwide?

REFERENCES

1. Lederer E. U.N. Pact on Disabled Rights Signed. *Associated Press Online* March 30, 2007. http://www.boston.com/news/nation/articles/2007/03/30/un_pact_on _disabled_rights_signed/. Accessed on July 29, 2008.

2. The Division for the Advancement of Women. Beijing Declaration. Fourth World Conference on Women, Beijing, China. September 1995. http://www.un.org /womenwatch/daw/beijing/beijingdeclaration.html. Accessed April 28, 2008.

3. United Nations Development Program. *Human Development Report 1995.* New York, NY: Oxford University Press; 1995.

4. Licuanan PB. Celebrating gains-confronting persistent and emerging issues. Plenary paper presented at: Asia Pacific NGO Forum Beijing + 10; June 30–July 3, 2004; Bangkok, Thailand.

5. Ward MJ, Merves ES. The picture of college freshman in greater focus: an analysis of selected characteristics by types of disabilities. Heath Resource Center, American Council on Education Web site. http://www.heath.gwu.edu/node/293. Accessed July 29, 2008.

6. National Organization on Disability. Landmark disability survey finds pervasive disadvantages. NEC Foundation Web site. http://www.necfoundation.org/news /news_show.htm?doc_id=650981. Accessed July 29, 2008.

7. Profile of U.S. Postsecondary Institutions 1999–2000: Statistical Analysis Report. *National Center for Education Statistics.* July 2002.

8. National Center for Education Statistics. Beginning postsecondary students longitudinal study. http://nces.ed.gov/programs/digest/d07/tables/dt07_181.asp? referrer=list. Accessed May 9, 2008.

9. Wagner M, Newman L, Cameto R, Levine P, Garza N. An overview of findings from wave 2 of the National Longitudinal Transition Study-2 (NLTS2). Washington, DC: National Center for Special Education Research; 2006. NCSER 2006-3004. http://eric.ed.gov/ERICDocs/data/ericdocs2sql/content_storage_01/0000019b /80/29/e3/86.pdf. Accessed July 30, 2008.

10. National Council on Education. People with disabilities and postsecondary education 2002. http://www.ncd.gov/newsroom/publications/2003/education.htm. Accessed March 21, 2008.

11. United Cerebral Palsy. 2004 Harris Survey finds people with disabilities still face

pervasive disadvantages. http://www.ucp.org/ucp_generaldoc.cfm/1/8/33/33-12262/5616. Accessed November 1, 2004.

12. Garza NM. Engagement in postsecondary education, work, or preparation for work. http://www.nlts2.org/reports/2005_04/nlts2_report_2005_04_ch3.pdf. Accessed July 30, 2008.

13. National Council on Education. People with disabilities and postsecondary education 2002. http://www.ncd.gov/newsroom/publications/2003/education.htm. Accessed March 21, 2008.

14. National Center for Education Statistics. Baccalaureate and beyond longitudinal study, first follow-up. http://nces.ed.gov/surveys/b&b/. Accessed May 1, 2008.

15. Higher Education Research Institute. CIRP—The Freshman Survey. http://www.gseis.ucla.edu/heri/cirpoverview.php. Accessed April 15, 2008.

16. National Science Foundation. Women, minorities and persons with disabilities in science and engineering: 2002. http://transcoder.usablenet.com/tt/www.nsf.gov/statistics/wmpd/employ.htm. Accessed March 24, 2008.

17. Barkley R, Murphy K, Fischer M. *ADHD in Adults*. New York, NY: The Guilford Press; 2008.

18. National Institute on Disability and Rehabilitation Research. Chartbook on women and disability: access to disability data. http://www.infouse.com/disabilitydata/womendisability/. Accessed March 19, 2008.

19. US Department of Education. National Postsecondary Student Aid Survey: data analysis system. 2002. http://www.nces.ed.gov/surveys/npsas/das.asp. Accessed July 30, 2008.

20. Licuanan PB. Celebrating gains—confronting persistent and emerging issues. Plenary paper presented at: Asia Pacific NGO Forum Beijing + 10; June 30–July 3, 2004; Bangkok, Thailand.

21. O'Brien R. *Crippled Justice: The History of Modern Disability Policy in the Workplace*. Chicago, IL: University of Chicago Press; 2001.

22. Harrison T. Has the Americans with Disabilities Act made a difference? *Policy, Polit Nurs Pract.* 2001;3(4):333-346.

23. National Organization on Disabilities. Education and disability statistics: a historical perspective. 2001. http://www.nod.org/index.cfm?fuseaction=feature.showFeature&FeatureID=109&C:\CFusionMX7\verity\Data\dummy.txt. Accessed July 30, 2008.

24. Kaye HS. *Improved Employment Opportunities for People with Disabilities*. Washington, DC: Department of Education National Institute on Disability and Rehabilitation Research; 2003. Disabilities Statistics Report 17.

25. Disability World. UN study of violence against women finds 50% of disabled women experience abuse. 2007. http://www.disabilityworld.org/01_07/abuse.shtml. Accessed July 30, 2008.

26. National Organization on Disability/Harris. Employment rates of people with disabilities. 2001. http://www.nod.org/index.cfm?fuseaction=page.viewPage&pageID=110. Accessed May 6, 2008.

27. US Census Bureau. Disability and American families: 2000. http://www.census.gov/main/www/cen2000.html. Accessed July 30, 2008.

28. The Center for an Accessible Society. Employers reluctant to hire workers with disabilities, study says. 2003. http://www.accessiblesociety.org/topics/economics-employment/restrictedaccess.html. Accessed March 19, 2008.

29. The formation of disability studies. In: Albrecht G, Seelman K, Bury M, eds. *Handbook of Disability Studies*. Thousand Oaks, CA: Sage Publications; 2001.

30. Groce E. *Everyone Here Spoke Sign Language*. Cambridge, MA: Harvard University Press; 1985.

31. Parkinson A. Sterilisation of children with intellectual disabilities. 2007. http://www.disabilityworld.org/01_07/sterilisation.shtml. Accessed July 30, 2008.

32. Ingstad B. Disability in the developing world. In: Albrecht G, Seelman K, Bury M, eds. *Handbook of Disability Studies*. Thousand Oaks: CA: Sage Publications; 2001.

33. Weiss M. Ethical reflections: taking a walk on the wild side. In: Sheper-Hughes N, Sargeant C, eds. *Small Wars: The Cultural Politics of Childhood*. Berkeley, CA: University of California Press; 1987.

34. Ingstad B, Whyte S. *Disability and Culture*. Berkeley, CA: University of California Press; 1995.

35. Qiu Q. New major targets disabled. *China Daily Online*. http://www.chinadaily.com.cn/English/doc/2004-05/24/content333507.htm. Accessed May 4, 2004.

Being blind means that your liberty is ceased; you live on Earth, but in a different world not part of Earth. Now, the family can come to me with their problems for me to give advice, but when I was blind, one could never remember that I was important to the family. I want to give my thanks and appreciation to all those who are working with Unite For Sight that made me important again.

—Jayne, Unite For Sight Patient
at Buduburam Refugee Camp, Ghana

The provision of eye care, and the consequences of blindness, is often overlooked in communities worldwide. There are an estimated 45 million blind people and 135 million visually impaired individuals in the world.[1] The World Health Organization (WHO) indicates that 90% of people who are blind live in developing countries, and 80% of blindness is curable or preventable.[1] Blindness affects both morbidity and mortality in developing countries. It is estimated that 3.1% of deaths worldwide are directly or indirectly related to leading causes of preventable or curable eye diseases: cataracts, glaucoma, trachoma, and onchocerciasis (river blindness).[2] Furthermore, 60–80% of children who become blind die within 1–2 years.[3]

A multitude of barriers prevent those with deteriorating vision and blindness from seeking treatment: education and awareness, expense, distance and transportation, as well as poor quality of services by untrained or undertrained doctors. Africa has one ophthalmologist per million people.[4] The west African country of Ghana, for example, has one of the highest numbers of ophthalmologists in Africa, with a total of 48 trained doctors. However, approximately 50% live and work in the capital of Accra, leaving the rest of the country with little access to care. Many other African countries have only a handful of ophthalmologists for the entire population of millions of people. In contrast, the United States has an estimated 59,146 eye doctors for the population, though patients in the United States also continue to become blind from preventable eye

CHAPTER 28

Blindness and Social Stigma in Women and the Girl-Child

Jennifer Staple, BS

Jennifer Staple, BS, is Founder, President, and CEO, of Unite For Sight, based in Newton, CT. Ms. Staple is recipient of the Golden Brick award, and a winner in Young Epidemiology Scholars Competition. She also received the 2004 Global Youth Action Network's Global Youth Action Award from the International Youth Foundation and Nokia for leading positive change throughout the world.

diseases due to lack of access to care, despite the relative prevalence of doctors.[5]

Patients in developing countries are often unaware that their blindness may be curable or preventable. Leading causes of blindness include cataracts, glaucoma, and trachoma. Approximately 18–24% of blindness worldwide is due to trachoma,[6] while 66.8 million people have glaucoma,[7] and 25 million eyes become blind due to cataracts annually.[8] Oftentimes, blindness is believed to be intrinsically linked with old age, and it is thought that eyes naturally become grey (with cataracts) when one's hair turns grey. Cataract is the leading cause of blindness in the world,[9] yet a 15-minute operation by an ophthalmologist can usually fully restore sight. The global need for cataract operations is at least 30 million per year, yet only 10 million cataract surgeries are performed annually.[10] Cataract patients in remote locations of the developing world, however, are unaware that their sight can be restored, and it is often impossible for them to access the sight-restoring eye care that they require. Dr. Seth Wanye, the only ophthalmologist for 2 million people in the northern region of Ghana, said in an interview (November 2007) with Unite For Sight, "These people are usually in the rural areas. Even if we asked them to come to the hospital, it is virtually impossible, because they don't have the means to come there. There are places where there are no vehicles in the village. Someone who is blind in both eyes, we cannot expect those persons to come to the hospital that is several hundred kilometers away."

There are a variety of nonprofit charity organizations throughout the world that focus on providing eye care to patients in the developing world. Unite For Sight, for example, is a nonprofit organization based on the premise that eye care is a fundamental right that should be available to all, regardless of a patient's ability to pay, or proximity to an eye doctor. The mission of the organization is to empower communities worldwide to improve eye health and eliminate preventable blindness. The communities where Unite For Sight works did not previously have access to eye care. Unite For Sight's model is unique among global health and eye care organizations in that it involves local and visiting volunteers who serve as support staff to eye doctors in the field. The eye clinic's eye doctors and Unite For Sight volunteers jointly provide community-based screening programs in rural villages, refugee camps, and slums. The clinic's eye doctors diagnose and treat eye disease in the field, and surgical patients are brought to the eye clinic for surgery. Patients receive free surgery funded by Unite For Sight so that no patient remains blind due to lack of funds. The Unite For Sight-sponsored patients receive surgical care in the same facilities as the private patients who are able to pay for their own surgeries. The goal of Unite For Sight is to create communities free of eye disease and to achieve the vision 2020 goals of WHO and the International Agency for Prevention of Blindness.

While providing eye care services to more than 600,000 patients thus far, including more than 12,000 sight-restoring cataract surgeries through the end of 2007, Unite For Sight has also been in the unfortunate position to identify patients who are permanently blind with incurable or degenerative eye conditions without the hope of restored sight. Those experiencing blindness in the developing world are frequently stigmatized, sometimes deemed pariahs due to their inability to work and their reliance on family members. Blindness prevents otherwise healthy individuals from engaging in a job to help support their family, often leading to increased poverty for the family. Ghanaian ophthalmologist Wanye describes the burden of blindness on families:

> When we talk about healthcare needs in the government sector, it is all about killer diseases. The government's attention is on these diseases that actually cause immediate death. It is assumed that eye diseases do not kill, resulting in resources being channeled to other areas of health care. However, I have a different opinion. If you have someone who is blind, then someone else will have to forgo his or her activities in order to take care of this person. Oftentimes, you have a child who is supposed to go to school, but he is instead guiding a blind man around the house and directing him wherever he wants to go. This child could have gone to school, study, and become somebody in the future to help the family.

> We often see very young people who are blind, many times younger than the age of

40. They become blind during their productive years; they could have been working and helping to contribute toward building wealth in the country. Instead, the blindness results in a financial loss to the nation because these people are not able to contribute to building the nation. We have therefore been trying to advocate to policy makers so they understand that even though eye diseases do not kill, they do result in financial losses to the nation. We must see this as an emergency issue. I see eye care as a very important area, and I love to do what I am doing now, to try to help people who I think would benefit from the services that we provide (interview, November 2007).

A 49-year old patient living in a remote village near Accra, Ghana, for example, was referred for surgery by the Unite For Sight outreach team to ophthalmologist Dr. James Clarke, an ophthalmologist and medical director of Crystal Eye Clinic. Having lost her husband shortly before her 12-year old daughter was born, her daughter remained the only person available to accompany her to her eye exam. Prior to becoming blind, the patient worked as "house help" and utilized her income to support herself and to pay her daughter's school fees. After becoming blind in both eyes, she was no longer able to work to support her family, nor to support her daughter's school fees, which led her daughter to drop out of school. The burden of supporting the family was transferred to her 12-year old daughter, who worked daily to round plait women's hair. "My daughter sometimes comes home weeping because some people she had worked for refused to pay her. I'm helpless because I cannot see to go and demand money for my daughter. I'm very grateful to Unite For Sight for making it possible to regain my sight. I hope to now find work and will try to encourage my daughter to go back to school" (Interview, January 2008).

Another patient referred to Clarke was a 45-year old woman, whose husband was 60 years old and a peasant farmer. The woman's husband explained to Clarke that he was most grateful when his wife regained sight because she could assist once again on the farm. Due to his advanced age, he could no longer work as hard as needed. Addi-

tionally, his oldest child had to stay with his blind mother, so the daughter, too, was removed from assisting on the farm. These factors reduced the farm's output, thereby lessening the family income and advancing their poverty. After having surgery, the woman and oldest child were again available to assist on the farm, leading to significantly improved income and living conditions.

Social Parameters and Consequences of Blindness in Ghanaian Rural Villages

Unite For Sight provides daily outreach programs to remote, rural villages, in an effort to make eye care a basic human right for all patients, regardless of their ability to afford or access care. In the region surrounding Accra, Ghana, ophthalmic nurses Robert Dolo and Kartee Karloweah visit on a daily basis a variety of Ghana's most impoverished villages located within a one to five hour radius of Accra. They provide on-site eye care in the villages and refer surgery patients to the Crystal Eye Clinic in Accra.

Ophthalmic nurse Dolo reported the story of a 71-year old patient who described herself as a burden to her family. She was diagnosed with bilateral mature cataracts, meaning that she was fully blind in both eyes. Until her eye examination by Dolo, she was unaware of the eye disease that caused her blindness. She was a fishmonger until her visual impairment forced her to stop working. As a fishmonger, she would go to the beach daily to purchase fish in order to later sell it at market. After becoming blind, however, she explained to Dolo that she was confined to her home, no longer able to cook, wash, dress herself, or go to the toilet without assistance. "I feel forgotten in the community and dehumanized or insulted if people in the community do not call me by my name, but rather 'Blind Woman'," she stated. The mother of six living children and three grandchildren, her youngest daughter cared for her, which affected her daughter's personal obligations and ability to work. She told Dolo that she tried to find a solution to her blindness, visited clinics and hospitals in the region, but she could not undertake the cost of the cataract operation until Unite For Sight provided the surgery free of charge.

A 70-year old patient seen by ophthalmic nurse Karloweah was blind in both eyes for 5 years. Like Dolo's patient, Karloweah's patient, too, was a fishmonger:

My sight loss has affected my life in so many ways. I can no longer see the surroundings, and everything appears dark. I don't work anymore to earn money, and I have to rely on the people to give me money, usually through begging. I don't have privacy taking shower, going to toilet, and even attending nature (urinating). I am usually led by my 9-year old granddaughter to go around the environment. I don't go to any gatherings or public places for meetings. This has made me feel very useless since my movement has been restricted thanks to my sight. Friends also do not come to visit me since I'm considered as a living dead. Most people live from their toils, and children have to go to school, so during the daytime, I'm left all to myself, but when people are around, I do get assistance from family, but hardly from the community. Having my sight restored will mean the whole world to me since it will bring back my old life, which was very active, useful, and independent (interview, January 2008).

Ghanaian patients who are not living in extreme poverty also face social stigma that, in many ways, is comparable to the stigma faced by blind patients in remote villages. One of Dr. Clarke's private, paying patients, for example, is a 70-year old woman. In Ghana, Clarke explains that blind patients often beg for alms by the roadside. "Though this brings a lot of embarrassment to the family, the family is helpless because it has no other means of support for the blind." The 70-year old woman reported that her children requested that she remain indoors because they feared that she might beg for alms, while they looked for funds to bring her to surgery. In addition to the embarrassment of begging, there was further embarrassment to the family if the community became aware that they had a blind member of the family who could not receive care due to lack of available funds. Clarke's patient told him that remaining indoors was "most unpleasant," and it took several months for her children to raise the money to cover the cost of surgery. When the family had the approximately $100 to fund her surgery, she reported that she was "very happy" because surgery allowed her to associate with people outdoors once again. "I feel that my social status has changed, and I can now lead a normal life," she told Clarke.

Blindness as Experienced by Women at a Refugee Camp

Unite For Sight operates the first and only eye care program provided to the refugees at Ghana's Buduburam refugee camp. The 120-acre refugee camp has a population of 45,000, and is located one hour from Ghana's capital city in Accra. The refugee camp was established in early 1990 by the government of Ghana to host a population of Liberian refugees fleeing the civil war. The camp continues to have more than 40,000 resident refugees from Liberia, Sierra Leone, and the Ivory Coast. Many who currently live at the refugee camp suffered human rights abuses by rebels when the civil war began in Liberia during 1989. They experienced crimes against humanity, including brutal killings, mass rape, torture, limb amputation, and eye trauma.

Ghanaian ophthalmologist Clarke provides examination, diagnosis, treatment, and surgery to the patients living at the refugee camp. A group of 10 local refugee Unite For Sight volunteers participated in Unite For Sight eye education programs and received training from Clarke. For the past three years, they have participated daily to identify patients with potential eye disease, and the patients are subsequently examined by Clarke's ophthalmic nurse Margaret Duah-Mensah, who visits the refugee camp several times per month. Those requiring treatment and surgery are brought to the Crystal Eye Clinic, with all of their eye care funded by Unite For Sight. The program at the Buduburam refugee camp in Ghana is so necessary and successful that patients from the neighboring country of Liberia—a country with only one ophthalmologist for the entire population of 3.5 million—have been reported to travel to the refugee camp solely to have their sight restored through the eye care program. Patients whose sight was restored often speak about the stigma that they faced during their blindness and the change in their lives once their sight is restored.

Fifty-four year old Liberian refugee Jayne* became blind in Ghana after fleeing Liberia in 1995. "Being blind means that your liberty is ceased; you live on Earth, but in a different world not part of Earth. Now, the family can come to me with their problems for me to give advice, but when I was blind, one could never remember that I was important to the family." After Jayne's grandson took her to the Unite For Sight eye clinic, she was brought to Crystal Eye Clinic for cataract surgery. She explained that her sight was perfect again the day after surgery, which brought enormous joy to her. "I want to give my thanks and appreciation to all those who made me important again."

Another woman who fled Liberia during the civil war first moved to the Ivory Coast before moving to Ghana. Starting in 2005, her vision began deteriorating, and she reported that with her extremely low vision, "everyone that ever showed me the best of love never again regarded me as important any longer. I was the most beautiful queen, but no one called me the best woman among all women and the most beautiful women ever." Her vision loss caused relatives and friends to reject her. She said that going to the bathroom was one of the biggest troubles she had in her life. "When there is no one to help, I felt that now was the end of my life. One thing that I never forgot in my life was a daily prayer to God. God sent his angel, that angel was my aunt. She came and asked to look into my eyes, and then she took me to Unite For Sight." She was diagnosed with cataracts and sent to Crystal Eye Clinic for her first surgery, subsequently returning to the clinic the month after to have surgery on her other eye as well. "My life has changed. I now have the respect of people who rejected me, and they are my friends."

Some refugee patients at the Buduburam refugee camp also face blindness and debilitation due to trauma. An 18-year-old, for example, was hit in the eye by a rock after she and her friends engaged in a fight at a school dormitory. After this accident, she felt a terrible pain that lasted for more than a week. Her mother purchased eye drops from

a local drug store, but only an eye doctor would have the skills to examine her and determine the best course of treatment. For a full month, her injury prevented her from reading, going to class, and she was no longer able to go anywhere by herself. After a month of visual impairment, however, she learned from a neighbor about Unite For Sight's program at the Buduburam refugee camp and was subsequently rushed to Crystal Eye Clinic, where surgery was performed by Dr. Clarke. The following day, she could see once again and is now able to continue her education. During her month of blindness, she explained that most of her friends would no longer identify with her, causing her to feel lonely and neglected. She expressed her thanks and appreciation for having her sight restored and said that she otherwise would have been forced to end her education.

Another Liberian refugee went to Ghana in 2003 as a result of the Liberian civil war. After rebel troops attacked her town, she escaped to Ghana by way of the Ivory Coast. She lost her sight in 2004, and she could see nothing but blackness by 2005. Her daughter brought her to an eye clinic in the capital city of Ghana, where she was diagnosed with cataracts, but she was told that she had to pay $150 for sight-restoring surgery, which was well beyond her financial capability. After returning to the refugee camp, she met a woman in the bus station who advised her to visit Unite For Sight's clinic at the camp. The following day, she was reexamined, her cataract diagnosis was confirmed, and she was scheduled for surgery at Crystal Eye Clinic. One day after surgery in each eye, her sight was fully restored. "If my daughter had not been around, I don't think I could live up to the point of surgery since she never had any concern with what others said about me. Today, I can see and can do my work and go places without anyone's help."

While sight has been restored to thousands of patients at the refugee camp, others have also been informed by the ophthalmologist that their blindness is permanent. When Unite For Sight began its work at the Buduburam refugee camp, many patients presented with complicated eye diseases that were uncommon in most other locations: macular scarring, corneal scarring, and uveitis. Patient interviews revealed that these conditions were mostly caused by physical abuse in Liberia prior to arrival at Buduburam Refugee

---

* The names of all patients have been changed. Patient stories and quotes were provided by the ophthalmic staff in Ghana and India.

Camp. Corneal scarring, constituting 35% of those with inoperable eye conditions, resulted from physical abuse to the eyes and face. Macular scarring was caused by a unique form of abuse that has received little, if any, documentation. As part of their war crimes and human rights abuses, rebels in Liberia forced the civilians to stare at the sun, which is described as brutally painful. Staring at the sun causes severe, irreversible retinal damage and macular scarring, and Unite For Sight determined that 14% of those with inoperable eye conditions had macular scarring that was likely the result of this form of abuse.

One of the refugees who volunteered as a Unite For Sight eye health educator was permanently blind due to these human rights abuses. He and his wife worked tirelessly for years to educate their community members about eye diseases and ways to prevent blindness:

> Presently, I cannot see. The eyes all started during the war. I was not born like this. I was attacked brutally, my family and I, on the ninth of the year 1990. When the rebels go to the house, they commanded everyone out of the house early in the morning. People started running away. We never left; we stayed in the community, while people were running away. When they brought us outside, we found out why we were dead, they were ill treating us. After they busted the door, they entered the house by force. They pulled everyone of us out. Because why, the only reason why they were doing these things somebody was with them, they knew I was working with the National Democratic Party office as a registrar prior to the war. So what they decided to do? They decided to kill us. Because why? It started with a tribal war. But later on they started to put it on all those that were affiliated or those who worked for the government. They don't mind your position; you can even be a sweeper. In as much, they find out that you work with the government. They all were killing people. Just like that. To my utmost surprise, they started to beat me and my children. They knocked me on the ground and told me to face the sun, look at the sun. For each time

I look at the sun like that, I bow my eye small. I closed my eyes. They get mad; they come and step into my eyes. That's how I started with the injury. Stepping into my eyes. When I look at the sun again, they do the same thing again. Just like that.[11]

Blindness as Experienced By Girls in Patna, Bihar, India

The social stigma of blindness also afflicts young children. The city and surrounding areas of Patna, India, are served by three ophthalmologists at AB Eye Institute: Dr. Ajit Sinha, his son Dr. Satyajit Sinha, and his daughter-in-law Dr. Pooja Sinha. They work daily from 7 a.m. to 10 p.m., which includes a full afternoon every day providing free care for 40–60 poor patients in charity clinics.

The Sinha family not only eradicates blindness and eye disease, they also founded and operate Bihar Netraheen Parishad, the only school in Bihar exclusively for blind girls. The goal of the school is to reduce stigma and to provide them with a quality education. The school was founded after Dr. Ajit Sinha wondered what the future would hold for those patients that he examined who were permanently and irreversibly blind. He sought to found a school to improve opportunities for blind girls. Dr. Sinha explained:

> The girls started enjoying the school campus atmosphere. It is unbelievable, but these girls did not like to go back home during long vacation of the school because they did not get that love and affection from their parents they got from the school teachers and the house warden. It was a great stigma in the family—*a blind girl*. Nobody wanted to extend sympathy to the blind girl, and that is why she enjoyed the school atmosphere more than the home atmosphere.

> These blind students are never prevented in going to perform in social functions, and they consider themselves no less than the sighted students. The school encourages them to take up other courses besides the

school curriculum for the classrooms, such as music, Braille short hand typing, computers, and general typing and sports (interview, January 2008).

One of the students at Bihar Netraheen Parishad told Dr. Sinha:

When I grew up, I wanted to go with my brother to different places, and they did take me there, but at times they left me alone in the house and went away. When my brothers used to go to school, I used to cry to go with them, but then my mother used to scold me and said that a blind person cannot read and write. When other children used to play, I also wanted to play with them, and again my family members scolded me and said that I could not play as I would get hurt.

After being enrolled in the Bihar Netraheen Parishad School, the young girl quickly gained confidence and important skills. "Often my parents visited me, and they were surprised to see how I was able to read and write. Now my parents are proud of me," she explained.

At present, I am in Class 9, and I want to take up teaching after completing my university education. With full facility extended to the blind, I can achieve all feats of life like the sighted. I am very grateful to the president of this school, Dr. Ajit Sinha, who is a noted eye surgeon and is working hard for the rehabilitation of the blind (interview, January 2008).

Another girl at the school explained to Dr. Sinha that she grew up in an impoverished family. Her parents sold vegetables in an effort to support the family. She was born blind and said that "It was a great misfortune for my parents. My parents tried to get me treated, but to no avail, and then they lost attention on me." During a public health ophthalmic survey, volunteers from Bihar Netraheen Parishad spoke to her parents about educational opportunities. The girl explained that her parents did not believe that she, as a blind girl, could ever read and write: "They thought that I would engage in a begging profession." After visiting Bihar Netraheen Parishad, her parents were surprised and enthusiastic that the blind girls were

reading, and they decided to enroll her in the school. Unfortunately, however, she continues to experience stigma from her family and community. She told Dr. Sinha:

During long vacation in the school, I went home, but I was not received cordially. My parents used to scold me by saying "Why did you come home?" The thoughts about me in the family are still downtrodden. I am preparing for my grade 10 exams, and all expenses are being provided by the school. I wish to become a social worker and help such children who have no one to look after them. I wish to thank the President Office bearers and teachers of this school who have done so much for me and made my life worth living. But as much I have wept in my eyes, not even the river can weep so much (interview, January 2008).

The stigma experienced by the young blind girls can often be ostracizing. Another girl at the school who lost her sight due to dysentery and dehydration was considered by her family to be an outcast. "Nobody wanted to keep me. The world was dark for me all around." Girls at Bihar Netraheen Parishad gain confidence, skill, and help to change the perception of their family and community about blindness. After attending the school and learning to read and write, the girl found that her local community "changed their thoughts about blind girls. After seeing me, they thought that I was no less capable in doing anything less than a sighted girl. My mother has great hopes for me, and I think I will fulfill it thanks to Bihar Netraheen Parishad."

Similarly, Aparna lost her sight as a young child due to cholera. Her father sold his land for her treatment and then took a job as a bus conductor. After being admitted to Bihar Netraheen Parishad, she received proper food, medical care, and "most of all love and care from my teachers." In addition to a regular education, she is also learning music, typing, and computer training. "The other members of my family were very happy to see me studying and gaining confidence," she explained to Dr. Sinha. "I will be able to earn my livelihood and monetarily support the family. Now the family treats me very supportively."

Conclusion

Young girls in India discussed their dissatisfaction and experiences with social stigma related to their blindness, but this ostracism often continues, and is sometimes compounded, during adulthood. While many are blind from childhood, there are others who are previously sighted adult women who became blind during midlife, or when elderly, from eye conditions such as cataracts and macular degeneration. These newly blind patients frequently experience humiliation and dishonor from their community, and are considered to be a burden on their families because of their inability to contribute to the household.

In addition to the social parameters and consequences of blindness, there are dire mortality statistics as well. Those who are blind in Africa have a 40% higher mortality rate.[12] 60–80% of children who become blind die within one to two years.[13] Astonishingly, one child becomes blind every minute from diseases such as measles, congenital rubella, meningitis, premature birth, and vitamin A deficiency.[14]

DISCUSSION QUESTIONS

1. What are the social parameters and consequences of blindness in rural villages?
2. How might the consequences of blindness be different in developing countries for those living in extreme poverty and those who have more wealth?
3. How does blindness affect young blind girls?

REFERENCES

1. Global Initiative for the Prevention of Avoidable Blindness. Geneva, Switzerland: WHO; 1997. WHO/PBL/97.61.
2. Murray CJ, Lopez AD. Global mortality, disability, and the contribution of risk factors: Global Burden of Disease Study. *Lancet.* 1997;349:1436-1442.
3. Lewallen S, Courtright P. Blindness in Africa: present situation and future needs. *Br J Ophthalmol.* 2001;85(8):897-903.
4. Sommer A. Global health, global vision [editorial]. *Arch Ophthalmol.* 2004; 122(6):911-912.
5. Low-cost eyeglasses. The problem. http://www.lowcosteyeglasses.net/stuck .htm. Accessed July 22, 2008.
6. Zhang H, Kandel RP, Sharma S, MD, Dean D. Risk factors for recurrence of post-operative trichiasis: implications for trachoma blindness prevention. *Arch Ophthalmol.* 2004;122(4):511-516.
7. Quigley HA. Number of people with glaucoma worldwide. *Br J Ophthalmol.* 1996;80(5):389-393.
8. Foster A. Cataract—a global perspective: output, outcome and outlay. *Eye.* 1999;13:65-70.
9. World Health Organization. Magnitude and causes of visual impairment. http://www.who.int/mediacentre/factsheets/fs282/en/. Accessed July 22, 2008.

10. Foster A. Cataract—a global perspective: output, outcome and outlay. *Eye*. 1999;13:65-70.

11. Unite For Sight at Buduburam Refugee Camp [DVD]. Unite For Sight; 2005.

12. Taylor HR. Refractive errors: magnitude of need. *Community Eye Health J*. 2000;13(33):1-2.

13. Lewallen S, Courtright P. Blindness in Africa: present situation and future needs. *Br J Ophthalmol*. 2001;85(8):897-903.

14. Carrin M. The Millennium Development Goals and Vision 2020. International Agency for the Prevention of Blindness. 2006. http://www.iapb.org/newsletters /49_march-newsletter-2006.pdf. Accessed July 22, 2008.

CHAPTER **29**

Older Women's Access to Health and Human Rights

It is often said that time heals all wounds. When it comes to women and their access to health and other human rights, however, the opposite is often true. For the most part, time—or ageing—exacerbates many of the burdens and much of the discrimination women face their entire lives, and adds new obstacles to their well-being.

When speaking of ageing, people generally think of specific age groups, usually those older than 55 or 60. However, ageing is a lifelong process that begins before birth and continues throughout life. As the World Health Organization's (WHO) Global Commission on Women's Health has acknowledged, "Since the health of a woman in earlier periods of her life forms the basis of her health in later stages of her life, it is essential to consider the health of ageing women within a *life course* perspective."[1]

The fact is that simply getting older is a challenge for women in many parts of the world owing to systemic injustice, including poverty, lack of access to healthcare services, environmental hazards, and gender discrimination. Even where women can expect to have a longer life, they cannot necessarily anticipate a healthier one. Women are more likely than men to be affected by chronic disabling conditions characterized by increasing impairment.[2]

Most parts of the world, both developing and developed, have not adequately prepared to meet the needs of the increasing number of older women. According to the WHO[3]:

- In 2000, there were 600 million people aged 60 and over; there will be 2 billion by 2050.
- About two-thirds of older people live in the developing world; by 2025, it will be 75%.
- In the developed world, the very old (age 80+) is the fastest growing population group.

Ageing is not gender neutral, and societies must embrace and accommodate the differences to meet the special health and human rights needs of older women.

Monica Sanchez

Monica Sanchez is a Former Director of the Medicare Rights Center, New York, NY.

Women Face Lifelong Barriers to Healthy Ageing

Although more boys are born around the world, women survive better at all ages *if* they receive similar care. Girls are more resistant to infection and malnutrition, "perhaps because of sex differences in chromosomal structures and a slower maturing of boys' lungs due to the effects of testosterone."[4] Whatever their biological advantage, however, in many parts of the world, girls are at a social disadvantage that has a profound impact on their chance of survival. Children who live past their fifth birthday have a much greater chance of living to adulthood and old age, yet the World Bank reports that in cultures where parents prefer sons over daughters, particularly in Asia and Africa, mortality rates of children under five years of age are much higher for girls than for boys.[5]

The longer life expectancy of women is really only clearly evidenced as overall mortality falls. Women generally live between five to eight years longer than men in the countries with the highest life expectancies, but the difference goes down to zero to three years in countries where overall life expectancy is low.[6] In Europe and North America, the gap only started to grow as economic development and social change removed some of the major risks to women's health, including the risk of dying in childbirth.

Unfortunately, a woman's right to live and age is still far from guaranteed in most of the world. According to UNICEF's State of the World's Children 2007, "Women and girls are disproportionately affected by the AIDS pandemic. Many girls are forced into child marriages, some before they are 15 years old. Maternal mortality figures remain indefensibly high in many countries. In most places, women earn less than men for equal work. Around the world, millions of women and girls suffer from physical and sexual violence, with little recourse to justice and protection."[7]

The 2004 World Health Report found that the leading causes of death for women around the world are HIV/AIDS, pregnancy and childbirth, malaria, and tuberculosis,[8] which primarily affect poor women. While adult mortality fell throughout the developing world from the 1960s to the 1990s, on average by about 1% a year for men and 2% a year for women,[9] the HIV/AIDS epidemic is taking a devastating toll. Life expectancy at birth has fallen by more than 10 years in the countries most affected by HIV/AIDS.[10]

In addition, gender discrimination in many parts of the world combined with poverty means that girls and women are more likely to be malnourished. Some "traditions" force women and girls to eat last and least, consuming what is left over after the men and boys are finished. Often the men and boys in the family will consume twice as many calories, despite all the heavy work women and girls undertake. Because of their poor diet, many women suffer from severe vitamin and mineral deficiencies, which expose them to serious health risks, including maternal and infant death, and a higher vulnerability to diseases.[11]

A further obstacle to women's survival is lack of access to appropriate medical care throughout their lifetime. The World Bank reports that in cultures where parents prefer sons over daughters, boys receive a larger share of the limited family resources. They get more food and better health care, including immunizations.[5] This phenomenon was also reported in an article on women's health published in the *British Medical Journal*, which found that in many countries in Asia and north Africa girls are less likely to receive childhood immunizations, especially if a fee is required for treatment.[4]

Lower educational attainment by women, whether due to poverty or gender bias, also affects their health in later life. According to the WHO, "Socioeconomic status, literacy, and access to health services have a strong impact on the development of noncommunicable disease and the delivery of health care.... Populations that undergo a major increase in social capacity (defined as the linkage between individual life course and institutional conditions favourable to health such as increasing the level of education among a population) are likely to experience a substantial decline in the burden of disease."[12]

An even more disturbing barrier to women's survival into old age is violence against women. Female infanticide is still practiced in many parts of the world, both through direct violence and intentional starvation.[13] Amartya Sen, the 1998 Nobel laureate for economics, estimated in 1992 that more than 60 million women were "demographically missing" from the world, especially from Asia and north Africa, as a result of the "comparative neglect of female health and nutrition, especially—but not exclusively—during childhood. . . . Considerable evidence exists of neglect of female children in terms of health care, admission to hospitals, and even feeding."[14] In a 2003 update, Sen states that while the previous problems had not improved a great deal, a new radical disadvantage to female survival had begun in the past decade—sex-specific abortions aimed against the female fetus.[15]

Infanticide of girls has been practiced throughout human history, but advances in medical technology have made it easier to kill unwanted female offspring even before they are born. While medical testing for sex-specific abortions has been outlawed in China, India, and the Republic of Korea, it remains commonplace. China's 2000 census puts the ratio of newborns at 100 girls to 119 boys—much higher than the biological norm of 100 to 103. The 2001 census in India found a similar discrepancy of 927 girls for every 1000 boys under 6 years old, a decline from 962 girls 20 years earlier.[16]

Health Challenges Faced by Older Women

Women who do manage to survive into old age continue to face much of the same gender bias they encountered throughout their lives with the added burden of the natural physical deterioration of old age. Older women have a higher risk of chronic illness and disability and spend a larger proportion of their lives in poor health than older men. While these differences are true in all countries, the impact is greater in poor countries, since health status and standard of living there are generally lower. The overall disadvantage women face is not caused solely by the fact that they live longer than men. Many older women's health problems are rooted in the discrimination they experienced earlier in life.[17] For example, in both developed and developing countries, working outside the home generally does not lessen a woman's workload inside the home, a double burden on women that often takes a toll on their health.[2]

In addition, women who were malnourished in the womb and early childhood are more likely to suffer from a variety of diseases as they age. According to the WHO, "Vitamin and other nutritional deficiencies may lead to adult diseases such as blindness, anemia, bone disease, and brain damage. Low weight gain in childhood, particularly during the first year of life, is associated with increased risk of cardiovascular disease and diabetes in adulthood. It is also linked to changes relating to the ageing process, including cataracts, lower hearing acuity, and reduced muscle strength. Malnutrition in childhood increases the risk of acquiring infectious diseases, particularly respiratory and diarrheal infections, which contribute to chronic disease in adult life."[18]

If they receive equal care as men, women can benefit from their biological advantage for a longer life expectancy until menopause, as hormones seem to protect them from certain diseases, such as ischemic heart disease.[9] While men are more likely to suffer from heart disease and stroke when they are younger, these diseases become the major causes of death and disability for women too as they age and their protective hormones decrease. As women age, they are more likely than men to be affected by such chronic disabling conditions as diabetes, osteoporosis, osteoarthritis, obesity, urinary incontinence, and Alzheimer's disease.[2]

According to a report on gender inequity in health prepared for the WHO Commission on Social Determinants of Health, "When taking into consideration HIV, reproductive infections, and cancers, the disability-adjusted life years (DALYs)* lost by women are 1.22 times those for men. In terms of reproductive cancers alone, women lose seven times more DALYs than men. If women's morbidity, disability, and mortality related to maternity, accounting for 42,173,635 DALYs, are added to this calculation, women lose 2.19 times more DALYs than men. Other areas where women lose more DALYs than men, as indicated by female-to-male ratios, include those related to eye sight (trachoma, cataracts, age-related vision disorders, glaucoma), migraine, mental health (posttraumatic stress disorder, panic disorder, unipolar depressive disorder, insomnia, obsessive compulsive disorder), muscle and bone strength

---

* Disability-adjusted life years (DALY) is a measure of the effects of chronic illness in time, both time lost due to premature death and time spent disabled by disease. One DALY is equal to one year of healthy life lost.

(rheumatoid arthritis, osteoarthritis, other musculoskeletal disorders, multiple sclerosis), ageing (Alzheimer and other dementias), nutrition (other nutritional disorders, iron-deficiency anemia, vitamin A deficiency), and burns."[19]

The most natural difference between men and women as they age is menopause. The end of a woman's ability to bear children has many cultural, physical, and psychological dimensions that vary around the world. Generally, women in developing countries tend to view menopause and its symptoms as a natural process. They know little about health issues related to menopause and do not think they require medical care for its symptoms.[20] Their reluctance to seek treatment has been reinforced by healthcare systems that focus on fertility and marginalize older women.[21] This traditional view of menopause is beginning to change, however, as educated women from developing countries begin to follow the example of developed countries, where menopause has come to be seen as a deficiency condition that should be medically treated.

This view of menopause has led to the widespread use of hormones in pill form to replace those naturally declining with age. Despite conflicting data (some research suggests benefits and other studies demonstrate harm), hormone replacement therapy (HRT) soon became one of the most prescribed group of drugs in the United States. By 1995, approximately 38% of postmenopausal women in the United States used HRT in the hopes of treating the symptoms of menopause and preventing chronic conditions such as heart disease and osteoporosis.[21] This large uptake in the use of HRT has been linked to the profit motive of the pharmaceutical industry.

As explained by Arthur Caplan, chair of the Department of Medical Ethics, University of Pennsylvania School of Medicine, and Carl Elliott, associate professor at the Center for Bioethics at the University of Minnesota:

> First, the manufacturers of enhancement technologies will usually exploit the blurry line between enhancement and treatment in order to sell drugs. Because enhancement technologies must be prescribed by physicians, drug manufacturers typically market the technologies not as enhancements, but as treatments for newly discovered or underrecognized disorders. . . .

Estrogen replacement therapy was initially marketed as a risk-free way for women to extend their youthfulness. But when a 1974 study found that estrogen replacement therapy was associated with an increased risk of endometrial cancer, the manufacturers added progesterone, renamed the combination "hormone" replacement therapy, and recast it as a treatment for medical problems associated with menopause such as osteoporosis.[22]

In 1998, the first major study to challenge the use of HRT for the prevention of heart disease was published in the *Journal of the American Medical Association*. Commonly referred to as the HERS study, it found that women with heart disease who used HRT had worse outcomes than those who did not take hormones.[23] Mounting evidence about the dangers of HRT has led to a reconsideration of its use for the prevention of chronic conditions. "The serious harms of HRT, including breast cancer and cardiovascular disease, appear to outweigh measurable benefits such as prevention of fractures."[24]

Even the idea that menopause should be treated as a medical condition has come under attack. A study published in the *International Journal of Health Services* argues against the medicalization of menopause. By examining mortality and morbidity statistics across countries, over time, and between genders, the study found no evidence that menopause puts women at increased risk of heart disease, osteoporosis, or Alzheimer's disease. The study's author further argues that there are six major consequences of medicalizing menopause:

1. It leads to unequal approaches to disease prevention for men and women, with research and interventions for women focused on hormone use at the expense of more important lifestyle factors.

2. It allows for the widespread acceptance of hormone use as a primary prevention strategy without proof of efficacy from large-scale, long-term randomized clinical trials.

3. It encourages women to accept the adverse consequences of hormones, such as an increased risk of breast cancer.

4. It further medicalizes women's lives, as other drugs are prescribed to

counter the adverse effects of estrogen use.

5. It diverts attention from real factors affecting women's health, such as the environment, socioeconomic status, and violence against women.

6. It harms women psychologically and socially by implying that women's bodies are flawed.[25]

Some medical experts have concluded that most women do not require treatment for menopausal symptoms. Instead they advocate using perimenopause—the time when women are most likely to experience the hot flashes and other symptoms commonly associated with menopause—as an opportunity for healthcare providers to discuss changes in sexual function, psychological effects of menopause, osteoporosis, and cardiovascular disease. They believe it is also an appropriate opportunity to counsel women on smoking, exercise, diet, calcium intake, weight maintenance, stress reduction, and other lifestyle changes that can minimize future health problems.[26]

The following is an overview of some of the most common health problems women face as they age.

Malnutrition

Older people are particularly vulnerable to malnutrition and frequently consume diets that are poor in both quality and quantity. This vulnerability has resulted in undernutrition among older people in all countries, but especially in developing ones.[27] Chronic undernutrition is common among older women in Latin America and the Caribbean, South Asia, and Africa. In both rural and urban settings, years of childbearing and sacrificing their own nutrition for that of their families can cause chronic undernutrition and anemia in women.[28] Older men generally receive larger portions of a desirable food while older women get a disproportionately small share. Animal products, desirable for their protein, are often first distributed to adult males and small children.[29]

The health consequences of undernutrition and poor micronutrient status in older people are considerable. While the average woman's lean body mass is always less than a man's, a woman suffers a fast decline in old age. Loss of lean muscle mass influences muscle strength, gait, and balance, contributing to the risk of falls, frailty, and proneness to infection in older persons.[30]

Among the types of disability, mobility disability, in particular walking disability, is currently acknowledged as one of the most important quality of life and public health concerns of older women. Slow walking speed is a risk factor for falls and other accidents, resulting in fractures, further disability, and loss of independence. In developing countries, losing the ability to walk can be even more devastating as walking is often the most common means of transportation.[31]

Independent of body weight, there is growing evidence that subclinical micronutrient deficiencies in older people are associated with declines in immune function and cognitive ability.[27] One of the most common micronutrient deficiencies is iodine deficiency, which is a major public health problem throughout the world. Iodine deficiency is the greatest cause of preventable brain damage in childhood.[32] Iodine deficiency impairs mental functioning and can cause goiter (a swelling of the thyroid gland) and hypothyroidism (a condition marked by fatigue and weakness). Yet, at least 130 countries have serious pockets of iodine deficiency disorders.[33] Women who are not getting enough iodine in the diet risk severe iodine deficiency through pregnancy as the fetus depletes the mother's stores. That may be one of the reasons there is a higher prevalence of goiter and thyroid disorders in women than in men.[34]

Older persons are also vulnerable to protein-energy malnutrition (PEM), which is one of the main public health problems in most low-income tropical and subtropical countries with largely rural populations.[30] PEM is a potentially fatal body-depletion disorder that occurs when consumption of protein and energy (measured by calories) is insufficient to satisfy the body's nutritional needs for healthy tissue formation and organ function.

Poverty, of course, is directly related to hunger, so the many older women living in poverty are at greater risk of malnutrition. This is true in developing as well as in developed countries. According to Global Action on Ageing, nearly 10% of people over the age of 65 in the United States lived in poverty in 2004.[35] However, poverty is not the only cause of malnutrition in developing countries. The problem can be exacerbated by limited knowledge and traditional views about what older persons should or should not eat. Migration of older adults or of their children may also play a role in worsening malnutrition among older persons since it takes away their traditional support systems. Older persons faced with these problems may also eat too much of the wrong foods. "The result is an increasingly common global paradox, the concurrent presence of chronic diseases such as obesity, diabetes, cancer, and other chronic illnesses associated with combined forms of undernutrition."[30]

Diabetes

The total number of people with diabetes is projected to rise from 171 million in 2000 to 366 million in 2030. While the prevalence of diabetes is higher in men than women, there are more women with diabetes than men.[36] Being older and having diabetes increases the risk of complications from the disease, including heart disease, kidney disease, stroke, and blindness.[37]

In both developing and developed countries, low socioeconomic status is associated with a higher risk of diabetes. There is substantial evidence that maternal malnutrition and obesity are associated with subsequent diabetes in the offspring.[38] The move of large numbers of people from rural to urban environments in search of jobs has led to changes in diet and lifestyle that have increased the prevalence of type 2 diabetes in developing countries.[39] Poverty has been linked to diabetes risk in developed countries as well. A study by Johns Hopkins researchers found that older adolescents in the United States who lived in poverty were 50% more likely to be overweight than their more affluent counterparts. Since being overweight is a major risk factor for diabetes, the researchers concluded that poverty is a risk factor for the disease.[40]

In addition, even in developed countries, women often have worse outcomes and receive less adequate care than men. According to the US Centers for Disease Control and Prevention, diabetes is a more common cause of coronary heart disease among women than men; and among people with diabetes, the prognosis of heart disease is worse for women than for men—women have poorer quality of life and lower survival rates than do men.[41] One study of women in the United States with heart disease and diabetes found they were less likely to receive several types of routine outpatient medical care than men who have similar health problems. For example, women with diabetes were less likely than men to have cholesterol levels within recommended ranges, and they were prescribed ACE inhibitor drugs for chronic heart failure and beta blocker drugs following a heart attack less often than men. These differences in care were found among women even though they generally see a doctor or other healthcare provider more often than men and even after researchers accounted for socioeconomic factors that may influence care.[42]

Diabetes has a broader impact on women than just their personal health. Women often take on the care of family members with diabetes. This can have a significant impact on women's own health and opportunities. In many cases women who are sick themselves cannot get treatment because they are overwhelmed with caring for others. Research has also shown that the social consequences for women and men can vary greatly. In some parts of the world, women are discriminated against if it becomes known that they have diabetes: they may find it impossible to find a husband or, if already married, may be deserted, leaving them in difficult economic circumstances, which make it harder for them to get adequate treatment and care.[37]

Osteoporosis

Osteoporosis and its major complications, hip and spine fractures, affect one in three postmenopausal women and is posing an increasing problem in developing countries as the proportion of the older population increases.[20] Risk factors for osteoporosis include low body mass index, low calcium intake, little physical exercise, smoking, and alcoholism.[43] Since osteoporosis in women has been linked to the decline in hormones after menopause, the disease tends to be overly medicalized, which can divert attention from other potentially more important social factors influencing women's vulnerability to osteoporosis and its complications, such as malnutrition in early childhood,[18] isolation among elderly women, and poor public and private infrastructures.[19]

Osteoporosis and the fractures it causes are a major cause of illness, disability, and death. It is estimated that the annual number of hip fractures worldwide will rise from 1.7 million in 1990 to around 6.3 million by 2050. Women suffer 80% of hip fractures. While a woman's lifetime risk for fractures due to osteoporosis is 30–40%, the risk for men is only 13%.[43]

Osteoarthritis

Osteoarthritis is one of the most common forms of musculoskeletal disease in all countries. It is the fourth most common predictor of health problems worldwide in women.[44] Osteoarthritis of the knee is a major cause of mobility impairment, particularly among women. Risk factors for osteoarthritis include age, family history, obesity, diabetes mellitus, hysterectomy, and activities requiring repeated knee bends. One study found that farming poses the greatest relative risk for osteoarthritis of the hip.[45] Due to financial insecurity, many older people, particularly in developing countries, work in agricultural production until very late in life. A large proportion of these are women, as many agricultural activities are inseparable from domestic tasks, including crop production and animal husbandry.[2]

Heart Disease and Stroke

Cardiovascular diseases are the number one cause of death globally: more people die annually from them than from any other cause. Heart disease and stroke are the major causes of death and disability in ageing women, accounting for close to 60% of all adult female deaths. Half of all deaths of women over 50 in developing countries are due to these conditions.[31]

The most important causes of heart disease and stroke are unhealthy diet, physical inactivity, and smoking. There are also a number of underlying determinants of cardiovascular diseases, including globalization, urbanization, population ageing, poverty, and stress.[46] Socioeconomic status has also been shown to influence the prevalence of the disease. In the 1970s, research showed that in British civil servants, the lower their status the higher the mortality from coronary heart disease.[47] Similar results were found in a study nearly 20 years later that did an age-adjusted comparison of people in the highest job grade (administrators), to people in the lowest grade (clerical and office support staff). It found a higher risk of heart dis-

ease in men and women in the lower job grades. Of the factors examined, the largest contributor to the difference found was little or no control over their work.[48]

Breast Cancer

While the incidence of breast cancer is generally lower in developing than developed countries, rates are rising because of the ageing of the population as well as reproductive, lifestyle, and socioeconomic changes. Age is the single most important risk factor for breast cancer, but other risk factors include starting menstruation at an early age, starting menopause at an older age, having a first child at an older age, short duration of breastfeeding, family history of breast disease, use of oral contraception or hormone replacement therapy, exposure to radiation, alcohol consumption, and possibly diet and exercise.[20]

The International Agency for Research on Cancer (IARC) estimates that in 2002 there were approximately 1.15 million newly diagnosed breast cancer cases and approximately 411,000 deaths. Incidence, mortality, and survival rates vary four-fold across the world's regions because of underlying differences in known risk factors, access to effective treatment, and the influence of organized screening programs. Incidence and mortality rates (the ratio of the total number of deaths to the total population) tend to be higher in high-resource countries and lower in low-resource countries. Conversely, fatality rates (the total number of deaths) tend to be higher in low-resource countries.[49]

Urinary Incontinence and Other Gynecological Problems

Studies in developing countries have found that women have a high incidence of gynecological and urinary problems. This is in large part due to complications of pregnancy and childbirth in less developed countries. About half of the nearly 120 million women who give birth each year experience some kind of complication during their pregnancies, and between 15 million and 20 million women develop disabilities lasting months, years, or even a lifetime. Generally, maternal disabilities are caused by lack of access to medical care during labor and immediately after the birth. Only about half of all births in less developed countries are attended by a trained healthcare provider.[50]

Common problems include menstrual disorders, urinary and reproductive tract infections, stress urinary incontinence, cervicitis, and uterine prolapse. A labor that is obstructed for several days leads to the most serious problems, including fistulas, bladder problems, pelvic inflammatory disease, amenorrhea, infertility, and nerve damage. Fistula is a condition that often develops during obstructed labor, when a woman does not have access to medical care and thus cannot get a Caesarean section. The prolonged pressure of the baby's head against the mother's pelvis cuts off the blood supply to the soft tissues surrounding her bladder, rectum and vagina, leading to tissue death.[51] Women are turned into social outcasts by the loss of fecal and urinary control created by fistulas. Not being able to bear children also leads to high divorce rates among women with fistulas.[20]

Social Challenges Faced by Older Women

Many of the human rights abuses women experience throughout their lifetime are intensified as they age, and they face new forms of maltreatment, violence, and neglect. For millions of women around the world, ageing means an escalation in poverty, institutionalized gender and age discrimination, and societal neglect.

Poverty

In all countries, inequalities in income and wealth in earlier life mean that older women tend to be poorer than older men. This is true in both developing and developed countries. In the United States, for example, older women are almost twice as likely to live in poverty as men, and minority older women are even more vulnerable. Among white American women 65 and older, 11.1% lived at or below the poverty line, while 30.2% of African American women and 25.3% of Hispanic American women that age did.[52]

The risk of falling into poverty is greater for older women than for older men since most social security systems are based on continuous salaried employment and on the amount earned. Women often do not fulfill this requirement, either because of career breaks for childbearing and the skewed division of unpaid work, or because they worked most of their lives in the "informal sector." According to the International Labor Organization, the informal sector consists generally of "small-scale, self-employed activities, with or without hired workers." This includes usually low-wage occupations, like selling street food and domestic work.[53] The informal sector is the primary source of employment for women in most developing countries. In some countries in sub-Saharan Africa, virtually all of the female nonagricultural labor force is in the informal sector. In India and in Indonesia, the informal sector accounts for 9 out of every 10 women working outside agriculture. In 10 Latin American and 4 East Asian countries, half or more the female nonagricultural workforce is in the informal sector.[54] In addition, even in developed countries women are often paid less than their male counterparts for the same work.[55] Such lower wages throughout most of their lives affects the amount older women receive in social security retirement allowance.

Institutionalized Discrimination

Individuals and institutions often discriminate by age because of the misconception that older people are "worthless" and economically inactive. As people age they face increased discrimination and are pushed into more menial and badly paid work. Many older people, especially in the developing world, support themselves and others through work in the informal sector.[2] For example, in Latin America many older people collect plastic bottles and cardboard from the streets for recycling and are paid US $0.05 for every kilo of rubbish collected.[56]

Informal discrimination includes institutional policies and societal norms that make it harder for older people to participate fully in society. For example, older people are regularly barred from getting loans because of their age, and in humanitarian crises they are excluded from livelihood rehabilitation programs.[56] In South Asia, restrictions on mobility and association make it hard for older women to overcome isolation once they are widowed.[17] In the Ukraine, Human Rights Watch found that age specifications openly set by employers adversely affected the participation of older women in the labor force.[57]

More formal discrimination against women can be found codified into law. In a number of countries women still lack independent rights to own land, manage property, conduct business, or even travel without their husbands' consent.[55] For example, women's inheritance rights are restricted in many countries. Family resources, including the house, the land, and all the money, must be left to a male relative, often along with the widow herself. Widows also suffer a loss of status, leaving them vulnerable to social isolation and depression along with discrimination and even physical violence. The very design of most social security pension programs around the world discriminate against women since people who have been working in the informal economy, predominantly women, qualify for little or no benefits. Even where some assistance is available, older people often encounter obstacles in obtaining it, ranging from transport difficulties to bureaucratic barriers. For example, in Egypt, where a social security system was set up in 1950, few people know how to access its provisions.[17]

Older women also face difficulty accessing the care they need because of poverty and institutional discrimination. Simply getting to medical services is a problem for women in rural and remote areas.[17] Healthcare systems can be biased against providing services for older people, and social barriers can exclude older women from receiving care. Many health professionals view ageing as an ongoing process of decline and do not understand the difference between the processes of normal ageing and disease, which leads them to dismiss older patients' complaints and symptoms. In addition, modern healthcare systems are more geared toward curing acute illnesses than managing chronic ones. Since chronic conditions are much more common among older people—women in particular—physicians and other healthcare providers often fail to provide the type of care that could improve their older patients' quality of life.[58]

In many countries, access to health care is tied to coverage by national health insurance systems that, like pension programs, are linked to employment in the formal sector of the economy. As many older women in developing countries have worked all of their lives in the informal sector or in unpaid activities, access to health care often re-

mains unaffordable and difficult at best.[31] Medicare in the United States and other social security health insurance systems in developed countries also discriminate against women through their benefit structure. Men and women suffer different health problems as they age. Men tend to suffer more from acute illnesses that require hospitalization, while women often suffer more from chronic diseases that may be disabling and require more help with activities of daily living. In some developed countries, medical coverage pays for hospital stays and for institutional care in a nursing home, but is very limited in terms of home healthcare assistance. That benefit structure ignores the needs of older women who might be better served by home health care than hospitalization or going to live in a nursing home.[59]

Research by HelpAge International found other barriers to access of healthcare services by older people in developing countries. By monitoring access to health services for older people in Kenya, Tanzania, and Bolivia the organization found:

> Attitudes of hospital staff toward older people can be disrespectful, with older people often at the back of the queue at medical clinics. Older people in rural communities often travel long distances to access health facilities and are therefore less likely to do so on a regular basis. Rather than travel long distances for immediate treatment, some older people prefer to rely on traditional healers. Medicines can be expensive and therefore unaffordable for older people with no fixed income. Old age is seen as a disease, with sickness a part of the disease, and without documents, such as birth certificates, proving an older person's age can be difficult and can mean that they are denied the free health care to which they are entitled.[60]

Increasing Family Responsibilities

Even as women live longer, their caregiving duties do not end or even lessen. Traditionally, older women are the ones that care for ailing spouses or relatives. In many developing countries with less established healthcare systems, older women act informally as nurses and midwives within their communities. Women in rural areas are frequently left to care for grandchildren as their own children migrate to the cities in search of work.[17] In communities severely affected by HIV and AIDS, around 50% of older people care for orphans and vulnerable children. Older women are more likely to take on caring roles than men and are twice as likely to have to do so alone.[56] Compounding the problem, the adult children that would have cared for them in their older years have died.[59]

Even in developed countries, family members—mostly women—are increasingly shouldering the majority of care.[61] In the United States, for example, the Census Bureau reported that in 1994, 1.6 million children were living with a grandparent with no parent present.[62]

Social Isolation

The social isolation of older people, particularly women, is an increasing problem around the world. Shifts in living arrangements are due partly to delayed marriage and changing roles for women, but also to increasing divorce rates and growing numbers of older people whose spouses have died. The trend is not limited to developed countries. In Burundi, for example, an examination of United Nations (UN) data showed that the largest number of older persons live in one-person households. Between one-fifth and one-third of older people in some Caribbean countries live alone, similar to levels in some European countries.[17]

Widowhood is an important factor in the isolation of older women. Because women live longer than men, they are also more likely to become widowed. This is compounded by the fact that most women marry older men. Throughout the developing world, typically half or more of women over age 60 are widowed.[63] In India and Bangladesh, for example, where care for older widows is the duty of their children, a rapid increase in elderly abandoned women has become a critical issue in urban areas. Women who never married or had children are even worse off. In Kenya, for example, traditional norms require women to have at least two sons in order to be "worthy of support." Those without children are often forced to leave their homes to avoid accusations of witchcraft.[17]

The worldwide trend toward smaller nuclear families also affects the care and isolation of older women.[63] In the United States, older people living alone make up a large and growing proportion of the elderly. Nearly 80% of all older people living alone are women. Widowhood and the geographic mobility of children both contribute to the growing number of older women living alone.[52] The most vulnerable older people are those who have no family or other support network—they are the ones that die first. In camps for displaced people in Darfur, Sudan, social isolation is a key indicator of vulnerability. Socially isolated older people are less visible to service providers and less likely to have ration cards or access to health services.[56]

Physical and Psychological Abuse

Older women everywhere can face abuse and violence. Most often, the abusers are family members and primary caregivers, but abuse also occurs in institutional care facilities. Since most developing countries have only recently become aware of the problem, information on the rate of elder abuse has relied on five surveys conducted in the past decade in five developed countries. The results show a rate of abuse of 4% to 6% among older people if physical, psychological, and financial abuse and neglect are included.[64] Those most at risk are older women with mental or physical impairments. Poverty, childlessness, social isolation, and displacement also put older women at risk for abuse, as do dependency and loss of autonomy.[17]

Although elder abuse was first identified in developed countries, where most of the existing research has been conducted, anecdotal evidence and other reports from some developing countries shows that it happens everywhere.[64] According to the Tanzanian government, for example, 17,220 women were abused between 1998 and 2001 as a result of witchcraft allegations; 10% of them were killed. Across the nine project districts in Tanzania where HelpAge International works, there have been 444 killings as a result of witchcraft accusations in the last 5 years. Of these, all except nine were older women.[56]

Conclusion: Towards Healthy Ageing for Women

To ensure older women have a dignified life, women must be assured equal and fair access to education, economic opportunity, health care, and political power throughout their lives. The UN recognizes this in its International Plan of Action on Ageing 2002, which states, "While recognizing that the foundation for a healthy and enriching old age is laid early in life, the Plan is intended to be a practical tool to assist policy makers to focus on the key priorities associated with individual and population ageing."[65] The recommendations made by the UN seek to ensure that people around the world will age with security and dignity and be able to participate fully in society. The top priorities include involving older persons in the development process, advancing health and well-being into old age, and providing supportive environments.

The ageing of populations worldwide requires that governments create strategies to care for the growing numbers of older citizens. This trend started over a century ago in more developed countries, where government-sponsored support systems, such as pensions and health care, have been developed. Today most elderly rely on such formal systems.[17] However, women have less access to formal pensions. The pension systems must be modernized to recognize the unique contributions of women and reward them with income security in their old age.

Similarly, developing countries must institute social security systems that include all sectors of society. The many decades of social security experience in developed countries has proved that a collective approach to ensuring income security and health care for older persons works.[2] Currently, a number of developing countries are considering making contributory pension schemes available to all workers, including those in the informal sector. However, making even small contributions to such a system would be impossible for the poor in many countries. Universal noncontributory pension programs, on the other hand, can be made accessible to everyone, including unpaid caregivers, primarily women, and women working in the informal sector.[17] HelpAge International is calling for a universal social pension for all people over 60 years of age, arguing that a universal pension—paid to everyone over a certain age—is more effective at reaching the poorest people than a means-tested pension (paid only to older people living below a defined poverty level). According to HelpAge, more than 70 countries across the world provide a social pension, including at least 50 low- and middle-income countries. Their experience shows that social pensions are affordable and feasible and that they contribute to economic growth.[66]

In addition, older women must be ensured access to affordable, supportive, unbiased, and informed health care:

- Healthcare providers must be trained to understand and recognize the special healthcare needs of older women, including screening for and treating gynecological disorders, counseling women about menopause and a healthy lifestyle, and managing chronic diseases.

- Effective public health initiatives to address the needs of older women must include an emphasis on the care and coverage of chronic illness and support for family caregivers.

- Outreach activities and public awareness campaigns also are essential to educate older women about their health. The 2002 Global Summit Consensus Conference on International Breast Health Care has recommended that early detection efforts in low-resource settings begin with public education and awareness activities.[46]

- In many poor countries expensive treatment for the major diseases that affect older women, such as diabetes, heart disease, and cancer, is not a viable option; more effective prevention and early detection strategies directly involving communities must be developed.

Finally, a great deal of research has been done to document how all segments of society hold negative attitudes toward ageing and older people. The literature also shows that the attitudes of others appear to affect the older person's self-image, feelings of adequacy and usefulness, and attitudes toward living. Negative views of ageing, life in general, and the self may result in an unwillingness or inability to seek needed services, health care, and other types of help.[67] For women, these negative attitudes towards the aged are compounded by gender bias.

Such discriminatory attitudes and beliefs at the interpersonal level must be combated with education and positive images. Institutionalized discrimination must be outlawed in both the public and private arena. For example, employers must not be allowed to discriminate against older workers, and governments must pass laws that protect the inheritance rights of women. All countries should strive to achieve the standards outlined in the UN Convention on the Elimination of All Forms of Discrimination Against Women (CEDAW). Often described as the international bill of rights for women, the document defines what constitutes discrimination against women and sets an agenda for national action to end such discrimination.

The ageing of the global population must be seen as the great human achievement that it is. Instead of being feared, it must be embraced and societal adjustments made to ensure that older women are rewarded for their lifelong contributions to their families and to society as a whole.

DISCUSSION QUESTIONS

1. What feeling or emotion do you experience when you think of ageing?
2. Do you believe the effects of ageing should be treated as a medical disorder?
3. Which obstacles to the health and human rights of older women discussed in this chapter did you find most surprising and why?
4. What similarities are there in the health and human rights of older women in developed and developing countries?

REFERENCES

1. Bonita, R. *Women, Ageing and Health: Achieving Health Across the Life Span*. Geneva, Switzerland: World Health Organization, Global Commission on Women's Health; 1998.
2. *Ageing: Exploding the Myths*. Geneva, Switzerland: WHO Ageing and Health Programme; 1999.
3. Kalache A. Ageing and life course. World Health Organization: Family and Community Health Cluster (FCH). http://www.who.int/fch/depts/alc/en/. Accessed May 8, 2008.
4. Craft N. Women's health: life span: conception to adolescence. *BMJ*. 1997; 315:1227-1230.
5. World Bank Group Development Education Program. Life expectancy. http://www.worldbank.org/depweb/english/modules/social/life/index02.html. Accessed May 6, 2008.
6. World Bank Group Development Education Program. Life expectancy. http://www.worldbank.org/depweb/english/modules/social/life/index02.html. Accessed May 6, 2008.
7. The State of the World's Children 2007, Women and Children: The Double Dividend of Gender Equality. UNICEF. http://www.unicef.org/sowc07/. Accessed May 7, 2008.

8. *The World Health Report 2004*. World Health Organization. http://www.who.int /whr/2004/en/. Accessed May 7, 2008.

9. Hill, K. Adult mortality in the developing world: what we know and how we know it. Training Workshop on HIV/AIDS and Adult Mortality in Developing Countries. United Nations Secretariat, Department of Economic and Social Affairs, Population Division. 2003. http://www.un.org/esa/population/publications /adultmort/HILL_Paper1.pdf. Accessed May 7, 2008.

10. *The HIV/AIDS Epidemic and its Social and Economic Implications*. New York, NY: United Nations Secretariat, Department of Economic and Social Affairs, Population Division; 2003.

11. Gender equality: key to every MDG. The Hunger Project. http://www.thp.org /women/index.html. Accessed May 6, 2008.

12. WHO. *Noncommunicable Disease and Poverty: The Need for Pro-Poor Strategies in the Western Pacific Region—A Review*. Geneva, Switzerland: WHO; 2006.

13. WHO. Addressing Violence Against Women and Achieving the Millennium Development Goals. Geneva, Switzerland: WHO; 2005.

14. Sen A. Missing women. *BMJ*. 1992;304:587-588.

15. Sen A. Missing women—revisited. *BMJ*. 2003;327:1297-1298.

16. Women in an Insecure World: Violence Against Women—Facts, Figures and Analysis. Geneva, Switzerland: Geneva Center for the Democratic Control of Armed Forces; 2005.

17. United Nations Department of Economic and Social Affairs and Women. *Gender Dimensions of Ageing*. New York, NY: UN; 2002.

18. Stein C, Moritz I. A life course perspective of maintaining independence in older age. World Health Organization. 1999. http://whqlibdoc.who.int/hq/1999 /WHO_HSC_AHE_99.2_life.pdf. Accessed May 12, 2008.

19. Sen G, Östlin P, for World Health Organization Commission on Social Determinants of Health. Unequal, unfair, ineffective and inefficient, gender inequity in health: Why it exists and how we can change it. 2007. http://www.who.int /social_determinants/resources/csdh_media/wgekn_final_report_07.pdf. Accessed May 12, 2008.

20. PATH, Reproductive Health Outlook. Older women. 2004. http://www.rho.org /html/pdfs.html. Accessed May 18, 2008.

21. Keating NL, Cleary PD, Rossi AS, Zaslavsky, Ayanian JZ. Use of hormone replacement therapy by postmenopausal women in the United States. *Ann Intern Med*. 1999;130:545-553.

22. Caplan A, Elliot C. Is it ethical to use enhancement technologies to make us better than well? *PLos Med*. 2004;1(3):172-175.

23. Hulley S, Nelson HD, Humphrey LL, Nygren P; et al. Randomized trial of estrogen plus progestin for secondary prevention of coronary heart disease in postmenopausal women. *JAMA*. 1998;7:605-613.

24. Nelson H, Humphrey LL, Nygren P, Teutsch SM, Allan JD. Postmenopausal hormone replacement therapy. *JAMA*. 2002;288:872-881.

25. Meyer VF. The medicalization of menopause: critique and consequences. *Int J Health Serv*. 2001;31(4):769-792.

26. Clinical challenges of perimenopause: consensus opinion of the North American Menopause Society. *Menopause*. 2000;7(1):5-13.

27. Dangour AD, Ismail SJ. Aging and nutrition in developing countries. *Trop Med Int Health*. 2003;8(4):287-289.

28. Young ME. Health problems and policies for older women: an emerging issue in developing countries. Human Resources Development and Operations Policy

(HRO). 1994. www.stpt.usf.edu/~jsokolov/agewom1.htm. Accessed May 9, 2008.

29. WHO. *Anthology on Women, Health and Environment*. Geneva, Switzerland: World Health Organization; 1994.

30. *Keep Fit for Life: Meeting the Nutritional Needs of Older Persons*. Geneva, Switzerland World Health Organization, Tufts University School of Nutrition and Policy; 2002.

31. Women, ageing and health. World Health Organization Web page. 2000. http://www.who.int/mediacentre/factsheets/fs252/en/. Accessed May 9, 2008.

32. Iodine status worldwide: WHO global database on iodine deficiency. World Health Organization Web page. 2004. http://whqlibdoc.who.int/publications /2004/9241592001.pdf. Accessed May 19, 2008.

33. Ransom EI, Elder LK. Nutrition of women and adolescent girls: why it matters. Population Reference Bureau Web site. 2003. http://www.prb.org/Articles /2003/NutritionofWomenandAdolescentGirlsWhyItMatters.aspx?p=1. Accessed May 19, 2008.

34. Glinoer, D. Thyroid regulation and dysfunction in the pregnant patient. Thyroid Disease Manager, Endocrine Education, Inc. Web page. 2007. http://www .thyroidmanager.org/Chapter14/ch01s03.html. Accessed May 19, 2008.

35. Global Action on Aging. *Old Age Hunger in the United States* [fact sheet]. New York, NY: Global Action on Aging; 2006.

36. Wild S, Roglic G, Green A, Secree R, King H. Global prevalence of diabetes: estimates for the year 2000 and projections for 2030. *Diabetes Care*. 2004;27(5):1047-1053.

37. Hannan C. Moving forward on women, gender equality and diabetes. Presentation at: Expert Group Meeting on Diabetes, Women and Development Organized by the Global Alliance for Women's Health (GAWH), WHO, and the World Diabetes Foundation; April 8, 2008; New York, NY.

38. Jovanovic, L. Nutrition and pregnancy: the link between dietary intake and diabetes. *Curr Diabetes Rep*. 2004;4:266-272.

39. Rashad, H. Promoting global action on the social determinants of health. *Diabetes Voice*. 2006;51(3):33-35.

40. Miech R, Kumanyika SK. Trends in the association of poverty with overweight among US adolescents, 1971-2004. *JAMA*. 2006;295(20):2385.

41. National Agenda for Public Health Action: A National Public Health Initiative on Diabetes and Women's Health. Atlanta, GA National Center for Chronic Disease Prevention and Health Promotion, Division of Diabetes Translation; 2005.

42. Bird CE, Fremont AM, Bierman AS. Does quality of care for cardiovascular disease and diabetes differ by gender for enrollees in managed care plans? *Women's Health Issues*. 2007;17(3):131-138.

43. Lau EMC. Osteoporosis—a worldwide problem and the implications in Asia. *Ann Acad Med*. 2002;31(1):67-68.

44. Brooks P. Inflammation as an important feature of osteoarthritis. *WHO Bull*. 2003;81(9):689-690.

45. Symmons D, Mathers C, Pfleger B. Global burden of osteoarthritis in the year 2000. In: *Global Burden of Disease 2000*. Geneva, Switzerland: World Health Organization; 2006.

46. Cardiovascular diseases. World Health Organization Web pages. 2007. http://www.who.int/mediacentre/factsheets/fs317/en/index.html. Accessed May 10, 2008.

47. Marmot MG, Rose G, Shipley M, Hamilton PJ. Employment grade and coronary heart disease in British civil servants. *J Epidemiol Community Health*. 1978;32: 244-249.

48. Marmot MG, Bosma H, Hemingway H, Brunner E, Stansfeld S. Contribution of job control and other risk factors to social variations in coronary heart disease incidence. *Lancet*. 1997;350:235-239.

49. Smith RA, Caleffi M, Albert US, et al. Breast cancer in limited-resource countries: early detection and access to care. *Breast J*. 2006;12(Suppl1):S16-S26.

50. Ashford L. Hidden suffering: disabilities from pregnancy and childbirth in less developed countries. MEASURE Communication Policy Brief. Washington, DC: Population Reference Bureau; 2002. http://www.prb.org/pdf/HiddenSuffering Eng.pdf. Accessed May 7, 2008.

51. Addressing obstetric fistulas [UNFPA fact sheet]. New York, NY: United Nations Population Fund; 2002.

52. Older women. Administration on Aging Web page. http://www.aoa.gov/naic /may2000/factsheets/olderwomen.html. Accessed May 8, 2008.

53. Sigg R. A global overview on social security in the age of longevity. Presented at: Expert Group Meeting on Social and Economic Implications of Changing Population Age Structure, Population Division, Department of Economic and Social Affairs, United Nations; Mexico City, 31 August – 2 September 2005

54. Chen MA. Women in the informal sector: a global picture, the global movement. World Bank Web page. 2002. http://info.worldbank.org/etools/docs/library /76309/dc2002/proceedings/pdfpaper/module6mc.pdf. Accessed May 8, 2008.

55. King EM, Mason AD. Engendering development through gender equality. *World Bank Group Dev Outreach*. 2001;Spring. http://www1.worldbank.org /devoutreach/spring01/article.asp?id=109. Accessed May 19, 2008.

56. Discrimination and role in society. HelpAge International Web page. 2008. http://www.helpage.org/Researchandpolicy/Stateoftheworldsolderpeople /Discriminationandrole. Accessed May 7, 2008.

57. Women's work: discrimination against women in the Ukrainian labor force. *Human Rights Watch*. 2003;15(5)(D).

58. Uhlenburg P, Hamil-Luker J. Age Discrimination. In: David J. Ekerdt (ed.) *Encyclopedia of Aging*. Macmillan Reference USA; 2002.

59. Older women: perpetual helpers in need of help. United Nations Second World Assembly on Ageing Web page. 2002. http://www.un.org/swaa2002/prkit /olderwomen.htm. Accessed May 8, 2008.

60. World Health Day and health needs of older people. HelpAge International Web page. 2007. http://www.helpage.org/News/Latestnews/1119021210. Accessed May 7, 2008.

61. Gibson MJ, Gregory S, Pandya S. Long-Term Care in Developed Nations: A Brief Overview. Washington, D.C. AARP Public Policy Institute; 2003.

62. Kreider RM. *Current Population Reports, Living Arrangements of Children: 2004, Household Economic Studies*. Washington, D.C.US Census Bureau; 2008.

63. State of the world's older people 2000. HelpAge International Web page. http://www.helpage.org/Resources/Policyreports/main_content/1118337662-0-11/SOTWOPeng.pdf. Accessed May 8, 2008.

64. World Health Organization. Abuse of the elderly. In: Etienne G. Krug, Linda L. Dahlberg, James A. Mercy, Anthony B. Zwi, Rafael Lozano (eds.) *World Report on Violence and Health*. Geneva, Switzerland: WHO; 2002.

65. Madrid International Plan of Action on Ageing, 2002. United Nations Web site. http://www.un.org/ageing/madrid_intlplanaction.html. Accessed May 8, 2008.

66. Practical issues in ageing and development, social pensions. *Ageways*. 2008;70. http://www.globalaging.org/pension/world/2008/Ageways.pdf. Accessed May 8, 2008.

67. Glass C Jr, Knott ES. Middle age: a time for thinking about being old. *J Extension*. 1984;22(1). http://www.joe.org/joe/1984january/a4.html. Accessed May 8, 2008.

The right to health is affirmed in the Universal Declaration of Human Rights and is part of the World Health Organization's (WHO) core principles.[1,2] The affirmation of equal and universal rights to health for all people, irrespective of economic class, gender, race, ethnicity, caste, sexual orientation, disability, age, or location are part of this declaration and the efforts of many WHO and other multilateral organizations' programs. Studies and reports demonstrate vast inequalities in access to health care prevalent among socioeconomic groups, between men and women, children and adults, and among other groups. And although there are no published studies specific to inequalities and palliative care, it can be inferred that if such inequalities exist in the availability of and access to health services in general, these are also prevalent in palliative care.

This chapter will describe the basic components of palliative care and how they relate to human rights, specifically in terms of access to pain relief, the prevailing differences among developed and developing countries, and special populations, especially women and children.

CHAPTER 30

Palliative Care and End-of-Life Issues

Liliana De Lima, MHA;
Peter Selwyn, MD, MPH

Liliana De Lima, MHA, is the Executive Director of the International Association for Hospice and Palliative Care and President, Latin American Association for Palliative Care, Houston, TX.

Peter Selwyn, MD, MPH, is Professor and Chairman in the Department of Family and Social Medicine for the Montefiore Medical Center, Albert Einstein College of Medicine, New York, NY.

Socioeconomic Issues

Controlling the burden of disease and suffering is a fundamental goal of economic development as the link of health to poverty reduction and long-term economic growth has been demonstrated. Low-income countries are home to 3.5 billion people, especially the countries in sub-Saharan Africa with almost 650 million people. These populations have far lower life expectancies and higher mortality rates than the rest of the world. Countries with the highest rates of life expectancy are all developed, while the ones with the lowest years of life expectancy at birth are all very poor countries in sub-Saharan Africa.[3]

More importantly, the HIV epidemic is killing individuals at their time of most economic productivity, leaving behind children and elderly unable to provide, produce, and care for themselves. Health is therefore a priority goal as well as a core issue in economic development and poverty reduction. On a worldwide basis, women make up approximately 50% of all cases of HIV/AIDS; in sub-Saharan Africa, women make up 61% of cases.[4] Significant changes are happening to the family structure in developing countries in addition to the increase in the number of children who are left orphaned in Africa as a result of the HIV/AIDS epidemic. In many countries widows have become ill themselves or are left alone to assume all the economic burden of running their households with little or no income. Most of the burden of care at home falls on women and girls as they often give up their jobs or drop out of school to be caregivers. A recent study demonstrated that 68% and 86% of primary caregivers in South Africa and Uganda respectively, were female.[5] Globally, HIV infection rates for women continue to rise disproportionate to rates of HIV infection in men. In 2005, 17.5 million women were living with HIV, an increase of over 1 million from 2003.[6] In fact, women and girls now represent 57% of all people in sub-Saharan Africa currently living with HIV/AIDS.[7] Rates are particularly high among young women in sub-Saharan Africa; young women between 15 and 24 years old are at least three times more likely to be HIV-positive than young men.[6] In addition, in many countries, after a man's death, wives lose their homes because they have no legal rights to ownership. Children without a birth certificate lose access to the estate and may be unable to attend school because they lack school fees. These factors can all combine to reinforce women's vulnerability and dependency, as they may both suffer disproportionately from certain diseases as well as facing the additional challenges of being caregivers for ill family members and dependent children. If in addition they are sick and do not have access to appropriate curative or maintenance treatments, the probability is that they will not have access to pain relief and palliative care at the end of their lives.

A critical aspect that determines access to care is the availability of resources for health care. The level of health spending in low-income countries is insufficient to address the health challenges they face. The proportion of public spending in developing countries is approximately half of the cost of care, while in the developed countries it is 70%. In most developing countries poor people pay on average 85% of the total health services they receive.[8]

There are three problems with the current health financing arrangements of low-income countries: First, there are insufficient levels of health spending per capita. In the least-developed countries health spending per capita averages approximately $13 per person per year, of which the public budget contributes only $7. The other low-income countries average approximately $24 per person per year, of which $13 comes from the public sector. Second, the proportion of total public healthcare spending in developing countries is much lower than in the high-income countries (55% versus 71%). Since public-sector spending on health is needed to provide critical public goods and to ensure adequate resources for the poor to gain access to health services, the small size of public spending exacerbates the problem of the overall insufficiency of resources. Third, private spending tends to be out of pocket rather than prepaid, so there are very little insurance elements and risk pooling built into private spending.[9] Such private spending tends to be inefficient and usually pays for high-priced medications, unnecessary and futile treatments, and poorly trained practitioners with little or nothing spent in palliative care. Governments in developing countries need to increase the amount of share for health care to ensure adequate access by increasing the domestic resources they mobilize for the health sector but especially, adopt the necessary measures to use the limited resources more efficiently.

Burden of Disease

Chronic diseases—mainly cardiovascular disease, cancer, chronic respiratory diseases, and diabetes—were estimated to cause more than 60% (35 million) of all deaths in 2005; more than 80% of these deaths occurred in low- and middle-income countries. In studies of 15 selected countries where death registration data are available, the estimated age-standardized death rates for chronic diseases in 2005 were 54% higher for men and 86% higher for women than those for men and women in high-income countries.[10] According to data from WHO, there are currently 24.6

million people living with cancer, and it is estimated that the incidence of cancer will double to 24 million new cancers per year by 2050.[11] This will add an additional 24 million/year to the existing numbers. In developed countries, the probability of being diagnosed with cancer is more than twice as high as in developing countries. However, in rich countries, some 50% of cancer patients die of the disease while in developing countries, 80% of cancer victims already have late-stage incurable tumors when they are diagnosed, emphasizing the need for much better detection programs and palliative care. More than 50% of the world's cancer burden, in terms of both numbers of cases and deaths, already occurs in developing countries where only 5% of the resources for cancer treatment reside.[11] Approximately 7.6 million people die from cancer each year; breast cancer is the leading cause of women's deaths from malignant diseases worldwide with more than 500,000 deaths. Every year about 500,000 women get cervical cancer and 250,000 die despite the fact that it is a preventable and curable condition.[12]

Given these numbers, the 58th World Health Assembly (WHA) in May 2005, adopted a resolution asking the WHO member states to develop and incorporate cancer control plans in their countries, which include the four components of care: prevention, early detection, curative treatment, and palliative care.[13]

Palliative Care

Palliative care is defined by the WHO as "an approach that improves the quality of life of patients and their families facing the problems associated with life-threatening illness, through the prevention and relief of suffering by means of early identification and impeccable assessment and treatment of pain and the physical, psychosocial and spiritual problems."[11]

The WHO definition expands the following about palliative care:

- Provides relief from pain and other distressing symptoms
- Affirms life and regards dying as a normal process

- Intends to neither hasten nor postpone death
- Integrates the psychological and spiritual aspects of patient care
- Offers a support system to help patients live as actively as possible until death
- Offers a support system to help the family cope during the patient's illness and in their own bereavement
- Uses a team approach to address the needs of patients and their families, including bereavement counseling, if indicated
- Will enhance quality of life, and may also positively influence the course of illness

According to WHO, of the 58 million people dying annually, at least 60% will have a prolonged advanced illness and would benefit from palliative care. Palliative care is applicable early in the course of illness, in conjunction with other therapies that are intended to prolong life, such as chemotherapy, radiation therapy, or highly active antiretroviral therapy (HAART), and includes those investigations needed to better understand and manage distressing clinical complications. About 80% of the dying would benefit from palliative care to alleviate pain and suffering in their final days of life. Yet, in countries such as India, only around 1% of them are able to access such care.

It is important to recognize that the approach to the patient with life-limiting conditions is never either all curative or all palliative, and that it always includes a shifting balance of both types of interventions. Figure 30-1[14] represents the inappropriate approach between curative and palliative care, which leads to poor quality of care for patients and families. The full range of patients' needs throughout the course of illness, including medical, psychological, and social problems for patients and families, needs to be evaluated and addressed at the moment of diagnosis. Figure 30-2[14] illustrates the more comprehensive and effective approach that needs to be advocated for patients with life-threatening conditions. As indicated in the figures, palliative care may predominate late in the course of illness, while curative or disease-specific therapy may predominate in the earlier phases of chronic disease. However, it is important to note that there should never be an either/or approach to palliative and curative care, and that

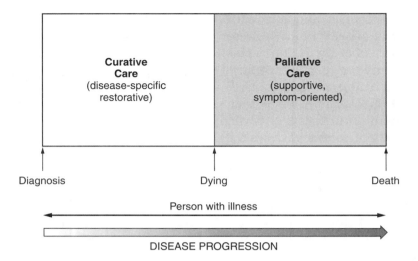

FIGURE 30-1 Traditional Dichotomy of Curative and Palliative Care for Chronic Progressive Illness. From WHO. *Cancer Pain Relief and Palliative Care,* Report of WHO Expert Committee. Publication # 1100804. Geneva, Switzerland: World Health Organization, 1990.

both of these approaches can and should coexist to different degrees along the course of illness. In addition, it should be noted that while the availability and access to curative therapies may be limited in developing countries, one may still seek the same balance and integration of disease-specific and palliative therapies. It must be emphasized that the existence of international—and domestic—variations in resources and health services should never lead to a system that endorses curative therapy for those with resources and palliative care for the poor. In any setting, policy and health advocacy must seek to obtain the best available curative treatments in whatever manner is feasible,

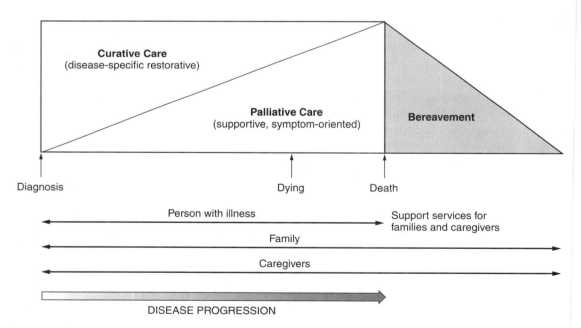

FIGURE 30-2 Integrated Model Including both Curative and Palliative Care for Chronic Progressive Illness. From WHO. *Cancer Pain Relief and Palliative Care,* Report of WHO Expert Committee. Publication # 1100804. Geneva, Switzerland: World Health Organization, 1990.

at the same time as seeking to obtain accessible and effective palliative care services for all those who may need them.

Palliative Care and Suffering

Suffering may be defined as the distress associated with events that threaten the intactness or wholeness of the person.[15] The causes of suffering may be grouped by their physical, psychological, social, cultural, or spiritual origin. For patients with advanced disease, suffering may result from any or all of the various causes, and the effects are additive. The term *total suffering* is used to describe the sum of a patient's suffering, which is addressed in palliative care.

The components of palliative care follow from the causes of suffering, and each has to be addressed in the provision of comprehensive palliative care. Treatment of pain and physical symptoms are usually addressed first because it is not possible to deal with the psychosocial aspects of care if a patient has unrelieved pain or other distressing physical symptoms. In addition, cultural factors and religious concerns may be the source of considerable suffering. All patients with a terminal illness experience some spiritual (or existential) suffering that in the presence of unrelieved pain or physical symptoms may go unsaid or unheard. The various aspects of suffering are interdepen-dent. Untreated or unresolved problems relating to one cause of suffering may cause or exacerbate other aspects of suffering.

Pain Relief

Pain relief lies at the core of palliative care. Pain is one of the most common symptoms in palliative care, resulting from disease progression, treatment, or surgery.[16] A significant majority of patients experience severe pain that requires the use of potent analgesics, such as morphine. In 1986, the WHO and its Expert Committee on Cancer developed an effective analgesic method for the relief of cancer pain. The method relies on the permanent availability of opioid analgesics, including morphine, codeine, and others. Known as the Three-Step Analgesic Ladder (see Figure 30-3),[17] it has been widely disseminated throughout the world, and it has been demonstrated to be safe and effective for the vast majority of patients in pain.

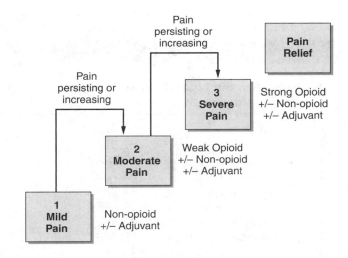

FIGURE 30-3　The WHO Analgesic Ladder Adapted from WHO. *Cancer Pain Relief.* Geneva, Switzerland: World Health Organization, 1990.

Both codeine and morphine are included as analgesics in the WHO Model List of Essential Medicines.[18] In addition, the IAHPC List of Essential Medicines for Palliative Care[19] includes morphine as well as oral methadone, oral oxycodone, and transdermal fentanyl as analgesics for the third step of the WHO Ladder. In spite of this recognition, it is estimated that 80% of patients in pain do not have access to pain-relieving medications.[20] Patients in the developing world suffer much more than those in the developed world. A review done by the Pain and Policy Studies Group (PPSG), a WHO Collaborating Center for Policy and Communications in Cancer Care of the University of Wisconsin, revealed that of the 2006 International Narcotics Control Board (INCB) morphine data reported by governments, seven high-income countries (United States, France, Canada, United Kingdom, Germany, Austria, and Australia) accounted for nearly 84% of medical morphine consumed in the world. These seven countries comprise less than 12% of the world's population.[21] Specific country data showing the countries with the highest and lowest consumption is included in Table 30-1.[22] These reports and figures point to the large and continuing disparity in morphine consumption among countries and provide further evidence of the inadequate global treatment of pain, especially in low- and middle-income countries. Some of the reasons why opioids are unavailable in developing countries are

TABLE 30-1

Countries with the highest consumption (mg/capita)			Countries with the lowest consumption (mg/capita)		
1	Austria*	153.5171	145	Congo	0.0039
2	Canada	62.0103	146	Angola	0.0030
3	U.S.A.	57.8888	147	Burundi	0.0019
4	Denmark	55.7115	148	Eritrea	0.0018
5	Australia	52.2852	149	Burkina Faso	0.0017
6	New Zealand	49.8354	150	Dem. Rep. of the Congo	0.0013
7	France	43.4565	151	Togo	0.0010
8	Portugal	38.7767	152	Malawi	0.0005
9	Norway	31.5411	153	Lao Peop. Dem. Rep.	0.0004
10	Switzerland	30.9566	154	Ethiopia	0.0002

Countries with the Highest and Lowest Consumption of Morphine in 2006[21]

Global mean: 5.9847 mg/capita

* Austria uses morphine in treatment of drug dependence.
Source: Pain and Policy Studies Group. Global, Regional and National Consumption Statistics for 2006. http://www.painpolicy.wisc.edu/news/international.htm#041508.

poverty, insufficient knowledge on how to asses and treat pain, high cost of opioids, and excessively restrictive laws and regulations that impose limits on the dosages and the duration of treatment.[20] In several developing countries where opioid analgesics are available, misconceptions and lack of education in pain management continue to be a hindrance. The WHO and the INCB have asked governments to ensure availability and accessibility of opioid medications to satisfy the needs of the population.[23]

Palliative Care as a Human Right

Palliative care embraces human rights that are already recognized in national laws, international human rights documents, and other consensus statements.[24] Health is defined in broad terms in the United Nations documents and declarations, and although there is no express right to palliative care in any of these documents, health includes the health of people at the end of their lives or with life-limiting conditions. The needs and desires of the terminally ill are often overlooked and not considered a priority in health systems that are usually focused on developing policies for acute and epidemic conditions. The most fragile, such as patients in end of life, tend to be abandoned by the main stream of care with arguments such as "nothing else that can be done." It is within this framework that palliative care advocates work for the relief of suffering based on the needs of the patients.

Palliative care rights include the right to the following[25]:

- Pain relief
- Symptom control for physical and psychological symptoms
- Access to essential medicines for palliative care
- Spiritual and bereavement care
- Family-centered care
- Care by trained palliative care professionals
- Receive home-based care when dying and to die at home if desired
- Treatment of disease and to have treatment withheld or withdrawn
- Information about diagnosis, prognosis, and palliative care services
- Name a healthcare proxy for decision making
- Not be discriminated against in the provision of care because of age, gender, socioeconomic status, geographic location, national status, prognosis, or diagnosis

Palliative Care in Children and Special Populations

Children with life-limiting conditions or in end-of-life are usually not offered palliative care, including in developed countries. Too often, children with fatal or potentially fatal conditions and their families fail to receive competent, compassionate care and are committed to pursuing only curative and life-prolonging options. This intensive but limited focus can expose children and families to unnecessary suffering, particularly if inadequate attention is paid to the children's physical and emotional distress. Children with life-threatening conditions and their families should have access to palliative care that offers physical, emotional, and spiritual comfort from the time of diagnosis through death and into bereavement—if death is the outcome. These principles also apply to other vulnerable populations, including the elderly, people with disabilities, ethnic groups, transgender populations, and prisoners who face additional barriers and discrimination.

Conclusion

Where diagnosis and prognosis differences interact with social determinants, policy efforts must address these different situations. Significant advocacy is required to raise attention and sustain support for other services that address the specific health needs of patients with life-limiting conditions and those who are also in their end of their lives. Special provisions need to meet the needs of patients in low-income countries, reducing their vulnerability to unnecessary suffering and guaranteeing that treatment can be accessed by children, women, and men without bias.

However, even with more efficient allocation and greater resource mobilization, the levels of funding necessary to cover essential services are far beyond the financial means of many low-income countries as well a few middle-income countries. Coordinated actions by the pharmaceutical industry, governments of high-income countries, philanthropists, and international agencies are needed to ensure that the world's poor have access to essential medications and appropriate healthcare services, including palliative care. Palliative care needs to be incorporated in the public healthcare policy to ensure its continuity and financial stability. Nations, individuals, and policy makers should learn from the lessons of others that relief of unnecessary pain and suffering will contribute to a better quality of life for all.

DISCUSSION QUESTIONS

1. Discuss the socioeconomic factors that influence palliative and end-of-life care globally.
2. "Palliative care is a human right." Do you agree with this statement?
3. What measures can be taken by the global health workforce in expanding and increasing access to palliative care?

REFERENCES

1. United National. Universal Declaration of Human Rights, Article 25. http://www.un.org/Overview/rights.html. Accessed October 28, 2008.

2. WHO. Constitution of the World Health Organization. New York, NY: UN: 1946.

3. WHO. *The World Health Report 2002*. Geneva, Switzerland: WHO; 2003.

4. UNAIDS. *AIDS Epidemic Update: December 2007*. Geneva, Switzerland: WHO; 2007. UNAIDS/07.27E/JC1322E.

5. Sen G, Östlin P. Unequal, Unfair, Ineffective and Inefficient Gender Inequity in Health: Why It Exists and How We Can Change It: Final Report to the WHO Commission on Social Determinants of Health. Stockholm, Sweden: Women and Gender Equity Knowledge Network; 2007.

6. United Nations. Taking Action: Achieving Gender Equality and Empowering Women Task Force on Education and Gender Equity. New York, NY: UN; 2005.

7. UNAIDS. *Report on the Global AIDS Epidemic, 2006*. Geneva, Switzerland: UNAIDS; 2006.

8. WHO. Supporting National Responses to the Commission on Macroeconomics and Health: Possible Elements of an Action Plan. Geneva, Switzerland: WHO; 2002.

9. De Lima, L, Hamzah E. Socieconomic, cultural and political issues. In: Bruera E, Wenk R, DeLima L, eds. *Palliative Care in Developing Countries: Principles and Practice*. Houston, TX: IAHPC Press; 2004.

10. Abegunde DO, Mathers CD, Adam T, Ortegon M, Strong K. The burden and costs of chronic diseases in low-income and middle-income countries. *Lancet*. 2007;370(9603):1929-1938.

11. WHO. *Cancer Control Program: Policies and Managerial Guidelines*. Geneva, Switzerland: WHO; 2002.

12. WHO. *The World Health Organization's Fight Against Cancer: Strategies that Prevent, Cure, and Care*. Geneva, Switzerland: WHO; 2007.

13. World Health Assembly. 58th resolution on global cancer and control. http://www.who.int/gb/ebwha/pdf_files/WHA58/WHA58_22-en.pdf. Accessed October 28, 2008.

14. WHO. *Cancer Pain Relief and Palliative Care, Report of WHO Expert Committee*. Geneva, Switzerland: WHO; 1990. Publication 1100804.

15. Woodruff R. Palliative care: basic concepts. In: Bruera E, Wenk R, DeLima L, eds. *Palliative Care in Developing Countries: Principles and Practice*. Houston, TX: IAHPC Press; 2004.

16. Solano JP, Gomes B, Higginson IJ. A comparison of symptom prevalence in far-advanced cancer, AIDS, heart disease, chronic obstructive pulmonary disease and renal disease. Journal of *Pain Symptom Manage*. 2006;31(1):58-69.

17. WHO. *Cancer Pain Relief, with a Guide to Opioid Availability*. Geneva, Switzerland: WHO; 1996.

18. WHO. *WHO Model List of Essential Medicines*. 15th ed. Geneva, Switzerland: WHO; 2007. http://www.who.int/medicines/publications/EML15.pdf.

19. De Lima L, Krakauer EL, Lorenz K, Praill D, MacDonald N, Doyle D. Ensuring palliative medicines availability: the development of the IAHPC List of Essential Medicines for Palliative Care. *J Pain Symptom Manage*. 2007;33(5):521-526.

20. WHO. Access to controlled medications programme. http://www.who.int/medicines/areas/quality_safety/access_to_controlled_medications_brnote_english.pdf. Accessed October 28, 2008.

21. Pain and Policy Studies Group. Global, regional and national consumption statistics for 2006. http://www.painpolicy.wisc.edu/news/international.htm#041508. Accessed October 28, 2008.

22. Pain and Policy Studies Group/WHO Collaborating Center for Policy and Communications in Cancer Care. Morphine consumption data for 2006: Countries with the highest and lowest consumption. Madison, WI: PPSG; 2008.

23. International Narcotics Board. UN drug control body concerned over inadequate medical supply of narcotic drugs to relieve pain and suffering [press release]. Vienna, Austria: INCB: 2000.

24. Brennan F. Palliative care as an international human right. *J Pain Symptom Manage*. 2007;33(5):494-499.

25. Open Society Institute and Equitas. *Palliative Care and Human Rights: A Resource Guide.* New York, NY: OSI and Equitas; 2007.

Effects of Cultural Practices, Environment, and Migration on Women and the Girl-Child

Culture, environment, and migratory practices have profound impacts on the lives of women in every walk of life. This section attempts to highlight the harmful effects cultural practices and environmental factors have on the health and well-being of women and the girl-child and discuss strategies in place and what we can do as a global community to improve their health and well-being.

What culture worth the name would deny women the right to safe motherhood? What value system would send young people ignorant into the world, when a little knowledge might save their lives?

*—Dr. Nafis Sadik,
former UNFPA Executive Director*

CHAPTER 31

INTRODUCTION

Breastfeeding: A Biological, Ecological, and Human Rights Imperative for Global Health*

Health is a human right. This chapter provides the reader with background on the intergenerational reproductive health and nutrition continuum, with breastfeeding as the keystone preventive health practice. Breastfeeding is an essential component of much of the program and policy needed to improve maternal and child nutrition, health, and survival worldwide. Our health and nutrition is also dependent on the state of the world in which we live; environmental concerns are affected by our feeding choices as are our food choices affected by environmental concerns, and our food availability is affected by the environment. Therefore, this chapter highlights the role of breastfeeding as a right and breastfeeding-related programs and policies, but also explores food and our environment. The objectives are that the reader will:

■ Understand the concepts of intergenerational health and nutrition.

■ Understand the role of breastfeeding in protecting the environment as an essential part of the reproductive health continuum.

■ Have a better understanding of breastfeeding as a reproductive right.

■ Outline a course of action for policy and program changes that would enable women to succeed in optimal breastfeeding for their health and the health of their children.

Miriam Labbok, MD, MPH, FACPM, IBCLC, FABM; Erica Nakaji, BA

Miriam Labbok, MD, MPH, FACPM, IBCLC, FABM, is a Professor of the Practice of Public Health and Director of the Center for Infant and Young Child Feeding and Care, in the Department of Maternal and Child Health, School of Public Health, The University of North Carolina at Chapel Hill at Chapel Hill, NC. Dr Labbok is a consultant for UNICEF, USAID, WIC, WHO, and the World Bank. She is recipient of the Healthy Child Achievement Award and the USAID Science & Technology in Development Award.

Erica Nakaji, BA is affiliated with the Department of Maternal and Child Health, School of Public Health, The University of North Carolina at Chapel Hill, Chapel Hill, NC.

Breastfeeding Is a Biological, Ecological, and Human Rights Imperative

Breastfeeding is a woman's right as well as a biological imperative that must be fully supported by multisectoral policy and programming if we wish to achieve sustainable intergenerational health, nutrition, development, and survival.

* Sections of this chapter are drawn or modified from previous work by the author:

Labbok M. Breastfeeding: a woman's reproductive right. *Int J Gynaecol Obstet.* 2006;94(3):277-286.

UNICEF Innocenti Research Centre. *1990–2005 Celebrating the Innocenti Declaration on the Protection, Promotion and Support of Breastfeeding: Past Achievements, Present Challenges and Priority Action for Infant and Young Child Feeding.* Florence, Italy: Innocenti Research Centre; 2007.

Breastfeeding: A Biological Imperative

Is breastfeeding nutrition or health? In fact, breastfeeding is the intergenerational link in nutrition and health. Breastfeeding is a biological imperative if we truly want to achieve sustained global health. Breastfeeding must not be seen as just one of the many optional interventions, but rather must be accepted and supported as the essential link in the intergenerational health continuum that it is.

While it takes a village to raise a child, there is little argument that the mother generally serves the role and has the responsibility to be the child's primary healthcare provider and primary educator when allowed and enabled to do so. By breastfeeding optimally, she is carrying out both of these responsibilities. She is also serving her own biological need for the physical resolution of her pregnancy and other reproductive health norms. Maternal health issues are also addressed with breastfeeding.

Exclusive breastfeeding in the early months is a biological imperative, especially in light of the changing picture of endemic diseases. We know that exclusive breastfeeding reduces the risk of infectious disease, but particularly it appears to reduce the risk of retroviral infections, such as HIV, compared to mixed feeding, which is defined as feeding other liquids or foods in addition to breastfeeding. This very special nature of exclusive breastfeeding deserves ongoing attention.

Breastfeeding: An Ecological Imperative

Breastfeeding has direct and indirect impacts on the environment.[1] Breastfeeding has a direct role in the rate of population growth, an essential environmental correlate. Indirectly, breastfeeding reduces the need for dairy production, plastics and packaging, pharmaceuticals, and fossil fuel use and energy consumption, all of which are necessary for the production and use of commercial infant formula. In 1992, US Vice President and global environmental lobbyist Albert Gore noted in his treatise on the environment that breastfeeding "simultaneously improves the health of children and suppresses fertility."[2]

A new nutrition-related area for consideration for recognizing breastfeeding as an imperative is the reality that it is a "slow food." The term *slow food* refers to food that is, simply put, "good, clean, and fair."[3] Slow Food emerged in the 1980s as a social movement against the fast-food industry and globalization, and has since evolved into an international organization.[4] It encourages people to know the origin of the food they consume, and to honor the food traditions of the geographical region and their culture. This movement supports the notion that food should be viewed as more than something that is simply eaten, but rather as "happiness, identity, culture, pleasure, conviviality, nutrition, local economy, survival."[5] Slow Food urges people to assume a larger role, viewing themselves as coproducers—not just consumers—who play an active part in the food cycle by making deliberate, responsible food choices that affect the food system and the environment positively. Slow Food supports environmental sustainability, including local agriculture and small-scale farming practices that are ecologically sound, protecting biodiversity and tightening the relationship between people and what they eat. The words *pleasure* and *gastronome* are seen frequently in Slow Food literature, and while the movement believes in the enjoyment of food, it more broadly promotes a conscious responsibility about the food people choose. Clearly, in this parlance, breastfeeding is slow food, and should be part of this social movement.

Breastfeeding: A Human Rights Imperative

Why is breastfeeding to be considered a woman's right? Because it is a human right. Later in this chapter, we discuss the rights continuum, but first it is important that we understand that the right of mothers to breastfeed their infants deserves to be accepted as a human right.[6] In his treatise on this issue, Dr. Michael Latham notes that Article 12 of the *International Covenant on Economic, Social, and Cultural Rights* describes "the right to health," and health is defined as "the enjoyment of the highest attainable standard of physical and mental health." The 1978 WHO/UNICEF *Declaration of Alma Ata* reminds us that health is a human right, and defines health as "complete physical, mental, and social well-being, and not mainly the absence of disease or infirmity." Further, the 1990 *Innocenti Declaration on the Protection, Promotion, and Support of Breastfeeding* recognizes that maternal milk provides ideal nourishment without equal for the infant, that it contributes to the health of the mother and infant, and has many other social, health, and psychological advantages. In sum, because there are health and other disadvantages to the mother and the child resulting from not breastfeeding, then obstacles to breastfeeding are also obstacles to the mother's and infant's human rights.

Why Breastfeeding? A Keystone in the Biological, Ecological, and Rights-Sensitive Reproductive Health Continuum

The Biological and Health Continuum

Breastfeeding is necessary for optimal maternal and child health, as well as the child's lifelong development and survival. Reproductive health may be defined as the successful production of a next generation that will successfully reproduce. Breastfeeding contributes to this biological and health continuum as the intergenerational link, helping the mother's body recover from the pregnancy, and delaying the next pregnancy until this child has achieved a level of maturity, thus ensuring the best start on life for the next generation.

It is estimated that breastfeeding currently saves about 5–6 million children's lives annually from common infectious diseases.[7] The *Lancet Child Survival Series* estimates that 1.3 million additional lives could be saved annually if women were enabled to achieve six months exclusive breastfeeding with continued breastfeeding thereafter.[8] Early breastfeeding for thermal regulation and continued breastfeeding with complementary feeding could save an additional 800,000 lives. Stated another way, 3500 unnecessary child deaths occur every day because support for exclusive breastfeeding is not forthcoming, contributing to a total of 5750 deaths that occur daily for lack of optimal infant and young child feeding.

Only breastfeeding, and breastfeeding alone, without other foods or liquids, provides the ideal nourishment for infants for the first six months of life, as breast milk contains all the water, nutrients, antibodies, and other factors an infant needs to thrive. Its components constantly adapt to the child's needs and environmental challenges. There are many well-recognized risks of not breastfeeding.[9,10] Lack of breastfeeding is associated with an increased incidence of acute ear infections, diarrheal episodes, and severe lower respiratory tract infections. Breastfeeding is associated with in-creased intelligence scores and is known to help overcome developmental delays.

Breastfeeding also reduces chronic diseases and developmental problems, including asthma in young children, obesity, type 1 and 2 diabetes, childhood leukemia, and sudden infant death syndrome (SIDS), all these factors contribute to global infant and child mortality rates. Universal breastfeeding would reduce postneonatal mortality in the United States by at least 21%. And, exclusive breastfeeding multiplies the benefits of breastfeeding; it has been estimated that exclusive breastfeeding would lower global child mortality by at least 13%, and early and exclusive breastfeeding may lower neonatal mortality by more than 50%.

Mothers who do not breastfeed suffer from increased risk of type 2 diabetes, breast cancer, ovarian cancer, and maternal postpartum depression. Additional risks of not breastfeeding include bone calcium depletion[11] and more rapid return to fertile status, significantly shortening birth intervals where family planning methods are less available and accessible. The mother who does not breastfeed also has been shown to suffer from slower recovery postdelivery, increased maternal stress[12] and blood loss[13] postpartum, less vigorous uterine involution,[14] and increased risk of cancer of the ovaries.[15] Immediate postpartum breastfeeding seems to enhance the bonding between mother and child, decreasing the chances of desertion.[16]

The Ecological Continuum

The availability of quality foods supports optimal health outcomes, and the availability of quality human milk bridges the generations. Human milk provides sufficient energy and protein to meet requirements during the first six months of infancy. However, some micronutrients are dependent on maternal stores.[17] A mother's nutritional status at her own birth and her nutritional status prior to her pregnancy are both associated with the birth weight of her children. The mother's prepregnancy nutrient stores can also influence the micronutrient composition of breast milk. During pregnancy and lactation, mothers should have about 500 additional calories every day, so in areas where resources are scarce, mothers may need longer birth intervals to allow the time to rebuild their nutritional stores prior to another pregnancy. Birth spacing of about three years also give the child time to mature sufficiently to be able to eat and properly utilize family foods. While the current recommendation is at least two years spacing between births, recent studies may indicate the need to update this recommendation to be closer to three years birth spacing for optimal outcomes for both mother and child.[18,19] However, spacing births alone is not sufficient for maternal nutrition and associated reproductive health. Proper nutrition throughout the life cycle for the girl child, and delay in age of the first pregnancy to at least 18 years of age, are also associated with improved birth outcomes.

Proper nutrition is more than food. Nutritional status depends not only on calories, but on the mix and balance of protein, calories, and micronutrients. Not all foods are equal, and often produce that is heartiest for agrobusiness is not the most nutritious by the time it reaches the dinner plate. As we look to the future, there are several arguments for using local foods for nutrition. Breast milk is clearly a "local" food. In considering sustainable nutrition, economics play an important role. Buying locally supports and improves the local economy. Just as buying locally preserves farmland and discourages its development into nonagricultural uses, breast-milk preserves resources. Small farmers—and mothers—are more likely to be able to maintain their production with the support of the community, which in turn will want to protect the source of its food for all age groups. Just as with breastfeeding, there are fewer environmental impacts with sustainable farming practices in contrast to the impact of some agro-industries. Organic farming does not use chemical fertilizers and pesticides, as seen in industrial agriculture, which damage the soil, water, and air. In addition, buying local uses fewer fossil fuels in transport, since the distance the food travels is significantly decreased.

Local foods, just like the human milk during breastfeeding, are typically of higher quality in terms of freshness, since they travel a shorter distance, have no preservatives, and are consumed more quickly. Purchasing directly from the farmer also has the advantage of creating a closer relationship between consumer and producer.[20] The consumer becomes educated in things that the postindustrial age has erased from his or her knowledge, such as where and how their food was grown. Slow Food argues that people should know the source of their food, which requires "shortening the chain along which a product passes from field to table."[21] All of these factors apply to breastfeeding as well.

Breastfeeding is not as yet specifically recognized by the Slow Food movement, but it follows the principles of the movement. While breastfeeding's ease of transport and accessibility may technically deem it a "fast" food, socially speaking, it is more aptly placed under the slow food label. Breast milk is local, and it is green. The factors in a mother's milk that provide immunizations are produced based on the local environment in which she and the baby live. Breastfeeding provides unprocessed milk, a renewable resource, which produces no waste as with the packaging used in infant formula. There is also no wasted milk with breastfeeding, as breast milk is produced in response to a child's suckling.[22]

Like the decrease in biodiversity associated with large-scale farming practices, such as monocropping, lactation will diminish if it is insufficiently practiced.[23] As the food industry has severed the connectedness people feel to the land and their food sources, so have the infant formula companies separated children from their mothers' intimacy and their breast milk. Breast milk provides nutrients and ever-changing antibodies that industrial infant formula cannot replace. Breastfeeding also serves as a bonding mechanism between mother and child through the skin-to-skin contact that bottle feeding cannot achieve. As long as infant formula is marketed strongly and the actions of the infant formula companies are not monitored, some mothers will ultimately choose formula over breastfeeding.

The Continuum of Human Rights

While breastfeeding may be considered a human right, the rights of women often are given a second place status to those of children and men. Breastfeeding as a woman's right has been explored in an annual report of the Federation of Gynecologists and Obstetricians[24] and in a series of symposia entitled Breastfeeding and Feminism.[25] However, breastfeeding is an area where one might perceive a potential for conflict between the woman's and the child's rights.[26] As confirmed by the Convention on the Rights of the Child, children have a right to the best start in life with the best chance for health.[27] But why is this is also a woman's right? In countries throughout the world, women's autonomy frequently has been limited in the name of ensuring children's well-being, thus subordinating women's rights to children's rights.

However, framing the issue as a woman's right to choose and succeed with breastfeeding makes it the responsibility for the family, society, and workplace to recognize and support her in her right to do what is best. Biological considerations indicate that, indeed, the right to breastfeed is a woman's right for her own health. Since women who breastfeed have improved postpartum recovery; less iron loss; delayed fertility return; lowered incidence of breast, ovarian, and uterine cancers; and apparently better bone status in older age, it is indeed her right to health that must be considered as well. Two international conventions, the Convention on the Rights of the Child and the Convention on the Elimination of All Forms of Discrimination against Women (CEDAW)[28] support this right for both the child and mother. Both conventions place substantial obligations on each nation to enable accommodation of childbearing and childrearing roles, among other roles.

What Has Been Done to Enable Women to Succeed in Their Efforts to Breastfeed Optimally?

There have been a series of international policy and program efforts to further enable women everywhere to practice optimal feeding.

During the decade of the 1990s, as the number of scientific studies demonstrating the importance of breastfeeding for mothers and children increased, two primary programmatic approaches were supported by the global community: The Baby-friendly Hospital Initiative (BFHI) and the International Code of Marketing of Breast-milk Substitutes.

The BFHI was developed based on studies in the 1970s and 1980s that identified healthcare workers and hospital delivery as risk factors strongly associated with difficulties in breastfeeding and the later use of artificial feeding. However unwittingly, health services frequently contributed to lower breastfeeding rates either by failing to support and encourage mothers to breastfeed or by introducing routines and procedures that interfere with the normal initiation and establishment of breastfeeding. To increase knowledge, skills, and supportive behaviors among healthcare providers, the BFHI included changes in policy, staff training, and strengthening and linkage with community support for breastfeeding, based on the "Ten Steps to Successful Breastfeeding"[30] as seen in Table 31-2. Step 10 asks hospital staff to "foster the establishment" of community support groups for breastfeeding, underlining that responsibility to support breastfeeding extends beyond the walls of health facilities.

TABLE 31-1

The Innocenti Declaration

Following on the messages of the Alma Ata meeting, a group of technical staff from WHO, UNICEF, USAID, and SIDA gathered to assess how to raise the profile and action related to breastfeeding as an important child survival intervention.[29] This group planned and executed a series of meetings that culminated in the Innocenti meeting.

The Innocenti Declaration of August 1, 1990, offered four operational targets for global support for breastfeeding, calling upon all nations to:

1. Appoint a national breastfeeding coordinator with appropriate authority, and establish a multisectoral national breastfeeding committee composed of representatives from relevant government departments, nongovernmental organizations, and health professional associations.
2. Ensure that every facility providing maternity services fully practices all the "Ten Steps to Successful Breastfeeding" set out in the WHO/UNICEF statement on breastfeeding and maternity services.
3. Give effect to the principles and aim of the International Code of Marketing of Breast-milk Substitutes and subsequent relevant Health Assembly resolutions in their entirety.
4. Enact imaginative legislation protecting the breastfeeding rights of working women and establish means for its enforcement.

Source: Innocenti Declaration, 1990.

TABLE 31-2

Ten Steps to Successful Breastfeeding

1. Have a written breastfeeding policy that is routinely communicated to all healthcare staff.
2. Train all healthcare staff in skills necessary to implement this policy.
3. Inform all pregnant women about the benefits and management of breastfeeding.
4. Help mothers initiate breastfeeding within one-half hour of birth.
5. Show mothers how to breastfeed and maintain lactation, even if they should be separated from their infants.
6. Give newborn infants no food or drink other than breast milk, unless medically indicated.
7. Practice rooming-in—that is, allow mothers and infants to remain together 24 hours a day.
8. Encourage breastfeeding on demand.
9. Give no artificial teats or pacifiers (also called dummies or soothers) to breastfeeding infants.
10. Foster the establishment of breastfeeding support groups and refer mothers to them on discharge from the hospital or clinic.

Source: WHO/UNICEF. *Protecting, promoting, and supporting breastfeeding: The special role of maternity services.* Geneva, Switzerland: WHO;1989.

Today, as may be seen in Figure 31-1, more than 20,000 maternity wards have achieved Baby-friendly status; however, there are no data available on how many have maintained these important practices.

The International Code of Marketing of Breast-milk Substitutes was adopted by the World Health Assembly (WHA) in 1981, and has been reaffirmed and reinforced by subsequent WHA resolutions. It was a natural party to Baby-friendly hospital practices; pending its enactment as national law or binding regulations, all artificial feeding product companies were obligated, by the terms of the code, to comply with its provisions regardless of whether it had yet been implemented by political processes. The only code element that was specifically incorporated into the BFHI global criteria was the prohibition of free and low-cost supplies of breastmilk substitutes, bottles, and teats accepted by or distributed through the healthcare system.

The main provisions of the International Code of Marketing of Breast-milk Substitutes may be found in brief in Table 31-3.[31]

The text of the code itself commits manufacturers and distributors of products under its scope to ensure that their conduct in all aspects of their work complies with all provisions of the code. Unfortunately, few countries have fully introduced the code into law (see Figure 31-2).

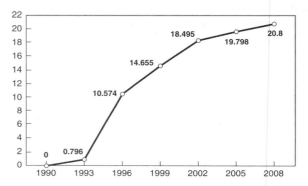

FIGURE 31-1 Progress in Implementing the Baby-friendly Hospital Initiative: Maternities ever certified as Baby-friendly, in 1990–2000's, worldwide (2008 estimated)
From Labbok M. Developed with UNICEF Data and presented in multiple venues. 2008.

Maternity protection in the workplace is supported by the International Labour Organization (ILO), which sets international standards for the workload adjustments needed by women in the formal workplace. There are three Maternity Protection Conventions (No. 3, 1919; No. 103, 1952; No. 183, 2000) and two recommendations (No. 95, 1952; No. 191, 2000). There is also some consideration of the woman employed in atypical forms of dependent work. Fifty-nine nations have ratified at least one of the three conventions.

TABLE 31-3

Basic Concepts Found in the WHO International Code of Marketing of Breast-milk Substitutes and Subsequent WHA Resolutions

- No advertising of breastmilk substitutes, feeding bottles, and teats to the public.
- No free samples to mothers.
- No promotion in healthcare facilities, including no free or low-cost supplies.
- No company personnel to contact mothers.
- No gifts or personal samples to health workers. Health workers should never pass samples on to mothers.
- No pictures of infants, or other words or pictures idealizing artificial feeding, on the labels or on brochures about the products.
- Information to health workers should be scientific and factual.
- Information on artificial feeding, including that on labels, should explain the benefits and superiority of breastfeeding and the costs and dangers associated with artificial feeding. Unsuitable products, such as sweetened condensed milk, should not be promoted for babies.

Source: Clark D, UNICEF Legal Advisor. Presentation on the International Code of Marketing of Breast-milk Substitutes. 2002.

Most countries have, however, developed national legislation that ensures that women workers are granted a paid leave before and/or after birth. Table 31-4 illustrates the durations of leave granted by countries in various regions.[32]

The Millennium Project

The single most important global development activity of this period is, arguably, the UN Millennium Project. At the Millennium Summit in 2000 world leaders adopted the UN Millennium Declaration: a new global partnership to reduce extreme poverty in its many dimensions—income poverty, hunger, disease, lack of adequate shelter, and exclusion—while promoting gender equality, education, and environmental sustainability. This project also builds on basic human rights: the rights of each person on the planet to health, education, shelter, and security. These targets, with a deadline of 2015, have become known as the Millennium Development Goals (MDGs).[33]

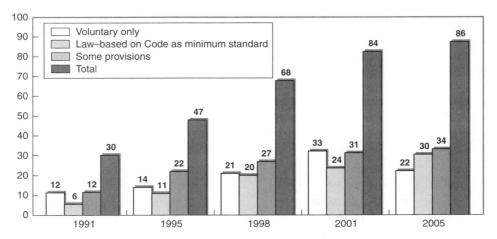

FIGURE 31-2   Progress in Implementing the International Code of Marketing of Breast-milk Substitutes
From UNICEF Innocenti Research Centre. 1990–2005 *Celebrating the Innocenti Declaration on the Protection, Promotion and Support of Breastfeeding: Past Achievements, Present Challenges and Priority Action for Infant and Young Child Feeding.* Florence, Italy: Innocenti Research Centre, 2007.

TABLE 31-4

Status of Maternity Protection by Region: Maternity Leave, in Weeks								
	<12	**12**	**13**	**14**	**15**	**16**	**17**	**>26**
Africa (39 countries)	5	15		18	1			
Western Pacific (13 countries)	7	5		1				
Southeast Asia (7 countries)	1	6						
Americas (31 countries)	3	18	3	1		2	1	3
Europe (28 countries)	2	4	1	3	1	9		8
Eastern Mediterranean (20 countries)	12	5		2		1		

Source: UNICEF Innocenti Research Centre. *1990-2005 Celebrating the Innocenti Declaration on the Protection, Promotion and Support of Breastfeeding: Past Achievements, Present Challenges and Priority Action for Infant and Young Child Feeding.* Florence, Italy: Innocenti Research Centre; 2007.

The Millennium Project was commissioned to develop an action plan to achieve the MDGs. In 2005, the final recommendations were presented to the UN Secretary-General as a synthesis volume: *Investing in Development: A Practical Plan to Achieve the Millennium Development Goals.*[34] The bulk of the project's work was carried out by 10 thematic task forces,[35] each of which also presented its own detailed recommendations. The task forces included researchers and scientists; policy makers; and representatives of NGOs, UN agencies, the World Bank, IMF, and the private sector. After the presentation of the Millennium Project's final reports, attention turned to supporting developing countries' national development strategies to achieve the MDGs. Among these goals are improvements in maternal and child survival, which demand improvements in breastfeeding. However, it is important to note that improved breastfeeding behaviors would contribute to the achievement of each of these goals (see Table 31-5).

The Global Strategy for Infant and Young Child Feeding

The activities called for in the Global Strategy for Infant and Young Child Feeding include increased attention to support for the mother's nutritional and social needs. It added five additional operational goals to those of the Innocenti Declaration, emphasizing comprehensive policy on infant and young child feeding in the context of nutrition, child and reproductive health, and poverty reduction; exclusive breastfeeding for six months and continued breastfeeding up to two years of age or beyond while providing women access to the support they require; timely, adequate, safe, and appropriate complementary feeding with continued breastfeeding; guidance on feeding infants and young children in exceptionally difficult circumstances; and creation of new legislation or other suitable measures in support of the *International Code of Marketing of Breast-milk Substitutes*. Finally, the Global Strategy for Infant and Young Child Feeding fosters multisectoral collaboration. There are many existing groups already working in partnership that could be called upon to collaborate further towards the best outcomes for children.

Innocenti + 15

Held in Florence, Italy, in 2005, this gathering celebrated the progress made since the original declaration and spelled out action programs needed to achieve breastfeeding goals. The report of this meeting contributed greatly to the material available in this chapter.[36]

Policy Associated with the HIV/AIDS Pandemic

The HIV/AIDS pandemic has had repercussions on many health issues, including infant feeding. WHO/UNICEF has recommendations for counseling mothers to help them reduce mother-to-child

TABLE 31-5

The Role of Nutrition and Infant and Young Child Feeding in Addressing the Millennium Development Goals

Goal Number and Targets	Contribution of Infant and Young Child feeding
1. **Eradicate extreme poverty and hunger.** Halve, between 1990 and 2015, the proportion of people: ■ Whose income is less than $1 a day ■ Who suffer from hunger	Breastfeeding significantly reduces early childhood feeding costs, and exclusive breastfeeding halves the cost of breastfeeding. Exclusive breastfeeding and continued breastfeeding for two years is associated with reduction in underweight and is an excellent source of high-quality calories for energy.
2. **Achieve universal primary education.** Ensure that by 2015, children everywhere, boys and girls alike, will be able to complete a full course of primary education.	Breastfeeding and adequate complementary feeding are prerequisites for readiness to learn. Breastfeeding and quality complementary foods significantly contribute to cognitive development.
3. **Promote gender equality and empower women.** Eliminate gender disparity in primary and secondary education, preferably by 2005 and in all levels of education no later than 2015.	Breastfeeding is the great equalizer, giving every child a fair start on life. Most differences in growth between sexes begin as complementary foods are added into the diet, and gender preference begins to act on feeding decisions. Breastfeeding is uniquely a right of women, and should be supported by society.
4. **Reduce child mortality.** Reduce by two-thirds, between 1990 and 2015, the under-five mortality rate of children.	Infant mortality could be readily reduced by about 13% with improved breastfeeding practices alone, and 6% with improved complementary feeding. In addition, about 50–60% of under-five mortality is secondary to malnutrition, greatly caused by inadequate complementary foods and feeding following on poor breastfeeding practices.
5. **Improve maternal health.** Reduce by three-quarters, between 1990 and 2015, the maternal mortality ratio.	The activities called for in the Global Strategy include increased attention to support for the mother's nutritional and social needs. In addition, breastfeeding is associated with decreased maternal postpartum blood loss; decreased breast cancer, ovarian cancer, and endometrial cancer; as well as the probability of decreased bone loss postmenopause. Breastfeeding also contributes to the duration of birth intervals, reducing maternal risks of pregnancy too close together.
6. **Combat HIV/AIDS, malaria, and other diseases.** Have halted by 2015 and begun to reverse the spread of HIV/AIDS.	Based on extrapolation from the published literature on the impact of exclusive breastfeeding on mother-to-child transmission (MTCT), exclusive breastfeeding in an otherwise untested breastfeeding HIV-infected population could be associated with a significant and measurable reduction in MTCT.
7. **Ensure environmental sustainability.**	Breastfeeding is associated with decreased milk industry waste, pharmaceutical waste, plastics and aluminum tin waste, and excess use of firewood and fossil fuels.
8. **Develop a global partnership for development.**	The Global Strategy for Infant and Young Child Feeding fosters multisectoral collaboration, and can build upon the extant partnerships for support of development through breastfeeding and complementary feeding. In terms of future economic productivity, optimal infant feeding has major implications.

Source: Adapted from UN Standing Committee on Nutrition Working Group on Breastfeeding and Complementary Feeding; 2004.

transmission (MTCT) via breastfeeding. In the past, the recommendations had emphasized replacement feeding and avoidance of breastfeeding.[37] Recent studies, however, indicate that the result of exclusive breastfeeding, as opposed to mixed feeding, is both improved child survival in general, as well as reduced MTCT,[38] and that exclusive breastfeeding support can be successfully implemented in field studies. As a result, WHO has modified its guidance to emphasize the need for exclusive breastfeeding support in all countries, including HIV-endemic countries, and notes that where sanitation, functioning household refrigerators, stoves, lighting systems, and literacy are limited, exclusive breastfeeding is good, if not better than replacements, stating:

> The most appropriate infant feeding option for an HIV-infected mother depends on her individual circumstances, including her health status and the local situation, and should consider the health services available and the counseling and support she is likely to receive. Exclusive breastfeeding is recommended for HIV-infected women for the first 6 months of life unless replacement feeding is acceptable, feasible, affordable, sustainable, and safe for them and their infants before that time. When replacement feeding is acceptable, feasible, affordable, sustainable, and safe, avoidance of all breastfeeding by HIV-infected women is recommended.[39]

Blueprints for Action on Breastfeeding

Both the United States[40] and the European Union[41] have developed blueprints, designed for countries, communities, and healthcare workers, that provide the background research, outline the public policy needs, and encourage community and health system actions. In addition, in many countries legal protection for the mother to breastfeed, wherever and whenever the infant is hungry, has increased. Television and other media are far reaching, albeit with sometimes conflicting messages concerning infant feeding: on one hand, breastfeeding is more frequently being mentioned on the air; on the other hand, advertising by the formula industry remains convincing to many.

What Has Been the Result?

As a result of these numerous changes and efforts, exclusive breastfeeding increased more than 10% worldwide during the 1990s, and from 1990 to 2004, there was a 20% increase over baseline (see Figure 31-3).

This increase in exclusive breastfeeding has, arguably, prevented millions of child deaths from infectious diseases alone, and prevented many times that number of serious and debilitating diseases. The following assumptions are used for this estimate: the increase in the numbers exclusively breastfed was linear; the increases in exclusive breastfeeding were matched by increases in some (i.e., partial) breastfeeding; there was a steady rate of 100 million births annually; nonbreastfed infants have about six times the mortality of exclusively breastfed infants in the first month or two; about 40–50% of the infant mortality rate (IMR) occurs in the first month of life; and nonbreastfed infants have about two times the mortality of breastfed infants in the remaining months of the first year of life. Using these assumptions, it is a conservative estimate that about 45 million additional children

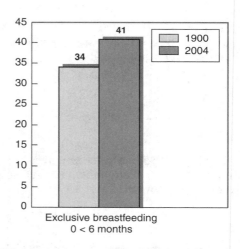

FIGURE 31-3 Trends in exclusive breastfeeding: Percent of mothers of children 0 < 6 months of age who are exclusively breastfeeding at the time of the survey. Adapted from UNICEF Innocenti Research Centre. *1990–2005 Celebrating the Innocenti Declaration on the Protection, Promotion, and Support of Breastfeeding: Past Achievements, Present Challenges and Priority Action for Infant and Young Child Feeding.* **Florence, Italy: Innocenti Research Centre, 2007. (Based on data from 37 countries covering 60% of the developing world population.)**

were exclusively breastfed over 15 years or so, with the concomitant reduction in mortality.

The decreased outlay in developing countries for imported and manufactured artificial foods is estimated at the level of more than a US $1 billion worldwide. This estimate is conservative, assuming only a three month decrease in the need for infant formula, and is derived from Food and Agriculture Organization (FAO)[42] and WHO[43] figures, developed by multiplying the cost of formula for three months times the number of children changed to exclusive breastfeeding. In addition, this increase will have affected fertility rates in many countries,[44] especially with the limited funding available for family planning in the last 15 years or so.

Despite these advances, much remains to be accomplished, especially in those countries with the highest rates of child mortality. As perhaps the most important preventive child survival intervention, early and exclusive breastfeeding with appropriate complementary feeding costs relatively little. Recent international analyses confirm that interventions to enable women to succeed in optimal feeding are among the most cost-effective and cost beneficial.[45] Nonetheless, this message has not been fully heard or accepted by decision makers in the countries that need it most. Although there are vulnerable populations in every country, the countries with the highest infant mortality rates share an especially heavy disease burden as well. However, with a coordinated multisectoral effort to support families, improve health systems, and enhance social norms through legal and regulatory efforts as well as social marketing, a revolutionary shift in child survival and well being could occur.

What Must Be Done Now? Programs and Policy Needed to Enable Women to Breastfeed

Nearly two decades since the launch of the Innocenti Declaration, much remains to be accomplished if we are to achieve its vision of "An environment that enables mothers, families, and other caregivers to make informed decisions about optimal feeding, which is defined as exclusive breastfeeding for six months followed by the introduction of appropriate complementary feeding and continued breastfeeding for up to two years of age or beyond."[46]

How Can This Vision Be Achieved in a Practical, Affordable, and Sustainable Way?

In every country that has seen significant improvements in breastfeeding, an active decision was made that saving children's lives is worth the time and energy to truly support women in making an informed and unbiased choice in feeding their children, and then to provide them with the support they need to succeed. In some settings, the government led the way; in others the medical professions acted first; while in still others, a gradual social revolution of behavior change took place. In all instances, however, comprehensive ongoing support is needed to achieve sustainable results. The institutionalization of protection, promotion, and support into law, health systems, and health professional training, as well as allocations for ongoing research and program evaluation, will presage real changes that will, in turn, allow the children of the world to achieve their full potential through optimal infant and young child feeding and care.

Today, the biggest threat to optimal infant feeding may be complacency or message fatigue.[47] The job is only partly completed: marketing practices continue that mislead and distract, healthcare workers have limited skills, and the issue remains misunderstood by many HIV/AIDS program planners and counselors. Further, the failure to recognize maternity rights in the private sector and in nonformal work remains a largely unaddressed issue.

The necessary activities are clear: coordinated, comprehensive strengthening of national oversight and health system reform—including health worker training, inclusion of feeding in health information systems, and Baby-friendly activities—as well as community and societal support for the breastfeeding mother. To ensure continued progress with breastfeeding, active programming and resource allocation must increase.

Support for optimal infant and young child feeding has been part of UN agency efforts for many years and now is endorsed or supported by the following: the MDGs, the Convention on the Rights of the Child, the 2002 WHO/UNICEF Global Strategy for Infant and Young Child Feeding, the new Partnership for Maternal, Newborn, and Child Survival, and the UN HIV and Infant-Feeding Framework for Priority Action. In addition, all rights-based, life-cycle sensitive approaches, as well as those emphasizing the most vulnerable populations and the lifetime impact of the interventions planned, must support optimal infant and young child feeding, and associated nutrition for mothers, to succeed.

The following indicators have been proposed as targets for the year 2015, the target date for MDGs, but remain to be endorsed or rejected by the international community:[48]

- At least 60% of children less than six months of age exclusively breastfed (to be increased from about 30% in the early 1990s)

- At least 75% of children 20–23 months of age still breastfed (to be increased from about 40% in the early 1990s)

- Skin-to-skin and early breastfeeding initiation increased to about 60% (to be increased from less than 30% in the early 1990s)

Figure 31-4 illustrates the country levels of exclusive breastfeeding for which data are available from UNICEF. Clearly, to achieve the stated goals by 2015, much action is needed.

Innocenti +15: Lessons Learned and Next Actions

The Innocenti +15 process included collaboration by many multilaterals and NGOs to assess the accomplishments of the past and to outline a series of proposed actions, summarized below. Perhaps most important was the confirmation of the impact of the initiatives outlined in the 1990 Innocenti Declaration, and the following:

- Every mother deserves, and should receive, adequate support and counseling to make an informed infant feeding decision, and to succeed with her decision.

- Comprehensive, multisectoral, and multiple contact approaches are necessary to achieve marked and sustainable improvements in infant and young child feeding.

- Child survival strategies must include active promotion, protection, and support of early, exclusive, and continued breastfeeding with age-appropriate complementary feeding, since these practices will prevent about 20% of

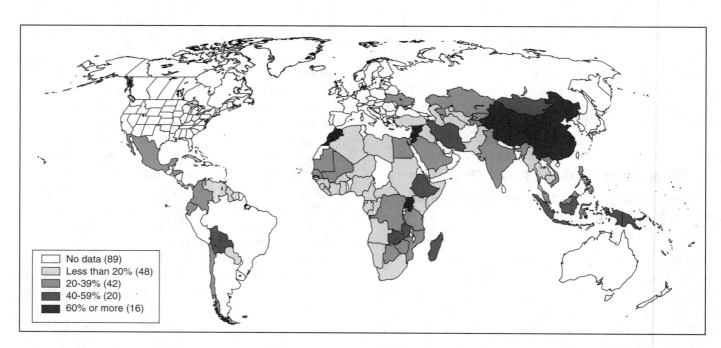

FIGURE 31-4 **Levels of exclusive breastfeeding among children 0-6 months of age**
From UNICEF Innocenti Research Centre. 1990-2005 Celebrating the Innocenti Declaration on the Protection, Promotion and Support of Breastfeeding: Past Achievements, Present Challenges and Priority Action for Infant and Young Child Feeding. Florence: Innocenti Research Centre, 2007

under-five deaths per year in the countries with the highest proportion of worldwide child deaths.

- Sustainable behavioral change is dependent on ongoing multiple contacts with the mother and community using multiple approaches, including legal protection, health system support, and community and peer involvement.

- The HIV/AIDS epidemic need not interfere with the promotion of optimal breastfeeding practices. Support for exclusive breastfeeding in the general population also helps women with HIV if choosing to exclusively breastfeed.

- The Baby-friendly Hospital Initiative can be expanded, modified, and incorporated into other facilities, and it continues to be an important catalyst for breastfeeding action. Ongoing monitoring and quality assurance of these efforts is vital.

- The implementation of the *International Code of Marketing of Breast-milk Substitutes* and subsequent relevant WHA resolutions as a minimum requirement for all countries, coupled with adequate enforcement mechanisms, is an essential component of a sustainable comprehensive approach to the protection of breastfeeding.

- Sustained efforts necessitate inclusion in national budgets as a permanent line item.

Innocenti +15 then went on to outline opportunities that have arisen since 1990 and actions needed, noting the importance of the Global Strategy for Infant and Young Child Feeding, and the emerging government and partner commitment to achieving the MDGs.

Innocenti +15 also outlined the need for emphasis on accountability mechanisms, partnerships, alliances, collaboration, and community involvement as an integral part of health system strengthening. The document also emphasized that the need to actively address these challenges demanded acceptance of breastfeeding as an essential activity within other ongoing efforts, including the essential nutrition action approach, emergency response, the integrated management of childhood illness (IMCI), and integrated management of pregnancy and childbirth (IMPAC), and within all partnerships to advance mother and/or child health and welfare. In sum, the Innocenti +15 document confirmed that there are well-established, effective, low-cost, low-

technology interventions to improve infant feeding, outlined in the Innocenti Declaration, and expanded on in the Global Strategy.

Proposed Next Actions: International Agencies and Governments, the Food and Nutrition Movements, Health Systems, and Health Workers and Community Involvement

The 2005 Innocenti +15 document reconfirmed the need to implement the strategies outlined in the 1990 Innocenti Declaration and the Global Strategy for Infant and Young Child Feeding (see tables above), noting that achieving implementation will demand the following:

- Advocacy, coordination, and establishment of multisectoral, comprehensive policy, and oversight of national efforts to be initiated by alliances of member states and international organizations.

- Policy and legislation, including implementing the *International Code of Marketing of Breast-Milk Substitutes,* maternity protection, and maintenance of oversight, to be initiated by national governments.

- Health system strengthening, including revitalizing and updating of Baby-friendly work, updating health worker core curricula, and establishing infant feeding data collection systems.

- Community and social mobilization, including mother-to-mother, peer counseling, baby-friendly communities, grandmother leagues, as well as community support and social marketing of various complementary feeding approaches.

These activities can be enacted through global support, national government commitment, and civil society advocacy and action.

Public health policy makers' and health workers' responsibilities are an essential component, and include the need to do the following:[49]

- Ensure that basic education and training for all health workers cover lactation physiology, exclusive and continued breastfeeding, complementary feeding, feeding in difficult circumstances, meeting the nutritional needs of the infants who have to be fed on breastmilk substitutes and the *International Code of Marketing of Breast-milk Substitutes* and related legislation.

■ Train all health workers in how to provide skilled support for optimal infant and young child feeding in neonatal, pediatric, reproductive health, nutrition, and community health services.

■ Promote achievement and maintenance of Baby-friendly hospital status.

■ Observe their responsibilities under the *International Code of Marketing of Breast-milk Substitutes* as a minimum, and national measures that strengthen these responsibilities.

■ Encourage the establishment and recognition of community support groups and refer mothers to them.

Conclusion

To achieve intergenerational health and nutrition, there must be increased attention to supporting and enabling mothers to succeed with optimal infant and young child feeding. We have the tools and the roadmaps in existing documents, such as the Innocenti Declaration and the Innocenti +15 document, as well as in the Global Strategy for Infant and Young Child Feeding. It is the responsibility of the global public health community to ensure that skills and practices are up to date. As part of the international community, it is our responsibility to know what to do, and to do it now, *with urgency.*

DISCUSSION QUESTIONS

1. How does breastfeeding contribute to global health and global development?

2. What are some of the individual, public health, and ecological risks of feeding infants commercial infant formula?

3. What is the relationship between nutrition and the environment?

REFERENCES

1. Labbok MH. Breastfeeding as a women's issue: conclusions and consensus, complementary concerns, and next actions. *Int J Gynaecol Obstet.* 1994;47(Suppl):S55-S61.

2. Gore A. *Earth in the Balance: Ecology and the Human Spirit.* New York, NY: Houghton Mifflin Co; 1992:314.

3. Slow Food International. Our Philosophy Web page. http://www.slowfood.com /about_us/eng/philosophy.lasso. Accessed June 13, 2008.

4. Slow Food International. http://www.slowfood.com/. Accessed June 13, 2008.

5. Petrini C. *Slow Food Nation.* New York, NY: Rizolli Ex Libris; 2007.

6. Latham MC. Breastfeeding—a human rights issue? Special Issue on Food and Nutrition Rights. *Int J Children's Rights.* 1997;5(4):397-417.

7. Saadeh R, Labbok M, Cooney K, Koniz-Booher P, eds. *Breast-Feeding: The Technical Basis and Recommendations for Action.* Geneva, Switzerland: WHO; 1993.

8. Jones G, Steketee R, Black R, Bhutta Z, Morris S, and the Bellagio Child Survival Study Group. How many child deaths can we prevent this year? Child survival II. *Lancet.* 2003;362:11-17.

9. Ip S, Chung M, Raman G, et al. Breastfeeding and Maternal and Infant Health Outcomes in Developed Countries. Evidence Report/Technology Assessment

No. 153 (Prepared by Tufts-New England Medical Center Evidence-based Practice Center, under Contract No. 290-02-0022). AHRQ Publication No. 07-E007. Rockville, MD: Agency for Healthcare Research and Quality. April 2007.

10. Horta BL, Bahl R, Martinés JC, Victora CG. Evidence on the long-term effects of breastfeeding: systematic reviews and meta-analysis. http://www.who.int/child-adolescent-health/publications/NUTRITION/ISBN_92_4_159523_0.htm. Accessed June 15, 2008.

11. Ward KA, Adams JE, Mughal MZ. Bone status during adolescence, pregnancy and lactation. *Curr Opin Obstet Gynecol.* 2005;17(4):435-439.

12. Mezzacappa ES, Kelsey RM, Katkin ES. Breast feeding, bottle feeding, and maternal autonomic responses to stress. *J Psychosom Res.* 2005;58(4):351-365.

13. Bullough CH, Msuku RS, Karonde L. Early suckling and postpartum haemorrhage: controlled trial in deliveries by traditional birth attendants *Lancet.* 1989; 2(8662):522-525.

14. Negishi H, Kishida T, Yamada H, Hirayama E, Mikuni M, Fujimoto S. Changes in uterine size after vaginal delivery and cesarean section determined by vaginal sonography in the puerperium. *Arch Gynecol Obstet.* 1999;263(1-2):13-16.

15. Tung KH, Wilkens LR, Wu AH, et al. Effect of anovulation factors on pre- and postmenopausal ovarian cancer risk: revisiting the incessant ovulation hypothesis. *Am J Epidemiol.* 2005;161(4):321-329.

16. Buranasin B. The effects of rooming-in on the success of breastfeeding and the decline in abandonment of children. *Asia Pac J Public Health.* 1991;5:217-220.

17. Butte N, Lopez-Alarcon MG, Garza C. *Nutrient Adequacy of Exclusive Breastfeeding for the Term Infant During the First Six Months of Life.* Geneva, Switzerland: WHO; 2002.

18. Rutstein SO. Effects of preceding birth intervals on neonatal, infant and under-five years mortality and nutritional status in developing countries: evidence from the demographic and health surveys. *Int J Gynaecol Obstet.* 2005;89(Suppl 1):S7-S24.

19. Conde-Agudelo A, Belizan JM, Norton MH, Rosas-Bermudez A. Effect of the interpregnancy interval on perinatal outcomes in Latin America. *Obstet Gynecol.* 2005;106(2):359-366.

20. Berry W. *The Art of Commonplace.* Washington, DC: Shoemaker & Hoard; 2002.

21. Petrini C. *Slow Food Nation.* New York, NY: Rizolli Ex Libris; 2007.

22. Radford A. The ecological impact of breastfeeding. http://reducepackaging.com/breastfeeding.html. Accessed November 20, 2008.

23. Tseng M. Breastfeeding: Part of the slow food movement? *Public Health Nutrition.* 2006;9(6):667-668.

24. Labbok M. Breastfeeding: a woman's reproductive right. *Int J Gynaecol Obstet.* 2006;94(3):277-86.

25. Labbok M, Smith P, Taylor E. Breastfeeding and feminism: a focus on reproductive health, rights and justice. *Int J Breastfeeding.* In press.

26. Johnson M. How *Can the Tensions Between Women's Rights and Children's Rights Be Resolved? Something to Think About.* . . . New York, NY: UNICEF; 2005. Bulletin No. 32.

27. United Nations. Convention on the Rights of the Child. 1990. http://www.unhchr.ch/html/menu3/b/k2crc.htm. Accessed June 15, 2008.

28. United Nations. Convention on the Elimination of All Forms of Discrimination against Women. 1979. http://www.un.org/womenwatch/daw/cedaw/text/econvention.htm. Accessed May 15, 2008.

29. Saadeh R, Labbok M, Cooney K, Koniz-Booher P, eds. *Breast-Feeding: The Technical Basis and Recommendations for Action.* Geneva, Switzerland: WHO; 1993.

30. WHO/UNICEF. *Protecting, Promoting, and Supporting Breast-Feeding—The Special Role of Maternity Services.* Geneva, Switzerland: WHO; 1989.

31. Van Esterik P, Clark D, Labbok M, eds. *1990–2005: Celebrating The Innocenti Declaration on the Protection, Promotion and Support of Breastfeeding Past Achievements, Present Challenges, and the Way Forward for Infant and Young Child Feeding.* Florence, Italy: UNICEF/Innocenti Centre; 2005.

32. International Labour Organisation. *Conditions of Work.* Vol. 13. Geneva, Switzerland International Labour Organisation; 1994.

33. United Nations. Millennium Development Goals (MDGs) Web pages. http://www.unmillenniumproject.org/goals/index.htm. Accessed June 15, 2008.

34. Sachs J (ed.). Investing in development: a practical plan to achieve the Millennium Development Goals. http://www.unmillenniumproject.org/reports/fullreport.htm. Accessed June 15, 2008.

35. United Nations. Millennium Project Task Force reports. http://www.unmillenniumproject.org/reports/rep.orts2.htm. Accessed June 15, 2008.

36. UNICEF Innocenti Research Centre.*1990–2005 Celebrating the Innocenti Declaration on the Protection, Promotion and Support of Breastfeeding: Past Achievements, Present Challenges and Priority Action for Infant and Young Child Feeding.* Florence, Italy: Innocenti Research Centre; 2007.

37. WHO/UNICEF. *HIV and Infant Feeding: A Guide for Health Care Managers and Supervisors.* Geneva, Switzerland: WHO:2004.

38. Iliff PJ, Piwoz EG, Tavengwa NV, et al., and ZVITAMBO study group. Early exclusive breastfeeding (EBF) reduces the risk of postnatal HIV-1 transmission and increases HIV-free survival. *AIDS.* 2005;19(7):699-708.

39. WHO. Child and adolescent health—HIV and infant feeding. http://www.who.int/child_adolescent_health/topics/prevention_care/child/nutrition/hivif/en/. Accessed June 15, 2008.

40. Office of Women's Health, USDHHS. *Blueprint for Action on Breastfeeding.* Washington, DC: United States Government; 2001.

41. European Union. *Blueprint for Action on Breastfeeding.* EU Project on Promotion of Breastfeeding in Europe. Protection, promotion and support of breastfeeding in Europe: a blueprint for action. European Commission, Directorate Public Health and Risk Assessment, Luxembourg, 2004 Luxembourg http://europa.eu.int/comm/health/ph_projects/2002/promotion/promotion_2002_18_en.htm Accessed November 21, 2008.

42. Food and Agriculture Organization of the United Nations. The economic value of breast-feeding. *Food Nutr Pap.* 1979;11:1-89.

43. UNICEF/WHO/UNAIDS UNFPA. *HIV and Infant Feeding: A Guide for Health-Care Managers and Supervisors.* Geneva, Switzerland: WHO; 2003.

44. Becker S, Rutstein S, Labbok M. Estimation of births averted due to breastfeeding and increases in levels of contraception needed to substitute for breastfeeding, *J Biosoc Sci.* 2003;35:559-574.

45. Adam T, Lim S, Mehta S, et al. Cost effectiveness analysis of strategies for maternal and neonatal health and developing countries. *BMJ.* 2005;331;1107-1136.

46. Innocenti Declaration, UNICEF. Innocenti Declaration: On the protection, promotion and support of breastfeeding http://www.unicef.org/programme/breastfeeding/innocenti.htm Accessed November 21, 2008.

47. Labbok M, Clark D, Goldman A. Breastfeeding: maintaining an irreplaceable immunological resource, *Nature Immunol.* 2004; 4(7):565-572.

48. UN Standing Committee on Nutrition, Breastfeeding and Complementary Feeding Working Group, Meeting Report, New York, NY: UN; 2004.

49. WHO/UNICEF. *Global Strategy for Infant and Young Child Feeding.* Geneva, Switzerland: WHO; 2003.

CHAPTER 32

Gender Equality Is Not Just a Women's Issue, but a Development and Human Rights Issue

In many poor countries, gender equality and women's rights are considered a mere whim of rich countries or, worse, an expression of Western decadence.[1]

Here is a small sample of what the "decadent" denounce:

- Of the nearly 137 million illiterate youths in the world, 63% are female.

- In no region of the world do women have a presence in national parliaments that exceeds 20%.[2]

- Women account for 70% of the world's poor.

- Worldwide, only about 1% of all loans are granted to women.[3]

- Forty-three million school age girls are not enrolled in school—most of them from socially excluded groups.[4]

- A greater volume of goods in sub-Saharan Africa is transported on the heads of women than on the backs of trucks.[5]

- The so-called missing women phenomenon, where there are fewer women than would be expected on the basis of biological norms, is also indicative of the continuing discrimination against women.[6]

This chapter complements others in the book; it gives a quick overview of and elaborates on where the People's Health Movement (PHM) stands vis-à-vis the linked issues of gender discrimination and gender inequality.[7] The text, here, particularly (and only) focuses on the social, cultural, and economic determinants of gender discrimination and inequality, and hints at pathways the solution to the problem will eventually have to follow.

Claudio Schuftan, MD

Claudio Schuftan, MD, is a consultant in public health and nutrition based in Ho Chi Minh City, Vietnam.

Discrimination as a Human Rights Violation

In many poor countries, the sharp differences between men and women in access to assets and to opportunities restrict women from their freedom to choose and, at the same time, have negative implications for the well-being of their families and their communities, and this is a flagrant discrimination.

Discrimination against women and girls is not only a flagrant violation of human rights and a negation of democracy, but it is also crippling in terms of economics. This is doubly important, because sustained gender discrimination shackles any economy. In other words, upholding women's rights helps an economy to thrive. Therefore, gender equality is a sensible goal also in business terms. Poor countries in particular cannot afford not to tap this potential.[8]

Nondiscrimination is an *immediate* obligation as considered in the UN Charter of Economic, Social, and Cultural Rights (ECOSOC, General Comment No.3, paragraph 2.2). The progressive realization of women's rights does, therefore, *not* apply to discrimination against women. Action is needed *now*.

Economic Marginalization of Women in the Context of Culture

Because of the traditional position of women in most societies, women face barriers in their access to assets and to opportunities not only for economic, but also most importantly, for cultural reasons.[9]

If traditional ideas, customs, and mores that denigrate the status of women—and that have been handed down for generations—do not match human rights standards and violate people's rights (and openly or indirectly discriminate against women), they simply have to be done away with; that may sound controversial, but there is no alternative. In that sense, separating church and state is fundamental for the universal upholding of human rights.*

It is said that in the European and North American culture gender equality has achieved a great deal. But has it? Not really as much as is to be expected. Still today, women in the North need to be given equal economic, senior management, and political chances.

Gender Inequality

At the global level, despite the fact that the heads of state at the Millennium Summit made gender equality and the empowerment of women a top priority worldwide (MDG 3), nothing much has happened in this domain since then.[10] It is perhaps because women's rights are often neglected and not prioritized by policy makers and heads of state.

The key elements to tackle in gender inequality are disparities in educational and health outcomes (the latter of particular concern to PHM), and disparities in the access to productive resources, to credit, to capital, to new technologies, and to other social and legal services.

Therefore, to promote gender equality, policies need to address inequalities as they pertain to rights, to the access to resources, and to the voice of women as claim holders:

- *Rights*—Gender equality primarily (but not only) refers to equality under the law (whether customary or statutory).

- *Resources*—Gender equality refers to equal access to human capital investments and to equal chances to own property, control productive resources, and markets.

- *Voice*—Gender equality refers to the ability of men and women to equally influence and contribute to the political discourse and the development process.[11]

---

* Countries that furthermore try to make people outside their culture or faith observe such discrimination, violate international human rights laws twice over—and it is the state's duty to protect the rights of those minorities.

In short, gender equality is to be understood as equal access to the opportunities that ultimately avoid deprivations in development outcomes. As a corollary, the promotion of women must not be confined to health and education alone. For instance, as much as literacy effectively empowers men and especially women, it is just one step of many in the right direction.[12]

Women's Projects

It is well known that most development projects do not contribute to empowering women; at best, they create a few earning opportunities for them. Gender equality cannot be achieved merely using financial credit. As a matter of fact, in addition, women that successfully borrow are often at risk of increased domestic violence if projects do not include measures to change male attitudes.[13]

Unfortunately, women's projects often only benefit small elite groups of women (a handful of the more entrepreneurial ones). The gap thus widens with a growing number of poor widows and teenage mothers being left behind. Credit and related support programs for women thus do not guarantee that the people most in need will be those to actually benefit. Furthermore, what is too often overlooked is that economic support targeted solely to women can and does exacerbate the trend of men reducing their financial contributions to household budgets. Therefore, this gender-targeted support does not contribute meaningfully to improve the situation of women and their families.[14][13]

Conclusion: Normative Considerations

Reducing gender inequalities indeed creates a fairer society.[14] The active participation of women has been proven to positively affect the lives and the self-determination of women.[15]

Looking at where governments put their money is indeed a good way to judge the impor-

tance they attribute to gender equality. Since there is no such a thing as gender-neutral government budgets, one way to pinpoint policies needed to reduce gender disparities is to embark in *gender budgeting*, which involves the systematic examination of budgets and policies for their potential impact on women and girls.[14,16] Because we need a more gender-responsive public financial management, this technique can influence the budgeting process to ensure it focuses on public policies that can truly help reduce gender disparities and thus can improve overall economic outcomes.

Basically, we need to support the advancement of women. The complementary effort to support this advancement is that other gender aspects are considered as well, meaning men also becoming systematically involved. For example, at the domestic level, as long as child care and housework remain a female preserve (i.e., are entirely considered women's tasks), the chances of women living up to their potential are limited. Hence, whoever fails to consider power relations in marriage in any given culture, automatically fails to reckon with the critical men's issues in gender streamlining.[13]

Moreover, gender-specific barriers must be removed to ensure a more level playing field for males and females. For example, women must simply be given viable economic chances.[17] Also, extra incentives are needed for more investments in girls' human capital formation and for aggressive gender-balanced education policies. Gender-informed investments in human capital formation are central (but not sufficient) to promoting gender equality.[18] Additionally, women need equal access to land, to the full range of social and financial services, as well as to infrastructural services, at the same time that they need a more enabling legal environment.[15,19]

To benefit the entire family, programs for women can and will only succeed if and when they address power relations. This implies that we need to get involved in gender mainstreaming rather than in exclusively empowering women.[20] Note that the use of the concept of *gender mainstreaming* is on its way out; it is being replaced by *full integration of women and men (and boys and girls)*.

Ultimately, the most effective way to achieve all the above is to, without further delay, start advancing women so they are quickly promoted to positions where more of them are put in charge of planning and executing development projects and programs.

Whimsical or decadent, progressive or premonitory, visionary or risqué, revolutionary or utopian, novel or repetitive, these are roughly the pathways PHM thinks gender equality proponents will have to travel for gender equality to become a reality in the decade(s) to come.

DISCUSSION QUESTIONS

1. What are the contributory factors to gender inequality?
2. How can the global community work to address this issue at various levels of society?

REFERENCES

1. Dembowski H. Equal opportunity a la Wolfowitz [editorial]. *Dev Cooperation Intl J*. 2007; 34(5)178.
2. Buvinic M, King M. Smart economics: more needs to be done to promote the economic power of women. *Finance Dev*. 2007;44(2)7-11.
3. World Bank. *World Development Indicators*. Washington, DC: World Bank; 2006.
4. Lewis MA, Lockheed ME. Getting all girls into school. *Finance Dev*. 2007;44(2)16-19.
5. Wieczorek-Zeul H. Without women, no sustainable development. *Dev Cooperation Intl J*. 2007; 34(5)188-190.
6. Stotsky JG. Budgeting with women in mind. *Finance Dev*. 2007;44(2)12-15.
7. PHM. People's charter for health. 2000. http://www.phmovement.org. Accessed January 8, 2009.
8. Kyte R. An unaffordable luxury. *Dev Cooperation Intl J*. 2007;34(5)191-193.
9. Stotsky JG. Budgeting with women in mind. *Finance Dev*. 2007;44(2)12-15.
10. Wieczorek-Zeul H. Without women, no sustainable development. *Dev Cooperation Intl J*. 2007; 34(5)188-190.
11. World Bank. *World Development Report 2006: Equity and Development*. New York, NY: World Bank and Oxford University Press; 2005.
12. Yeboah-Afari A. Literacy empowers. *Dev Cooperation Intl J*. 2007;34(5)199-201.
13. Trautmann R. Benefits for entire families. *Dev Cooperation Intl J*. 2007;34(5)196-198.
14. Stotsky JG. Budgeting with women in mind. *Finance Dev*. 2007;44(2)12-15.
15. Wieczorek-Zeul H. Without women, no sustainable development. *Dev Cooperation Intl J*. 2007; 34(5)188-190.
16. Wallace L. A woman's touch [editorial]. *Finance Dev*. 2007;44(2)1.
17. Dembowski H. Equal opportunity a la Wolfowitz [editorial]. *Dev Cooperation Intl J*. 2007; 34(5)178.
18. Buvinic M, King M. Smart economics: more needs to be done to promote the economic power of women. *Finance Dev*. 2007;44(2)7-11.
19. Okonjo-Iweala N. Stuck at the small-scale level. *Dev Cooperation Intl J*. 2007;34(5)194-195.
20. Kyte R. An unaffordable luxury. *Dev Cooperation Intl J*. 2007;34(5)191-193.

CHAPTER 33

Water and Sanitation

Cathey Eisner Falvo, MD, MPH

Cathey Eisner Falvo, MD, MPH, is the President of Physicians for Social Responsibility, NYC Chapter, New York, NY.

INTRODUCTION

Air, water, and food are essential for life. Humans can live three to four minutes without oxygen (air), three to four days without water, and four weeks without food. Therefore, potable water must be considered a human right. To have consistent availability of potable water requires concomitant sanitary removal of human and animal waste as well as chemicals and heavy metals from industrial by-products and nature.

The World Health Organization (WHO) estimates that 20 litres of fresh water is the minimum amount needed per person per day. The range of actual consumption in the world varies. Within countries in Asia, Latin America, and Africa some rural or slum areas have six or less litres per person per day while wealthy urban dwellers use hundreds of litres per person per day. Over a billion people in developing countries lack adequate access to water, and at least twice that number lack access to sanitation.[1]

Water Use

General

Although two-thirds of the Earth's surface is covered with water, less than 3% of the planet's water exists as freshwater needed for human use. More than two-thirds of the freshwater is frozen in glaciers, and almost all of the rest is in groundwater. Most people get their daily drinking water from rivers or lakes, a minuscule percentage of the Earth's freshwater.[2]

Water is also essential for economic development. Globally, agriculture uses about 70% of available water supplies and industry uses 22% leaving just 8% for human use.[2] Industry, agriculture, and humans all need clean water, yet each tends to add contaminants that may cause serious threats to themselves and the other users.

Water availability in any one place is affected by its use along the rest of its course.[1] Much water crosses political boundaries—often placing its availability beyond the control of the local community. Forty percent of the earth's people live in these transboundary water basins. The number of transboundary water basins has increased over the years as the number of sovereign nations has increased. In 1978 there were 214 international basins, in 2006 there were 262.[1]

Amount

The United Nations Children's Fund (UNICEF) and the WHO have set 20 litres per person per day of clean water available within 1 km from home as the minimum standard. However, to meet usual needs including bathing and laundry, 50 litres per person per day are needed. Most people categorized as lacking access to clean water use about five litres a day. In Europe the average is 200 litres per person per day, and in the United States it is more than 400 litres per person per day. Water is considered clean when it comes from an improved water source: in-house connection, standpipe, pumps, or protected wells.[1,3]

The ability to obtain water of any quality varies from having piped potable water (household service) available at all times from any of several faucets in one's house to walking miles to find a highly contaminated gallon. In Africa, only one in four people have household service. About half of the population of Asia enjoys household service. In Latin America and the Caribbean just two out of every three people have household water service.[2]

Costs

Urban poor not connected to a municipal system get water from many sources including rivers and streams, vendors via water trucks, private standpipes, kiosks, and agents. These water sources are often of poor quality and more expensive than municipal network sources. In Barranquilla, Colombia, utility water prices averaged $0.55 per cubic meter versus $5.50 from truckers.[4] Dakar standpipe users paid 3.5 times that paid by households connected to the municipal network.[5] In addition to the basic cost of water, the cost to connect to the network is very high: for the poorest quintile of the population the cost varied from about three months income in Manila to six months in Kenya and more than a year in Uganda.[1]

The results of these costs as well as the cost of sanitation were confirmed by analyses done for the UNDP 2006 report. In developing countries 85% of the richest quintile of the population has piped water while only 25% of the poorest quintile has piped water. In those same countries 75% of the richest quintile and 50% of the next quintile have sanitation. In Colombia nearly 100% of the richest quintile have flush toilets while for the poorest quintile 40% have flush toilets, another 20% have pit latrines, and 40% have no facilities.[1]

Women's Role

In parts of Africa, women, who usually are responsible for all household chores, spend an average of 15–17 hours per week collecting water. During the dry season they may have to walk 10 km to find a source. Ugandan households spend on average 660 hours per year collecting water. This is equal to two months full-time labor.[1] Studies by Parker and Skytta[6] of time spent collecting water by women versus men found that in Benin in 1998 urban women spent 16 minutes per day versus 6 minutes per day by men, rural women 62 minutes per day versus 16 minutes per day by men, and nationally the difference was 45 minutes per day by women versus 12 minutes per day by men. Findings in Guinea in 2002–2003 were similar: urban women spend 10 minutes per day versus 3 minutes per day by men, rural women 28 minutes per day versus 6 minutes per day by men, and nationally women spend 23 minutes per day versus 5 minutes per day by men. Estimates suggest some 40 billion hours a year are devoted to collecting water in sub-Saharan Africa. This is a year's labor for the entire work force in France.[7]

Sanitation

Achieving potable water for all cannot be achieved without having sanitation. Sanitation refers to the safe removal of sewage and other human waste from households as well as individual hygienic measures and safe discharge of chemicals and other waste from industry. Sir John Snow's studies of cholera in England during the 1800s clearly documented that exposure to water contaminated with human excreta was the principle means by which cholera spread.[8] Flies and other insects breeding or landing on excreta in open sewers or on the ground help spread disease as do people walking through contaminated areas. Each year 1.8 million child deaths are related to unclean water and poor sanitation. Recurring diarrhea and other impure water diseases in childhood cause ongoing developmental deficit and lifelong deficit in functioning (chronic malnutrition damages the brain, and so on).[1] According to the WHO, diarrhea and related illnesses account for 60 million disability-adjusted life years (DALYs)[9] lost each year–4% of the total.[10]

Social Considerations

Around the world, 2.6 billion people lack basic sanitation, defined by the WHO as having a pit latrine. Social mores in some cultures deem that defecation by females must be done in private. This further complicates sanitation and the situation for girls and women. If no facilities are provided, they can go only after dark.[1] One-half of girls in sub-Saharan Africa drop out of primary school because of poor water and sanitation. Pubescent girls won't go to school if there are no sanitary facilities. A UNICEF program run between 1990 and 2000 to supply sanitation to schools in Bangladesh increased girl attendance by 11%.[1] The arduous task of fetching water and managing the illnesses caused by poor-quality water deprives many women and children of educational and economic opportunities that could help them to escape the cycle of poverty in which they live.[2]

Health Considerations

Combining piped water to homes with flush toilets improves health. Piped water in the house decreased diarrhea incidence by almost 70% in Ghana and more than 40% in Vietnam; flush toilets reduced the risk more than 20% in Mali, Nicaragua, and Egypt.[1,11] In Peru, urban installation of pit latrines decreased diarrhea by 50% and flush toilets decreased it by 75%.[1] It is estimated that the diarrhea reduction achieved by meeting the Millennium Development Goals[12] (MDGs) will gain 272 million school days attendance, with particular improvements in sub-Saharan Africa.[1]

In offering sanitation as part of a potable water plan to a community two considerations are paramount. First, the need for sanitation has to be understood. The benefits of sanitation are not as widely understood as the benefits of clean water; it is not apparent to everyone that defecating in a stream negates the possibility of obtaining clean water from that stream.[13] Second, the community must be involved in the planning to be sure the suggested technology is accessible and acceptable (pour flush latrines where water is scarce won't be used readily or correctly).

Cost

The cost to achieve the MDG for sanitation—halving the number of households without basic latrines by 2015—is $10 billion and will still leave 1.3 billion households without sanitation. The cost to achieve flush toilets with sewer connections would be $34 billion.[14] In planning to achieve water and sanitation for all, nations need a strategy to enlist public support as costs would affect much of the population, especially the poor. In Latin America 20–50% of households would be stressed to pay the costs of accessible potable water, and in sub-Saharan Africa 70% of households would be stressed if complete recovery of potable water delivery costs were required of them; poverty in Mozambique would increase by 7%.[1] Adding the cost of installing sanitation markedly increases these numbers.

Solutions

Where public sewer systems are not available or impractical, a variety of latrines that are relatively easy and inexpensive to build can solve this problem. Septic tanks allow hook ups to flush toilets in homes and avoid the odors of latrines, but the cost and complexity is considerably greater than any of the latrine models. For urban areas more complex sewer systems are indicated. The pros and cons of each type and specific directions for building and maintaining them can be found in the WHO document *A Guide to On-Site Sanitation*.[15]

Sufficient water for human needs is not always available. Scientists arbitrarily consider that 1700 cubic meters per person per year is needed to meet human needs of individual use, agriculture, industry, and maintaining the environment. One thousand cubic meters is the lower limit for sufficiency, and below 500 cubic meters is absolute scarcity. On average the annual water cycle makes available 6900 cubic meters per person, much of which is unusable because it comes in the form of floods or is in inaccessible places such as the ice caps; but more than 1700 cubic meters is available.[16] Water availability refers to rainfall that returns to ground water. Water that soaks into the ground and then evaporates is not included.[1]

Water Availability

In developing countries, especially those already lacking sufficient water (water stressed), there is a continuing decline in water available for human use. In sub-Saharan Africa, the percentage of water-stressed countries will increase from 30% to 85% by 2025. In North Africa and the Middle East 90% of the population will be—in the next two decades—living in water-stressed areas.[1] Overextraction of river water; overdraft of groundwater; pollution of rivers, streams and aquifers; along with climate change, will create additional problems. The Aral Sea is a case in point. The sea is shared by Uzbekistan and Kazakhstan, but its water use also affects Turkmenistan, Tajikistan, and Kyrgyzstan. Beginning in 1960 when the Aral Sea was the world's fourth largest lake, covering 26,250 square miles, agricultural demands deprived it of enough water to sustain itself, and it has shrunk rapidly—volume has decreased by 75%, its surface area by 50%, and the shoreline has receded up to 120 km from its former shore. Uzbekistan, Kazakhstan, and other Central Asian states use this water to grow cotton and other export crops despite widespread environmental consequences including fisheries loss, water and soil contamination, and dangerous levels of polluted airborne sediments. As the Aral Sea shrank, its salinity increased. By the early 1980s commercially useful fish had been eliminated, shutting down an industry that had employed 60,000 people. Irrigated agriculture in the feeding rivers' deltas used large amounts of pesticides resulting in high contaminant concentrations in the sea.

Overirrigation caused salt buildup in many agricultural areas.[17,18,19]

Groundwater overdraft is a problem in many places. China, despite huge rivers, has a 25% groundwater overdraft rate, and in parts of India it is 56%.[20] Unfortunately, there is only limited ability to trade or transfer water from areas of abundance to areas of scarcity. Dos Pueblos, the New York–Tipitapa Sister City Project, is a nonprofit organization that partners with Asociación Coordinadora Municipal De Proyectos De Ciudades Hermanas De Tipitapa (COMPALCIHT), a local Nicaraguan community-based organization, to supply material aid to development projects in Tipitapa, Nicaragua. One of the project areas supported is providing potable water supplies for barrios within Tipitapa. In 2006 the community of Los Coleros requested help to bring municipal water to each household. The community had a well but a free-trade zone factory opened on land adjacent to the barrio and installed a high-power water pump in its well. The factory drew so much water the only time the community could use its well was between midnight and 5 AM. Los Coleros worked with the local government and COMPALCIHT to arrange that all the work be done locally. New York raised the funds to buy the pipes.[21] In India, soft-drink companies extract ground water causing wells to dry up.[21–23] The availability of water must be included in planning economic development and be added into the cost of finished items.

Natural contamination of groundwater is also a potential problem. Arsenic leaching into ground water from the surrounding rock poses a growing global health risk as large numbers of people consume unsafe levels. Naturally occurring arsenic poisoning affects nearly 140 million people in more than 70 countries according to new research presented at the annual Royal Geographical Society meeting in London. There is a very important connection between arsenic in water and arsenic in food. Food crops absorb arsenic, along with other heavy metals and chemicals, when it is in the irrigation water. Bangladesh has been affected the most. Industrial activities such as mining can also lead to contamination.[24]

Agriculture uses about 70% of available fresh water. Use across crops is not even. When planning land use for agriculture, thought should be given to which crops raised or animals grazed would be most efficient and effective in an area.

To produce 3000 calories of food, 3500 litres of water are needed, and 2000 to 5000 litres of water are needed to grow a kilo of rice.[25]

The following lists how much water it takes to make each item from start to finish.

- 1 cup coffee (250 ml)—280 litres (74 gallons)
- 1 microchip (2 gm/0.07 oz)—32 litres (8.5 gallons)
- 1 hamburger with the works (150 gm/5.3 oz)—2400 litres (634 gallons)
- 1 slice bread (30 gm/1.60 oz)—40 litres (10.6 gallons)
- 1 glass wine (125 ml/4.23 fl oz)—120 litres (32 gallons)
- 1 sheet paper (81/2″ × 11″)—10 litres (2.6 gallons)
- 1 cotton t-shirt (medium 500 gm/17.6 oz)—4100 litres (1083 gallons)
- 1 tomato (70 gm/2.5 oz)—13 litres (3.4 gallons)
- 1 pair cowhide leather shoes—8000 litres (2014 gallons)[26]

Surface water sources almost always need to be purified whether for human, agricultural, or industrial use. Agricultural runoff, industrial discharge, and proximity of human discharges to a source of water cause contamination. Use of untreated wastewater for irrigation is one of the ways through which heavy metals, toxic chemicals, and microbial agents can enter into the food chain. Many of the poorer countries lack resources to treat either municipal or industrial wastewater.[27]

Most water from deep aquifers and some from shallow wells can be used directly. These waters should be tested periodically for toxic chemicals that leach from the containing strata as well as unexpected microbial incursions. After floods many wells that usually produce clean water become contaminated.

Water Treatment

The treatment of surface water is fairly standard. First, large objects such as fish and sticks are removed by large filters and then chemicals (coagulants) are added to the water to coagulate tiny suspended particles into larger particles ("flocs"). These flocs are further treated (flocculation) to create large flocs. Once the flocs are large and heavy enough to settle, the water is moved into basins so the flocs can settle to the bottom. After sedimentation, some form of filtration through sand or membranes occurs. Finally, disinfection and then chemicals to adjust pH to prevent corrosion of the pipes in the distribution system or to prevent tooth decay takes place. There are several choices for disinfection: chlorine, chloramine, ozone, or ultraviolet light. Chlorine is the most common, but each has pros and cons including price, availability, effectiveness against the microbial agents and other contaminants in the water supply, maintenance, and by-products from the reaction of the disinfecting agent with the organic and inorganic compounds in the water.[2]

Once the water is in the distribution system, there are additional opportunities for drinking water to be contaminated. If pipes are not successfully protected from contaminants, the quality of drinking water suffers. Extra disinfectant should be added at the end of the water purification process to neutralize the small foci of contamination that develop in pipes over time. All too often money was saved by digging one ditch for both sewer and water delivery pipes. Over time the pipes develop leaks and cross-contamination occurs. Improper storage can also result in unsafe drinking water.[2]

Where public potable water systems are not available alternate means of purifying water are needed. Boiling water is one option, but in many areas fuel is scarce. If boiling is used, a vigorous boil should be maintained for one minute. At altitudes greater than 6562 feet (> 2000 m), water should be boiled for three minutes or a chemical disinfectant used after the water has boiled for one minute.[28]

Collecting rain water into covered barrels or cisterns and covering wells is an improvement over using open water sources, but they may become contaminated if care is not taken. Wells frequently become contaminated when flooding occurs. Exposure of water to sunlight in clear plastic or glass containers for several hours will kill most microbial agents. A number of small, inexpensive water filter systems have been developed. They use gravity filtration through sand, ceramic, pots activated charcoal, or a combination of the three. Water can be filtered through fairly porous material including a clean cloth to remove larger size impurities and then treated with a disinfectant such as chlorine bleach or iodine because viruses can pass through almost all filters available although they do adhere to some.[29,30]

Conservation

Over millennia societies have developed ways to preserve water in areas or seasons of scarcity. Collecting rain water into cisterns above or below ground and damming rivers are documented in ancient cultures. Even desert nomads have methods of collecting and storing water during the rare rainfalls. More recently the need to keep collected water covered to keep it clean and to prevent mosquitoes from breeding has been appreciated.

Building dams on rivers has some advantages for maintaining available water at a constant level and controlling floods, but at costs to displaced communities and obliteration of species. Research has shown that small dams cause much less environmental and human disruption and are more efficient and effective than large dams in both preserving water flow and preventing flooding.[31] A new worry has arisen. The volume of glacial-fed rivers is increasing now from increased ice melt caused by the warming of global climate change. Winter snow is not replacing all the summer glacial melt so glacier-fed rivers will dry up in coming years.

Water can be used multiple times before being discarded. The water used for rinsing fruits and vegetables subsequently can be used for washing clothes and then to water the garden. The typical "kitchen garden" where food for the family was grown was so placed for just this reason. The pails of used household water did not have to be carried very far. Bath water can be used to flush toilets. Large amounts of water would be saved if all pipe leaks and faucet drips were fixed promptly.[25,31]

Waste water from sewer systems and industrial facilities should be processed to remove toxic chemicals and microbial agents before being flushed into lakes and rivers. Guidelines for waste water processing are available from many sources including WHO,[16] the US Environmental Protection Agency,[32] national, regional, or municipal departments for protecting the environment, or university sources.[33]

More efficient use of water by agriculture includes rain-fed methods, check dams, and drip irrigation. Rain-fed crops produce about one-half the yield of irrigated crops and use more water yet are the primary irrigation method for many.[1,31,34] Drip systems using computer-determined needs are most effective and efficient but using buckets with drip kits works well.[35] Every $1.00 invested in drip kits gave $2.00 after all costs except labor were calculated, and water use was decreased by 30–60% while crop yield increased by 5–50%.[36]

In many areas women are the chief providers of local food crops. Improved and expanded education for them to use these methods is needed.[37] Along with improving water use and preservation, improvement of soil so that it can more effectively hold the water available needs to be addressed.

Future Issues

Fresh potable water is not equitably distributed in the world, and availability will decrease over the coming years from a combination of continued population growth, climate change, and the continuing degradation of the quality of water supplies because of lack of sanitation, unregulated industrial discharge, and agricultural runoff. Government intervention will be needed to assure that the minimum quantity of potable water (20 litres per person per day) is available. Private water vendors are not likely to undertake the costs of water delivery infrastructure including maintenance if collection of fees in rural areas, informal settlements, or large urban slums is not assured. As there is little competition supplying water, and it is essential that quality and quantity be maintained for health and development, government oversight is essential. The regulation of all water providers needs to be independent and have penalty powers.

Conclusion

Water and sanitation is a shared right and a shared responsibility. To best achieve water for all, the community and all individuals in it need to be involved in the process from the initial assessment of needs to implementation and continuing maintenance. But, having the right to participate in decisions is not the same as having the ability to participate. This is particularly true for women. In studies in developing countries, 4–5% of women feel they will be heard if they speak in a community meeting, but their words will not make a difference in village decision making.[38,39,40] The initial community assessment should consider its uses, practices, and beliefs concerning water and then discuss how the health and well-being of the community's members are affected by their findings.

Achieving ample supplies of fresh water and sanitation for all is a long-term project. It is an inter- and intraborder process requiring continuous involvement by both international and local governments. Maintaining essential support for these activities from the international community, given the decidedly unappealing nature of the subject, will be difficult, but it must happen.

DISCUSSION QUESTIONS

1. Enumerate essential uses of water (at least three).
2. What are the sources of water for human use?
3. Enumerate potential means of contaminating or decreasing availability of otherwise potable water (at least three).
4. List ways in which obtaining water for family use particularly affects the lives of women and the girl-child.

REFERENCES

1. Watkins K, ed. *Human Development Report 2006—Beyond Scarcity: Power, Poverty and the Global Water Crisis*. Hampshire, UK: Palgrave McMillan; 2006.
2. National Academy of Science. Safe drinking water is essential. http://www.drinking-water.org/html/en/Overview/Cost.html. Published 2008. Accessed October 11, 2007.
3. WHO/UNICEF Joint Monitoring Programme. Meeting the MDG Drinking Water and Sanitation Target: the urban and rural challenge of the decade. http://www.wssinfo.org/pdf/JMP_06.pdf. Published 2006. Accessed January 1, 2008.
4. Kariuki M, Schwartz J. *Small-Scale Providers of Water Supply and Electricity*. Washington, DC: World Bank; 2005. Policy Research Working Paper 3727. http://siteresources.worldbank.org/EXTWSS/Resources/337301-1147283808455/2532553-1149858231928/Kariuki&Schwartz_SmallScalePSP.pdf. Accessed January 2, 2008.
5. Rosenberg CE. *The Cholera Years: The United States in 1832, 1849, and 1866*. Chicago, IL: University of Chicago Press; 1962.
6. Parker R, Skytta T. *Rural Water Projects: Lessons from OED Evaluations*. World Bank Working Paper. http://www-wds.worldbank.org/external/default/WDSContentServer/WDSP/IB/2000/11/04/000094946_00102111465146/Rendered/PDF/multi_page.pdf. Published March 2000. Accessed January 2, 2008.

7. Blackden M, Wodon Q. Gender, time use, and poverty in sub-Saharan Africa. World Bank. http://www4.worldbank.org/afr/ssatp/Resources/HTML/Gender-RG /Source%20%20documents/Technical%20Reports/Gender%20Research/TEGE N1%20Gender,%20Time%20Use%20Poverty%20SSAfr%20WB%20%2005.pdf. Published 2006. Accessed January 1, 2008.

8. Snow J. *On the Mode of Communication of Cholera.* London, England: John Churchill; 1855. http://www.ph.ucla.edu/EPI/snow/snowbook.html. Accessed February 5, 2008.

9. WHO. Health statistics and health information systems. http://www.who.int /healthinfo/boddaly/en/. Published 2008. Accessed February 14, 2008.

10. Hutton G, Haller L. 2004. Costs and benefits of water and sanitation improvements at the global level (Evaluation of the). World Health Organization. http://www.iwmi.cgiar.org/Publications/IWMI_Research_Reports/PDF/pub084 /RR84.pdf. http://www.who.int/water_sanitation_health/wsh0404/en/. Accessed January 2, 2008.

11. Fuentes R, Pfuetze T, Seck P. *Does Access to Water and Sanitation Affect Child Survival? A Five Country Analysis.* Human Development Report 2006, Human Development Report Office Occasional Paper. New York, NY: UNDP; 2006. http://hdr .undp.org/hdr2006/pdfs/background-docs/Background_papers/Fuentes %20et%20al%20A.pdf. Accessed January 2, 2008.

12. United Nations. Millennium Development Goals. http://www.un.org/millennium goals/. Accessed February 23, 2008.

13. Phan KT, Frias J, Salter D. 2004. Lessons from market-based approaches to improved hygiene for the rural poor in developing countries. http://www.danidadev forum.um.dk/NR/rdonlyres/E617F287-36D0-44BD-A426-E18E2F3AD29A /0/LessonsMarketbasedHygiene.pdf. Accessed February 3, 2008.

14. Winpenny J. Financing water for all. World Water Council, Secretariat of the 3rd World Water Forum and Global Water Partnership. http://www.worldwater-council.org/fileadmin/wwc/Library/Publications_and_reports/CamdessusReport.pdf. Published 2003. Accessed January 6, 2008.

15. Rijsberman FR. Sanitation and water. The challenge paper on water and sanitation. http://www.copenhagenconsensus.com/Default.aspx?ID=228#895. Accessed January 2, 2008.

16. WHO. 1992. A guide to on-site sanitation. http://www.who.int/water_sanitation_health/hygiene/envsan/onsitesan.pdf. Accessed February 5, 2008.

17. Calder J, Lee J. ARALSEA: Aral Sea and Defense Issues. ICE Case Studies, Number 69, 1995. http://www.american.edu/ted/ice/aralsea.htm. Accessed February 5, 2008.

18. The Aral Sea. http://visearth.ucsd.edu/VisE_Int/aralsea/index.html. Accessed February 5, 2008.

19. Regional Partnership for Prevention of Transboundary Degradation of the Kura-Aras River Basin—UNDP. http://www.undp.org.ge/Projects/kura.html 2002. Accessed January 1, 2008.

20. World Bank. Reengaging in agricultural water management. http://sitere-sources.worldbank.org/INTARD/Resources/DID_AWM.pdf. Published 2006. Accessed January 1, 2008.

21. Dos Pueblos, New York City-Tipitapa, Nicaragua Sister City Project. http://www.tipitapa.org/index.html. Accessed December 10, 2007.

22. Molle F, Berkoff J, eds. *Irrigation Water Pricing: The Gap Between Theory and Practice Comprehensive Assessment of Water Management in Agriculture.* Wallingford, UK:

CABI; 2007. Series 4. http://www.iwmi.cgiar.org/assessment/Synthesis/Water PricingBook_000.htm. Accessed January 2, 2008.

23. Molle F, Berkoff J. *Cities versus Agriculture: Revisiting Intersectoral Water Transfers, Potential Gains and Conflicts.* International Water Management Institute. CA Research Report 10, 2006. http://www.iwmi.cgiar.org/assessment/files_new /publications/CA%20Research%20Reports/CARR10.pdf. Accessed January 2, 2008.

24. REUTERS. Arsenic in drinking water said to be rising risk. *New York Times.* August 30, 2007. http://www.nytimes.com. Accessed August 30, 2007.

25. Rijsberman FR, Manning N, de Silva S. Increasing green and blue water productivity to balance water for food and environment. Presented at: Fourth World Water Forum; March 2006; Mexico City. http://www.worldwaterforum4 .org.mx/uploads/TBL_DOCS_83_29.pdf. Accessed January 1, 2008.

26. American Museum of Natural History. Water facts: a drop of water information from the AMNH. http://www.amnh.org/exhibitions/water/facts.php. Accessed November 15, 2007.

27. SPRU—Science and Technology Policy Research. Contaminated irrigation water and food safety for the urban and peri-urban poor. http://www.pollutionand food.net. Accessed February 15, 2008.

28. Centers for Disease Control and Prevention. Travel. http://wwwn.cdc.gov/travel /contentWaterTreatment.aspx. Accessed February 5, 2008.

29. Centers for Disease Control and Prevention. Parasites. http://www.cdc.gov /ncidod/dpd/parasites/cryptosporidiosis/factsht_crypto_prevent_water.htm. Accessed February 5, 2008.

30. Narain S. *Community-led Alternatives to Water Management: India Case Study.* Occasional Paper. New York: UNDP; 2006. Human Development Report 2006.

31. Fox P, Rockström J. Supplemental irrigation for dry-spell mitigation of rain-fed agriculture in the Sahel. Natural Resources Management, The Netherlands. http://www.sciencedirect.com/science/article/B6T3X-47X6SVH-1/2/58e0 aa83552e495a615af238f567e65e. Published 2002. Accessed February 5, 2008

32. US Environmental Protection Agency.. http://yosemite.epa.gov/water/owrccatalog .nsf/EPATitle?OpenView&StartKey=W&Count=385&e=&CartID=8521-064907. Accessed January 7, 2009

33. Wastewater Treatment Methods and Disposal http://water.me.vccs.edu/courses /ENV149/methods.htm. Accessed January 7, 2009

34. Botha JJ, van Rensburg LD, Anderson JJ, et al. Evaluating the sustainability of the in-field rainwater harvesting crop production system. http://www.fao.org/ag /agl/aglw/wh/docs/botha.doc. Accessed February 5, 2008.

35. Shah T, Keller J. 2002. Micro-irrigation and the poor: A marketing challenge in smallholder irrigation development. In Sally H, Abernethy CL, eds. *Private Irrigation in Sub-Saharan Africa.* Regional Seminar on Private Sector Participation and Irrigation Expansion in Sub-Saharan Africa; October 22-26, 2001; Accra, Ghana. Colombo, Sri Lanka: IWMI, FAO, ACP-EU Technical Centre for Agricultural and Rural Cooperation; 2001:165-183.

36. Shah T, van Koppen B, Merrey D, de Lange M, Madar S. 2002. Institutional alternatives in African smallholder irrigation. News of the Progress and Impact of IWMI's Research, May 2002. http://72.14.205.104/custom?q=cache:1P5N_smSa-cJ: www.iwmi.cgiar.org/News_Room/Newsletters/Research_Updates/PDFs /ResearchUpdateJune2002.pdf+t+shah&hl=en&ct=clnk&cd=89&gl=us&client= google-coop-np. Accessed January 1, 2008.

37. Rijsberman FR. Water Scarcity: Fact or fiction? Presented at: 4th International Crop Science Conference, September 2004; Brisbane, Australia. http://www .cropscience.org.au/icsc2004/plenary/1/1994_rijsbermanf.htm. Accessed January 2, 2008.

38. Lipton Ml. Approaches to rural poverty alleviation in developing Asia: role of water resources. IWMI. http://www.sussex.ac.uk/Units/PRU/iwmi_irrigation.pdf. Published 2004. Accessed January 2, 2008.

39. Meinzen-Dick R, Zwarteveen MZ. Gender dimensions of community resource management: the case of water users' associations in south Asia. In: Agrawal A, Clark C, eds. *Communities and the Environment: Ethnicity, Gender, and the State in Community-Based Conservation*. New Brunswick, NJ: Rutgers University Press; 2001: 63-88.

40. Faysse N. An assessment of small-scale users' inclusion in large-scale water user associations of South Africa. IWMI Research Report 84. http://www .iwmi.cgiar.org/Publications/IWMI_Research_Reports/PDF/pub084/RR84.pdf. Published 2004. Accessed January 2, 2008.

CHAPTER **34**

Society, Exercise, and Women

Physical activity, as defined by the Centers for Disease Control and Prevention (CDC) is "any bodily movement produced by the skeletal muscles that result in an expenditure of energy."[1] The physical, social, and mental health benefits of engaging in moderate amounts of physical activity, preferably daily, are well researched and numerous. Being physically active helps reduce the risk of developing a number of chronic illnesses such as coronary heart disease (CHD), diabetes, obesity, and various forms of cancer. Regular exercise can help maintain healthy bones, muscles, and joints and has been shown to reduce symptoms associated with arthritis. Studies have found that in conjunction with estrogen replacement therapy, physical activity may even help decrease bone loss after menopause. An association between exercise and reduced symptoms of anxiety and depression has also been fairly well researched finding that activity improves overall feelings of well-being.[2] This may be of particular note for women given that the depression rates for females are nearly double that of males in both developing and developed countries.[3]

It has been estimated that worldwide physical inactivity causes about 1.9 million deaths yearly, including 10–16% of diabetes mellitus cases and breast, colon, and rectal cancers, and about 22% of ischemic heart disease.[2] The risk of developing cardiovascular disease (CVD) is nearly 1.5 times greater for those who do not engage in proper amounts of physical activity.[2] In the United States, over 60% of women are not physically active enough, and over 25% are not physically active at all.[3] The sad truth is that women and girls tend to be less physically active than men and boys. Across spans of varying cultures and geographical distributions, females are consistently less active than their male counterparts.[4] Explanations for this global health concern are as diverse as the people who populate the planet.

Amy Ansehl, RN, MSN, FNPC;
Marly B. Katz, MPH;
Padmini Murthy, MD, MPH, MS, CHES

Amy Ansehl, RN, MSN, FNPC, is Executive Director for the Partnership for a Healthy Population and Assistant Professor and Practicum Coordinator for the New York Medical College School of Public Health, Valhalla, NY.

Marly B Katz, MPH, is based in Yonkers, NY.

Padmini Murthy, MD, MPH, MS, CHES, is an Assistant Professor in the Department of Health Policy and Management as well as the Director of the Global Health Program at New York Medical School of Public Health in Valhalla, NY. She is the Medical Women's International Association NGO Representative to the United Nations, New York, and Robert F Wagner Public Service Scholar, New York University.

Barriers and Limitations

To help promote physical activity, it is important to try and understand some of the barriers that may be preventing people, women specifically, from being active. Common barriers include culture, socioeconomics, time, motivation, accessibility, education, and health or physical conditions.

Cultural factors are often important barriers preventing women from engaging in proper amounts of physical activity. For example, women of south Asian descent believe the majority of their time should be spent caring for their families and that exercising for personal benefit is to be considered a selfish behavior.[5] Additionally, language barriers, or the inability to speak or understand the local language, may deter women from participating in public exercise facilities.

People of low socioeconomic groups tend to be less active than those who are more affluent. People with low income have less money available to devote to exercise; for example, there are often costs associated with accessing physical activity facilities. People with low incomes are also more likely to list lack of transportation as a barrier to exercise. It is important to note that the income of women is often lower than that of men, which would make it more difficult for an average female to afford these costs. Women with higher incomes, however, tend to cite lack of time and motivation as their greatest limitations in scheduling exercises regularly.[6]

Time, or the lack thereof, is an important issue for many people since demands related to employment, studies, or familial obligations tend to take priority over exercising.[7] Additionally, when there is a lack of motivation, or the inner desire to engage in physical activity, people may have difficulty focusing on the importance of exercising or might more easily be distracted by other activities.[8] Limited access to areas where one can safely exercise, such as open spaces, gymnasiums, sidewalks, or playgrounds, may also prevent people from being physically active.[2]

Studies have found that education is positively related to physical activity levels. Less educated people tend to be less physically active than those with higher levels of education. Researchers have attributed this association to differing levels of perceived control over the relationship between behavior and outcomes. Those who are less educated have less confidence over their own abilities and are thus less likely to believe in the personal benefits of exercise.[9]

Biological factors and health conditions may also behave as barriers to physical activity for women. Women who perceive their health to be poor are less likely to be physically active than those who perceive their health to be good. Those women with better health perceptions also tend to have more positive attitudes about being active. Women will also often cite medical conditions or illness as reasons for not engaging in exercise, such as general or specific pain and chronic disease.[10] Many women are not aware of the importance of remaining physically active even when suffering from a medical condition. This lack of knowledge may suggest a lack of access to healthcare providers that offer information on how to exercise properly under certain situations. Women with medical conditions, such as heart disease or diabetes, can benefit greatly from exercising regularly. It is important for women to consult their physician about proper techniques and guidelines for exercising with a disease or medical condition.[11]

Other conditions specific to women that may act as barriers to exercising are menstruation and pregnancy. In a number of cultures, women and girls are discouraged from participating in physical activity while menstruating and are instead encouraged to relax and take it easy. Throughout the course of pregnancy, levels of activity tend to decrease with a number of cited reasons including feeling unwell or tired, being too busy, and feeling uncomfortable while exercising (this one is often listed later in the pregnancy). Additionally, a number of women are concerned over the safety of their baby and are not of aware of the importance of remaining physically activity even while pregnant. Therefore it is important to distribute information to pregnant women regarding ways they can exercise safely and comfortably throughout the pregnancy.[12]

A Global Picture

Cultural aspects of physical activity among women worldwide vary continent to continent, country to country, and region to region. Barriers preventing women from obtaining the recommended amounts of exercise are often dependant on societal roles and social pressures and expectations. By exploring specific limitations for women in varying lands and cultures one would be better equipped to paint a bigger picture of global health.

South Africa

In South Africa, it is a common belief among black women that being overweight is a reflection of wealth and happiness. Many women residing in urban areas perceive body weight as an indication of their husband's ability to provide for their family. Being thin, on the other hand, is often undesirably equated with the HIV/AIDS virus infection.[13]

Nearly half of all adult women in South Africa do not engage in enough exercise.[14] Historically, women remained active while performing chores such as fetching water, tending to the animals, and walking long distances.[13] Many of these labor-intensive activities have been replaced due to the introduction of motorized transport and the mechanization of labor, in addition to increases in sedentary leisure activities such as television viewing.[14]

Morocco

The Sahraoui people of Morocco used to live as nomads; however, because of environmental conditions such as desertification and increased aridity they are being urbanized. This process has been rapid, and in conjunction there have been numerous lifestyle changes including alterations to diet and physical activity levels. Sahraoui women traditionally engage in sedentary activities including tea drinking and afternoon naps. They do not participate in sports either, since in their culture females are not considered physically capable enough to participate in such competitions. Being overweight is also considered beautiful.[15]

India

Despite being a poor country with high rates of malnutrition, the prevalence of overweight women in India has increased suggesting a nutritional and behavioral shift. Poorer women living in slum areas maintain relatively active lifestyles due to physically demanding household chores and less access to mechanized transportation and television than more affluent women. The poor women of India cite lack of priority as the most common barrier to physical activity, compared to time constraints and lack of willpower among the more affluent. Overall, the levels of obesity in India are relatively low; the evidence pointing to a shift in activity levels means that health campaigns promoting healthy behaviors will be required soon in order to prevent future problems.[16]

Australia

In Australia, women are about half as likely as men to be adequately active.[17] One study identified the most common barriers preventing women from exercise. Among younger women, motivation, time, and cost were listed as the most important limitations, whereas among women with children the lack of social support was the most restricting barrier.[18]

Israel

In general, the Israeli population lives a relatively sedentary lifestyle. This varies among subgroups suggesting the need to develop different strategies and group specific approaches. Splitting the Israelis into two populations, the Jews and the Arabs, can offer some insight to the cultural differences and perspectives of the people living in Israel.

Studies have found that the Jews tend to be more active than their Arab neighbors. In both populations, the more educated people engage in more physical activity than those who are less educated, and those who are single tend to be more active than those who are married. Additionally, the women exercise less than the men. The margin of difference between the physical activity habits among men and women within the Arab population, however, is much greater than that within the Jewish population. This may suggest a greater difference between the genders in the Arab population than in the Jews.

The more religious Jews tend to be less active than the less religious ones, but there does not seem to be an association between the level of religiousness and physical activity among the Arabs. Physical inactivity among the Jews has also been found to be associated with other unhealthy behaviors or risk factors such as smoking and obesity whereas there is no such association among the Arab population. These differences may partly be explained by the current social status of physical activity amongst the two populations. The Jews may be more physically active because there is an awareness of the health benefits, whereas the Arabs may still be undergoing the process of Westernization and have yet to adopt the recommended healthy lifestyle.[19]

Iran

When in public, Iranian women are required to cover up their hair and bodies by dressing in loose, uniform garments so that men cannot see their body shape. Since body shape and cosmetic-related media images and fashion advertisements were banned in 1979, the women tend to have less social-related pressure in terms of conforming to any ideal body image. Women are also less likely to engage in physical activity due to religious and social restrictions.[20]

Canada

As is the general trend globally, women in Canada are less physically active than men. About 57% of the women are physically inactive compared to about 50% of men. For Canadian women, the most commonly cited barrier preventing them from exercising is the lack of time due to family responsibilities, which includes child care, cooking, cleaning, and other household chores. Other cited barriers include lack of motivation and self-efficacy, poor perception of health, and the lack of social support.

Among ethnic minorities, cultural barriers may include the lack of community support, differing social norms, lack of knowledge of the importance of exercise, culturally dictated family roles, and language barriers.[21] In Canada, the official languages are English (59%) and French (23%); however, there are other languages spoken including Chinese (2.9%), Italian (1.7%), and German (1.5%), which may provide limitations for non-English or non-French speaking people.[22]

United States

According to the 1994 Behavioral Risk Factor Surveillance System (BRFSS), about 33% of women in the United States reported having had no leisure time physical activity (LTPA) in the previous month at all, compared to 28% of men. There are a number of factors associated with physical activity levels among women including sociodemographic, psychological, and environmental.[10]

One sociodemographic factor that seems to influence physical activity among women in the United States is race. Research has found that minorities, including Black, Hispanic, Asian, or Native American women, tend to be less physically active than White women. The 1994 BRFSS estimated that 46% and 33% of Black and Hispanic women, respectively, are not physically active compared to 30% of White women.[10] One particular study found that with regard to body image, White women tend to be less satisfied with their bodies than Black or Hispanic women due to differing perceptions of beauty.[23] The concept of a perfect, beautiful body seems to vary depending on cultural influences.

In terms of geographic location, rural women tend to be less active than their urban counterparts. Women living in rural settings experience more severe barriers than urban women preventing them from engaging in healthy activities. These barriers include higher levels of poverty, greater distances from health services or exercise facilities, and lower levels of education. Rural residents also tend to have less interest in becoming more physically active.[24]

Psychological factors often greatly influence physical activity levels. One important concept to understand is self-efficacy, which is the confidence in one's abilities to do specific activities. There is a positive association between self-efficacy and exercise, meaning a person is more likely to be physically active if they have high self-efficacy. Additionally, women who perceive the benefits of physical activity to be greater than the barriers are more likely to be active. Other barriers related to attitudes and beliefs include lack of time and motivation, fatigue or lack of energy, being self-conscious about one's appearance, receiving discouragement from others, the fear of injury, high levels of stress, and lack of knowledge about the benefits of regular physical activity.[10]

Environmental factors include social support from friends and family, professional support, and family structure. Research consistently demonstrates a positive association between support from family and friends and physical activity levels. This kind of support can increase enjoyment and adherence of exercise programs and improve the likelihood of program adoption. Likewise, professional support from a physician or other health professional is associated with greater activity levels. In terms of family structure, women who have children are more likely to be physically inactive than those who do not have children.[10] This may be due partly to time constraints from familial obligations.

Research has found a few barriers unique to minority women in the United States. Black women are likely to cite sweating and messing up one's hair as barriers preventing them from being physically active. They also tend to value rest over physical activity or hard labor. Native American women often feel that planning time to participate in recreational activities does not fit in with the identity of Native American women. Asian women feel that by completing their daily tasks, for example housework or walking for transportation, they engage in enough exercise. Additionally, they believe physical activity should have a purpose, and they should be active when completing some kind of chore instead of just following an exercise video.[10]

Special Needs

Refugee and Immigrant Women

Women of south Asian descent living in the UK, including Pakistani, Indian, Bangladeshi, and Sri Lankan have been identified as being less physically active than Europeans. According to the research, these people participate in far less recreational physical activity. These women cite a number of barriers preventing them from being ac-

tive including religious modesty, the fear of going out alone, and the avoidance of mixed-gender exercise. Those who could not speak English also reported that as a limitation. Additionally, they believe engaging in physical activity beyond that which involves everyday work contributing to the care of their families or the house income as selfish activity. None of their relatives participated in sports; instead, they remained active through household chores, including the care of their children and other relatives, and through their work.[5]

European women living in the United States identify a number of barriers preventing them from participating in physical activity including time constraints, an unaccommodating schedule, the consequences of physical activity, environmental barriers, and individual barriers. Time constraints are cited to include familial situations and obligations such as taking care of the children, having to cook dinner, and being up early for work. An unaccommodating schedule is defined as everyday activities including work or shopping that limits engagement in physical activity. Women also cite the lack of an exercise routine, inadequate time management skills, and the lack of variety in repetitive exercises as being barriers directly related to their schedules. Consequences of physical activity include possible negative outcomes such as injuries. An unsupportive environment involves issues surrounding work, for example a desk job reducing motivation to be physically active, and the climate, including changes in daylight hours and temperature. There are a number of internal or individual factors that influence the lack of physical activity among European women in the United States including insufficient knowledge, lack of commitment, lack of motivation, physical inability, and poor body image.[8] For Latina immigrant women living in the United States, the greatest barriers to physical activity are the lack of companionship while exercising and the absence of other female figures to watch over their children.[25]

Women with Disabilities

In 2005 about 19.6% of all adults suffered from a disability. The Behavioral Risk Factor Surveillance System (BRFSS) 2005 estimated that only about 37.7% of people with disabilities meet the recommended amounts of physical activity, compared to about 49.4% of adults without a disability, and that 25.6% were physically inactive, compared to about 12.8% of those not disabled.[26] As a result of their disabilities, behavior, lifestyle, or environment, people with disabilities are at greater risk of developing secondary health conditions including obesity and depression. There are a number of barriers preventing people with disabilities from engaging in proper amounts of physical activity including physiological limitations as a result of the disabling condition itself, lack of transportation to fitness centers, lack of information on available and accessible facilities and programs, lack of accessible exercise equipment, and the perception that facilities are not disability friendly.[26] Additionally, attitudes assuming people with disabilities cannot or need not exercise are often discouraging and misleading. To develop a more disability-friendly facility, health clubs should have accessible parking, wide aisles, automatic doors, and accessible showers, lockers, and pools.[27]

In the United States, about one in five women suffer from some kind of disability; this includes more than half of women over the age of 65. The most common disabilities are associated with chronic conditions including arthritis, heart disease, respiratory problems, and back disorders.[28] In other areas of the world, a disability is thought of as a curse or punishment from God. People with disabilities are often hidden from society and deemed unfit to participate in mainstream activities. Additionally, women and girls suffering from a disability may be denied access to health services, education, and employment.[29]

Elderly Women

Older women tend to be less active than their younger counterparts. There are a number of barriers associated with increased age that is limiting for the elderly population including the lack of knowledge regarding the benefits of physical activity, lack of access, fear of falling, lack of social support, and environmental conditions such as a lack of safe areas to exercise and poor weather. Many elderly women also perceive themselves as being too old to be physically active, and often blame their declining health as a reason for not engaging in exercise.[21]

Children and Adolescents

About 23% of children never participate in any free-time physical activity.[30] Leisure time activities are becoming increasingly more sedentary, and children are spending more time watching television, playing video games, and using the internet.[31] Girls are less physically active than boys, which may suggest a difference in attitudes toward exercise and social stereotypes regarding the active female body.[21] Children are less likely to participate in sports or exercises if they perceive their skills to be low in comparison to their peers. If the girl does not believe that she can do it, the likelihood that she will is very small.[32] Inactive girls are more likely to be dissatisfied with their looks and weight, and tend to suffer from lower self-esteem. This lowers their confidence in their physical abilities and discourages them from participating in certain activities. The media is a huge influence on what girls perceive to be the ideal body shape and size. In addition to lowering self-esteem, media images lead to mental conditions such as depression and eating disorders such as anorexia and bulimia. Counseling and encouragement can help increase a person's self-efficacy and self-esteem, and thus increase the probability of success.[33]

Young girls often define being healthy as "the absence of illness or of unhealthy activities or symptoms." They believe they are healthy as long as they do not perceive themselves as being over- or underweight, do not have diseases, and are not addicted to any harmful substances such as alcohol, drugs, or cigarettes. Appearances and fitting in with peers is usually viewed with greater importance than diet or exercise. They desire to look and act like the accepted social norm, or be "normal healthy." Being too active is thought of as "extremist" behavior. Girls also tend to become less active with age, preferring to spend more time on the computer, watching television, talking on the phone, and associating with friends.[34] In a study published in 2008, researchers estimated a decrease of about 41 minutes of moderate to vigorous physical activity per year of age between the ages of 9 and 15. They found that among 9 year olds, about 90% engage in at least a couple of hours of exercise most days; whereas among 15 year olds, less than 3% do.[35] The *Wall Street Journal* brought attention to this growing epidemic of physical inactivity among young American children and emphasized the health and financial implications of this kind of behavior following into adulthood.[36]

In South Africa, the physical activity levels of children seem to be directly related to a number of factors. Those living in families of higher socioeconomic status tend to watch less television and are more physically active than those of lower socioeconomic status. Mothers with higher levels of education are more likely to have physically active children than those of lower education. Additionally, White children are more likely to be physically active, participate in physical activity classes in school, and watch less television than Black children.[37]

Physical activity levels and attitudes toward exercise among adolescent girls in Mexico as compared to adolescent girls in Spain are rather different. This demonstrates how varying geographic and cultural aspects can influence behavior. Mexican girls tend to be more physically active and are more likely to participate in sports outside of school than Spanish girls. The girls in Spain spend about half as much time exercising as the Mexican girls and engage in less nonspecified physical activities such as gymnastics. For the girls in Mexico, there seems to be more pressure from family and friends to be thin than for the girls in Spain.[38] Being more active is certainly healthier; however, exercising for the sake of fitting into the socially designed concept of beauty may contribute to poorer mental health and emotional disorders.

Further Limitations

Throughout the world, many women face sexual discrimination over multiple aspects of life. Some are discriminated against in their own homes, requiring the permission of males to pursue extracurricular activities. Those participating in professional sports are pressured by the media to appear more attractive while playing. In 2004, Sepp Blatter, the president of the Federation International Football Association (FIFA), suggested that female soccer players wear tighter shorts while competing in order to look more feminine, much like the women volleyball players.[39] A number of Christian writers blame feminists for women being able to participate in professional sports. They believe

such competitions make women appear more masculine and less attractive as they sneer, wince, push, and fight like men.[40]

The lack of campaigns and policies promoting exercise for women in various countries is a huge limitation preventing improvements in health worldwide. Social, environmental, and physical factors acting as barriers for women are often dependant on culture and location. More research needs to be conducted so that all women of the world may partake in the benefits of being more physically active.

Conclusion: Opportunities

There are a number of ways women can be encouraged to excel in physical activity, minimizing the false conceptions and notions of exercise while at the same time promoting education and self-efficacy. All over the world, there are women who feel uncomfortable exercising in public for various reasons. It may therefore be beneficial to offer separate health facilities for men and women and to provide equipment specially guided for women.

Workplace promotions for physical activity may be a good way to help provide opportunities for women to be active. For many people, a good portion of the day is spent being sedentary at a workplace. A number of well-known national and multinational companies are involving themselves in the promotion of a healthy lifestyle amongst their employees and surrounding communities. Examples of promotions offered by US companies include on-site fitness centers, subsidized gym memberships, on-site child care, telecommuting, paid sabbaticals, and compressed workweeks. Some companies also sponsor walks or special days where employees and their families can participate in physical activities. Others offer cash incentives or less expensive health insurance to employees who participate in health screenings or presentations.[41,42,43]

Public health focuses on enhancing the health status of the population. Reducing health disparities is essential to public health practice. To provide meaningful interventions, the public healthcare workforce must have an understanding of the multicultural factors influencing women's physical activity both locally and globally.

DISCUSSION QUESTIONS

1. Discuss the links between culture and physical activity in women.
2. Do certain cultures promote physical activity in women more than others?
3. Should public health professionals and providers consider their patients' cultural perspectives when promoting physical activity?
4. Can you give some examples of differences across cultures in the way women look at physical activity and implement it in their daily lives?
5. Is their a benefit from taking a culturally specific approach to promoting physical activity in women?

REFERENCES

1. Centers for Disease Control and Prevention. Physical activity for everyone. http://www.cdc.gov/nccdphp/dnpa/physical/everyone/index.htm. Accessed July 8, 2008.
2. Centers for Disease Control and Prevention. A report of the Surgeon General—physical activity and health. http://www.cdc.gov/nccdphp/sgr/sgr.htm. Accessed May 1, 2008.
3. World Health Organization. Health and development through physical activity and sport. http://libdoc.who.int/hq/2003/WHO_NMH_NPH_PAH_03.2.pdf. Accessed May 1, 2008.
4. World Health Organization. Physical activity and women. http://www.who.int/dietphysicalactivity/factsheet_women/en/. Accessed July 3, 2008.
5. Sriskantharajah J, Kai J. Promoting physical activity among South Asian women with coronary heart disease and diabetes: what might help? *Fam Pract.* 2007; 24(1):71-76; doi:10.1093/fampra/cml066.
6. Chinn DJ, White M, Harland J, Drinkwater C, Raybould S. Barriers to physical activity and socioeconomic position: implications for health promotion. *J Epidemiol Community Health.* 1999;53:191-192.
7. Andajani-Sutjahjo S, Ball K, Warren N, Inglis V, Crawford D. Perceived personal, social and environmental barriers to weight maintenance among young women: a community survey. *Int J Behav Nutr Phys Activity.* 2004;1(1):15. PMID 15462679.
8. Nies MA, Vollman M, Cook T. Facilitators, barriers, and strategies for exercise in European American women in the community. *Public Health Nurs.* 2001;15(4): 263-272.
9. Droomers M, Schrijvers CTM, Mackenbach JP. Educational level and decreases in leisure time physical activity: predictors from the longitudinal GLOBE study. *J Epidemiol Community Health.* 2001;55:562-568.
10. Eyler AE, Wilcox S, Matson-Koffman D, et al. Correlates of physical activity among women from diverse racial/ethnic groups. *J Women's Health Gender-Based Med.* 2002;11:239-253.
11. American Council on Exercise. Exercising with heart disease. http://www.acefitness.org/. Accessed May 15, 2008.

12. Duncombe D, Wertheim EH, Skouteris H, Paxton SJ, Kelly L. Factors related to exercise over the course of pregnancy including women's beliefs about the safety of exercise during pregnancy. *Midwifery*. 2007. PMID: 18063253.

13. Puoane T, Bradley H, Hughes G. Obesity among black South African women. *Hum Ecol*. 2005;13:91-95.

14. Joubert J, Norman R, Lambert E, et al. Estimating the burden of disease attributable to physical inactivity in South Africa in 2000. *S Afr Med J*. 2007;97:725-731.

15. Rguibi M, Belahsen R. High blood pressure in urban Moroccan Sahraoui women. *J Hypertens*. 2007;25:1363-1368.

16. Griffiths P, Bentley M. Women of higher socio-economic status are more likely to be overweight in Karnataka, India. *Euro J Clin Nutr*. 2005;59:1217-1220.

17. Wen LM, Thomas M, Jones H, et al. Promoting physical activity in women: evaluation of a 2-year community-based intervention in Sydney, Australia. *Health Promot Int*. 2002;17:127-137.

18. Andajani-Sutjahjo S, Ball K, Warren N, Inglis V, Crawford D. Perceived personal, social and environmental barriers to weight maintenance among young women: a community survey. *Int J Behav Nutr Phys Activity*. 2004;1:15. PMCID: PMC524367.

19. Baron-Epel O, Haviv A, Garty N, Tamir D, Green M. Who are the sedentary people in Israel? A public health indicator. *Isr Med Assoc J*. 2005;7:694-699.

20. Maddah M, Eshraghian MR, Djazayery A, Mirdamadi R. Association of body mass index with educational level in Iranian men and women. *Euro J Clin Nutr*. 2003;57:819-823.

21. Bryan S, Walsh P. Physical activity and obesity in Canadian women. *BMC Women's Health*. 2004;4:S6. http://www.biomedcentral.com/1472-6874/4/S1/S6. Accessed April 2, 2008.

22. Canadian Heritage. Official languages. http://www.patrimoinecanadien.gc.ca/progs/lool/pubs/census2001/tdm_e.cfm. Accessed July 18, 2008.

23. Sanchez-Johnsen L, Fitzgibbon ML, Martinovich Z, Stolley MR, Dyer AR, Van Horn L. Ethnic differences in correlates of obesity between Latin-American and Black women. *Obes Res*. 2004;12:652-660.

24. Wilcox S, Castro C, King AC, Housemann R, Brownson R. Determinants of leisure time physical activity in rural compared with urban older and ethnically diverse women in the United States. *J Epidemiol Community Health*. 2000;54:667-672.

25. Thornton PL, Kieffer EC, Salabarria-Pena Y, et al. Weight, diet, and physical activity-related beliefs and practices among pregnant and postpartum Latino women: the role of social support. *Matern Child Health J*. 2006;10(1):95-104

26. CDC. Physical activity among adults with a disability—United States, 2005. *MMWR*. 2007;56(39):1021-1024. http://www.cdc.gov/mmwR/preview/mmwrhtml/mm5639a2.htm. Accessed May 16, 2008.

27. CDC. Physical activity for women with disabilities. http://www.cdc.gov/ncbddd/women/physical.htm. Accessed May 28, 2008.

28. CDC. Women with disabilities. http://www.cdc.gov/ncbddd/women/default.htm. Accessed May 28, 2008.

29. Finnish Disabled People's International Development Association. Disability and development. http://www.fidida.fi/. Accessed June 15, 2008.

30. American Heart Association, Robert Wood Johnson Foundation. *A Nation at Risk: Obesity in the United States, A Statistical Sourcebook*. Dallas, TX: American Heart Foundation; 2005.

31. Prevention of pediatric overweight and obesity. *Am Acad Pediatr*. 2003;112(2):424-430.

32. Pivarnik, J, Pfeiffer, K. The importance of physical activity for children and adolescents. http://michiganfitness.org/Publications/documents/Adolescents.pdf. Accessed March 10, 2007.

33. Hogan, M. Media education offers help on children's body image problems. *Am Acad Pediatr*. http://www.aap.org/advocacy/hogan599.htm. Accessed March 16, 2007.

34. Schoenberg J, Salmond K, Fleshman P. Girl Scouts of the United States of America. The new normal? what girls say about healthy living. New York: Girl Scouts of the USA; 2006.

35. Nadir PR, Bradley RH, Houts RM, McRitchie SL, O'Brien M. Moderate-to-vigorous physical activity from ages 9 to 15 years. *JAMA*. 2008;300(3):295-305.

36. Children sharply cut back on exercise once they're teens. *Wall Street Journal*. July 16, 2008. http://online.wsj.com/article/SB121617562658757025.html. Accessed July 25, 2008.

37. McVeigh JA, Norris SA, de Wet T. The relationship between socio-economic status and physical activity patterns in South African children. *Acta Paediatrica*. 2004;93:982-988.

38. Toro HJ, Gomez-Peresmitre G, Sentis, J et al. Eating disorders and body image in Spanish and Mexican female adolescents. *Soc Psychiatry Psychiatr Epidemiol*. 2006;41:556-565.

39. Christenson M, Kelso P. Soccer chief's plan to boost women's game? Hotpants. *The Guardian*. http://www.guardian.co.uk/uk/2004/jan/16/football.gender. Accessed July 12, 2008.

40. Jonas S. Should women play sports? http://www.jesus-is-savior.com/Womens%20Page/christian_women_and_sports.htm. Accessed June 1, 2008.

41. 100 best companies to work for 2008. *Fortune*. http://money.cnn.com/magazines/fortune/bestcompanies/2008/full_list/index.html. Accessed June 12, 2008.

42. The Horizon Foundation. Horizon-Chamber collaboration brings wellness to the workplace. http://www.thehorizonfoundation.org/ht/d/sp/i/1152/pid/1152. Accessed July 17, 2008.

43. Owen M. Case managers play important part in employers' culture of health. *Case Manager*. 2006;15(3):53-55.

A Woman's Sexuality

Jean L. Fourcory, MD, PhD, MPH

Women's health status is affected by complex biological, social, and cultural factors, which are interrelated and can only be addressed in a comprehensive manner. Reproductive health is determined not only by the quality and availability of health care, but also by socioeconomic development levels, lifestyles, and women's positions in society.[1]

The question of a woman's sexuality must be understood within the confines of her culture and environment. Culture as well as social and religious mores play an important role in the acceptance and achievement of normal sexual function for both men and women. Culture dictates a woman's freedom during her entire life span, from marriage, pregnancy, and menses and postpartum. Cultural mores identify specific customs that should or must be followed. Thus tradition, law, education, and the status of women are important indicators of sexual health. Sexuality is a right for every woman, and it should be on her own terms.[2–4] In responding to a woman's problems one must try to understand the role of the culture she lives in, the religion that controls her, and the violence that surrounds her. These factors are essential in responding to her needs; they are essential to understanding her needs.

Jean Fourcroy MD, PhD, MPH, is Staff Urologist at Walter Reed Army Medical Center and The Uniformed Services University of Health Sciences. Dr. Fourcroy is an honored physician in the National Library of Medicine exhibit on women physicians that have "changed the face of medicine" and a recipient of the Camille Mermod Award from the American Medical Women's Association.

The Right to Reproductive and Sexual Health

Sexual health is a state of physical, emotional, mental, and social well-being related to sexuality; it is not merely the absence of disease, dysfunction, or infirmity.[5] Sexual health requires a positive and respectful approach to sexuality and sexual relationships, as well as the possibility of having pleasurable and safe sexual experiences. A sexual experience must be free of coercion, discrimination, and violence. For a large number of women discrimination and violence are part of their lives. For sexual health to be attained and maintained, the sexual rights of all persons must be respected, protected, and fulfilled.[2] Sexual rights embrace human rights that are already recognized in international human rights documents, national laws, and other consensus documents. These include the right of all persons to be free of coercion, discrimination, and violence. Education of women may be the most important socioeconomic piece of the puzzle to preserve the sexual health of women.[6–8] Many cultures and religions, often unconsciously, control women, limit their options, and make them subordinate to men. A serious approach to reproductive health has to have this cultural perspective to liberate women.[9]

Sexual health assumes that each individual is able to do the following:

■ Receive the highest attainable standard of health in relation to sexuality, including access to sexual and reproductive healthcare services

■ Seek, receive, and impart information in relation to sexuality

■ Have sexuality education

■ Have respect for bodily integrity

■ Have a choice of partner

■ Decide whether to be sexually active or not

■ Have consensual sexual relations and/or marriage

■ Decide whether or not, and when, to have children

■ Pursue a satisfying, safe, and pleasurable sexual life

The responsible exercise of human rights requires that all persons respect the rights of others.[10]

Cultural issues and social mores play an important role in the acceptance and achievement of normal sexual function for both men and women. Tradition, law, education, and the status of women are important indicators of the reproductive function of and freedom of women.[11-13] Cultural mores dictate women's freedom during her entire life span. A woman's expectations for her body beauty may affect her ability to have a meaningful sexual life. Sexual self-consciousness can affect a woman's sexual arousability and pleasure.[14]

Female Genital Cutting or Female Genital Mutilation (FGC/FGM)

FGC has been called the "Three Feminine Sorrows": the sorrow on the day of the mutilation, that of the wedding night, and that with the birth of a baby. These sorrows relate to pain associated at each point of time in a woman's life.[15]

To understand the impact of a cultural custom on a woman's sexuality one must understand the origin, perpetuation, and prevalence of the custom as well as an understanding of the procedure itself. Only then can one begin to understand the impact of this procedure on a woman's sexuality. One important example is female genital cutting. Does female genital cutting or female genital mutilation (FGC/FGM) affect female sexuality? The current preferred term is *female genital cutting* (FGC), but both female genital mutilation (FGM) and female circumcision (FGC) can be and are used interchangeably.

What Is FGC/FGM?

The origin of female cutting rituals cannot be traced but appears to have been practiced as early as the time of the Egyptian pharaohs. Even though FGC/FGM is practiced in mostly Islamic countries, it is not an Islamic practice and does not appear to have a religious connection. FGC/FGM is practiced by Muslims and non-Muslims alike residing in sub-Saharan countries and throughout Africa and the Middle East.[16]

FGC/FGM is thought to preserve a family's honor and prevent promiscuity and immorality. Virginity of the girl-child is economically important and probably dates back to the days of a nomadic existence. However, it is claimed that the custom is perpetuated because a circumcised woman would provide[s] more sexual pleasure for her husband. In a given community when the majority of women have been circumcised, those who are not are considered abnormal by themselves or their families. It is a mark of cultural identity. Within a culture FGC/FGM is a powerful marker and affirms a woman's identity in that culture. To be circumcised is to be normal. Belonging to the culture has tremendous significance in terms of the desirability of a young woman for marriage, which provides a major means for achieving economic strength and independence; thus, being unsuitable for marriage affects the ability of her family to prosper. The procedure is believed to ensure cleanliness, chastity, and to minimize the sexual appetite of women and thus reduce the likelihood that they will bring shame on themselves or their families through sexual indiscretions. These guarantees of a young woman's purity further enhance her attractiveness to potential suitors.[16-19]

The term *female circumcision* is clearly inaccurate and refers to the removal of part of the male prepuce. The World Health Organization (WHO) has defined FGC/FGM as all procedures that involve the partial or total removal of the female external genitalia and/or injury to the female genital organs for cultural or any other nontherapeutic reasons.[2] FGC/FGM refers to a spectrum of surgical excisions from partial to complete clitoridectomy including the removal of labia minora and/or majora, scarifying the remnants, and even, at times, inserting a match stick to maintain a sufficient opening for urination. The cutting is usually done in infancy or before puberty but varies from tribe to tribe even within a country. It is a rite of passage and a physical marking of a woman's marriageability, the insurance of virginity, and the formation of a chastity belt of her own tissue. The perpetuation of this custom is difficult to understand since the risks to the health of women are so great but harm is not the intention.

The procedure can be classified according to the extent of the excision: Type I, often referred to as "Sunna circumcision"' involves the removal of only the clitoral prepuce, which would be similar to a male circumcision, but is very difficult in a small girl. More traditional are Types II, III, and IV excisions that are more damaging to the external genitalia. Extensive genital excisions may require that the girl remain with her legs bound together from hip to ankle for a period of one month and longer to ensure the adequate formation of scar tissue around the raw edges of the labia.[5,15,20-29] Associated complications can be either immediate or delayed. At the time of the procedure hemorrhage, shock, infection, and even septicemia and death are possible; severe pain because of the lack of anesthesia can contribute to shock and death. Urinary retention is often an immediate result of the procedure.

Although the age of circumcision ranges from newborn to adult years, it is primarily a prepubertal custom done while the child is held down by a family member. Most girls undergo FGM when they are between 7 and 10 years old. However, FGM seems to be occurring at earlier ages in several countries because parents want to reduce the trauma to their children. They also want to avoid government interference and/or resistance from children as they get older and form their own opinions. Some women undergo FGM during early adulthood when marrying into a community that practices FGM or just before or after the birth of a first child.[30,31] When one considers the anatomy of the underdeveloped prepubertal female external genitalia, one can begin to understand the associated adverse events. It is a procedure done without anesthesia, sterile instruments, or visual accuracy. Miscalculations are disastrous. The clitoris, like the penis, is rich in vascular, lymphatic, and neural supply and extensive bleeding is common.

Classification of the procedures includes the following:

- Type I, also known as "Sunna," involves the excision of the prepuce and partial or total clitoridectomy.
- Type II involves removal of the clitoris and partial or total excision of the labia minora.
- Type III, also known as "pharonic," involves clitoridectomy, excision of the labia minora and majora. Infibulation is the reapproximation of the cut ends.
- Type IV involves other forms of genital manipulation, such as burning, pricking, or piercing.

Where Is It Practiced?

FGC/FGM is practiced in at least 26 of 43 African countries; the prevalence varies from 98% in Somalia to 5% in Zaire. A review of country-specific demographic and health surveys (DHS) shows FGM prevalence rates of 97% in Egypt, 94.5% in Eritrea, 93.7% in Mali,[10] 89.2% in Sudan,[11] and 43.4% in the Central African Republic. FGM is also found among some ethnic groups in Oman, the United Arab Emirates, and Yemen, as well as in parts of India, Indonesia, and Malaysia.[32] It is important to remember that within one country tribes or cultures may vary in the practice or the type of cutting that they practice.[33]

A review of country-specific demographic and health surveys defines the FGC/FGM prevalence rates globally which is maintained by the US State Department.[34] FGC/FGM has become an important issue in Australia, Canada, England, France, and the United States due to the continuation of the practice by immigrants from countries where FGC/FGM is common. Patterns of immigration have spread this ritual worldwide. Estimates of the prevalence of FGC/FGM in the United States have been made based on prevalence of these families throughout the country. It was estimated in 1990, that nearly 168,000 immigrant women and girls in the United States had either undergone FGC/FGM or were at risk for this practice.[32,33,36] Although US (Federal Prohibition of Female Genital Mutilation Act of 1996) and Canadian law as well as many state laws prohibit the circumcision of any woman under the age of 18 years, there are still many women in this country who have undergone this ritual procedure.[18,34,36]

Why Is It Practiced?

The proponents of FGC/FGM believe the following:

- The ritual reinforces a woman's place in her given society.
- The ritual establishes eligibility for marriage.
- The ritual initiates a girl into womanhood.
- Female genitals are unhygienic and in need of cleaning.
- Female genitals are ugly and will grow unwieldy if not cut back.
- The ritual safeguards virginity.
- The ritual prevents maternal and infant mortality.
- The ritual improves fertility.
- The ritual enhances a husband's sexual pleasure.

Reasons for supporting FGM include the beliefs that it is a "good tradition," a religious requirement(s), or a necessary rite of passage to womanhood; that it ensures cleanliness or better marriage prospects, prevents promiscuity and excessive clitoral growth, preserves virginity, enhances male sexuality, and facilitates childbirth by widening the birth canal.

Does It Alter Her Sexuality?

There are many complications following FGC/FGM. Some are immediate, such as death, while others appear later. The occlusion superior to the imperforate hymen can be a most disastrous complication when a girl presents with an enlarging abdominal mass and apparent amenorrhea, when virginity was the goal of the procedure. The urological complications are related to the extent of the adnexal damage from infection, bleeding, or wideness of the excision of the clitoris and adnexal labia. Either incontinence, because of loss of sphincter function, or urethral stenosis and inability to void appropriately can result. Delayed gynecological complications include hematocolpos, menstrual disorders, vaginal stenosis, and future infertility or sterility. The latter will be associated with increased urinary infections because of the relative or complete obstruction. Obstetrical complications include prolonged labor and fistula formation between the vagina and the bladder or urethra because of the prolonged labor secondary to the altered birth canal.[28,30,37-40] Late appearing scars include dermoid inclusions, neuromas, vulvar cysts and abscesses, and keloid formation.[41-43] All of these are especially troublesome and painful when nerve endings become entrapped. Sexual scars also include the pain and fear that may accompany intercourse and can lead to marital problems. Depression and other psychiatric complications may be secondary to a system built on distrust. The person holding the child at the time of the procedure was usually a trusted family member such as the mother; this break in trust has long-term effects on child and parent.

I know of no other cultural mandate so harmful to children and women. One example was foot binding of women in China which was swiftly abandoned. Today it is more appropriate to have a festival rite of passage, not a virginity procedure or hymen clean job. The Kuna Indians of San Blas Islands have a festival, not a cutting, marking the maturation of their girls. Are there other surgical procedures that should be considered? Cosmetic beautification or the quest for the perfect body image is not a new phenomenon; however, the surgical utilization of this desire has exploded. Is there a desperate quest for physical transformation—transformation to the dream world?[44,45] Most of the body beautification schemes are built on cultural expectations. Hymenography is illegal in most Arab countries, but it is performed unofficially; specialists undertake five or six procedures weekly. The trade in hymen repairs maybe justifiable in certain circumstances when the woman would otherwise suffer disgrace or worse. Nonvirgin brides may be killed by their brothers, uncles, or even father. It is a cultural custom.

Does FGC/FGM Allow Women to Have a Normal and Fulfilling Sexual Relationship?

The complications of FGC/FGM can obviously affect a woman's sexuality. However, there is little research on the effects of these procedures on a woman's sexuality. The removal of a woman's external sexual organs (such as the clitoris), and infibulation may leave the woman with little sexually sensitive genital tissue. Although FGC/FGM does not affect the hormones that contribute to sexual arousal, the missing structures and tissue can have a negative effect on sexual desire, arousal, pleasure, or satisfaction. Other sexually sensitive parts of the body, such as the breasts, nipples, lips, neck, and earlobes, may become increasingly sensitive in women who have undergone FGC to make up for the lack of clitoral stimulation.[7,46]

The type and depth of the genital cut also affect sexual responsiveness. Each of these factors plays an important role in the sexual life of women with FGC/FGM. Although Type 1 may be practiced in one culture, the cutter may have lost aim with a screaming child. It has been reported that women with Type I were unaffected while those with Type III were significantly affected.[46] Anecdotal reports confirm some of the problems. One woman is reported as saying: "When I make love with my husband, I can't handle it. I don't want to see him because I have a lot of pain."[18,27] Women with extensive FGC/FGM may find vaginal intercourse impossible. Women are fertile although

sexual intercourse is impeded. Childbirth also requires appropriate care, including anesthesia and a midlongitudinal cut to avoid extensive tearing and obstetrical delay.[28,47] Nour notes that the two main causes of infertility are anatomic and psychologic barriers.[28] Women with type III have infertility rates as high as 25–30%. Dyspareunia and the inability to achieve penetration can create stress and frustration in a couple's sexual life.

Gruenbaum[23] concluded "The effect of female circumcision on sexuality is not uniform or sufficiently well understood." It would appear that the various forms of female circumcisions are not equally devastating to female sexuality. There can be no doubt that many of the circumcision practices do affect physical well-being, including the woman's sexual responsiveness. Psychological aspects of sexuality must also affect sexual responses. The trauma of circumcision may always influence a woman's sex life. Lightfoot-Klein reported that "close to 90% of Sudanese women interviewed claimed to achieve, or had at some time in their lives, achieved orgasm."[25,48] It should be observed that orgasmic responses may vary according to the amount of tissue removed and variation in erogenous stimulation as well as cultural expectations.

Coital frequency has been used as a surrogate marker of normal sexual function; unfortunately, there is no way to identify in these studies who initiated the act.[38] In one study, Nigerian women attending family planning and antenatal clinics were given a structured questionnaire that asked the frequency of orgasm achieved during sexual intercourse and symptoms of reproductive tract infections. Forty-five percent of the women were circumcised including 71% with Type I and 24% with Type II. The researchers found no significant differences between cut and uncut women in the frequency of reports of sexual intercourse, the frequency of reports of early arousal during intercourse, and the proportions reporting experience of orgasm during intercourse. Uncut women were significantly more likely to report that the clitoris was the most sexually sensitive part of their body while cut women were more likely to report that their breasts were their most sexually sensitive body parts. Cut women were significantly more likely than uncut women to report having lower abdominal pain and vaginal discharge. Female genital cutting in this group of women did not attenuate sexual feelings. However, female genital cutting may predispose women to adverse sexuality outcomes including early pregnancy and reproductive tract infections. Depression may be an important sequelae of FGC/FGM and would also be an important marker on the perception of a women's sexuality. No research has been done to determine the effect of depression on sexuality in these women.

Do Male Expectations Determine the Prevalence of FGC/FGM and the Sexual Response of the Woman?

"If men say they don't want the external genitalia then women won't want to have it."[23] An important aspect of assumed male sexual pleasure is the culturally defined anatomical appearance. Male preference is for smoothness of the vulva in cultures practicing female circumcision, and there is an added fear that a husband may find one's body distasteful if the vulva is not smooth. Female sexual desires may reflect the cultural norm set by men. In many of these cultures the fidelity of the partners will be an important aspect of a woman's sexuality. Does the presence of multiple partners outside the home effect a woman's sexual response? Partner reduction has been an important part of HIV reduction.[49] The acceptance and availability of prostitutes in a particular country will also be important determinants.

The role of FGC/FGM in the normal cycle of sexuality is unclear. It is also difficult to look with Western eyes to understand. Although FGC/FGM is supposed to control sexuality before marriage, these same women are expected to be sexually responsive to their spouses in marriage. Coital difficulty or inability to have vaginal intercourse at all because of stenosis of the vagina may affect up to 35% of pharaonically circumcised women, and dyspareunia may be common. It is probable that sexual pain disorders may play a role and have an indirect effect on desire, arousal, and orgasmic sexual responses. Sexual dysfunction is highly associated with negative experiences in sexual relationships and overall well-being. Sexual complications include the pain and fear that may accompany sexual intercourse, which can lead to marital problems. Variations in sexual behavior may well be unrelated to the type of FGM, but instead reflect differences in the social characteristics of the participants.[31]

Cultural sensitivity in addressing these problems with a circumcised woman is critical. Most immigrant women do not feel comfortable discussing intimate problems with healthcare workers they view as strangers. Toubia[7] cautions healthcare workers to first assume that satisfactory sexual and emotional relationships exist in couples regardless of the degree of the women's genital cutting. In interviews with genitally cut women it was found they have experienced orgasm at some time. Their statements were "qualified by the fact that they were not always sexually satisfied and it was the nature of the relationship and the sensitivity of the partner that made the difference." Many couples can have a fulfilling relationship because of the deep emotional bond, camaraderie, and social compatibility even if the sexual aspect is missing.

In many of the cultures practicing FGC/FGM a dry vagina is also deemed important. The role of agents thought to dry and tighten a woman's vagina and serve as love potions to attract sexual partners and ensure their faithfulness is unclear. It is presumed that these agents draw out moisture, but such astringent agents may be important to reduce secretions from vaginal infections.[50-53]

> The Qur'an does refer to the sexual relationship in marriage as one of mutual satisfaction that is considered a mercy from Allah.[16]

Does Religion Play a Role in Her Enjoyment?

There is little information on the role of religion in control of a woman's sexuality and pleasure. We are reminded that the opening chapters of Genesis, according to some readers, establish woman as second in creation and thus inferior to man and also the first to disobey. This reading fosters the perception that women are intrinsically disruptive, disorderly, and unclean. Recent feminist reinterpretations of Genesis have not influenced those most comfortable with a male-oriented theology and a hierarchically structured marriage. Without suggesting that such attitudes about women's place, duty, and nature condone violence, these interpretations can make violence seem tenable as a vehicle to subdue what the man might interpret as disorder.[54]

It is important to acknowledge the tremendous diversity of beliefs, teachings, and traditions that exist among the many religions of the world. Whether Roman Catholic, Jewish, Protestant, Orthodox Christian, Muslim, Buddhist, Hindu, Native American, First Nations, as well as many others, religion is an important part of a woman's culture and environment and must be considered. A comprehensive exploration of the relationship between religion and violence against women is beyond the scope of this chapter. Yet, there are some basic issues, questions, teachings, and new interpretations to minimize the roadblocks and maximize the resources for religiously identified women. No woman should ever be forced to choose between her safety and her religious community or tradition. She should be able to access the resources of both community-based advocacy and shelter *and* faith-based support and counsel. For her to do so, she needs these two resources to work collaboratively so that they can provide consistent advocacy and support for victims and survivors and participate in the process of holding perpetrators accountable. Among the many world religions, Christianity, Judaism, and Islam, for example, incorporate beliefs and practices that vary greatly in their impact on women and their choices. Are there specific religious laws that tell her when she must be submissive, when she can have enjoyment—how she participates and what pleasure she must give only to the man?

> Countless women remain in harsh constraint established by religions, families, doctors, husbands, the police, needy children, the court of public and private opinion, their own beliefs, and prejudice. [55]

What Is the Aftermath of Physical and Mental Control or Violence?

The most important global health issue for women is violence. As a result of violence it is thought that women are not reaching their full potential. Violence is a commonplace phenomenon. There are too many ways that violence can hinder or prevent a woman's enjoyment. Violence can occur as part of childhood abuse, as rape as a weapon of war, or by her intimate partner. Four million women are believed to be battered every year by their partners. At least one-fifth of all women will be physically assaulted by a partner or ex-partner during their lifetime. There is no universally accepted def-

inition of violence against women. However, a group of international experts convened by WHO in February 1996 agreed that the definition adopted by the United Nations General Assembly provides a useful framework for the organization's activities. The Declaration on the Elimination of Violence against Women (1993) defines violence against women as "any act of gender-based violence that results in, or is likely to result in, physical, sexual, or mental harm or suffering to women, including threats of such acts, coercion, or arbitrary deprivation of liberty, whether occurring in public or in private life." This encompasses, inter alia, "physical, sexual, and psychological violence occurring in the family and in the general community, including battering, sexual abuse of children, dowry-related violence, rape, female genital mutilation, and other traditional practices harmful to women; nonspousal violence and violence related to exploitation; sexual harassment and intimidation at work, in educational institutions, and elsewhere; trafficking in women; forced prostitution, and violence perpetrated or condoned by the state."[56]

In different parts of the world, between 16% and 52% of women suffer physical violence from their male partners, and at least one in five women suffer rape or attempted rape in their lifetimes. It is also well known that rape and sexual torture are systematically used as weapons of war. Violence negates women's autonomy and undermines their potential as individuals and members of society. Domestic violence is believed to be the most common cause of serious injury to women and accounts for more than 40% of female homicide cases. Women of every age face the threat of violence, abuse, and assault. Current estimates indicate that 1 of 5 girls is sexually abused, and the peak ages of such abuse are from 8 to 12 years of age. Violence has no class or age boundaries. At every age in the life span, females are more likely to be sexually or physically assaulted by father, brother, family member, neighbor, boyfriend, husband, partner, or ex-partner than by a stranger or anonymous assailant. Violence and abuse knows no economic or cultural barriers. [57-65]

The need for more research on the connection between human rights, legal and economic issues, and the public health dimensions of violence is clear. A rapidly growing body of evidence demonstrates that women's experience of violence has direct consequences not only for their own well-being, but also for that of their families and communities. In addition to broken bones, third-degree burns, and other bodily injuries, abuse can have long-term mental health consequences, including depression, suicide attempts, and post-traumatic stress disorder. Violence involving sexual assault may also cause sexually transmitted diseases, unwanted pregnancies, and other sexual and reproductive health problems. For girls, the health consequences are carried into their adult lives. Violence against women can also have intergenerational repercussions. For example, boys who witness their mothers being beaten by their partners are more likely than other boys to use violence to solve disagreements in their own adult lives. Girls who witness the same sorts of violence are more likely than other girls to become involved in relationships in which their partners abuse them. Thus, violence tends to be carried over from one generation to the next.

The healthcare system has an important role to play along with many other sectors, such as the judicial, police, and social services. However, those systems are largely ill prepared to deal with the consequences of violence or even recognize the signs. Healthcare workers must be trained to recognize both the obvious and the more subtle signs of violence, and to meet women's health needs in this regard. From a public health perspective, it is equally important that strong prevention programs and well-coordinated legal and social support services are in place. Mandatory reporting systems are present in many states and were initiated to provide a better system for the providers and the abused; however, the very act of reporting may put the abused at a greater risk.

Both worldwide and in the United States, violence to women robs half of our population of achieving their full potential. Why are we missing so much, and how can we change it in the future? The Constitution of the World Health Organization declares that "the enjoyment of the highest at-

tainable standard of health is one of the fundamental rights of every human being." Yet worldwide mortality and morbidity data suggest that this right has not been achieved by the half of the world's population that are women. Some of the reasons for this are *abuse, assault, battering, beating, betrayal, control, the Sequelae squeal of trauma,* and *posttraumatic stress syndrome.*

Conclusion

A woman's sexuality must be understood within the confines of her culture and environment, although we have minimal scientific research to help us. Providing health and sexual rights for women and girls is fundamental to achieving lasting humane and equitable development. It is necessary to provide women and girls with better access to health, education, and financial resources to break the cycle of poverty that entraps them, their families, and their communities. Women and girls should not be experiencing violence in any form. When working with women and girls we must remember: An estimated 1600 women die every day from complications caused by pregnancy and childbirth, 99% in developing countries. Each year, approximately 2 million girls are at risk of female genital mutilation. About 70,000 women die every year from unsafe abortions, and many more suffer infections and other consequences. Domestic violence, rape, and sexual abuse are a significant cause of disability among women.[9]

I am reminded that the body mends soon enough. Only the physical scars remain. Unfortunately the wounds inflicted upon the soul take much longer to heal. Throughout her life, her culture, environment, and past experiences affect a woman's expectations. As providers we must remember this when working with women around the world.

DISCUSSION QUESTIONS

1. Are sexual rights human rights, and how should they be recognized internationally?
2. Is a woman's sexual health altered by the culture or religion she lives in?
3. What is a woman's sexual health?

REFERENCES

1. International Monetary Population fund. http://www.imf.org/external/index.htm. Accessed April 8, 2008.
2. World Health Organization. Constitution and fact sheets: FGC/FGM. http://www.WHO.int. Accessed March 25, 2008.
3. Basson R, Leiblum S, Brotto L, et al. Definitions of women's sexual dysfunction reconsidered: advocating expansion and revision. *JPsychosom Obstet Gynaecol*. 2003; 24(4):221-229.
4. Fourcroy JL. Customs, culture, and tradition—what role do they play in a woman's sexuality? *J Sex Med*. 2006;3:954-959.
5. Cook RJ. *Women's Health and Human Rights*. Geneva, Switzerland: WHO;1994.
6. Okonofu FE, Larsen U, Oronsaye F, Snow RC, Slanger TE. The association between female genital cutting and correlates of sexual and gynaecological morbidity in Edo State, Nigeria. *BJOG*. 2002;109(10):1089-1096.
7. Rainbo. Health and Rights for African women. http://www.rainbo.org. Accessed April 8, 2008.
8. United Nations Web site. http://www.un.org. Accessed April 8, 2008.
9. United Nations Population Fund. Women—the right to reproductive and sexual health. http://www.un.org/ecosocdev/geninfo/women/womrepro.htm. Accessed April 8, 2008.
10. World Health Organization. Sexual health. http://www.who.int/reproductive-health/gender/sexualhealth. Accessed April 8, 2008.
11. Osaku, GI, Martin-Hilber A. *Women's Sexuality and Fertility; Nigeria Breaking the Culture of Silence. Negotiating Reproductive Rights: Women's Perspectives Across Countries and Cultures*. New York: Zed Books;1998:180-216.
12. Petchesky, RP, Judd K. *Negotiating Reproductive Rights*. London: ZED; 2001.
13. Wolff B, Blanc AK, Gage, A, et al. Who decides? Women's status and negotiation of sex in Uganda. *Culture, Health Sex*. 2000;2:303-322.
14. Odoms-Young A. Factors that influence body image representations of black Muslim women. *Soc Sci Med; 66* (12); 2008:2573-2584.
15. Fourcroy JL. The Three Feminine Sorrows. *Hosp Pract. 33* 1998:15-21.
16. Muslim women's League http://www.mwlusa.org/publications/positionpapers/fgm.html. Accessed April 8, 2008.
17. Fourcroy JL. L'eternal couteau: review of female circumcision. *Urology*. 1983; 22:458-61.
18. Morris RJ, Gulino C, eds. *Curriculum—Reproductive Health Promotion in Special Populations. Presentations and preparation*. San Diego, CA: San Diego State University; 2001.

19. Wasunna A. Towards redirecting the female circumcision debate: legal, ethical and cultural Considerations. *McGill J Med.* 2000;5:104-110.

20. Elchalai U, Ben-ami B, Brzezinski A. Female circumcision: the peril remains. *BJU Int.* 1999;83(Suppl 1):103-108.

21. El Saadawi N. *The Hidden Face of Eve. Women in the Arab World.* Boston: Boston Press; 1980.

22. World Health Organization. Regional Office for the Eastern Mediterranean. Background papers to the WHO Seminar. Traditional practices affecting the Health of women and children. WHO/EMRO Technical Publication no. 2, vol. 2. Alexandria, Egypt: WHO; 1982.

23. Gruenbaum E. *The Female Circumcision Controversy. An Anthropological Perspective.* Philadelphia: University of Pennsylvania Press; 2001.

24. Lightfoot-Klein H. *A Woman's Odyssey into Africa.* New York: Haworth Press; 1992.

25. Lightfoot-Klein H. *Prisoners of Ritual. An Odyssey into Female Genital Circumcision in Africa.* Binghamton, NY: Haworth Press; 1989.

26. Morris R. The culture of female circumcision. *Adv Nurs Sci.* 1996;19(2):43-53.

27. Morris R. Female genital mutilation: perspectives, risks, and complications. *Urologic Nurs.* 1999;19(1):13-19.

28. Nour NM. Female genital cutting: clinical and cultural guidelines. *Obstet Gynecol Surv.* 2004;59(4):272-279.

29. Toubia N. Female circumcision as a public health issue. *N Engl J Med.* 1994;331:712-716.

30. Slanger TE, Snow RC, Okonofua FE. The impact of female genital cutting on first delivery in southwest Nigeria. *Stud Fam Plann.* 2002;33(2):173-184.

31. Van Rossem R, Gage AJ. The effects of female genital mutilation on the onset of sexual activity and marriage in Guinea. *Arch Sex Behav.* 2007(2):113-20.

32. PATH. http://www.path.org/africa.php. Accessed April 8, 2008.

33. The Female Genital Cutting Education and Networking Project. http://www.fgmnetwork.org. Accessed April 8, 2008.

34. US Department of State. http://www.state.gov. Accessed April 8, 2008.

35. Jones WK, Smith J, Kieke B Jr, Wilcox L. Female genital mutilation. Female circumcision. Who is at risk in the U.S.? *Public Health Rep.* 1997;112(5):368-377.

36. Federal Prohibition of Female Genital Mutilation Act of 1996. http://www.mgmbill.org/usfgmlaw.htm. Accessed April 8, 2008.

37. Banks E, Meirik O, Farley T, Akande O, Bathija H, Ali M. Female genital mutilation and obstetric outcome: WHO collaborative prospective study in six African countries. *Lancet.* 2006;367(9525):1835-1841.

38. Okonofu FE, Larsen U, Oronsaye F, Snow RC, Slanger TE. The association between female genital cutting and correlates of sexual and gynaecological morbidity in Edo State, Nigeria. *BJOG.* 2002;109(10):1089-1096.

39. Okonofua FE. Female circumcision and obstetric complications. *Int J Gynaecol Obstet.* 2002;77(3):255-265.

40. Rushwan, H. Female genital mutilation (FGM) management during pregnancy, childbirth and the postpartum period. *Int J Gynecol Obstetr.* 2000;70:99-104.

41. Fernandez-Aguilar S, Noel JC. Neuroma of the clitoris after female genital cutting. *Obstet Gynecol.* 2003;101(5 Pt 2):1053-1054.

42. Nour NM. Female genital cutting: a need for reform. *Obstet Gynecol.* 2003;101(5):1051-1052.

43. Yoong WC, Shakya R, Sanders BT, Lind J. Clitoral inclusion cyst: a complication of Type I female genital mutilation. *J Obstet Gynaecol.* 2004;24(1):98-99.

44. Goodman MP, Bachmann G, Johnson C, et al. Is elective vulvar plastic surgery ever warranted, and what screening should be conducted preoperatively? *J Sex Med*. 2007;4(2):269-276.

45. Logmans A, Verhoeff A, Bol Raap R, Creighton F, van Lent M. Should doctors reconstruct the vaginal introitus of adolescent girls to mimic the virginal state? Who wants the procedure and why. *BMJ*. 1998;316:459-460.

46. Thabet S, Thabet A. Defective sexuality and female circumcision: the cause and the possible management. *J Obstet Gynecol RES*. 2003;29:12-19.

47. Chen G, Dharia S, Steinkampf MP, Callison S. Infertility from female circumcision. *Fertility Sterility*. 2004;81(6):1692-1694.

48. Lightfoot-Klein H. The sexual adjustment of genitally circumcised and infibulated females in the Sudan. *J Sex Res*. 1989;26(3):375-392.

49. Epstein H. The fidelity fix. *New York Times* [magazine section]. 2004.

50. Brown, JE, Ayowa OB, Brown RC. Dry and tight: sexual practices and potential AIDS risk in Zaire. *Soc Sci Med*. 1993;37:989-994.

51. Brown RC, Brown JE, et al. Vaginal inflammation in Africa [letter]. *N Engl J Med*. 1992;327:572.

52. Brown RC, Brown JE, Ayopwa OB. The use and physical effects of intravaginal substances in Zairian women. *Sex Transm Dis*. 1993;20:96-99.

53. Dallabetta GA, Miotti PG, Chiphangwi JD et al. Traditional vaginal agents: use and association with HIV infection in Malawian women. *AIDS*. 1995;9:293-297.

54. The Park Ridge Center for Health, Faith and Ethics. http://www.parkridgecenter.org/Page385.html. Accessed April 8, 2008.

55. Tiger L. *The Decline of Males*. Golden Books Paperback. New York;1999.

56. United Nations. Declaration on the Elimination of Violence against Women. http://www.un.org/ecosocdev/geninfo/women/womrepro.htm. Accessed April 8, 2008.

57. CDC. Lifetime and annual incidence of intimate partner violence and resulting injuries—1995. *MMWR*. 1998;47(40):849-853.

58. IPPF. Violence against women. http://www.ippf.org/newsinfo/ma98/women.htm. Accessed April 8, 2008.

59. Crowell MA, Birgess AW. *Understanding Violence Against Women*. Washington, DC: National Academy Press; 1996.

60. Duffy SJ, McGrath, Meghan, Becker, Bruce et al. Mothers with histories of domestic violence in a pediatric emergency department. *Pediatrics*. 1999;103:1007-1013.

61. Elders MJ. Adolescent pregnancy and sexual abuse [editorial]. *JAMA*. 1998; 250:648-649.

62. Hinds A, Baskin LS. Child sexual abuse: what the urologist needs to know. *J Urol*. 1999;162:516-523.

63. McFarlane J, Malecha A, Watson K, et al. Intimate partner sexual assault against women: frequency, health consequences, and treatment outcomes. *Obstet Gynecol*. 2005;105(1):99-108.

64. Romans SE, Martin J, Morris E et al. Psychological defense styles in women who report childhood sexual abuse: a controlled community study. *Am J Psychiatry*. 1999;156(7):1080-1085.

65. Yehuda R, Friedman M, Rosenbaum TY, Labinsky E, Schmeidler J. History of past sexual abuse in married observant Jewish women. *Am J Psychiatry*. 2007; 164(11):1700-1706.

CHAPTER 36

INTRODUCTION

FGM—The Clinician's Perspective

This paper is an attempt to chronicle the author's experiences in the clinical management of women who have undergone female genital mutilation (FGM) for the past 25 years in northern Ghana. The experiences are made up of operations research into FGM, gynaecologic and obstetric clinical management of such women, psychological counselling of those women and their spouses, and the rehabilitation of the women. Though the term *female genital mutilation* has been in use for a long time, it has been recognized that this term could be judgmental and offensive to some groups, including women who have undergone the procedure. However, 30 years of clinical practice in an area where between 30% and 80% of women have undergone this form of surgery leaves no doubt in my mind that the term *female genital mutilation* is the most appropriate.

With support from the United Nations Population Fund (UNFPA), a rural project was set up between 1995 and 2000 to address the reproductive health needs of the population, especially those of adolescent girls and women in northern Ghana. Under this programme, an operations research was conducted into the gynaecological morbidity of women who had undergone FGM. Later, between 2001 and 2003 the author was the principal investigator for the Ghana portion of a multicountry prospective cohort study conducted in Ghana, Burkina Faso, Cameroon, Gambia, Kenya, Nigeria, and the Sudan. The study was commissioned by the Department of Reproductive Health and Research of the World Health Organization (WHO). The study's main objective was to determine the obstetric sequelae of women who had undergone FGM. The original study document, the sample size, power calculation, and other parameters were adjusted to suit conditions in Ghana and provide statistically significant results representing the situation in Ghana. A total of 6400 women were examined during the study.

The age at which the procedure of FGM is carried out varies from community to community. It is performed on infants, children and adolescents, and during pregnancy. Excision of the clitoris and the labia minora (FGM Type II) is the most common type and accounts for up to 80% of all cases,

Kwasi Odoi-Agyarko, MD, PhD

Kwasi Odoi-Agyarko, MD, PhD, is recipient of the 2002 United Nations Population Fund Population Award and Executive Director of Rural Help Integrated in Ghana.

while infibulation (FGM Type III) constitutes about 2% of all procedures.

Reasons Why FGM Continues in Northern Ghana

FGM is practiced for a variety of sociocultural reasons.

Tradition

Most people have no tangible reason to support the practice except to say that is has been their long-standing tradition and must therefore be maintained. FGM is regarded as a patriarchal legacy and any attempt to stop it may incur the wrath of the ancestors.

Sociological

Reasons vary from one community to the other. They include:

- Social pressure and ridicule from peers and rivals. This can weigh so heavily on the girls that some of them have actually run away from home to be circumcised without the knowledge of their parents.
- Uncircumcised women are considered inferior [in the society] and a child born to an uncircumcised woman is derogatorily called *clitoris child*.
- It is an initiation rite, which ushers young girls into adulthood (popularly referred to as puberty rites).
- FGM increases fertility and prevents the death of first-born babies.
- The clitoris is an extra load women carry and must be removed to lighten their burdens and enable them to work better during the farming season.
- The culture demands an elaborate funeral observance for a dead mother. Girls who are not circumcised are not allowed to perform those

rites, and it is believed that the girls who are unable to perform the funeral rites will endure hardships for the rest of their lives.

Psychosexual Beliefs

FGM is practiced in the belief that:

- The phallus represents masculinity and the presence of a clitoris in a woman suggests that she is a man. When such a woman dies her funeral and burial ceremonies are performed like that of a man and in extreme cases, the clitoris is removed before burial.
- The absence of the clitoris reduces a woman's sexual desire and thus reduces the chances of a woman leading a promiscuous life. Moral uprightness is so cherished that the penalty paid by an adulterous woman is drastic. The family is often involved in sharing the disgrace.
- Children born to uncircumcised women are stubborn and troublesome.
- The length of the clitoris may hamper easy access of the penis into the vagina during sex.
- Children will become blind if the clitoris touches their eyes or become dumb if the clitoris touches their tongue at the time of birth.
- Foreplay during sex is an act of prostitution and the clitoris should be removed to discourage it.

Hygiene

Uncircumcised women are regarded as unclean and must therefore be ignored in society.

Economic

The financial gain, reputation, and respect attached to the work of a circumciser are important, and no one would willingly let it go.

Certain plants have economic value (the gourd plant—a climbing plant that produces large, hard-skinned, fleshy fruit; the dried shell of the fruit used as a bowl, cup, etc.). Communities believe these plants become unproductive if they are touched or handled by uncircumcised women.

Religion

Some orthodox Muslim groups ignorantly practice FGM citing religious reasons.

Special Ceremonial Observances and Taboos

When the excision is performed as part of an initiation rite into womanhood, the girl is expected to be a virgin. They are confined in groups and given tutorials in womanhood, which include housekeeping and the preparation of meals, servitude, and obedience to the husband and the elderly; polygamy is widely practiced, and the girls are tutored in special ways to please a husband so that he may be monopolized.

During the compulsory confinement, uncircumcised women are not allowed to visit the victims; those who are known to have committed adultery in the community are also barred from visiting. The girls must abstain from eating certain foods, such as eggs and ground nuts, during the time of confinement. Later, toward the end of the confinement, the girls are force-fed with specially fattened lambs and dogs. This is a sort of "last supper" for the girls. In some areas of northern Ghana, women are traditionally not allowed to eat meat for the rest of their lives after puberty and the aim of the forced feeding of the fatty meats is supposed to render the girls nauseous to meat so as not to desire meat again in their lifetime.

The Surgeon

The surgeon (*Pokubga* in the Gruni language) is usually a male and a professional. It is a lifetime job. He inherits the practice, usually from his father, and would have served as an apprentice for a long time. It is believed that it is the fetish that chooses the one to inherit the practice, and if one is not chosen all excisions performed by the impostor will end in excessive bleeding and the death of the victim. It is a requirement to sacrifice to the fetish yearly and before and after each session of operations. Refusal to sacrifice or stop performing the excision will incur the wrath of the gods, which will lead to insanity, mysterious deaths in the family, or blindness.

Rarely women, and sometimes traditional birth attendants, perform the operation.

The Instruments

The surgical bag used by the surgeons contains three different kinds of locally made cutting blades. The first set is the shaving set used in shaving the vulva, the second set is the outline set used in marking out the area to be cut, and the third set is used for the actual cutting. There are usually three knives in each set and if the victims are more than three, the knives are reused without washing or cleansing. Some of the knives are never washed with water; they are cleansed with *kenaf* leaves, which are supposed to have antiseptic qualities. Razor blades and even surgical blades have been found in the bags of the operators. In babies under two weeks, fingernails are sometimes used as the cutting objects.

Cost of the Operation

Long ago, the usual cost of excision for a virgin was a basket of millet and a guinea fowl. These days a fowl and cash ranging from the equivalent in the local currency of US$ 1 to US$ 5 are paid for the operation. In the case of a nonvirgin, the normal fee mentioned above is paid with an additional penalty of a calabash and a goat.

Gynaecologic Morbidity

Overall, subjects living in rural areas have three times the risk of being cut (odds ratio [OR] 3.70, $3.28 < OR < 4.17$; relative risk [RR]: 2.91, $2.66 < RR < 3.20$) than subjects in the urban areas, because girls and young women in the urban areas are spared the sustained pressure that is put on them by the older women who are the custodians of the traditional practices and make sure that all girls are cut before marriage.

Girls who were cut were 2 times more likely to be sexually active (OR 1.72, 0.92<RR<1.85 at 95% confidence limit [CL]) and 10 times more likely to have been pregnant [or have been pregnant] at the time or before while in school (OR 10.61, RR 9.87, 1.72<RR<56.50 at 95% CL). This leads to the girls leaving school to become teenage mothers. Hitherto, FGM has not been mentioned as one of the factors leading to the high school dropout rates in northern Ghana.

Girls with no education and living in the rural area had a 77% chance of being cut compared with girls with a secondary-level education living in an urban area that had only 0.9% chance of being cut.

Girls and women who have been cut run five times the risk of having pain at urination (OR 5.09, RR 4.94, 0.53<RR<45.82 at 95% CL), four times the risk of bleeding during sexual intercourse (OR 3.94, RR 3.48, 1.26<RR<9.41 at 95% CL), and three times the risk of developing pain during sexual intercourse (OR 3.46, RR 3.17, 0.97<RR<10.35 at 95% CL, chi-square: 71.23).

Girls who have been cut run 16 times the risk of developing pelvic inflammatory disease.

Obstetric Morbidity

FGM had a direct relationship with caesarean section. FGM Type I and FGM Type II did not demonstrate any association. FGM Type III (OR 3.12, z-statistic: 3.76, P = 0.000, CI = 1.75 to 5.86) was significantly associated with caesarean section. The presence of the other factors such as religion, distance to hospital, previous stillbirths, poor health, and maternal height further increased the chances of a woman with FGM Type III undergoing caesarean section during delivery.

FGM had a direct relationship with postdelivery fistulas. The association between FGM Type I and FGM Type II was not significant, however, but FGM Type III (OR 33.08, P = 0.000, z-statistic = 4.00, CI = 5.95–184.09) was strongly associated with postdelivery fistulas. The presence of factors such as the general health of the woman and labour augmentation further influenced the outcome of the association between FGM and postdelivery fistulas.

FGM had a direct relationship with postdelivery wound infections. FGM Type II and Type III were significantly associated with postdelivery genital wound infection. FGM Type III (OR 38.03, P = 0.003, z-statistic = 2.94, CI = 3.36–430.85) was strongly associated with postdelivery genital wound infection. Other factors such as area of residence, antenatal attendance, and labour augmentation further increased the chances of a woman with FGM developing postdelivery genital wound infections.

FGM had a direct relationship with third-degree perineal tears. FGM Type II and FGM Type III were significantly associated with third-degree tears. FGM Type III (OR 453.16, P = 0.000, z-statistic = 5.77, CI = 56.65–3624.64) was strongly associated with third-degree tears. Other factors such as area of residence, parity, antenatal attendance, and labour augmentation further increased the chances of a woman with FGM sustaining perineal tears, especially third-degree tears during delivery.

FGM had a direct relationship with a low Apgar score. FGM Type III (OR 2.70, P = 0.003, z-statistic = 2.94, CI = 1.39–5.24) was significantly associated with low Apgar scores. Other factors such as distance to the health facility, area of residence, maternal age, previous stillbirths, antenatal attendance, and labour augmentation further increased the chances of a woman with FGM delivering a baby with a low Apgar score.

FGM had a direct relationship with prolonged labour when all the cases of the latter in the study was grouped together (OR 1.47, z-statistic = 4.18, P = 0.000, CI = 1.23–1.75). Prolonged labour as an indication for caesarean section accounted for 13.4% of all caesarean sections performed, and FGM Type 1 was significantly associated with prolonged labour when the latter was the indication for caesarean section. FGM Type II was also significantly associated with prolonged labour when it was an indication for caesarean section but in a different way. Statistically, the negative z-statistic and an OR of 0.05 meant that FGM Type II had a protective value and the event of FGM Type II causing prolonged labour as the indication for C-section was unlikely to occur. However, it was observed clinically that it was not the FGM Type II per se that provided the protection but a result of the widened vagina orifice caused by repeated perineal tears obtained during previous deliveries in multiparous women.

It is 4:00 in the morning; Abaane Akologo sacrifices a guinea fowl to one of the totem mounds in front of his thatched round house. He calls on his ancestors and says a short prayer: "May the day go well, may the journey be smooth, may you guide my hands and eyes and your sacrifice will be in abundance." He wears his talismans, one around his waist, one around his neck, and a third around his left wrist. He examines his surgical bag to make sure he has the necessary equipment and repacks them carefully. The bag contains the three different kinds of locally made cutting blades. The first set is the shaving set used in shaving the vulva, the second set is the outline set used in marking out the area to be cut, and the third set is used for the actual cutting. The other contents of his surgical bag are made up of a flint stone for sharpening the blades when they become blunt, and a specially made wand covered with the feathers of guinea fowls. A feather is stuck on the wand for each operation. The broad end of his magic wand is made of a receptacle filled with black powder. The bag also contains stitching needles of various sizes; different kinds of threads, ties, and rubber bands; and an apron made from jute strands and a piece of dirty linen cloth. Akologo is ready to go. He hangs a towel around his neck over his century-old-looking gown (fugu) and jumps onto his new bicycle.

Today he has five girls at Namoranteng, a village 16 kilometres away. After a ride of an hour and half he arrives and his presence is announced by the ringing of a bell tied to his surgical bag. The ringing of the bell drives away evil spirits.

Akologo is welcomed into the village by an elderly woman who has been waiting for over an hour on the outskirts of the village. She whispers to him, "They are eight instead of five." "That is the wish of the oracle," he replies. The eight girls, aged between 9 years and 16 years have been woken up at dawn and confined in a dark hut on the outskirts of the village, with three elderly women guarding them. Five of the girls are there by their own consent, and they assist the elderly women to confine the other three girls, all aged 9 years. The 9-year-olds do not know what is happening, but the older girls were being laughed at and called boys by their peers who were cut and so have volunteered for the cut.

Akologo is led to the "local theatre" a sacred grove shaded by big tall trees. It is in the rainy season, and the vegetation is lush. The early morning light breeze makes the place comfortable. A broad flat stone at one corner of the grove serves as the operating table. Akologo opens his surgical bag, spreads the dirty linen cloth on the ground and carefully arranges his surgical instruments on the cloth. He makes a final check of his surgical instruments and checks on what the elderly women had been instructed to supply and is satisfied. He removes his outer gown, ties a rope around his waist to keep his clothing out of the way, and says another short prayer to the ancestors, an incantation; "It is time. Your presence is solicited. Keep the evil spirits away. Guide my hands and your reward will be abundant." All is set. There are 12 elderly women in attendance.

The first girl is brought in with a wry smile on her face. She is placed naked on the stone, a cloth is tied around her waist, a stick is stuck into her mouth to prevent her from screaming aloud and her legs spread and held wide apart by four of the women. Two of the women hold the upper part of her body. One more holds and pins her pelvis down. The place is quiet. Akologo picks one of the shaving blades and carefully shaves the vulva. The girl is uncomfortable; she moves her pelvis a little and receives a cut from the shaving blade. There is a speck of blood, and Akologo says that it is a good omen. Akologo then mixes some fine sand and wood ash that the women have brought from home and sprinkles the mixture over the vulva. This is to render the vulval area dirty and uninviting so that Akologo, on looking at the girl's vulva, will not have a penile erection. A penile erection will demand a big sacrifice and the punishment of Akologo by the gods.

Akologo then picks one of the outline blades and carefully marks out the area to be cut. The extent of the cut depends on the traditions of the area. In this village only the clitoris is cut off. He takes one of his cutting blades and cuts the clitoris off with deft movement of the hands. There was some bleeding. An herbal paste made of *kenaf* leaves (a plant which grows wildly during the rainy season and is supposed to stop the bleeding and enhance healing) is immediately plastered onto the wound; a cotton pad is put over the herbal paste and held down for four to five minutes. The bleeding has stopped. Four cowries are tied around the waist of the girl. The operation is over. It all took eight minutes. The girl is asked to get up and walk without support. She is a brave girl. She is congratulated and led to another hut for confinement.

(continued)

The three 9-year-olds followed and uneventfully went through the same procedure. They screamed and resisted, but the women holding them overpowered them.

Akologo has four sets of blades. He has four more girls to cut. He asked for a pail of water, rinsed all the used blades, brought out his flint stone and sharpened all the blades, ready for reuse.

The fifth and the sixth cuttings went uneventfully. The seventh girl started struggling violently and she could not be firmly held down. Akologo lost his patience and started cursing the girl; the blade slipped and went beyond the intended cut. The right labia minora was sliced off and the left labia minora had to be removed to make it look as if that was the intended cut. The herbal paste was applied but bleeding could not be stopped. Black powder from Akologo's magic wand was mixed for her to drink, but the bleeding would not stop. Teni was not a virgin and her ultimate punishment was eventual death. Akologo was exonerated. He was paid fully for his work and departed for his village on his bicycle.

The confinement and the daily dressing of the wounds were the responsibility of the elderly women. This story does not end here.

As part of its advocacy programme, Rural Help Integrated, a nongovernmental organization (NGO) working in the area, has trained and sensitized the youth of the area to report such cases for a reward. Two days after the episode, two young boys from the village managed to make it to the capital town to report the incidence. A medical team was immediately mobilized to visit the village. Teni was almost dead when the team got there. Luckily she is still alive today. The other girls were also brought to the capital and admitted in hospital and managed until the wounds healed satisfactorily. Akologo was arrested by the police, arraigned before the law courts, and is now serving a six-year sentence.

FGM had only a mild association with postpartum haemorrhage (PPH), but the presence of other factors such as poor health, mode of delivery, and augmentation of labour increased the chances of a woman with FGM to bleed excessively during delivery to the level of PPH.

FGM had no direct relationship with cephalopelvic disproportion (CPD), but women with FGM who lived between 21 kilometres and 50 kilometres away from the health facility were more likely to undergo caesarean section with CPD as the indication.

FGM had no direct relationship with maternal death, but the presence of other factors such as the general health, number of antenatal attendances, parity, and the distance and time to reach the health facility increased the chances of a woman with FGM to die during delivery.

FGM had no direct relationship with extended stay in hospital after delivery, but the presence of factors such as the general health, the distance and the time to reach the health facility, episiotomies, labour duration, and labour augmentation increased postpartum morbidity and the resultant long hospital stay.

FGM had no direct relationship with low birth weight. However, adverse socioeconomic factors such as area of residence, maternal age, general health, previous stillbirths, antenatal attendance, and level of education increased the chances of a woman with FGM delivering a baby with low birth weight.

FGM had no direct relationship with stillbirth. However, adverse socioeconomic factors such as area of residence, maternal age, general health, previous stillbirths, antenatal attendance, and level of education will increase the chances of a woman with FGM delivering a baby with low birth weight.

The performance of FGM without sterilization of instruments, cigarette smoking (especially among Muslim women), the chewing of raw tobacco, alcohol consumption, unprotected sexual intercourse during pregnancy, and sexually transmitted infection during pregnancy may increase the risk of HIV transmission and mother-to-child transmission especially in women who have undergone FGM.

FGM and Legislation

Despite the law against the practice in Ghana, FGM still goes on. Article 39 of the Constitution of Ghana provides in part that:

(1) Whoever excises, infibulates, or otherwise mutilates the whole or any part of the labia minora, labia majora, and the clitoris of another person commits an offence and shall be guilty of a second degree felony and liable on conviction to imprisonment of not less than three years. (2) For the purposes of this section "excise" means to remove the prepuce, the clitoris, and all or part of the labia minora; "infibulate" includes excision and the additional removal of the labia majora.[1]

It is important to involve traditional authority, political and religious authority, local media practitioners, human rights groups, and the local police to form a coalition to enforce existing laws.

Human Rights and FGM

Several factors have, in the past, prevented FGM from being seen as harmful and as a human rights issue. Parents and family members who believe that it will have a beneficial consequence for their daughters later in life encouraged FGM. FGM and other violence against women and girls in the home or in the community were seen as a "private" issue. The practice was rooted in a cultural tradition, and outside intervention in the name of universal human rights risked it being perceived as cultural imperialism.

Today, however, the harmful effects of FGM on women and girls have been clearly demonstrated, and the human rights implications of FGM are clearly and unequivocally recognized at an international level. This recognition requires governments, local authorities, and others in position of power and influence to honour their obligations established under international law—to prevent, investigate, and punish all forms of violence against women, especially FGM.

Advocacy

Some men are rejecting their circumcised wives because they either find the vagina too small (Type III FGM) or too big (because of unsutured perineal tears sustained during deliveries by traditional birth attendants), which reduces friction for enjoyment during sexual intercourse. These days, FGM is being questioned not only by community leaders but also by ordinary people. They are asking why other ethnic groups in Ghana do not practice FGM and yet lead normal lives. They also wonder why some men from the north marry women from the south who are not cut. Through education of girls, the myths surrounding FGM are gradually being broken, and through the empowerment of female students through advocacy, the FGM beliefs are being demystified. There is a certain wind of change blowing through many communities in northern Ghana because of the intense behavioural change campaigns against violence and harmful practices against women and children by developmental NGOs.

There are a number of existing good practices that will accelerate the elimination of FGM in northern Ghana. These practices are as follows:

- Existence of appropriate laws against FGM
- Existence of a national plan of action against FGM
- Incorporation of the prevention and management of complications arising out of FGM into the national reproductive health service protocols
- Incorporation of the prevention and management of complications arising out of FGM into the curriculum of the medical schools
- Incorporation of the prevention and management of complications arising out of FGM into the curriculum of nursing and midwifery schools
- Training of community-based service providers in the management of complications of FGM in the remote areas

NGOs providing information, education, and communication (IEC), and behavioural change advocacy at the community level involve the following:

- Traditional authority
- Religious authorities
- Women and men groups
- Youth and youth groups

- Community in general
- The use of entertainment education—videos, film, songs, and drama especially for low-literacy areas at the community level
- Advocacy for the conversion of circumcisers
- Microcredit schemes for women at the community level for economic empowerment and to be assertive
- Research and dissemination of finding at all levels showing the harmful effects of FGM

Recommendations

Community Action

Education for all, especially the girl-child, poverty alleviation, modernizing traditional ancestral worship, and providing basic infrastructure at the community level to transform rural communities to urban communities are medium- and long-term issues that should be tackled at the governmental level.

Organizations dedicated to the elimination of FGM must include all interested parties in the design, planning, and implementation of programmes.

Programme designs should suit the work plan of the beneficiaries taking into account the diverse reasons in the different communities for practicing FGM.

Community-based workers such as community-based distributors, traditional birth attendants, village health workers, and community health animators should be recruited, retrained, motivated, and redirected to include gender issues, violence, and harmful practices in their communities in their day-to-day activity.

There should be repeated and frequent meetings with chiefs, opinion leaders, assemblymen and women, unit committee leaders, and members to persuade them to leave behind the outmoded customs in the communities.

Various men's group meetings, women's meetings, farmers meetings, and other such recognized community group meetings should be organized with the aim of gradually making all of them "change agents."

Community-based experts involved in gender-based violence programmes and services should facilitate these meetings.

International cross-border campaigns against FGM should be encouraged especially between countries that share boundaries.

Public health and community health nurses should be trained and mandated to examine the vulva of all infants as part of the normal examination during postnatal follow up, because of the recent reports that infants are being cut. Midwives and doctors should integrate health promotion on FGM into routine antenatal and postnatal care.

Other partners such as ministries of women's and children's affairs, ministries of information, NGOs, traditional and religious leaders, schools, and the media should work in partnership to organize outreach education for young people, adults, and communities.

Research

Studies are needed to do the following:

- *Investigate* the local traditional practices undertaken during the antenatal period to prepare women for childbirth and delivery and to assist in the preparation of appropriate educational programmes on FGM tailored to specific local needs.
- *Examine and document* the use of traditional birth attendants (TBAs) in health provision in resource-poor areas with a view to testing schemes for expanding their role; extensive involvement of trained and supervised TBAs may be the only viable means of reducing maternal mortality and morbidity in some of the most deprived areas. It is important for stakeholders including policy makers to assess the knowledge, attitudes, practice, and beliefs of health workers with respect to FGM at all levels.
- *Seek appropriate ways of studying and documenting* psychosexual problems caused by FGM in order to establish a well-designed protocol for research in this area.

Conclusion

FGM practice is a topic of grave concern, and all should be concerned because of its associated reproductive health consequences. The increased risk of adverse obstetric outcomes observed with FGM occurs against the background of increased maternal morbidity and mortality. This means that FGM is likely to be responsible for substantial numbers of additional cases of adverse obstetric outcomes.

In Ghana, FGM is not a national issue despite the fact that a law has been passed outlawing the practice. After all, it is prevalent only in the northern regions of the country. This geographical area of Ghana is periodically plagued by life-threatening epidemics such as cerebrospinal meningitis, cholera, measles, and yellow fever. Scarce resources are directed at containing these epidemics, and not much governmental support is given to efforts to eradicate FGM.

Most of the NGOs involved in the advocacy work to eradicate FGM are based in southern Ghana. In my opinion, for any real change to begin to take place, efforts should be redirected to tackle the problem at the source, which is at the community level. In rural areas where 60–80% of the population live but receive only 5–20% of resources, advocates for the eradication of FGM must be deceiving themselves that they are making an impact.

It is unacceptable that the international community remain passive in the name of a distorted vision of multiculturalism. Human behaviours and cultural values, however senseless or destructive they appear from the personal and cultural standpoint of others, have meaning and fulfill a function for those who practice them. However, culture is not static, but it is in constant flux, adapting and reforming. People will change their behaviour when they understand the hazard and indignity of harmful practices and when they realize that it is possible to give up harmful practices without giving up meaningful aspects of their culture.[2]

DISCUSSION QUESTIONS

1. What are the reasons for the widespread practice of FGM in certain geographic areas of the world?

2. What are the barriers faced by public health workers and other healthcare providers who are working to eliminate the practice of FGM?

3. Discuss the role of UN agencies, nongovernmental organizations, and community leaders in eliminating the practice of FGM.

REFERENCES

1. The Law on Female Genital Mutilation (FGM)—Ghana. The Criminal Code, 1960 (Act 29).
2. World Health Organization. Female Genital Mutilation. Give Up Harmful Practices. A Joint WHO/UNICEF/UNFPA statement. 1996. http://www.unfpa.org/swp /1997/box16.htm. Accessed July 22, 2008.

INTRODUCTION

Practice and Problems in Occupational Health for Women

There are three major factors that affect the practice and problems of occupational health for women workers. One problem is that the term *occupational health* is generally associated with health conditions that are affected by a working environment that is functionally and geographically different from the woman's home. In spite of the changes in workforces engendered by the globalization of the market economy, in many developing areas of the world, women have worked both at home and outside the home for generations. Because the actual tasks carried out by such women are difficult to differentiate—all of them being considered "traditional" women's work—there are little data and fewer studies examining the effect of "occupation" on health, or of health on "occupation."

The second major problem is that the history of women's work in the modern trades and industries is relatively short, a situation that leaves the epidemiologists with smaller numbers of study participants and shorter durations of exposures to those raw materials, products, and processes that contribute to the bulk of today's concerns about chronic disease occurrence caused by occupational exposures.

And finally, the third factor is the significant contribution to both morbidity and mortality from violence that occurs to women in the workplace. The objective of this chapter is to present some of these issues in light of recent efforts in several countries to better understand the factors that are common to the effects of work on health in women and men, as well as those that are different.

Robin C. Leonard, PhD

Robin C. Leonard, PhD, is Professor in the Department of Health for the College of Health Sciences, West Chester University, located in West Chester, PA.

Political Organizational Structures for Occupational Health

Practitioners of occupational health in the United States are usually supported by employers. Large companies often hire in-house medical and support staff, and frequently supplement these individuals with contract physicians and nurses located near the manufacturing or business sites.

Smaller companies seeking occupational health support for their employees take advantage of independent occupational health providers who provide contracted services to several client companies. Because of privacy regulations and societal concerns over confidentiality, it has not always been clear that such medical records and collected data can be used for research purposes. However, careful reading of the US Health Insurance Portability and Accountability Act (HIPAA) makes clear that research is considered a legitimate function of those who manage the health of workers and the data that enable that task. Conditions of data management, informed consent, and the deidentification of individuals are just a few of the issues that researchers need to address, but these conditions do not prevent the conduct of research in occupational health.

In the European Union, occupational health is generally considered to be a government responsibility and is managed through national health services organizations. The advantage to researchers in these countries derives from the consistent collection of data across industries and geographic areas and the centralized maintenance of many types of health data, including information about potential and actual workplace exposures to health risk factors. As in the United States, privacy and confidentiality are serious concerns; but, again, careful reading of the European Union Privacy Directive and individual national privacy regulations shows that research in occupational health is valued and can be conducted as long as safeguards are met concerning confidentiality, deidentification of individual data, and nontransport of identifiable data across national borders. In the developed countries, occupational health programs are not uncommon, are usually based on high medical practice standards, and retention of data for periods of 30 to 40 years is required by regulation. Why then would there appear to be a dearth of research concerning women's occupational health?

Nontraditional Workplaces for Women

Large Manufacturing Industries

One reason that many women's occupational health issues have not been addressed as thor-

oughly as those of men is the relatively recent hiring of women for the industrial and trade jobs that have been the primary focus of occupational health research for the last 60 years. Beginning with the discovery around the time of World War I that beta-naphthylamine could cause bladder cancer in dye industry workers,[1] the large US and European companies have focused on the risks of specific chemicals, processes, and products that cause chronic diseases—primarily cancer, but also respiratory and cardiovascular diseases. These industries have, until quite recently, primarily hired males to operate these line processes. Women are few in number and often restricted by size, physical strength, and lack of seniority to jobs that do not bring them in contact with large chemical batch processes or pipe and valve maintenance operations. In the modern chemical industry, for example, the potential for significant exposures are usually found only in these types of jobs. Given the amount of time and effort required to reconstruct historical exposures based on industrial hygiene data, job task descriptions, and process engineering changes, it is not surprising that cohorts for such studies are limited to those workers most likely to have had sufficient time in the tasks to accumulate exposures of measurable quantity and health consequence.

Thus, in the developed countries, the relatively small number of women employed in major manufacturing industries results in fewer studies conducted that have sufficient statistical power to examine health in working women. Epidemiology is a population science, and as such, relies heavily on large numbers of individuals in order to provide stable estimates of risk and adequately populated strata to control for confounders. In addition to the small numbers of women with sufficient job duration to provide information on chronic disease risk, there has been a tendency for many occupational health professionals interested in women's health to focus on the reproductive risks to women in the workplace. Pregnancy is, after all, the one characteristic that everyone can agree is unique to females, and in fact, places two individuals at risk for the "work of one." The manufacturing industries have in the past used several approaches to protect pregnant women in the workplace: (1) refusal to hire women of childbearing age into certain jobs, and (2) dismissal from work upon becoming pregnant.[2] In March of

1991, the US Supreme Court ruled that barring fertile females from jobs due to potential reproductive hazards was illegal sex discrimination.[3] Since then, the usual approach for many companies is to provide either reassignment to equivalent pay jobs, or paid temporary leave.

Potential adverse effects of work on reproduction are a major concern for many women; however, reproductive epidemiology studies are notoriously difficult and time consuming to conduct, with attendant high costs. The array of variables, the reliability and validity of qualitative interview data, the supporting biomedical screening data, and the review of historical medical records are just a few of the complex and time-consuming factors involved. An additional problem is the frequent reluctance of spouses or partners to participate in providing data for what remains a very personal and private arena. Sharing information about number and frequency of copulations, providing semen samples for sperm count, and discussing past successes or failures at reproductive attempts are not generally easy for many people. Another factor that makes reproductive studies difficult is the reversal of the "healthy worker effect" in women being studied for reproductive outcomes. In general, working women tend to have less successful reproductive histories than women who do not work outside the home.[4] Therefore, comparisons of working women to females in the general population will introduce some selection bias into the calculations of relative risk. This so-called unhealthy worker effect may be due to a combination of self-selection out of the workforce of women with several children as well as potential risk factors in the workplace that act against successful reproduction.[5]

Very few companies have the staff and research funding to conduct detailed reproductive studies, with the result that government grants or contracts to universities or consulting houses provide much of the support for this work. Decreases in funding for health research—either direct or due to uncompensated inflation—reduce further the chances that quality research in this area will be conducted. In spite of the difficulties in studying occupational risk factors for reproduction, there have been successes. Industry coalitions and some individual companies have supported large epidemiology studies on general and reproductive health for women in the semiconductor manufac-

turing industry.[6] Substantial literature exists on reproductive outcomes of working women that, while largely reassuring, has provided evidence for several occupational risk factors affecting reproductive health.[7] In addition, the US National Institutes of Health Women's Health Initiative has provided significant amounts of health research in women, which, while not designed primarily to address occupational issues, provides valuable data that provide both theory and context for occupational health research.[8]

In developing countries such as China, the drive to expand the economy as well as a gender-neutral approach to work that was instilled by early Marxist philosophy has resulted in large numbers of women employed in the large manufacturing industries. Again, as in the more developed nations, there has been emphasis on understanding reproductive risks from the assumption of these jobs by women. Several important reproductive studies on workers in the acrylonitrile industry in China were undertaken that suggested adverse reproductive effects on these women and their partners, many of whom also worked in the industry.[9] The lack of control for confounding factors, as well as anecdotal reports of exposures occasionally reaching levels capable of inducing acrylonitrile poisoning, has called into question whether these exposures were in fact targeting the reproductive system or causing general systemic toxicity. An additional complexity in the conduct of reproductive studies in China arises from the governmental requirement that each couple produce one child only. It is difficult to know how this could affect the ability to obtain accurate reproductive histories. It is possible, however, that a sociolegal policy that mandates that attempts at reproduction be approved, would in fact, motivate the couple to keep accurate records concerning dates of menstrual periods, body temperature changes indicating ovulation, and number of copulations per week. These kinds of detailed information are necessary for teasing out confounding or modifying effects of workplace factors by other genetic or environmental factors. A study of birth defects among the offspring of acrylonitrile workers in Hungary revealed no increased risk; however, the exposure metric was categorical rather than quantitative.[10]

Musculoskeletal complaints are another major occupational risk for female workers. A study in

Indian flight attendants—both female and male—indicated that about 73% suffered from back pain, due largely to awkward equipment and badly designed galley spaces.[11] The prevalence of musculoskeletal problems among male and female workers in the Norwegian seafood production industry were also studied. Female production workers showed significantly higher odds ratios for upper limb symptoms compared to males.[12] Eighty-two percent of women working in the salmon industry had musculoskeletal symptoms in the wrists and hands compared to 64% of males doing the same work. Cold work was a major factor in the prevalence of symptoms; however, the difference in male and female prevalence of symptoms may well involve height and width of work areas and tables, as well as tool design.

Professions and Small-Scale Enterprisers

The growing number of professional women—including physicians, nurses, academics, lawyers, and executives—has initiated several interesting studies. A study of work environment and mental health among female Japanese physicians revealed that several factors significantly contributed to risk for psychological distress. These factors were younger age, marital status, medical facility, working time, and working at night.[13] Similarly, hospice workers in South Africa have been found to be at high risk for burnout owing to the emotional intensity of their relationships with clients, organizational stressors, and social stressors related to family and community obligations.[14]

An investigation of prevalence and associations between self-rated health and working conditions for small-scale enterprisers was conducted in Sweden.[15] Questionnaires were completed by 340 males and 153 females. These responses were compared to those of 1699 employees in private companies. The frequency of health problems in males was higher in the enterprisers than in the company employed, while the frequencies of health problems among the females were not different between enterprisers and the company employed. The most common health complaints among the enterprisers, both male and female, were musculoskeletal and mental health problems. These problems were associated with poor

job satisfaction and poor physical work environment. Interestingly, adjustment for sex, age, and working conditions did not affect the association between poor general health and working as an enterpriser. These findings suggest that for males, but not females, working as enterprisers (or being self-employed) may be the result of poorer general health rather than the cause.

Traditional Workplaces for Women

Domestic Labor and Childcare as a "Second Job"

A particularly interesting aspect of women's occupational health is the effect of dual occupations. For many women, the paid work they do outside the home is in addition to the domestic chores and childcare that they do inside the home. A study conducted by the Women's Health Office of Tyrol, Austria, in 2004 examined 1083 women who were employed at the Innsbruck Medical Hospital.[16] The study population was divided into 98 medical doctors; 145 technical personnel; 667 nurses; 92 administrative personnel; and 81 other hospital workers, comprising primarily scientific personnel and psychologists. The first aim was to assess the physical and mental health status of a group of women employed by the same organization, but divided into different job categories. The second aim was to identify factors that affected health status and to determine if any of these were job specific.

Forty-three percent of the women reported doing one to four hours of domestic work and childcare every day; 14% spent more than four hours a day on domestic work. Higher age reduced all scores on the physical health metrics, but did not affect mental health. Domestic duties showed a stronger effect on general health than did age. Low satisfaction with their work schedules predicted low scores for physical and general health, vitality, and social functioning. Multivariable regression models indicated that low satisfaction with work schedules and high volume of domestic duties were significantly associated with poorer general health and mental health in all the occupational groups except the administrative workers. The authors speculate that this may be because administrative workers tend to have fixed hours during the daytime, and routines are more easily established to accommodate family and domestic responsibilities. In addition, better mental health among administrators may be due to the absence of the emotional as well as physical strain encountered in direct patient care and contact. The evidence from this and a few similar investigations suggests that women's occupational health has several dimensions, not all of which are directly connected to the paid workplace.

The previous studies provide examples of research that indicate an emerging theme in women's occupational health research. This theme supports tenets that were either denied or disparaged during the first phases of the modern feminist movement. It is now being accepted (albeit grudgingly by some) that women are, by and large, more often drawn to the caregiving professions; that women are more satisfied with less pay if there is greater personal commitment to the work they are doing; and that women have more difficulty balancing their work and home obligations than do men. As described by Killien, Habermann, and Jarrett, the responsibility for resolution of work–family interference is placed on the woman herself, usually at a high cost to her physical and mental health.[17] Systemic changes in the social environment that provide assistance with removing these interferences will benefit the individual women, their families, and the communities in which they live and work.

Violence in the Workplace

Work-related violence is an important problem worldwide; nurses, who are more often than not female, are at increased risk. A study identifying rates of workplace violence among 6300 nurses in Minnesota, United States, used a case-control approach to determine differences in perception of the workplace between those nurses who had experienced violent assault and those who had not.[18] Annual rates of physical and nonphysical assault per 100 nurses were 13.2 (95% CI: 12.2–14.3), and 38.8 (95% CI: 37.4–40.4), respectively. Those who were assaulted reported more job stress, higher expectation that risk of assault was part of the job, and witnessing more patient-perpetrated violence

within the last month. Those who had not been assaulted reported more trust, respect, and higher morale among coworkers, and that administrators took action against violent behavior.

Similar results were seen in a study in Ankara, Turkey, of approximately 622 nurses, 30% of whom reported physical abuse—largely from patients and patients' family members—and 91% reported episodes of verbal abuses, primarily from colleagues.[19] The most common reactions among the nurses to abusive behavior were anger, helplessness, humiliation, and depression. The authors particularly noted that the most common response to actions taken in response to verbal abuse was "did nothing." The apparent inability of the nurses to receive administrative support or respond in a positive, active way to the abuse suggests that the low status and power of the nurses contributed to a workplace that was damaging, both mentally and physically.

In addition to being at increased risk of becoming victims of violence in the workplace, nurses are also subject to secondary traumatic stress syndrome due to treating and caring for other women victims of violence.[20] Secondary traumatic stress syndrome results in emotional numbness, avoidance, and intrusive imagery that can seriously impact the ability of nurses to be professional, productive, and satisfied with their work. These effects also affect the women's abilities to cope with personal and family responsibilities. Hospital managers, as well as nursing educators, need to be aware of these issues and implement policies that assist nurses to cope with this additional stress due to "secondary violence." Aggression prevention training has been proposed as part of the student nurses' curriculum. Counseling and continuing education about the causes, responses, and treatment of intimate partner violence (IPV) should also be provided.

Women are more likely to be the victims of IPV than men. While most of these acts of violence occur in the domestic setting, women have been beaten and even murdered in the workplace by their intimate partners. The costs to the workplace of IPV have been studied. Not surprisingly, lifetime victims of IPV missed more hours of work due to absenteeism than nonvictims or current victims.[21] Current victims were more likely to be distracted at work than lifetime victims or nonvictims. It appears that victims of IPV cost organizations in terms of time lost and effectiveness, but the type of loss depends on the histories of the victims. It may be important to further quantify the costs to companies and other business organizations that are incurred due to domestic violence, whether the violence occurs in the home or in the workplace. Systemic changes are required to alter the cultures that tolerate such behavior, and economic benefits can often be powerful forces for such change.

While most of the research on the workplace effects of IPV has involved low-wage, low-status jobs, there is increasing interest in the effects of such violence among women in high-wage, high-status jobs. It has been suggested that women in high-wage, high-status jobs have more access to organizational benefits, such as employee assistance programs and leave of absence policies.[22] However, the current pressures imposed by traditional gender models for these kinds of jobs may prohibit women from taking advantage of such programs. The expectations of performance in the high-wage, high-status jobs are that the work demands are the first priority of the employee, regardless of personal or family responsibilities. Help-seeking behavior of any kind may be viewed as detrimental to continued performance and promotion.

Impact of Occupational Safety and Health Regulations

Legislation mandating adherence to occupational health and safety principles is more likely to be found in economically and politically stable countries with the political will and resources to provide their populations with reasonably safe and healthy workplaces. Perfect implementation of such legislation is a rarity, however, and the fewer resources available, the less likely is implementation. It has been estimated that only about 15% of the global workforce has access to any occupational health services. Several factors are involved in the derailment of regulations as they move toward implementation.[23]

Political and administrative organization can be a significant factor. In countries where the ministry (or department) of health and ministry (or department) of labor are not aligned, issues that affect occupational safety and health policy implementation are difficult to resolve, both in terms of priority and responsibility. In some countries, public health policies encompass occupational health issues within the same agency. In these situations, the breadth of the scope of that agency—which may include HIV/AIDS, malaria control, and provision of clean water—leaves little energy or resources for occupational health issues. It has been argued that it is not so much the level of resources allotted to occupational health that effects implementation as it is those who control those resources.[24] Another factor that appears to hamper implementation of workplace health and safety policies is weakness of trade or labor unions, especially in developing countries.

Recognition of the global disparities in implementation of occupational health policies led the World Health Assembly 2007 to endorse the Global Plan of Action of Workers' Health 2008–2017. This plan of action links occupational health to public health because it addresses several systemic approaches directed to the occupational arena that are also within the recognized mission of public health. These approaches include (1) primary prevention of occupational hazards, (2) promotion of health at work, (3) conditions of employment, and (4) improving the response of local and national health systems to workers' health. The primary objective of the Global Plan of Action of Workers' Health is to provide assistance to countries in developing their national plans by providing templates of action agendas that can be adapted to fit national priorities and specific circumstances.[25] Although no enforcement of these action plans is possible outside the individual national governments, the availability of structured regulations, guidelines, and protocols that have proven effective for other countries should expedite the development and implementation of occupational health requirements in countries that may have limited experience with introducing such policies on a national scale.

The difficulties encountered with implementation of occupational health regulations in many places has led to a growing conviction that the private and corporate sectors have a large role to play. The Bangkok Charter, adopted by the 6th Global Conference on Health Promotion in 2005, called on global corporations and businesses to make the promotion of health, especially occupational health, a requirement for good corporate practice.[26]

The social and ethical responsibilities of those who own and manage large companies are increasingly being met as companies headquartered in developed nations with stronger occupational health regulations and practices strive to provide "one standard" for all their worldwide employees.

Even in countries where good policies and regulations exist, there are significant national variations in the reporting of occupational health conditions between males and females. Women are less likely to be counted as having a workplace-induced health condition than men, even though a European Union Labor task force survey found that work-related conditions are more prevalent in women.[25] A 15-year prospective study in Denmark on disability pensions found that shift work was a significant predictor of disability in women, but not men. This significance remained when the model for calculating the hazard ratio included such factors as age, body mass index, general health and socioeconomic status, smoking habits, and ergonomic exposures.[27] As discussed, women are more often than men in healthcare jobs, most of which are 24-hour operations entailing either three 8-hour shifts or two 12-hour shifts. Women who work shifts that interfere with domestic and child care duties in environments with attendant risks of infection, needle-stick wounds, violence, musculoskeletal disorders, and sexual harassment are at high risk for reduced physical and mental health. Many of these cases, however, never get reported as occupationally related, let alone compensated. Equity in regulation does not guarantee equity in actuality.

Conclusion

The growing awareness that males and females respond to their work in different ways, both emotionally and physically, increases the probability that employers, and society in general, may become more willing to accommodate these differences. We have learned that one size does not fit all in terms of personal protective equipment, desks, workbenches, gloves, and tools. The value that societies place on work that many women prefer to do—the caregiving, nurturing, and "other-oriented" jobs so important to a healthy social structure—must increase to reflect the benefits to communities of the work and the people who perform that work, who are usually, but not exclusively, female. In addition, the recognition that domestic and childcare responsibilities constitute the full-time occupation of many women, and a second occupation for others, suggests that occupational health for women comprises effects from both the home and workplace environments. Often, these effects combine to reduce a woman's ability to achieve good physical and mental health. Occupational health policies and regulations generally address the paid workplace only; the recognition of the interactions of women's multiple social and economic roles may require accommodation and certainly demands further research.

DISCUSSION QUESTIONS

1. What are some of the factors that make reproductive studies among working women difficult to do in occupational settings?

2. Using criteria such as population prevalence, seriousness of outcome, and cost to society, how would you rank the health impact on women workers of intimate partner violence, secondary traumatic stress syndrome of caregivers, and dual occupations of paid work and domestic responsibilities?

3. Name some of the ways that governmental organization of public health agencies can affect occupational healthcare delivery to women workers.

4. What is the major limitation of the Global Plan of Action of Workers' Health?

REFERENCES

1. Veys CA. Bladder tumours in rubber workers: a factory study, 1946–1995. *Occup Med (Lond)*. 2004;54(5):322-329.

2. Frey GM, Ott MG, Messerer P, et al. Pregnancy protection program in a large chemical company: infant outcomes. *J Occup Environ Med*. 2007;49(5):519-525.

3. Claus CA, Berson M, Bertin J. Litigating reproductive and developmental health in the aftermath of UAW versus Johnson Controls. *Environ Health Persp*. 1993; 101(suppl 2):205-220.

4. McDonald A. Work and pregnancy. In: McDonald JC, ed. *Epidemiology of Work Related Diseases*. London, UK: BMJ Publishing Group; 1995:301-302.

5. Savitz DA, Whelan EA, Rowland AS, Kleckner RC. Maternal employment and reproductive risk factors. *Am J Epidemiol*. 1990;132(5):933-945.

6. Beaumont JJ, Swan SH, Hammond SK, et al. Historical cohort investigation of spontaneous abortion in the semiconductor health study: epidemiologic methods and analyses of risk in fabrication overall and in fabrication work groups. *Am J Indust Med*. 1995;28(6):735-750.

7. Figá-Talamanca I. Occupational risk factors and reproductive health of women. *Occup Med (Lond)*. 2006;56(8):521-531.

8. Women's Health. *Science*. 2005;308(5728, special section):1569-1594.

9. Wu W, Su J, Huang M. An epidemiological study on reproductive effects in female workers exposed to acrylonitrile. *Zhonghua Yu Fang Yi Xue Za Zhi*. 1995; 29(2):83-85.

10. Czeizel AE, Szilvási R, Timár L, Puhö E. Occupational epidemiological study of workers in an acrylonitrile using factory with particular attention to cancers and birth defects. *Mutat Res*. 2004;547(1-2):79-89.

11. Sharma L. Lifestyles, flying and associated health problems in flight attendants. *J R Soc Health*. 2007;127(6):268-275.

12. Aasmoe L, Bang B, Egeness C, Løchen ML. Musculoskeletal symptoms among seafood production workers in North Norway. *Occup Med (Lond)*. 2008;58(1): 64-70.

13. Hayasaka Y, Nakamura K, Yamamoto M, Sasaki S. Work environment and mental health status assessed by the general health questionnaire in female Japanese doctors. *Ind Health*. 2008;45(6):781-786.

14. Sardiwalla N, VandenBerg H, Esterhuyse KG. The role of stressors and coping strategies in the burnout experienced by hospice workers. *Cancer Nurs*. 2007; 30(6):488-497.

15. Gunnarsson K, Vingård E, Josephson M. Self-rated health and working conditions of small-scale enterprisers in Sweden. *Ind Health*. 2008;45(6):775-780.

16. Musshauser D, Bader A, Wildt B, Hochleitner M. The impact of sociodemographic factors vs. gender roles on female hospital workers' health: Do we need to shift emphasis? *J Occup Health*. 2006;48(5):383-391.

17. Killien MG, Habermann B, Jarrett M. Influence of employment characteristics on postpartum mothers' health. *Women Health*. 2001;33(1-2):63-81.

18. Nachreiner NM, Gerberich SG, Ryan AD, McGovern PM. Minnesota nurses' study: perceptions of violence and the work environment. *Ind Health*. 2007; 45(5):672-678.

19. Celik SS, Celik Y, Ağirbaş I, Uğurluoğlu O. Verbal and physical abuse against nurses in Turkey. *Int Nurs Rev*. 2007;54(4):359-366.

20. Gates DM, Gillespie GL. Secondary traumatic stress in nurses who care for traumatized women. *J Obstet Gynecol Neonatal Nurs.* 2008;37(2):243-249.

21. Reeves C, O'Leary-Kelly AM. The effects and costs of intimate partner violence for work organizations. *J Interpers Violence.* 2007;22(3):327-344.

22. Kwesiga E, Bell MP, Pattie M, Moe AM. Exploring the literature on relationships between gender roles, intimate partner violence, occupational status, and organizational benefits. *J Interpers Violence.* 2007;22(3):312-326.

23. Ivanov I, Kortum E, Wilburn S. Protecting and promoting health at the workplace. *Global Occupational Health Network Newsletter.* 2007-2008; Winter. http://www.who.int/occupational_health/publications/newsletter/gohnet_14e .pdf. Accessed May 23, 2008.

24. Navarro V. The new conventional wisdom: an evaluation of the WHO report Health Systems; Improving Performance. In: Navarro V, Muntaner C, eds. *Political and Economic Determinants of Population Health and Well-being: Controversies and Developments.* Amityville, NY: Baywood; 2004:163-172.

25. Lethridge J. Occupational health regulations and health workers: protection or vulnerability? Public Services International Research Unit (PSIRU). http://www .psiru.org. Accessed May 23, 2008.

26. The Bangkok Charter for Health Promotion in a Globalized World. Accessed June 1, 2008. http://www.who.int/healthpromotion/conferences/6gchp/hpr_050829 _%20BCHP.pdf.

27. Tüchen F, Christensen KB, Lund T, Feveile H. A 15-year prospective study of shift work and disability pension. *Occup Environ Med.* 2008;65(4):283-285.

Challenges and Progress

Globalization and rapid advancement in science and technology have resulted in great progress in many arenas for the global society. Unfortunately the lives of millions of women worldwide have not improved owing to a myriad of factors. This section attempts to discuss the challenges faced and the progress made in improving women's health and status in society. The long and difficult journey from Alma-Ata to Millennium Development Goals within a framework of women's global health and human rights is discussed.

We think sometimes that poverty is only being hungry, naked, and homeless. The poverty of being unwanted, unloved, and uncared for is the greatest poverty. We must start in our own homes to remedy this kind of poverty.

—Mother Theresa, Nobel Peace Prize Laureate

CHAPTER 38

Women's Engagement Essential to Building the Culture of Peace

Pervasive poverty and limited human, financial, technical, and institutional capacities in the developing countries not only breed conditions for conflict, but they also severely limit people and government's ability to deal with the consequences of war and conflict. Of course, not only does poverty breed conflict, but conflict also cultivates poverty. Massive displacement of civilians, destruction of social and physical infrastructure, and diversion of resources toward military activities—all combine to depress economic activity, deprive people of their livelihoods, and deny them basic services such as healthcare, education, food, and water.

The most victimized of this apparently intractable cycle of poverty and conflict are women. Women constitute 50% of the global population, but their participation and full engagement in building sustainable peace at national, regional, and global levels still remains rather minimal. Though in nearly every country and region of the world, we can point to areas in which there has been some progress in achieving gender equality and women's empowerment, that progress has been uneven and the gains remain fragile. Virtually nowhere are women's rights given the priority they deserve.

*Ambassador Anwarul K. Chowdhury, MA,
Former Under-Secretary-General
and High Representative of the UN*

Ambassador Anwarul K. Chowdhury, MA, is the former Under-Secretary-General and former President of Security Council and High Representative of the UN. He is also the recipient of the U Thant Peace Award and UNESCO Gandhi Gold Medal for Culture of Peace. He is an Honorary Patron of the Committee on Teaching About the UN (CTAUN), New York. In March 2003, the Soka University of Tokyo, Japan conferred on Ambassador Chowdhury an Honorary Doctorate for his work on women's issues, child rights, and culture of peace as well as for the strengthening of the United Nations.

Challenges Women Face

Volumes have been spoken and written about the role of women in development. However, one area of women's involvement that has not been adequately addressed is women's role in the area of peace and security. Their role in this crucial area has been ignored and undervalued for a long time.

Women are deeply affected by conflicts that they have had little or no role in creating. Women's interests have been neglected by the peace-making process, which has resulted in male-centered approaches to peace and security. Equally challenging is the growing violence against women and girls in armed conflict. In today's conflicts, they are not only the victims of torture and terror, displacement and destitution, they are directly targeted with rape, forced pregnancies, and assault as deliberate instruments of war:

- A statement from the Fourth World Conference on Women, in Beijing in 1995,[1] noted that women are to an alarming degree the main victims of war and violence. The culture of violence affects women in many ways—through direct physical and sexual violence, especially in war, which is the ultimate expression of the culture of violence. Women also suffer disproportionately from the neglect of social services due mainly to excessive military expenditure.

- But the statement also declares that "the dynamic movement toward a culture of peace derives inspiration and hope from women's visions and actions."[1,2] It further underscores that full respect for the human rights of women; the release of women's creative potential in all aspects of life; the equal participation of women in decision making; equal access to educational opportunities for woman and girls; the promotion of equality between women and men are all seen as prerequisites to attaining the culture of peace.

- The core message of this 1995 statement continues to be equally relevant today.

Role of UN Agencies, NGOs, and Governments

It is reassuring to note that during the last few years, there has been an increasing recognition by governments, international organizations, and civil society of the importance of gender equality and the empowerment of women in the continuing struggle for equality, poverty reduction, peace, security, democracy, human rights, and development. If enough efforts and resources were invested in fighting poverty through equality of participation by women and men, many of the costly conflicts we have experienced would probably not have occurred. Ensuring women's equality is therefore a wise investment in achieving the culture of peace and poverty reduction.

Nonviolence can truly flourish when the world is free of poverty, hunger, discrimination, exclusion, intolerance, and hatred. As a set of values, modes of behaviour and ways of life based on respect for life, human rights, nonviolence, and the economic and social well-being of each and every human person, the culture of peace can be a powerful tool in promoting a global consciousness that serves the interests of a just and sustainable peace. That is how women and men can realize their highest potential and live a secure and fulfilling life.[3]

The need to banish poverty and conflict has never been greater, given that with globalization, our destinies are becoming ever more intertwined. Human tragedies in one part of the world affect us all, be it through economic shocks, refugee flows and forced migration, or increased threats of terrorism.

A very far-reaching initiative in March 2000 resulted in the United Nations Security Council resolution 1325 of 2000.[4] It is a landmark decision that has taken into account, for the first time in 55 years, the unrecognized, underutilized, and undervalued contribution women can make to preventing war, building peace, and bringing individuals and societies back in harmony. That is when launching the initiative, as the president of the security council, I strongly emphasized that "Peace is inextricably linked with equality between women and men."

The potential of Resolution 1325,[5] its implications and its impact in real terms, are enormous. Women and men all over the world have been energized by such a resolution. Political support for its implementation by member states, international organizations, and, most importantly, civil society is growing, albeit slowly.

Some progress has been made in six broad areas, led by the UN:

1. Awareness of the importance of gender perspectives in peace support work

2. Development of gender action work plans in disarmament and humanitarian affairs

3. Training in gender sensitivity and deployment of gender advisers

4. Prevention and response to violence against women

5. Work on codes of conduct, including sexual harassment that resulted in significant Security Council deliberations in June 2008

6. Support to greater participation of women in postconflict reconstruction, postconflict elections, and governance

Much, nevertheless, remains to be done. Women are still very often ignored or excluded from formal processes of negotiations and elections.

That women make a difference when in decision- and policy-making positions is no longer in dispute. Gender equality needs to be a fundamental requirement of the development cooperation architecture. Gender-oriented programmes funded by donors should be aimed at empowering women in productive activities, improving their access to assets, providing them with equal opportunities, and increasing their role in decision making.

When women participate in peace negotiations and in the crafting of a peace agreement, they keep the future of their societies and their communities, in mind. They think of how their children and grandchildren will live in their country and how they will benefit from the peace agreement in a sustainable way. They have the greater and longer-term interest of society in mind. Whereas, historically in postconflict situations, men are interested in ensuring that, following the peace agreement, they will retain authority and power in the government or in the cabinet or in any other power structure.

The Mano River Women's Peace Network,[6] for example, brings together women in west Africa from Guinea, Liberia, and Sierra Leone. In pursuing their vision of peace, they rallied together to call for disarmament and played a crucial role in paving the way to solving the conflict by having the three heads of government sitting at the same table. This joint peace initiative by the women of the Mano River region was awarded the UN Prize for Human Rights for 2003 by the General Assembly in recognition of its outstanding achievement.

Women's distinctive experiences, perspectives, skills, and competence in conflict resolution and management, in opposing the use of force, in preventing violence, in healing and reconciliation, as well as women's potential for leadership, need to be recognized and enhanced. Effective mechanisms—both national and global—to fully implement and monitor women's rights and participation in peace processes need to be developed.

Peace is a prerequisite for human development. A lasting peace cannot be achieved without the participation of women and the inclusion of gender perspectives in peace processes. Informal peace initiatives by grassroots women's groups and networks, organized across party and ethnic lines, have carried out reconciliation efforts and have been increasingly recognized by the Security Council.

Conclusion

Gender perspectives must be fully integrated into the terms of reference of peace-keeping-related Security Council resolutions, reports, and missions. Peace support operations should include gender specialists, and consultations with women's groups and networks must be ensured. Full involvement of women in negotiations of peace agreements at national and global levels must be provided for, including training for women on formal peace processes. Gender perspectives should also be an integral part of postconflict reconstruction programmes. A no-tolerance approach must be used in cases of violation of the code of conduct in peace-keeping operations. Gender sensitivity training must be provided to the peace keepers before they arrive in the zones of conflict.

I would strongly emphasize the importance of women's equal participation in all efforts for peace and security—in the prevention and resolution of conflicts and in peace building. While women are often the first victims of armed conflict, they must also and always be recognized as a key to the solution. Women have an essential role to play in rebuilding war-shattered societies, not through token representation but as full-fledged participants in the process.

> For generations, women have served as peace educators, both in their families and in their societies. They have proved instrumental in building bridges rather than walls.
>
> —Kofi Annan, UN Secretary General

Sustainable peace is inseparable from gender equality. When women are marginalized, there is little chance for an open, participatory, peaceful society.

DISCUSSION QUESTIONS

1. Why is women's engagement vital to promote the culture of peace?
2. Discuss some of the factors that prevent women from enjoying their human rights.
3. Discuss the role of the United Nations in promoting women's health, human rights, and in promoting peace and security.

REFERENCES

1. Division for the Advancement of Women United Nations. Beijing Platform for Action adopted by the United Nations Fourth World Conference on Women, China 1995. http://www.un.org/womenwatch/daw/beijing/platform/plat1.htm. Accessed July 18, 2008.
2. United Nations Educational, Scientific and Cultural Organization. Statement on Women's Contribution to a Culture of Peace, Fourth World Conference on Women Beijing, China September 1995. http://www.unesco.org/cpp/uk/declarations/wcpbei.htm. Accessed July 18, 2008.
3. United Nations Educational Scientific and Cultural Organization. Asian Women for a Culture of Peace Conference Hanoi Declaration. December 9, 2000. http://www.unesco.org/cpp/uk/projects/wcpviet_declar.htm. Accessed July 18, 2008.
4. Chowdhury AK. *United Nations Security Council Resolution 1325: What Are the Challenges?* Presented at: Peace and Security: Implementing UN Security Council Resolution 1325; May 30–June 2, 2006; Wilton Park, UK.
5. Chowdhury AK. *Message for the GAPS UK event on SCR 1325 Implementation.* Presented at: Report on Involving Men in the Implementation of UN Security Council Resolution 1325 on Women, Peace and Security; May 13, 2007; London.
6. United Nations Treaty Series. No. 13608. Mano River Declaration Establishing the Mano River Union Between Liberia and Sierra Leone. 1973. http://untreaty.un.org/unts/60001_120000/9/14/00016661.pdf. Accessed July 29, 2008.

CHAPTER 39

Women's Health in a Multicultural World: Challenges and Progress in Africa

Culture, in the form of long-held views, taboos, and customs, lies behind the gender imbalance and the lower status given to women in practically all communities and nations, and is consequently of particular importance in the field of reproductive health. Internationally accepted human rights are frequently ignored, often in the name of culture or anachronistic laws and practices, and this is particularly so in Africa. While some traditions are beneficial, others are harmful or prejudicial.

This chapter argues that culture is dynamic and subject to external influences of various kinds. Several aspects of reproductive health are examined, including the reasons for high maternal mortality, unsafe abortion, sexually transmissible infections, and HIV/AIDS. Recommendations for improvements in reproductive health service provision and women's empowerment are made. The Africa Health Strategy agreed upon in April 2007 should be implemented. Steps should be taken to change adverse cultural practices in Africa by education and new laws where appropriate, and the medical profession should strive to advocate the good and eliminate the bad.

Whether one believes in biblical creation, intelligent design, or evolution, it is difficult to escape the conclusion that nature is biologically sexist. How else can the contribution of the male to human reproduction be reduced to such a few moments of ecstasy and the female tasked with such a long period of personal suffering and commitment and even death? Instead of mankind seeing to it that this reproductive vulnerability of the female is minimized through all possible means it has rather become a reason for the creation of all manner of structures, institutions, and laws aimed at keeping the female of the species down and denying her autonomy in many traditions and cultures.

Religion that supposedly should bring compassion, understanding, and assistance in case of need is even invoked in many instances to support the belief that women are inferior to men or that they should be made to suffer for original sin. The biblical curse on Eve for having led Adam astray is still quoted, in some circles, as a justification for this. Nor is this all. For many centuries, Western

Fred T. Sai, MB, BS, FRCP, MPH

Fred Sai, MB, BS, FRCP, MPH, is currently an advisor to the President of Ghana on Reproductive Health, HIV/AIDS; has been Professor of Community Health and Director of Medical Services in Ghana, Nutrition Advisor to the Africa region of FAO, Assistant Secretary General and later President of the International Planned Parenthood Federation (IPPF), and Population Advisor to the World Bank. He chaired the Main Committee of the ICPD (Cairo 1994).

Recipient of UN Population Award in 1993 and honorary fellowship of the ACOG & Royal College of Obstetricians and Gynecologists, for his promotion of women's health and rights.

societies believed that women's brains were physically smaller than men's, and therefore women were biologically inferior to men. Advances in medicine have proved this wrong, but getting rid of a basis for stigmatization is difficult. Women's smaller physical frame has also been interpreted as the weaker sex, until lifetime studies proved beyond all doubt that they are made for better longevity than men. Despite much proof, long-held views, taboos, and customs, often put together as culture, still lie behind the gender imbalance and the lower status given to women in practically all communities and nations.

Although culture is important in the entire health field it could be of particular nastiness in its application in the field of reproductive health. At this point let me try and give some working definitions of culture and then the accepted definition of reproductive health. These would form the basis for examining the relationships between the two.

Culture

Culture may be defined according to the Random House dictionary as "the total sum of ways of living built up by a group of human beings and transmitted from one generation to another." A more expansive definition given by Acsadi and Acsadi is:

Culture determines sources of authority and power and defines status. It is the reference for judicature and specifies who and what each member is and how others will react to and deal with her or him. It enhances or retards political stability, economic growth and, importantly, recognition of and respect for individual's human rights. Every aspect of the systematic maltreatment of women and girls has a cultural reference, is part of an institutionalized phenomenon. Consequently, amelioration of female-gender-determined sufferings and disadvantages will require alterations or banishment of elements of long-established cultural patterns.[1]

My only qualification would be that some of the patterns may not be that long-established. Changes in breastfeeding practices are an example of relatively recent changes. Secondly, culture is dynamic and subject to external influences of various kinds.

Reproductive Health

The International Conference on Population and Development (ICPD), held in Cairo in 1994, obtained a definition from The World Health Organization (WHO) which was agreed by consensus as follows:

Reproductive health is a state of complete physical, mental, and social well-being and not merely the absence of disease or infirmity in all matters relating to the reproductive system and to its functions and processes. Reproductive health therefore implies that people are able to have a satisfying and safe sex life and that they have the capability to reproduce and the freedom to decide if, when, and how often to do so. Implicit in this last are the rights of men and women to be informed and to have access to safe, effective, affordable, and acceptable methods of family planning of their choice for regulation of fertility that are not against the law, and the right of access to appropriate healthcare services that would enable women to go safely through pregnancy and childbirth and provide couples with the best chance of having a healthy infant. In line with the above definition of reproductive health, reproductive health care is defined as the constellation of methods, techniques, and services that contribute to reproductive health and well-being by preventing and solving reproductive health problems. It also includes sexual health, the purpose of which is the enhancement of life and personal relations and not merely counseling and care related to reproduction and sexually transmitted diseases."[2]

It comes as no surprise that such a very broad definition would confront culture, religion, and legal issues in its interpretation and implementation. In fact, such recognition led to the statement introducing the principles to the ICPD Program of Action as follows: "The implementation of the recommendations contained in the Program of Action is the sovereign right of each country, consistent with national laws and development priorities, with full respect for the various religious and ethical values and cultural backgrounds of its people, and in conformity with universally recognized international human rights."[3]

Unfortunately this well-crafted statement seems to be only partially accepted—to the extent that nations have the sovereign right to implement or not. The part referring to internationally accepted human rights is frequently ignored, often in the name of culture or some anachronistic laws and practices.

Culture itself covers a wide spectrum of human activities, beliefs, and practices about health and illness, laws, religion, and medical practices. Culture determines to a great extent the attributes of good health and the origins, prevention, and management of disease, including the definition of cure. In many traditional societies health and disease may depend on both organic and spiritual or magical causes. Many traditional societies strongly believe in the ability of certain specially endowed individuals to cause disease in others. There are gods whose anger or displeasure could create havoc with individuals and whole societies. Even accidents on the farm or on the road could be assigned to supernatural origins. Why else should the rare constellation of circumstances that lead to the situation occur? In clinical medicine we need to be acutely aware of the patient's beliefs about the illness if we are to cure the whole person.

Such beliefs and traditions are all parts of culture and could lead to the development of a whole series of practices of "dos and don'ts" that could be harmful, neutral, or helpful. Perhaps it is in the field of sexual and reproductive health that we encounter most of the sad outcomes of traditional and cultural practices that are harmful or prejudicial to the enjoyment and self-fulfillment of women—some of these are examined below.

Pregnancy and unsafe abortion are the leading causes of death among women of reproductive age in most African countries. The maternal mortality rate, which measures the death rate of women due to pregnancy and childbirth, is higher in Africa than on any other continent: 820 deaths per 100,000 live births for the continent as a whole in 2005, and an average of 900 for sub-Saharan Africa. In some countries it is believed to be as high as 2000 deaths per 100,000 live births.[4]

The high mortality rate masks an even higher morbidity rate: the same afflictions that kill hundreds of thousands of women maim and render sterile many millions more of their sisters. For every woman who dies, 50 to 100 others suffer short-, medium-, or long-term debilities from their pregnancies and deliveries. Vesicovaginal fistula is an example of the serious long-term problems.

These ratios do not give a true picture of the risk of death associated with pregnancy and childbirth. When we factor in the total numbers of births per woman we get the true lifetime risks, and these range from 1 in 22 for sub-Saharan Africa to 1 in 8200 for the UK.[5]

It has been rightly observed that the differences in the risk of death from pregnancy-related causes indicate the worst possible health environments which result from apartheid inter- and intra-country conflicts in the world. The major causes of maternal deaths are practically the same all over the world: hemorrhage, infection, pregnancy related hypertension, anemia, obstructed labor, and abortions. That these no longer kill in the advanced countries means the technologies and methods for their control and management exist. Why are we so far behind in applying the knowledge and technologies to save the African women? Is it because they are not considered worth saving?

The immediate reasons for these high mortality and morbidity figures are poor, inadequate, or inaccessible health and other services to handle pregnancy and its complications. No matter what is done, pregnancy and childbirth carry the risk of complications, the majority of which arise without any warning. But the situation is complicated and worsened by the context within which African women grow and form their families too.

Some Background Causes of High Maternal Mortality

Many girls are born prematurely or at low birth weight because their own mothers were malnourished, ill, or overworked. If she survives infancy, an African girl will most likely grow up on a diet that does not meet her minimum nutritional requirements. As a child she will have a heavy burden of household chores and may receive little or no schooling. She is likely to be married off young, especially if a good bride price is available. She is likely taught that her role in life is to bear as many children "as God brings." During pregnancy her needs for adequate rest, good nutrition, and healthcare are too often ignored. Poverty forces her to work through the final stages of pregnancy, and myths restricting the consumption of food generally and certain foods (such as eggs and vegetables) in particular, may further deplete the pregnant woman's strength at a time when she urgently needs a balanced diet. Fortunately many of these beliefs are changing, but such change, where it is happening at all, is often too slow.

There are many traditional practices that also increase the risks for women. There are societies in which women are forced into marriage at an early age. Such coerced marriage is usually followed by too early childbearing. There are societies that do not consider rape and defilement serious crimes against the female person. In some cultures men have such complete rights over the bodies of their wives that the police will not touch domestic violence, even when such violence is aimed at a pregnant woman. Ghana's recent effort to enact a domestic violence act should be a reminder of how strong some male positions could be. For two years or so, the bill was held up, until the clause on marital rape was removed. This led someone to observe that with the removal of that clause, men could continue beating their spouses into submission, even if they were bringing diseases home. Unfortunately, many African men today want these practices to continue in the name of culture.

Perhaps a cultural practice that directly influences maternal mortality is the husband or another male relation having exclusive right to decide whether a pregnant woman should seek outside help. This leads to delays that often prove fatal.

Many other forms of violence and denial of the reproductive and sexual rights of women persist in Africa. A practice known as *trokosi*, in Ghana, is particularly vicious. Young virgins, some of them mere babies, are assigned to shrines in atonement for some sin or crime allegedly committed by a member of their clan or even ancestor. These virgins become sex slaves for the shrine head. As soon as they menstruate they are ready for sex. They have no say whatsoever in what happens to their own bodies. These are extreme forms of denial of human and reproductive rights, and again

change, though happening, is very slow. Trafficking and subjugation of young women for sex and other nefarious purposes is on the increase.

We may ask why a damaging cultural tradition such as female genital mutilation or cutting, FGM or FGC, continues in so many societies. As well as being a way of repressing or lessening the sexual gratification of women, it can also cause obstetric and other physical damage, including deaths due to hemorrhage, infection, and tetanus that may follow the procedure. Nahid Toubia has claimed that 84 to 114 million women have had this procedure done on them, and that at least 2 million young girls are at risk of having FGM performed each year.[6] Across Africa the prevalence rates of the operation vary from a high of 90% in Ethiopia to a low of 5% in Uganda and Zaire.

Unsafe Abortion

Of the 66,500 abortion-related deaths occurring worldwide, well over half (35,900) occur in sub-Saharan Africa. The average percentage of maternal mortality due to unsafe abortion in Africa is around 14%.[7] In many countries the figures are 25 to 50%. In Ghana 20–30% of maternal deaths are caused by unsafe abortion, even though the law has been liberalized since 1985. In Nigeria, where abortion is legally restricted and permitted only to save the life of the pregnant woman, an estimated 610,000 abortions occur annually, with unsafe abortions contributing 40% of maternal mortality, estimated to account for 20,000 of the 50,000 maternal deaths occurring each year. Adolescents are claimed to account for more than half the recorded cases. And yet this is among the most preventable of conditions. Unsafe abortion is defined as abortion being performed by an unskilled person, under unsanitary conditions, or both. Such an abortion is usually being performed where there are legal restrictions to abortions, like we have in practically all countries in the African region. Tunisia and South Africa stand out as the exceptions.

It should not be forgotten that the restrictive abortion laws found in Africa today have been inherited from the colonial powers. These laws date from the mid-1800s, at a time when abortions were mainly done by the barber surgeons and abortion mortality rates were higher than those from carrying a pregnancy to term. Essentially the laws were meant to protect the lives of women. To me it is a cruel irony that these laws have been repealed in all of the countries that introduced them to Africa, and that those countries now have practically no deaths from unsafe abortions anymore, while African nations maintain them and see unsafe abortions killing their women.

Why?

One thing that is certain is that no level of restriction has ever succeeded in preventing abortion as a major cause of maternal mortality. In fact when a relatively liberal abortion law was replaced by a strictly restricted one in Romania, abortion mortality skyrocketed as did the maternal mortality figures. With a revolution and a change in government, the laws were again changed and the abortion and maternal mortality figures plummeted. All restrictions do is drive the practice underground and make victims of women. More upsetting is the fact that such laws become most discriminatory in their implementation. Usually the higher social classes, the moneyed, and the more highly educated get their abortions done safely, even if at a high financial cost. The poor, the illiterate, and the young resort to quacks, and pay with their health, their future and often, with life itself.

Sexually Transmissible Infections

Sexually transmissible infections (STIs) have been a major world health problem for a long time; yet, until the advent of HIV/AIDS, very few countries gave much attention to them. Perhaps this is because with the conquest of syphilis, they do less damage to men than to women. Certainly women's health is more seriously affected by STIs, causing a tremendous amount of suffering, such as pelvic inflammatory disease and infertility. STIs are estimated to be second only to maternal causes in the load of sickness and disability of women.

According to WHO, STIs have become the most common group of notifiable diseases in most countries worldwide, but prevalence rates are particularly high in developing countries. In 1990, WHO estimated the world prevalence at 250 million, in 1999 the figure was revised upward to 340 million new cases in persons aged 15 to 49 years. Among the more than 20 pathogens known to cause these infections the major ones are syphilis, gonorrhea, chlamydia, trichomoniasis, and chancroid. HIV has a place of its own. Ulcerative STIs increase the chances of transmission of HIV by a factor of 10. The following figures are presented just to give an idea of how serious these infections are. There are 12 million new cases of syphilis, 62 million of gonorrhea, 30 million of papilloma virus (a cause of many cervical cancers), 92 million of chlamydia, and 174 million of trichomoniasis. WHO estimated in 2001 that there are 69 million new cases of curable STIs (syphilis, gonorrhea, chlamydia, and trichomoniasis) every year in sub-Saharan Africa—the highest rate of new cases per 1000 population of any region.[8]

It has been claimed that among women, syphilis prevalence rates are 10 to 100 times higher in developing countries, gonorrhea rates 10 to 15 times higher. Untreated syphilis can lead to pregnancy wastage (abortions, stillbirths, neonatal deaths, or childhood abnormalities). The annual rate of new gonorrhea infection in some large African cities have been found to be as high as 3000 per 10,000 population. In Kenya the prevalence of gonorrhea was estimated at 1–10% with the highest prevalence among rural women. Chlamydia affected between 6% and 21%, and syphilis between 1% and 9%. Accurate figures are hard to get, but rates as high as 60% have been found in some populations, and a figure of 20% was found in some schoolgirls in Cameroon. A recent study in Ghana showed some 10% of junior secondary schoolchildren had had some type of STI in the previous 12 months.

Needless to say, women are more likely to catch STIs than men: transmission occurs more easily from male to female than vice versa. The risk of acquiring gonorrhea from a single act of coitus in which one partner is infectious is approximately 25% for men and 50% for women.

HIV/AIDS

In the beginning of the AIDS epidemic, at least in the US and western Europe, AIDS was found in homosexuals and intravenous drug abusers. This was unfortunate, in that it led to a sluggishness of response, if not outright denial that the infection could be of any consequence to general society, who behaved correctly and obeyed God's laws. By the time society realized that this was a serious threat to mankind as a whole, the infection could no longer be contained. Now the statistics are frightening, particularly for Africa.

In 2007, over two-thirds (68%) of all persons infected with HIV were living in sub-Saharan Africa—22.5 million. An estimated 1.7 million African adults and children became infected with HIV in 2007, more than in all other regions of the world combined. The 1.6 million AIDS deaths in sub-Saharan Africa represent 76% of global AIDS deaths. There are 13 million AIDS orphans in Africa—more than in the whole of the rest of the world.[9]

HIV/AIDS in Africa has demonstrated the extreme vulnerability of the African woman when it comes to the area of sexual and reproductive rights and health. Worldwide, the male:female ratio of infection is several men to one woman. In Africa the ratio is on average 1 man to 1.2 women. During the early period of the epidemic, in Ghana, the ratio was about six women to one man. This came down to two women to one man and now it is about 1.3 to 1, still a serious statistic of one-third more women. For younger women the situation is even graver. Among young people ages 15–24 years, women were found to be two and half times as likely to be infected as their male counterparts. For 15 to 19 year olds even worse figures have been found; in some studies six females to one male. While biological differences no doubt account for some of the differences, the majority must be due to environmental and societal factors related to femalehood and gender in sub-Saharan Africa.

That most women are powerless in gender relations is well known. A woman refusing a husband or man-friend his request for sex risks severe beatings or immediate termination of all rights in the relationship. But what should be an even greater cause for concern is the belief, in some areas and cultures, that sleeping with a virgin cures a sexually transmitted infection, or the equally heinous attitude of men sleeping with ever younger girls because they would be less likely to carry an infection. The recent news reports of increases in female child defilement must be abhorrent to all and not just to women. These acts are committed against the most vulnerable in society most of the time. Human and reproductive rights are being violated, often with impunity, just because the victims are girls or women.

Recommendations

Family Planning

Universal access to family planning must rank as the number one strategy for improving maternal health and reducing maternal mortality. A woman's ability to manage her fertility surely underpins her capacity to manage all other aspects of her life. Once pregnancy and childbirth can be confined to the appropriate age and in cognizance of personal development and other needs, there is freedom to pursue economic and developmental activities. It is not just a cliché to say that if one does not get pregnant one does not suffer maternal mortality; and the adverse risks are higher with unwanted, unplanned, or ill-timed pregnancies. The risks of complicated pregnancy are higher in the teens, in the over 40s, and in women with fertilities over four.

There are encouraging signs that things are beginning to change, but the tempo is still too slow. African governments are now worrying more specifically about the implications of high population growth rates: three-quarters of Africans now live in countries with governments that view their population growth rates as too high. In fact, one of the most significant population policy developments of recent years was the continued rise in the number of African governments that reported policies aimed at reducing the rapid growth of their population: 66% in 2005, up from 60% in 1996, 39% in 1986, and 25% in 1976.[10]

Family planning programs should pay special attention to the adolescent. This is a period of very rapid development of physical, psychological, and sexual attributes and orientation, a period in which dangerous experiments and practices may be pursued, practices that could create risks and vulnerabilities. Quality and realistic education and service programs developed with the involvement of the youth should be the ideal. Adolescent sexuality and reproductive health is an issue that makes some feel most uncomfortable. But such discomfort does not make the problem go away.

Religious fiats have not produced the desired effects in most cases. Evidence abounds of how to go about such programs, and we must endeavor to come to terms with the execution of such programs. Health workers in particular should not be moral judges over youngsters who have "gone astray."

Unsafe Abortion

The issue of unsafe abortion needs to be looked at as a public health issue. Many reproductive health programs now include postabortion care. This is good as far as it goes, but it is not enough. We should strive for comprehensive abortion care rather than simply trying to clear the mess after it has been created.

With modern technology and in the proper circumstances, abortion can be the safest of all medical procedures. If unsafe abortion is contributing 10–50% or more of the maternal deaths then what is the justification for not wanting safe abortion? Laws should protect the individual and safeguard personal rights, such as autonomy, the right to life, and the right to access suitable medical services. Restrictive abortion laws negate the enjoyment of these rights by women—and only women.

Eliminating unsafe abortion alone could reduce the maternal mortality rate in some African countries by 30–50%. In some countries it will minimize, if not completely remove, the very upsetting premature deaths of young females. Unfortunately many who take such a strong stand against pregnancy termination on any grounds are not privy to some of the heartrending cases that some doctors have to deal with.

Making Pregnancy Safer

The third major recommendation requires a holistic effort to make pregnancy safer, in other words safe motherhood programs. All pregnancies carry a risk, and the majority of the risks cannot be predicted. Therefore, apart from ensuring that women are properly prepared, in all ways to carry a pregnancy to term, proper arrangements must be made for handling the unexpected. In this the health system has the primary role, and this is to be played out among families and communities. From evidence collected during the last decade a holistic system for safer motherhood should consist of the services discussed in the following sections.

Antenatal or Prenatal Care   It is during the prenatal period that any existing condition that may interfere with the pregnancy or safe delivery is tackled. In much of Africa today anemia is common, as is malaria. Protocols for handling these exist. HIV, as stated, is highly prevalent in many countries; rates as high as 40% have been found in some regions. The antenatal visits give a chance for testing for the prevention of mother-to-child transmission if indicated and for the better care of the expectant mother. This is also the period for educating the woman, her spouse, and her family on what to expect and where her emergency and other medical needs can be met.

Delivery Care   Wherever the delivery is to take place it must be attended by a trained birth attendant. This could be a physician, a nurse, or a midwife. The traditional birth attendant, even with training, has not proven very good at saving the lives of pregnant women. They could perform a useful function of linking the pregnant women and their families with the health system.

As soon as an emergency threatens or occurs, the pregnant woman should be transferred to a health facility equipped and staffed to provide emergency obstetric care. More deaths occur around the time of delivery and immediately thereafter than at any other period. Therefore no delay in accessing care should be permitted at this time.

Three levels of fatal delay have been identified as contributing to the majority of maternal deaths. The delay in the decision to seek higher medical help occurs in the home or within the community in which the birth is occurring. Such a delay may be due to nonrecognition of danger signs by the woman, her family members, or even the birth attendant. Sometimes culture, beliefs, or tradition may be to blame. We all know that there are people who believe that prolonged labor is an indication of female infidelity and without confession the baby would not come out. There are cultures in which only the spouse or a male relative can allow evacuation for further treatment.

The appalling state of transportation in Africa means that even when the decision to seek higher help is taken, getting to the facility could itself be a problem. So any means of getting quick transportation or the use of two-way communication to get helpful direction on what to do can help. There are many examples of community transportation arrangements that have helped to overcome this delay, and these need to be expanded.

Even when the pregnant woman gets to a health facility it may be poorly equipped. It may lack appropriate drugs, blood, or transfusion fluids. It may be closed or the single trained person may be away or resting. A 24-hour, 7 days a week, fully functioning facility is the only one that will help finally to remove this last delay.

These measures can only function properly if the total health system is so revamped as to be accessible socially, culturally, geographically, and financially to those needing care. And therefore there is a need to look at how we make our health systems more responsive to the needs of women and to make the women appreciate and use them. Various small projects have shown the value of community involvement in transportation, payment for supplies and services, and even the purchase of some equipment. These provide examples that could be scaled up.

Women's Empowerment and Gender Issues

None of these improvements and reforms will work on their own if our women are not treated with equity, if they are considered as less than equal and if we do not accept them by our sides in everything. Each African country should ask itself how far it has come in implementing the consensuses on equal rights, human rights, and gender equality and equity. Efforts are being made, but these are in many cases small and slow. It is now time for African women as individuals and as groups to become even more aggressive in the fight for their human and sexual and reproductive rights. They should identify those practices, traditions, laws, and other socially approved actions or views that hold them down, and set out selectively to remove and/or correct them. Some of the traditional practices that govern marital relations have to go. Even so-called modern laws that tend to remove voluntariness from marital sex should be removed. Violence in the home should not be tolerated under any circumstance. And here let me

plead with our priests. It is not right to use the phrase, "Obey and be humble to your husbands" anymore. Intrahome relationships should not be a one-way street. It should be one of mutual love and respect.

Women should continue advocating for good-quality education even though many countries are now trying to achieve the basic minimum for all. We need to ask for secondary-level education. Education, up to secondary levels, not only empowers but makes women better at taking care of their own and their family's health. Economic emancipation is the ability to exercise one's autonomy. The participation of women in policy making and administration is still low in many African countries, and this must change.

We must do better at reforming and implementing our own policies and must ensure that the MDGs that capture the essence of our women and their health-related targets are met. Men of goodwill should be partners in this endeavor. Although many men tend to think anything giving power to women means taking power from men, the reality is otherwise. Complementarity of thinking and of action in the home as well as in national situations makes for a better aggregate.

Conclusion

Observers of maternal health and mortality in Africa, including Shiffman and Okonofua in a recent paper, have concluded that the major reason why African women are faring so badly is the lack of political will by African leaders and not the lack of knowledge, the lack of human resources, or even the lack of financial resources.[11] The subject is simply kept below the radar, as it were, because those most intimately concerned, the women themselves, are among the voiceless. Perhaps the time has come for the women of Africa to make their voices heard and heard loudly. There are many women's organizations in all of the countries; there are some Africa-wide ones. Sadly, so far, there is none specifically to fight this very cruel injustice. My suggestion is that there is a need for national women's organizations advocating gender equity to make sexual and reproductive health and rights a major focus of their work. A continent-wide federation should make this subject a priority campaign and get a mass movement employing all legitimate methods to make the continental and national leaders fulfill their promises to make life better for women.

In April 2007, the African Union Conference of African Health Ministers meeting in Johannesburg, South Africa, adopted the Africa Health Strategy: 2007–2015, which significantly incorporated the African Charter's Protocol on the Rights of Women. This protocol is groundbreaking in a number of respects, not least in the sphere of reproductive rights, and abortion rights in particular: it is the first international human rights instrument to explicitly provide for abortion as a right in cases of rape and incest and for the mental and physical health of the pregnant woman.[12]

The Africa Health Strategy also acknowledges in its introduction that, despite some progress, "Africa is still not on track to meet the health Millennium Declaration targets, and the prevailing population trends could undermine progress made." But it also notes that "while Africa has 10% of the world population, it bears 25% of the global disease burden and has only 3% of the global health workforce. Of the 4 million estimated global shortage of health workers, 1 million are immediately required in Africa. This crisis has developed as a result of long-standing neglect and unfavourable international development policies and practices."[13]

It is hoped this milestone strategy will lead to international recognition that, because family planning and reproductive health programmes are so important for health, demographic, and general development reasons, it is essential that more, not fewer, resources be invested in this area. Many programmes are new and will need substantial funding as they expand. The numbers of women in the reproductive age groups are increasing, as are the proportions of those women who want to use contraception: today there are nearly 1 billion women of reproductive age in the developing world (projected to rise to over 1.2 billion by 2010).

Finally, more needs to be done to change adverse cultural practices in Africa. Change of behaviour, individual or collective, takes a long time. Confrontation usually is unhelpful. Greater emphasis should be given to girls' education and programmes to foster gender equity and equality and the social and economic empowerment of women. There should be specific laws against FGM and other forms of mutilation. But while legal change is useful, it is not always the first need, nor is it enough by itself. Safe abortion, for example, could be carried out within the existing laws in many African countries. Education, implementation, and demonstration of need could be a more useful approach.

The medical profession, in this and in other ways, needs to take its responsibilities more seriously. Doctors should have the courage to refuse to accept laws that infringe on human rights. They should use the public health justification for doing good—or at least doing no harm—more frequently than they sometimes do. As doctors, we should educate ourselves about the cultural and traditional environments in which we operate, understand their interaction with our roles, and make appropriate choices as to which are bad, which are neutral, and which are good; with the community we should strive to advocate the good and eliminate the bad. In doing this we should have the humility of knowledge and the patience and empathy that in the end make our efforts acceptable.

DISCUSSION QUESTIONS

1. Compare and contrast the influence of culture on women's health in Africa with the situation in your own region or country.

2. Discuss the challenges faced by the girl-child and women in enjoying a complete state of health (as defined by the WHO) in Africa.

3. Discuss the progress made with regard to women's health in Africa since the International Conference on Population in Mexico in 1984.

REFERENCES

1. Acsadi GTF, Johnson-Acsadi G. *Socio-Economic, Cultural and Legal Factors Affecting Girls' and Women's Health and Their Access to Utilization of Health and Nutrition Services in Developing Countries.* Washington, DC: World Bank; 1993.

2. United Nations. *Population and Development. Volume 1. Program of Action Adopted at the International Conference on Population and Development, Cairo, 513 September 1994.* New York: United Nations; 1995. ST/ESA/SER.A/149.

3. Ibid.

4. UNFPA. *Maternal Mortality in 2005: Estimates developed by WHO, UNICEF, UNFPA, and the World Bank.* New York: 2007.

5. United Nations. *Population and Development. Volume 1. Program of Action Adopted at the International Conference on Population and Development, Cairo, 513 September 1994.* New York: United Nations; 1995. ST/ESA/SER.A/149.

6. Toubia N. *Female Genital Mutilation: A Call for Global Action.* New York, NY: Population Council; 1993.

7. World Health Organization. *Unsafe Abortion: Global and Regional Estimates of the Incidence of Unsafe Abortion and Associated Mortality in 2003.* Geneva, Switzerland: United Nations; 2007.

8. World Health Organization. *Global Prevalence and Incidence of Selected Sexually Transmitted Infections.* Geneva, Switzerland: United Nations; 2001.

9. WHO/UNAIDS. *2007 AIDS Epidemic Update.* Geneva, Switzerland: United Nations; 2007.

10. United Nations. *World Population Policies 2005.* New York: United Nations; 2006.

11. Shiffman J, Okonofua FE. The state of political priority for safe motherhood in Nigeria. *Int J Obstetr Gynaecol.* 2007;114(2):127-133.

12. *Protocol to the African Charter on Human and Peoples' Rights on the Rights of Women in Africa.* http://www1.umn.edu/humanrts/africa/protocol-women2003.html. Accessed December 2, 2007.

13. *Africa Health Strategy 2007–2015.* http://www.sarpn.org.za/documents/d0002494/Africa_Health_strategy_Apr2007.pdf. Accessed December 2, 2007.

CHAPTER 40

Being a Woman in Rural India

Because the purpose of this book is to help public health practitioners and social scientists understand the challenges facing women, this chapter seeks to explain the choices that a woman in rural northern India makes and why she makes those choices, including the choice of female feticide. It is based on this author's 25 years of experience of research in rural India and tries to describe the life of a woman in rural Uttar Pradesh (a state in north India and India's most populous state) to help the reader understand the context of her decisions, her life, and circumstances.

The phrase "perfect storm" originates from a book[1] that talks of a rare combination of meteorological factors that, taken individually, would be far less powerful than the storm resulting from their chance combination. This phrase aptly describes the storm that has been brewing in India for a couple of decades now, whose impact is already being felt but whose true force and brutality will be felt for many decades. This is the storm of a steadily worsening sex ratio such that India today has 934 girls in the 0–4 year age band for every 1000 boys.[2] This ratio is worse in urban areas (912) compared to rural areas (942). This storm has been precipitated by the coming together of four disparate factors—social values and norms regarding women, deep-rooted cultural value placed on a male heir, economic opportunities that have given rise to aspirations not seen in earlier decades, and technology that is being used for a purpose that it had never been designed for.

Until the mid-1980s, when ultrasound technology made it possible to determine the gender of a child by about 14 weeks after conception, girls continued to be born in roughly the same proportion as boys, and their birth was often regarded with worry, or even disappointment, given the strong son bias in India. With the availability of ultrasound technology and the socioeconomic pressure to have fewer children, that disappointment was substituted by the proactive choice to not give birth to an unwanted girl-child. Available data shows that a first-born girl-child has a very good chance of survival. If the first born is a boy and the second pregnancy shows a girl, this child also has a very good chance of survival. However, if the

Hema Viswanathan, MA, PGDBA

Hema Viswanathan, MA, PGDBA is affiliated with ICG Consultants of Mumbai, India.

first born had been a girl, the second female fetus has a significantly lower chance of survival.[3,4]

Each family that used this technology did so to create a family composition of their choice. They were not thinking of the national picture then or of what would happen to society if every family started opting for boys. They were only thinking of their own world and how they wished to shape it.

In an attempt to curb this misuse of ultrasound technology, the government of India outlawed the whole process of sex determination and sex-selective abortion. The Prenatal Diagnostic Techniques Act 1994 makes sex determination illegal and the provisions of the Medical Termination of Pregnancy Act prohibit sex-selective abortions. Despite many attempts to enforce these laws it is believed that these are being routinely violated.

The second factor that has contributed to the storm of a skewed gender ratio today is growing economic aspiration. This author's anecdotal observation across hundreds of villages points to the same story. The decision to have fewer girl-children is not a decision made in abject poverty—it is a decision that is more likely to be seen in a family that has managed to claw its way out of real poverty and has seen some of the fruits of economic well-being. Families that have started to breathe easy because they now have enough to eat and have something saved away for a rainy day can despair at the thought of how a new daughter can drag them back into poverty. In the current social scenario, a girl-child can spell disaster to a family that has worked hard to make ends meet.

In earlier times, when everyone around was poor and there was not much hope of working one's way out of poverty, the impact was probably not as strong as it is today when a good life is visible and tantalizingly within reach. India's economic growth of the last decade has increased the desire for more because more can be seen and can be imagined for oneself and one's family. This does not mean material goods alone, though they do have a role in an average family's aspirations. Some of the largest dreams are for the education of children, particularly of sons. Families save money to send their children to private English-medium schools with the hope that fluency in English will help their sons break through the language barrier and make a quantum leap in earnings and living standards. Aspirations are for the good life, a comfortable home, good and sufficient food everyday,

and entertainment brought home to them on a color TV and cable channels. Aspirations are for savings to fall back on and a worry-free existence.

All these aspirations can be dashed with the birth of a girl-child whose dowry and wedding expenses would require a family to forego today's dreams. In this scenario, when seen from the perspective of a family whose dreams of comfort might be finished, ultrasound technology would seem to offer a simple solution to a problem.

These are the new factors in the storm; the old factors are those of social and cultural beliefs and practices that make sons so critically important to a family and daughters so redundant. This paper seeks to explain the sociocultural context in which it has become acceptable to detect and kill an unborn female fetus. Traditional Indian society is at this tipping point where social and cultural issues rooted in the deep past have encountered an economic impetus and an unwitting technical ally to create a situation that needs immediate attention.

The Sociocultural Context

The sociocultural context with regard to the girl-child is so deep rooted and so all-pervasive* that very few Indians need to have it explained to them—they have an intuitive understanding of the boy-child/girl-child conundrum. Yet it must be explained because the roots of the imbalanced gender ratio that poses such a threat to the future peace and harmony of Indian society lie in these sociocultural beliefs and practices. It would be important to begin with an analysis of the life of a woman in rural north India, with specific reference to villages in Uttar Pradesh, the most populous state in India.

Childhood and Adolescence

It is no coincidence that in the agricultural belt of north India, farmer families have started destroy-

---

* The only minor exceptions are the very small pockets of matriarchal systems in India found in a couple of states.

ing male cattle over the last few decades. Once a valued asset, a bull has become redundant after the mechanization of agriculture. Other than stud duties, the bull is not worth using for any other productive work because tractors and other machines can do the job more efficiently and with greater comfort for the farmer. Therefore, a male calf is killed—or sent to the butchery. There is no point feeding the animal. The rationale with regard to the girl-child is the same.

In the highly patriarchal Hindu society that north India represents, a girl is fondly described as "someone else's property, given to her natal family in safekeeping till the day of her marriage." From the time of her birth, a girl is seen to be an outsider, someone who really does not belong to the family she is born into. More often than not, this statement is made with warm affection, and told to a little girl with a cuddle and a kiss, but most girls hear it as they grow up, on more than one occasion. This belief guides most decisions taken with regard to the girl-child, more so in the very traditional families.

Since society demands that a girl has to be married into the same caste and subcaste that she is born into (but not the same village), it is important for the family's reputation and for the welfare of society that the choice of her husband should not be left to her. Even traditionalists understand that young hearts can be wayward and will not necessarily choose within predefined boundaries of caste and community. It is therefore seen to be critically important that family elders select a partner for their daughter and as critically important that she should know that it is her duty is to marry where she is told to marry. Simultaneously, virginity is an absolutely critical precondition to marriage, more so in rural India. Families therefore focus on keeping the girl under cover, so to speak, and finding a marriage partner for her as soon as possible. In the larger scheme of things, nothing is seen to be more important than virginity and a suitable marriage, and these considerations guide almost all other decisions, whether or not these are explicitly stated as reasons for the decisions being taken. Thus, for example, a girl will be sent to a village school but will not be allowed to continue into secondary or high school if that school is not in the village. In the final analysis, as traditional families see it, education for a girl is nice to

have, but not critical. So it is an indulgence that is allowed, if possible, as long as it does not interfere with other considerations.

A girl is valued by the new family into which she marries for her virginity, an absolutely unblemished reputation, and her housekeeping skills. She is not valued for her school education, except in communities that belong to the higher rungs of the socioeconomic ladder. Not only does this make a school education quite redundant, it also carries the risk of contamination—not contamination of her body by disease but contamination of her mind with new ideas, assertiveness, and a sense of self-worth. All these could be dangerous in a social structure where a girl is expected to merge into a new family (as an old saying goes) "like sugar into milk, sweetening the milk while dissolving her own identity into that of her new family."

Further, education and age bring the risk of a developing personality that carries the risk of a thinking mind. It is in the interest of social equilibrium to keep a girl-child without independent thought. In fact, another aphorism says that "a daughter and a cow are alike; they will go as they are led." Docility, adaptability, and servility are desired attributes and bring praise of good upbringing to a family. Educating a girl in light of these desired qualities is often seen to be foolhardy—it not only amounts to swimming against the tide but also runs the risk of somehow tarnishing the family's reputation if the girl were to develop an interest in boys with growing age, with mobility in the course of going to school and with a thinking mind.

This fear of raging hormones is another factor in the desire to get a girl married as soon as possible, along with the desire to make an alliance with the best possible family within the community. The fear that an older girl will not get a good marriage proposal (all the good boys would have been taken, presumably) and the complete aversion to taking any risks whatsoever with virginity and reputation makes the answer very clear—keep a girl indoors, teach her the skills needed to run a house (while she also doubles up as an assistant to her overworked mother and a caregiver for younger siblings), save money on education and put it into the dowry fund, start the search for a suitable family, and get her married as soon as one is found.

Society understood and appreciated the fact that a prepubescent girl could not be subjected to sexual activity. Yet, it was important to grab the right match when it was available. This led to the creation of a concept called *gauna*, where a girl could be married at any age, even in childhood, but would only be sent to live with her husband and his family after she reached puberty. This prevented sexual assault on an immature body; once she was in her husband's home, however, there was no way of preventing motherhood in a still-immature mind and body. To date, no solution has been found for this in conservative rural societies because it is expected that *gauna* will be followed by childbirth, within the year if possible, as a proof of fertility. The 2004 NFHS survey found that "Overall, 12% of women age 15–19 have become mothers and 4% of women age 15–19 are currently pregnant with their first child. This means that one in six women age 15–19 have begun childbearing. The proportion of women age 15–19 that have begun childbearing is more than twice as high in rural areas (19%) as in urban areas (9%)."[5]

Marriage

Marriage in traditional India is not about individuals. It is a social contract between two families and an extremely important one because it brings two families together in a permanent bond. The individuals marrying each other only represent the living ends of two lineages that are being knotted together. As a carpet weaver weaving a complex and elaborate carpet would be concerned with the strength and color of the wool that he knots together (and does not concern himself with the two ends only) so also senior members of the family try to ensure compatibility between the two families, not the two individuals. Marriages are arranged between families that are similar to each other. Community, caste, and village of origin are the external flags that signal similarity—similarity of overt parameters such as religion, language, and food as well as inner parameters such as values and beliefs, customs and rituals, rules, norms, and priorities. When a family finds another that is well matched with their own and one that they would like to build a permanent bond with, they arrange a marriage between their daughter and the other family's son, or vice versa.

Marriage would mean dowry. Dowry as it exists today is the jagged remnant of a broken system that started with the decent thought of giving a girl her share of the family property, to help her during adverse times. In earlier days, this was known as *stree-dhan* (woman's wealth) and was meant to remain with the girl, for her protection. It was given to her at the time of marriage because in agricultural families where land was the chief and immovable asset, it was important to ensure that the land remained within the family. A girl merged into another family, and it would be unwise for a family to have to share land with another family, particularly since that other family would almost certainly be in some other village. Therefore, the girl would be given her share of movable assets, and with that a clean break would be made. There would be no further expectations from either side; the girl would expect nothing more from her parents, and parents would expect nothing more from their daughter.

Over centuries, this custom has morphed into an ugly one called dowry, something that is greedily demanded by a boy's family and which families of brides succumb to because of pressures of society, custom, and the immense fear of being excommunicated. So from the time a girl is born, a family will try and save for a good dowry, because a higher dowry would buy them a better family for their daughter and for their own status in their society. It made little sense to invest in the girl-child for all these reasons—she was soon to be given away and would forever thereafter, till the end of her life, belong to a different family; in theory, her natal family then has no rights over her, and she has no further duties toward them. When a girl's parents grow old or fall ill, they cannot expect their daughter to come over and look after them. In the same way, no matter what her troubles, her parents are unlikely to take a daughter back into their family. She visits them as a guest, and each time she goes back to her husband's home (especially in the early years of marriage) she goes laden with gifts of food and sweets for her in-laws. Conversely, when a girl's parents visit her at her married home, the most orthodox would not accept any food or drink since they honestly believe that they have no rights over their daughter or her hospitality.

There is a very good reason that nobody concerns themselves excessively about whether the two young people being married to each other are compatible or not, and that is that the two individuals are not going to spend much time with each other after they get married. The family of a young man *recruits* a young girl into their family through the route of marriage. She joins the family (read organization) at the lowest rung in the hierarchy, and is inducted into training to run an efficient household in the way that her husband and his family are accustomed to having it run. She reports to her mother-in-law and keeps a respectful (and often veiled) distance from all the men of the household, including her husband. In fact, the husband and wife would never be *seen* talking to each other at all—it would be considered brazen and shameless for them to do so. Any conversations they have would be in the privacy of their own room at night. If a young couple does develop a bond of affection over time, this public distance only adds piquancy to their budding romance; if not, the distance ensures comfort because there are other family members to bond with and two not-very-compatible individuals are not thrown into solitary confinement with each other. They get the space and time to develop an understanding of each other.

So this young teenage bride enters a family of strangers. Her mother would have spent many years preparing her for this role, for obedience, adjustment, decorum, politeness and even subservience. She joins the family, neither seen nor heard, but making every effort to be useful and to establish her credentials in the cooking and housekeeping departments. If she lets her hair down to laugh and chatter, it would be with the children of the family and with her husband's younger siblings. They become her friends and her companions. Her husband often remains, at least in the first few years, a distant stranger who is also her sexual partner—but nothing more in the initial period. Companionship develops over a slow time frame, over many years, and often after a couple of children have been born.

Authority and Power

The new family exerts control over the new daughter-in-law both as a measure of discipline and a symbol of their power over her. Having severed all ties with her natal family, the young bride is in a position of extreme dependence. Though families differ, and there are those who are kind and gentle, many families tend to be authoritative or even harsh in their dealing with the new addition to the family, essentially to keep her in her place and let her know who is in charge. The fo-

cus is on ensuring that the girl blends well into the family and learns their ways.

In 1997–1998, the International Centre for Research on Women funded a study on the unmet need for family planning in Uttar Pradesh, India.[6] This study tried to quantify autonomy by asking women (through a structured questionnaire, n = 799) if they were consulted on a variety of decisions, ranging from the menu for the day to health care and education of her children, household purchases, the amount of money to be spent on food, and marriage decisions of other members in the family. Responses were coded on a five-point scale where five represented complete autonomy. The study found that decision-making autonomy increased significantly among women after the age of 25, which would be roughly 10 years after her marriage and much after the birth of her first two or three children. The NFHS survey of 2004 asked a similar question and found that "participation in decision making increases steadily with age and is higher in urban than in rural areas. Notably, almost half (46%) of the women age 15–19 do not participate in any of the four decisions (own health care, major household purchases, purchases of daily household needs, and visits to her family or relatives), compared with 13% of women age 40–49."[7]

Similarly, the unmet need study looked into her freedom of movement and found that mobility was clearly higher for work within the village than outside the village. It also found that freedom of movement was directly linked to age, and that the majority of young women (less than 25 years of age) had very little independence of movement. Though freedom of movement was not well correlated with the woman's education, the study found that there was an inverse correlation with the husband's education level; the more educated husband tended to impose greater restrictions than one who was less educated! The NFHS survey asked similar questions in 2004 and found that "Freedom of movement, as indicated by being allowed to go alone to the three types of places (the market, health facility, outside the village), increases sharply with age; however, even among women age 40–49, only 51% of women are allowed to go alone to all three places. (Percentage allowed to go alone to all three places: age 15–19 years: 12.8%; 20–24 years: 23.1%; 25–29 years: 33.4%; 30–39 years: 43.6%; 40–49 years: 51.2%.)[7]

The unmet need study also looked into her experience of violence in her husband's home. While an earlier phase of detailed, in-depth interviews had found a large mention of violence, even these short and structured interviews found that nearly a third of the women had known physical violence in the form of being beaten at least once. Many others had been scolded or otherwise abused for small mistakes such as the food being badly cooked to behavioural errors such as giving cheeky retorts to the husband or mother-in-law. The NFHS 2004 study also examined the issue of violence. "Thirty-four percent of all women age 15–49 had experienced violence at any time since the age of 15. Nineteen percent of women age 15–49 had experienced violence in the 12 months preceding the survey. Rural women were more likely than urban women to have ever experienced physical violence since the age of 15, and to have experienced it in the past 12 months. As expected, almost all ever-married women who have experienced violence report a current or former husband as the person who inflicted violence."[7]

The picture that came together rings true for a large number of rural households across the country: that of a young married woman with little or no autonomy, low levels of freedom of movement, and with tight controls on her behaviour to ensure conformity and subjugation. These controls are highest on a new bride; they decrease with age, familiarity, conformity with household norms, and with her improved stature in the family hierarchy. This stature improves rapidly with the birth of sons.

Motherhood

In this highly stratified family where decorum and obedience separate the senior strata from the junior,[†] the young bride's first promotion comes with pregnancy and motherhood. Her status goes up a notch as soon as she gives birth to a child. If that first child happens to be a son, her status goes up dramatically and joyously. If that first child happens to be a daughter, no matter—every family does need a daughter, too. In addition to the warmth and love a daughter brings into the house, she also brings a special bonus. Hindu scriptures note that every man must perform the holy duty of giving a daughter in marriage. The act of "gifting a daughter" (*kanyadaan*) bestows blessings on the giver and therefore is a duty that every man hopes to perform at least once in a lifetime. Therefore, one daughter is desired and welcomed. However, real status for the young wife comes when she becomes the mother of multiple sons—two or more sons.

In village after village in Uttar Pradesh, when men and women were asked to describe an ideal family composition, the answer was the same each time: "An ideal family would have at least two sons." Some would add "and a daughter," but there was no doubt that in about two out of three cases, this addition was an embarrassed afterthought, something that they realized they should say. That does not mean it was a lie. A daughter would certainly be desired and valued, but only after the two sons had been secured and, ideally, only if the family's economic circumstances were good. But very few rural households, especially in the Hindi belt (as the central swathe cutting across India is widely known), can be said to have good economic circumstances. A girl-child for them is a nonperforming asset, one that drains the family of whatever meager means they have.

Some decades ago, when large families were considered to be a good thing, daughters were usually a by-product of the attempt to have many sons. As social and economic pressures made it impractical to have large families and a two-child family became the unwritten norm, the unrealistic hope was that a family could have two sons and stop at that. But not having a son was unacceptable. Therefore, families that were unfortunate enough to have two, three, or four daughters had little option but to keep trying till they could have two sons. The family grew larger than their income could afford, but that problem was of little importance when compared with the problem of not having sons.

A woman gains status in her new household if she gives birth to sons. Being the mother of two or more sons assures her a place of respect in the

---

[†] Typically, age and gender decide seniority, in that order. The oldest man of the house is the patriarch, and the unquestioned authority over family and business matters. The oldest woman (usually his wife or it could be his mother) has the final authority over household matters. Therefore, old + male ranks higher than old + female; but old precedes young, without question. Therefore, in the absence of an older man, an old matriarch would rule and her sons would listen to her, even though they may be middle-aged themselves.

household and a measure of equality with the other, senior women in the family. Without the mandatory son, a woman does not get respect in her youth and runs the risk of facing old age without the authority that would come from being a mother-in-law to new recruits into the family hierarchy; more importantly, she runs the risk of having to depend on the kindness of other family members in the absence of a son when she grows old—a position that is both undesirable and fraught with insecurity. If she had one or more sons, her old age would be secure as she could rightfully expect her sons to look after her, with respect and honour, till the end of her days.

When a woman becomes the mother of sons, she grows in stature and authority. If she has several sons, she can look forward to a day when each brings in a daughter-in-law; with many daughters-in-law, she could well end her days as an authoritative matriarch with more power than she ever dreamt of in her youth. She could be in the position that had seemed so awesome in her mother-in-law when she had herself first entered her new home as a bride. Conversely, a mother of many daughters but no sons develops a permanent look of apology and failure, fearful of being dependent on nephews and their wives in her old age.

Contraception

In this scenario of low power and low status that awaits a new bride in the first decade of marriage, accompanied by the fact that her husband is a virtual stranger and distanced from her by hierarchy and tradition, it is almost impossible for a young woman to discuss contraception to space her children or limit their number.

By the time a woman is able to gather up the courage to talk of limiting the family size, she would probably be the mother of a couple of children. The 2004 NFHS survey found that about four-fifths of women who had ever used contraception did so for the first time when they had three or fewer children. "The same age pattern is observed in urban and rural areas. However, at each age urban women are more likely to begin contraceptive use when they have fewer children."[7] Further, it is a lonely battle that she has to fight. Unless her husband is enlightened enough to take the initiative and/or support her intention,

she has to make a difficult choice. If a woman chooses to use a contraceptive method (about which she is likely to be fairly well informed, given the good reach of health workers across rural India) she must first contend with the disapproval of older family members. Assuming she goes ahead despite their disapproval, she must hope that the contraceptive method that she chooses works well without the slightest side effect or negative reaction. It would also ideally have to be a simple method that does not call for repeated expense or visits to the health centre.[‡]

If her choice of contraceptive method were to produce any negative reaction such as making her ill (and therefore incapable of work for a day or more) or, even worse, calling for a visit to a doctor and for expenses on treatment to correct the situation, the scolding and censure that would come her way would make sure that she never tried any such thing again.

Seen from her perspective, her choice is between two evils. On the one hand, the worst consequence of not using a contraceptive would be another pregnancy, which is in any case familiar territory. She had traveled that path before and knew what to expect. If she did become pregnant again, it was unlikely that she would be scolded by her family for that accident. She might instead receive care and support. If she produced a son, she would be congratulated for the same. If the pregnancy required medical expenses to be incurred, those would not be grudged.

On the other hand, if she tried to adopt a method of contraception she would be alone and on her own in that effort. Family support would be difficult to find. Any expense or time required for that would be questioned and allowed only grudgingly. If the contraception went awry and needed medical attention and expense, she could be sure that strong disapproval and scolding would follow.

It seemed easier by far to give in to the path of least resistance and have all the children that were wanted to complete the family. Contraception

---

[‡] Women in villages often ask urban women researchers if they know of any simple contraceptive method that they could use just once and in secret, that would be completely effective and produce no side effects. There is a strong desire among women with multiple children for a "magic bullet" that would protect them from unwanted pregnancies without the knowledge of the husband and his family.

could then be followed using terminal methods. The NFHS supports this with the finding that "Female sterilization accounts for two-thirds of total contraceptive use and 77% of modern method use. Eighty-one percent of sterilized women were sterilized before age 30. The median age at sterilization is 25.5 years."[7]

This then is the context of the life of a woman in rural Uttar Pradesh—a life of very little autonomy, even over her body or decisions pertaining to her life. From her viewpoint, the only hope of power and status lies in having sons. Conversely, giving birth to more than one daughter is a certain path to a lifetime of worry, apology, and a feeling of inferiority. Magically for her, about two decades ago, she learnt that it was possible for a doctor to do some test that would tell her in a few weeks after conception if she had conceived a girl and if so, she could easily abort that fetus. It is difficult to blame her for thinking that this was certainly an answer to her prayers!

Conclusion

This author has a deeply imprinted memory of a village near Rajkot in Gujarat state from the mid 1990s. It was a relatively prosperous village in a prosperous state, albeit a very patriarchal state. The streets of the village were full of playing children; it was a while before it became apparent that these children were all boys. There were just two girls playing in a group of over 20 boys. As the sun went down in the evening, the doors of many houses opened and many girls came out to collect water from the borewell at the centre of the village. For a minute, it seemed that all was well. There were girls in the village after all. Maybe they had just been staying indoors to be away from the scorching sun. However, a second look showed that all the girls at the well were teenagers or just a little short of entering their teens. The village had just two girls below the age of 12!! In the last twelve years, some 20 plus boys had been born in this village—but in the last twelve years, only two girls had been born. This cannot be explained by chance or any other act of nature. Such a skewed ratio can only happen when man-made methods interfere with the laws of nature.

The future looks very grim indeed if this situation were to continue. On an optimistic note, the one good that might come out of it would be the cessation of dowry. If brides are in short supply, it is possible that they will be gratefully accepted without the additional demands of dowry. Some signs to this effect are already evident. Anecdotal evidence has emerged from some communities in Gujarat that families are only willing to give their daughters into homes that have a daughter to give them in return as a bride for their son. This potentially leaves out of the marriage set those families who eliminated daughters from their lives two decades ago. Such a cartel formed by parents of daughters would be one good step in the right direction.

But there is not much room for optimism. The concept of even 70 men in a 1000 being left without a wife brings a new set of worries. There is a real fear that crimes against women could increase as a result of the distorted numbers. Stories filter in from some states about brides being asked to allow sexual access not just to their husbands but to all his unmarried brothers as well. Other stories pertain to brides being brought in from poor states to provide wives for the men in states that were early adopters of feticide. It is likely that these women will be little more than sexual and domestic slaves because the cultural basis of a traditional marriage would be missing. The impact of the sins of one community is being felt in other, poorer communities.

The need is for education of entire families on several issues such as: selective abortions, why dowries are a decadent practice that should be abolished, and that the misplaced fear families have that a girl child is a burden is very important for advocacy and bringing about empowerment and gender equity in societies. Behavior change communication has long focused on how a daughter can choose to pursue and be successful in a career in almost any field (i.e. to communicate that girls are as capable as boys). This might be misplaced emphasis, because social customs do not allow parents to benefit from the achievements of a daughter. A daughter's career prospects or earning prospects might be pleasant to think about, but not if they are only going to benefit the family that she has been married into. If a girl's earnings become nothing more than "dowry in many installments" then such a prospect gives no reason for a family to give birth to and invest in the education and health of a girl-child.

Communication must focus on questioning the social norms that turn a daughter into a stranger once she is married. Communication must focus on emphasizing the continued role of a daughter in the life of her parents so that they may look upon her as a support in life rather than a burden. There is a need for communication for social change in its deepest and most profound form, to bring about a change in the way society sees its daughters.

Tribal communities of India have an answer in the equal status that they accord their daughters. Research in one tribal community in Navapur district of Maharashtra showed that daughters were valued as much as sons were valued because the tribe did not have different rules for sons and daughters. A family would expect their daughter to look after her parents in their old age and to help them, financially or through caregiving, whenever they needed help. There was no stigma to an old man or woman living with the daughter—in fact, the tribal practice at the time of marriage is to ask for a bride price since the family will give away a productive asset to another family and expect to be compensated for this loss.

A paradigm shift is needed in the country on how people view their daughters. All modes of communication—film, television, literature, art, and commercial communication need to work together to bring about this much needed shift in attitude. It will have to be a relentless effort, accompanied by strong laws and even stronger enforcement of those laws. It will be a slow change, but it is an urgently needed change.

DISCUSSION QUESTIONS

1. When the birth of a son is so critical for a woman's own status in her family, for her sense of self-worth and for her future security, how can communication and education try to balance out the enormous value that a son brings to a woman?

2. What methods of surveillance could ensure that pregnant women get the benefits of technology without technology being used for purposes that damage the very fabric of society?

3. How can the worth of a daughter be increased in strongly patriarchal societies, and how can society be mobilized to bring the same customs of social ostracism to deal with families that kill female fetuses?

4. How can programs that work for women's health and human rights understand deep rooted sociocultural norms of a society that is not their own?

5. How can health programs invest in understanding a culture before they proceed to plan the program strategy?

REFERENCES

1. Junger S. *The Perfect Storm: A True Story of Men Against the Sea.* New York: Harper Paperback; 1998.
2. Census of India, 2001. Retrieved from http://www.censusindia.gov.in. Accessed December 30, 2008.

3. Francis Z, Francis AJ. Fertility decline and gender bias in northern India. *Demography.* 2003;40(4):788-790.
4. Jha P, Kumar R, Vasa P, Dhingra N, Thiruchelvam D, Moineddin R. Low male-to-female sex ratio of children born in India: national survey of 1.1 million households. *Lancet.* 2006; 367:211-218.
5. National Family Health Survey 2004. Fertility and Fertility. Retrieved from http://www.nfhsindia.org/data/ne/nechap4.pdf Accessed December 30, 2008.
6. Viswanathan H, Godfrey S,Yinger N. *Reaching Women: Unmet need for Family Planning in Uttar Pradesh, India.* Washington, D.C.: International Centre for Research on Women.1998.
7. National Family Health Survey 2004. Women's Empowerment and Demographic and Health Outcomes; 463. Retrieved from http://www.nfhsindia.org/india1.html Accessed December 30, 2008.

CHAPTER 41

From Alma-Ata to Millennium Development Goals: Status of Women's Health in the 21st Century

Gopal Sankaran, MD, DrPH

Gopal Sankaran, MD, DrPH, is a Professor in the Department of Health for the College of Health Sciences, West Chester University, located in West Chester, PA.

INTRODUCTION

The status of women's health in the 21st century raises an important and interesting question: Should those working tirelessly for the welfare of women throughout the world celebrate the progress made in the last century and the beginning years of the current century or feel disappointed that a lot more is yet to be done? In other words, should the progress made so far be viewed as a glass half full or half empty? Complicating this perspective is the fact that improvement in the status of women worldwide has not been uniform. There are several geographic areas in the world where women still have not benefited from the miracles of science and modern medicine or the life-altering positive changes brought about by technology. Even carefully thought out policy initiatives have not translated into programs and services for many women. Apart from the philosophical and social debate the initial question raises, the widespread acceptance of and commitment to Millennium Development Goals (MDGs) provide a unique opportunity to examine the stated question based on available evidence and to chart a course for the future. This chapter offers a brief history of the declarations and movements that have helped to enhance the women's health status throughout the world beginning with the Alma-Ata Declaration. Following the historical perspective, the current status of women's health is presented. Finally, the future course of action needed to realize the MDGs is addressed.

Why focus on the status of women's health? There are several reasons why women need special attention when framing an agenda for global health. First, women are different from men biologically and based on these differences have different needs throughout their lifespan. Second, women are treated differently in different cultures based on the norms set up, often by men, and prevalent in those societies. Third, women across the globe do not have uniform access to health and social services that would enable them to attain the highest possible level of health. Fourth, women are the primary caregivers of children and often shoulder a larger share of rearing them. Increasingly, women are being called upon to nurture and care for the elderly in their families. Finally, women's health status is closely associated with the development of their communities. Some of these reasons will be addressed in this chapter.

Evolution of Health as a Human Right

While human beings have been around for thousands of years, the notion of health as a human right is relatively new. The aftermath of World War II offered a time for reflection on the state of the world and a realization of the inevitable destruction of human life and property that a war entails. In the years immediately following the end of World War II, the League of Nations gave way to the United Nations with increased responsibility toward resolving conflicts, maintaining peace, and enhancing the lives of humans. It was within this spirit of cooperation and understanding the first steps toward identifying what would constitute human rights and how they need to be articulated were taken.

The General Assembly of the United Nations on December 10, 1948, adopted and proclaimed the Universal Declaration of Human Rights.[1] Article 1 of this historic declaration states "All human beings are born free and equal in dignity and rights. They are endowed with reason and conscience and should act toward one another in a spirit of brotherhood." This declaration laid the foundation for widespread recognition of human rights in the spirit of equality among sexes. While the language of some of the articles (including Article 1), such as the exclusive use of male pronouns, refers to the time period when the declaration was written, the articles themselves are clear in their intent and applicability to both men and women. Reference to health and well-being is made in Article 25.1, which states that "Everyone has the right to a standard of living adequate for the health and well-being of himself and of his family, including food, clothing, housing and medical care, and necessary social services."[1] Recognizing the special vulnerability of women and children, Article 25.2 spells out clearly that "Motherhood and childhood are entitled to special care and assistance."[1] Furthermore, the same article (25.2) adds that "All children, whether born in or out of wedlock, shall enjoy the same social protection."[1]

The Universal Declaration of Human Rights also recognized the importance of education to the individual. Specifically, Article 26.1 of the declaration states that "Everyone has the right to education." The declaration further adds that "Education shall be free, at least in the elementary and fundamental stages. Elementary education shall be compulsory." The same article (26) in a later section (26.2) specifies that "Education shall be directed to the full development of the human personality and to the strengthening of respect for human rights and fundamental freedoms."[1]

The declaration thus framed both health and education to be fundamental rights of human beings that are to be provided to individuals irrespective of their nation of origin or place of residence.

Health for All by the Year 2000: The Alma-Ata Declaration

Thirty years from the time of the Universal Declaration of Human Rights came the International Conference on Primary Health Care hosted by the World Health Organization (WHO) and the United Nations Children's Emergency Fund (UNICEF) at Alma-Ata, Kazakhstan, Union of Soviet Socialist Republics (USSR), in September 1978. This meeting brought together representatives from 134 member countries and 67 international organizations.[2]

The participants at this international gathering quickly recognized that making progress in the health arena needed concerted action wherein intersectoral and international cooperation was vital. The need for nations to develop and strengthen their own health systems in the face of increasing need for health services was understood by the participants. They adopted Primary Health Care as the core strategy to accomplish the goal of Health for All by the Year 2000.[3] While primary health care itself had multiple interpretations, there was consensus that every person in the world, irrespective of his or her ability to pay, had to have access to a basic level of healthcare services. Additionally, the responsibility to ensure that such a level of care is indeed available to all citizens of a nation (developing or developed) rested with the respective government of each nation. The Declaration of Alma-Ata was the culmination of this new paradigm that everyone should receive a basic level of healthcare services and that the care could be often provided using appropriately trained healthcare workers using appropriate technology.

The declaration stated that "Health, which is a state of complete physical, mental, and social well-being, and not merely the absence of disease or infirmity, is a *fundamental human right* [italics added]."[3] The assertion that health is a fundamental human right is important, as it provides for individuals to view and seek health care as a right and not merely a privilege. The declaration further stated that "the attainment of the highest possible level of health is a most important *worldwide social goal* [italics added] whose realization requires the action of many other social and economic sectors in addition to the health sector."[3] The declaration highlights health as a fundamental human right and advocates for an intersectoral approach that cuts across socioeconomic, cultural, educational, and geographic boundaries and promotes development in the spirit of social justice. Such a declaration that health is a human right and attainment of the highest possible level of health needs to be a social goal worldwide is one of the most important milestones in assuring improvement in women's health status.

Women as Constituents with Special Needs

While the years following the Declaration of Alma-Ata showed promise in the adoption of primary health care as a viable strategy for increasing access to care using innovative approaches, the progress was not uniform across nations. Women, in particular, continued to suffer because of their biologically determined sex and culturally determined social status and practices.

United Nations International Conference on Population and Development (ICPD)

The United National International Conference on Population and Development (commonly known as the ICPD) was held in September 1994 in Cairo, Egypt. The ICPD Programme of Action (sometimes referred to as the Cairo Consensus) tenable for the next 20 years was adopted by 179 representatives of governments.[4,5] The conference reaffirmed the interrelationship between population, sustained economic growth, and sustainable development. More importantly, from the women's health perspective, the conference emphasized the importance of gender equality, equity, and empowerment of women. The ICPD recognized that reproductive health and rights, as well as women's empowerment and gender equality, are cornerstones of population and development programs. The reproductive rights and reproductive health, particularly of women, were framed in the context of individuals rather than the time-honored tradition of viewing them as targets of population control at national levels. The ICPD identified the increased equality for the girl-child as a necessary first step in ensuring that women realize their full potential and become equal partners in development. The conference also recognized the power disparity between men and women and urged men to play a key role in bringing about gender equality.

Beijing Declaration and Platform for Action

Before making a leap into the Beijing Declaration and Platform for Action that culminated from the Fourth World Conference on Women, it would be useful to understand the objectives and outcome of the previous lesser known, but nonetheless equally important, three world gatherings with their exclusive focus on women and their welfare.

The First World Conference on Women,[6] held in Mexico City in the summer of 1975, identified three objectives in relation to three areas of focus—quality, peace, and development. These objectives were: (1) full gender equality and the elimination of gender discrimination, (2) the integration and full participation of women in development, and (3) an increased contribution by women toward strengthening world peace.[6]

The Second World Conference on Women[7] was held in Copenhagen in July 1980. The participants at the conference identified three objectives related to equality, peace, and development. They were (1) equal access to education, (2) equal access to employment opportunities, and (3) equal access to adequate healthcare services.[7]

The Third World Conference on Women[7] was hosted by Nairobi, Kenya, in June 1985. While women were expected to benefit from the action steps from the previous two world conferences, in reality only a small amount were benefiting from them. This called for new ways to overcome the barriers faced by the majority of women in achieving the objectives related to equality, peace, and development. The Nairobi Forward Looking Strategies for the Advancement of Women established the following three categories to measure the progress made in the future: (1) constitutional and legal measures, (2) equality in social participation, and (3) equality in political participation and decision making. The interconnectedness of gender equality with all areas of human activity was recognized and emphasized in the conference proceedings.[7]

The Fourth World Conference on Women,[8,9] held in September 1995 in Beijing, People's Republic of China, played a vital role in refocusing the world's attention on the plight of women and the yet unfinished agenda of equality and empowerment. The Beijing Conference has been hailed as "a landmark in policy terms, setting a global policy framework to advance gender equality."[9] The Beijing Conference ended with the adoption of the Beijing Declaration and Platform for Action[8] that was forwarded to the General Assembly of the United Nations at its 50th session. The Beijing Declaration[8] unequivocally stated that "Women's rights are human rights." Furthermore, the declaration[8] called for "men to participate fully in all actions toward equality," an important message to men who can either choose to serve as facilitators or barriers to women's progress and their achieving equality at home, at work, and in the society. The recognition that globally most of the resources are controlled by men, policies and programs for women are often designed and implemented by men, and the power imbalance between the genders favoring men were instrumental in calling upon men to do their part in ensuring equality for women.

The Beijing Declaration noted that while progress in women's health, gainful economic employment, and improvement in their social status has occurred, several critical areas of concern continued to persist. Alarmingly, these 12 areas of concern (see below) significantly impeded the progress of women and the declaration called for a Platform for Action to address quickly and effectively the identified areas of concern:[8]

1. Poverty: women facing persistent and increasing burden of poverty

2. Education and training: women having unequal access to both education and training, and even when available it is inadequate

3. Health care: women having unequal access to health care and other services including emergency care

4. Violence: women being targeted in interpersonal violence

5. Armed conflicts: women feeling the effects of armed or other kinds of conflict

6. Economic structure and policies: women continuing to have less access to resources and productive activities

7. Power sharing and decision making: women not having the same opportunities as men who have more power and often make decisions for them

8. Advancement: women having lesser opportunities than men to advance in their careers

9. Human rights: women receiving less protection and inadequate promotion of their human rights

10. Media: women experiencing stereotyping besides limited access to and participation in communication systems

11. Natural resources and environment: women feeling gender discrimination in the management of natural resources and in the safeguarding of the environment

12. Girl-child: the girl-child facing discrimination and often violation of her rights

The Beijing Platform of Action,[8] after careful assessment of the critical areas of concern, came up with strategic objectives and actions for each one of them. The specific actions recommended for implementation cut across the boundaries of equality, development, and peace, which were the goals of the Nairobi Forward-Looking Strategies for the Advancement of Women.[7] In reality, these three domains are interdependent and, hence the recommendation that specific actions overlap across boundaries for achieving success that is sustainable. The expected outcome was to benefit all women and particularly those who are the most disadvantaged in any society.

ICPD Plus Five

In 1999 the UN convened a special session, ICPD+5[10] to take stock of the progress made towards meeting the ICPD goals. The review identified several areas (such as reproductive health care, unmet needs for contraception, female education and literacy, maternal mortality reduction, and HIV/AIDS) to be problematic with inadequate progress and called for urgent action. The session reaffirmed the ICPD goals and set benchmarks for progress toward reaching them.[10]

The Millennium Declaration

In 2000, leaders from 189 member states of the United Nations came together and adopted the Millennium Declaration[11] and the eight MDGs.[12,13] The Millennium Declaration set 2015 as the target date for achieving most of the MDGs (see Table 41-1).[14]

TABLE 41-1

Millennium Development Goals (MDGs) and the Goal-Specific Targets

MDG 1: Eradicate extreme poverty and hunger
Target 1: Halve, between 1990 and 2015, the proportion of people whose income is less than one dollar a day.
Target 2: Halve, between 1990 and 2015, the proportion of people who suffer from hunger.

MDG 2: Achieve universal primary education
Target 3: Ensure that, by 2015, children everywhere, boys and girls alike, will be able to complete a full course of primary schooling.

MDG 3: Promote gender equality and empower women
Target 4: Eliminate gender disparity in primary and secondary education, preferably by 2005, and in all levels of education no later than 2015.

MDG 4: Reduce child mortality
Target 5: Reduce by two-thirds, between 1990 and 2015, the under-five mortality rate.

MDG 5: Improve maternal health
Target 6: Reduce by three-quarters, between 1990 and 2015, the maternal mortality ratio.

MDG 6: Combat HIV/AIDS, malaria, and other diseases
Target 7: Have halted by 2015 and begun to reverse the spread of HIV/AIDS.
Target 8: Have halted by 2015 and begun to reverse the incidence of malaria and other major diseases.

MDG 7: Ensure environmental sustainability
Target 9: Integrate the principles of sustainable development into country policies and programmes and reverse the loss of environmental resources.
Target 10: Halve, by 2015, the proportion of people without sustainable access to safe drinking water and basic sanitation.
Target 11: By 2020, to have achieved a significant improvement in the lives of at least 100 million slum dwellers.

MDG 8: Develop a global partnership for development
Target 12: Develop further an open, rule-based, predictable, nondiscriminatory trading and financial system.
Target 13: Address the special needs of the least developed countries.
Target 14: Address the special needs of landlocked developing countries and the small island developing states.
Target 15: Deal comprehensively with the debt problems of developing countries through national and international measures in order to make debt sustainable in the long term.
Target 16: In cooperation with developing countries, develop and implement strategies for decent and productive work for youth.
Target 17: In cooperation with pharmaceutical companies, provide access to affordable, essential drugs in developing countries.
Target 18: In cooperation with the private sector, make available the benefits of new technologies, especially information and communications.

Source: Adapted with permission from The Millennium Development Goals Report Statistical Annexe, 2007; United Nations.[14]

Several different perspectives have been provided in the published literature as to which of the MDGs relate directly to women and at times in their special social role as mothers. For example, the Partnership for Maternal, Newborn & Child Health in its joint statement highlights that health professional groups are key to reaching MDG 4 (Reduce child mortality) and MDG 5 (Improve maternal health), a notion reinforced by the Blantyre Declaration of Commitment to MDGs 4 and 5.[15] The Blantyre Declaration stemmed from the first Partnership for Maternal Newborn and Child Health Workshop for Health Care Professional Associations and their Role in Reaching MDGs 4 and 5 held in Blantyre, Malawi, in November 2007 and affirmed by representatives from Ethiopia, Malawi, Nigeria, Tanzania, and Uganda.[15] Grown, Gupta, and Pande[16] focus on improving women's health through gender equality and women's empowerment, as proclaimed in MDG 3 (Promote gender equality and empower women). Skolnik[17(p148)] in a chapter on women's health in his recent book, *Essentials of Global Health*, identifies and links MDGs 1 through 6 to be related to women's health.

However, this author's perspective is that all of the eight MDGs have an impact on women's health, some exerting more direct influence than others (see Table 41-2). Explanations of the linkage between the various MDGs and women's health are presented in Table 41-2.[14]

ICPD Plus Ten

The ICPD Programme of Action reached the midpoint of its clearly laid out 20-year plan in 2004 and was thus ready for a review. The United Nations Population Fund (UNFPA), through a survey, assessed the progress made on the ICPD Programme of Action by each signatory nation. Its review found that the first 10 years of ICPD had helped to build a solid foundation for the implementation of the Cairo Consensus. The review, Investing in People,[18] found that "continued efforts and commitment are needed to mobilize sufficient human and financial resources, to strengthen institutional capacities, and to nurture stronger partnerships across sectors and all stakeholders."

Beijing Plus Ten

In 2005, 10 years after the initial Beijing Conference, the United Nations' Commission on the Status of Women in an intergovernmental meeting (often referred to as the "Beijing Plus Ten" event) reviewed the progress made on the commitment to fulfill the Beijing Declaration and the Platform for Action.[19,20] As compared to the Beijing Conference, the Plus Ten event was focused on affirming what had been accomplished rather than developing new policies for implementation.[9]

A review[19] of the past accomplishments at that time received a mixed rating. Based on its review, the event identified five priority areas for future action. These included: women and poverty, education and training of women, women and health, violence against women, and women and armed conflict. Several member governments in the survey used in developing the review[19] had responded that they "saw the role of men and boys as critical for the achievement of gender equality and empowerment of women." They had elaborated plans for further work in this area.

2005 World Summit

The largest-ever gathering of world leaders at the World Summit at the United Nations in New York[21] lent their support to the full implementation of the goals and objectives of the Beijing Declaration and the Platform for Action. They identified that realization of the goals and objectives would help achieve world development goals and declared "We remain convinced that progress for women is progress for all."[21]

The gathered leaders agreed to promote gender equality and eliminate still prevalent gender discrimination. They agreed to take steps to (1) eliminate gender inequalities in schools, (2) ensure equal access to reproductive health, (3) promote women's equal access to work, (4) guarantee the free and equal right of women to own and inherit property, (5) eliminate all forms of discrimination and violence against women and girls, and (6) promote increased representation of women in decision-making bodies in the government.[21]

From the time of the Alma-Ata Declaration in 1978 to the World Summit in 2005, the special needs of women in different phases of their life have gained greater visibility and attention from the policy makers and service providers. The ICPD Programme of Action, the Beijing Declaration and Platform of Action, and the Millennium Declaration, among others, have been instrumental in

TABLE 41-2

Millennium Development Goals (MDGs) and their Linkages to Women's Health

Millennium Development Goal (MDG)	Linkages to Women's Health[a]
MDG 1: Eradicate extreme poverty and hunger	Poverty is associated with poor health. Poverty is also associated with hunger. Hunger is associated with poor nutritional status. Both poverty and hunger have adverse outcomes on the health and nutritional status of women with resultant adverse effects on the health of their babies.
MDG 2: Achieve universal primary education	Education is associated with the ability of women to improve their economic status. This, in turn, promotes positive health of women and helps them care better for their children.
MDG 3: Promote gender equality and empower women	Gender equality for women and their empowerment will lead to better access to education, enhance opportunities for economically gainful employment, equity in wages, and reduce chances of interpersonal violence against them.
MDG 4: Reduce child mortality	Women's health and nutritional status are linked to mortality among their children. Child mortality impacts a woman's fertility, which in turn can affect her health status.
MDG 5: Improve maternal health	This is directly linked to women's health status in their roles as mothers.
MDG 6: Combat HIV/AIDS, malaria, and other diseases	The feminization of poverty is often associated with greater risk of acquiring HIV and other sexually transmissible infections (STIs). HIV and some of the STIs have the potential for both vertical and horizontal transmissions that could adversely affect their families. Malaria is an important cause of anemia in developing countries which in turn could have deleterious consequences for women and their children.
MDG 7: Ensure environmental sustainability	Unsafe drinking water and inadequate basic sanitation have an adverse impact on a women's health by increasing the risk of acquiring infectious diseases with undesirable results.
MDG 8: Develop a global partnership for development	Women contribute significantly to the overall development of a society. Health is associated with productivity. Women's health, thus, is not simply a health issue but a development issue. Global partnership is essential for removing the many disparities noted in women's health status across the world.

Source: Adapted with permission from the Millennium Development Goals Report Statistical Annex, 2007; United Nations.[14]
[a]Author's perspective explaining the linkage between each MDG and women's health

keeping the focus on improving women's health and enhancing their lives. How much all these pronouncements, action plans, pro-women policies and programs have contributed to promoting gender equality and empowerment of women and at what pace is still debatable.

The Progress Made: Current Status of Women's Health

Given that multiple conferences and declarations have resulted in the reaffirmation of women's rights and needs in the health and other sectors, what progress has been made in terms of women's health status? One way to answer this question would be to see the progress made in the targets set for the MDGs especially as they pertain to women.

The *Millennium Development Goals Report*[13] and the *Statistical Annex*[14] for the Millennium Development Goals Report, both published in 2007, provide the most up-to-date information on the progress made so far on the MDGs. Select targets for each of the eight MDGs along with their indicators and progress made on those indicators are presented in Table 41-3.[14] Indicators have been chosen to allow for effective comparisons to be made (for example, between developing and developed regions, or over two calendar years, or to

TABLE 41-3

Progress Report on the Millennium Development Goals (MDGs) (over varying time periods[a])

MDG 1: Eradicate extreme poverty and hunger.
Target 1: Halve, between 1990 and 2015, the proportion of people whose income is less than one dollar a day.
Indicator 1: Population living below US $1 purchasing power parity (PPP) per day.

Percentage of population below US $1 PPP per day	1990	1999	2004
Developing regions (aggregate)	31.6	23.4	19.2
Sub-Saharan Africa	46.8	45.9	41.1

Target 2: Halve, between 1990 and 2015, the proportion of people who suffer from hunger.
Indicator 4: Prevalence of underweight children under five years of age

Percentage of children under five years of age who are underweight (total; both boys and girls)	1990	2005
Developing regions	33	27
Southern Asia	53	46

MDG 2: Achieve universal primary education.
Target 3: Ensure that, by 2015, children everywhere, boys and girls alike, will be able to complete a full course of primary schooling.
Indicator 6: Net enrollment ratio in primary education

Primary- and secondary-level enrollees per 100 children of primary-education enrollment age	1991	1999	2005
Developing regions	80.2	83.5	87.9
Sub-Saharan Africa	53.7	57.4	70.4

Indicator 7b: Primary completion rate

Gross intake ratio to last grade		1999	2005
Developing regions (boys)		84.0	88.6
Developing regions (girls)		76.7	83.4
Sub-Saharan Africa (boys)		55.1	65.9
Sub-Saharan Africa (girls)		46.2	55.6

MDG 3: Promote gender equality and empower women.
Target 4: Eliminate gender disparity in primary and secondary education, preferably by 2005, and in all levels of education no later than 2015.
Indicator 9: Ratio of girls to boys in primary, secondary, and tertiary education

	1999	2005
Developing regions (primary education)	0.91	0.94
Developing regions (secondary education)	0.89	0.93
Developing regions (tertiary education)	0.78	0.91

(continued)

TABLE 41-3

Progress Report on the Millennium Development Goals (MDGs) (over varying time periods[a]) *(continued)*

Indicator 11: Share of women in wage employment in the nonagricultural sector

Percentage of employees in nonagricultural wage employment who are women	1990	2000	2005
World	35.6	37.8	38.9
Southern Asia	13.1	16.7	18.1

Indicator 12: Seats held by women in national parliament

Percentage of parliamentary seats occupied by women	1990	2002	2007
World	12.8	13.8	17.1
Sub-Saharan Africa	7.2	12.0	16.6
Southern Asia	5.7	4.9	13.0

MDG 4: Reduce child mortality.

Target 5: Reduce by two thirds, between 1990 and 2015, the under-five mortality rate.
Indicator 13: Under-five mortality rate

Deaths of children before reaching the age of five per 1000 live births	1990	2005
Developing regions	106	83
Sub-Saharan Africa	185	166
Developed regions	12	6

Indicator 14: Infant mortality rate

Deaths of children before reaching the age of one year per 1000 live births	1990	2005
Developing regions	71	57
Sub-Saharan Africa	110	99
Developed regions	10	5

MDG 5: Improve Maternal Health

Target 6: Reduce by three-quarters, between 1990 and 2015, the maternal mortality ratio.
Indicator 16: Maternal mortality ratio

Maternal deaths per 100,000 live births	2000
Developing Regions	450
Sub-Saharan Africa	920
Developed Regions	14

Indicator 17: Births attended by skilled health personnel

Percentage of births attended by skilled health personnel	1990	2005
Developing Regions	43	57
Southern Asia	30	38
Commonwealth of Independent States, Europe	99	99

Indicator 19c: Contraceptive prevalence rate (moved from MDG 6 to 5 in March 2007)

Percentage using contraception among women aged 15–49 who are married or in union	1990	2005
Developing Regions	52.0	62.7
Sub-Saharan Africa	12.3	21.3
Developed Regions	69.8	68.4

MDG 6: Combat HIV/AIDS, malaria, and other diseases.

Target 7: Have halted by 2015 and begun to reverse the spread of HIV/AIDS.

(continued)

Table 41-3

Progress Report on the Millennium Development Goals (MDGs) (over varying time periods^a) (continued)

Indicator 18: HIV prevalence

Percentage of adults (15+ years of age) living with HIV who are women	1990	2002	2006
Developing Regions	47	50	50
Sub-Saharan Africa	54	58	59
Oceania	23	55	59
Developed Regions	16	30	30

Indicator 23: Incidence, prevalence, and death rates associated with tuberculosis

Number of new cases (incidence) per 100,000 population (excluding HIV infected)	1990	2000	2005
Developing Regions	148	150	149
Sub-Saharan Africa	148	253	281
Southeast Asia	272	231	215
Developed Regions	26	19	16

MDG 7: Ensure environmental sustainability.

Target 10: Halve, by 2015, the proportion of people without sustainable access to safe drinking water and basic sanitation.

Indicator 30: Population using an improved drinking water source

Percentage of population using an improved drinking water source	1990	2004
Developing Regions	93 (urban)	92 (urban)
	60 (rural)	70 (rural)
Sub-Saharan Africa	82 (urban)	80 (urban)
	36 (rural)	42 (rural)
Developed Regions	100 (urban)	100 (urban)
	99 (rural)	95 (rural)

MDG 8: Develop a global partnership for development.

Target 18: In cooperation with the private sector, make available the benefits of new technologies, especially information and communications.

Indicator 47: Telephone lines and cellular subscribers

Number of fixed telephone lines per 100 population	1990	2005
Developing regions	3.1	13.7
Sub-Saharan Africa	1.0	1.5
Southern Asia	0.7	5.0
Developed Regions	44.2	52.4

show regions that lag greatly on a particular indicator highlighting the challenges ahead).

It is important to note that only the averages for the various indicators or data for select areas are provided in Table 41-3. For details about a particular region or a nation, the reader is directed to visit the online database MDG Info.[22] A visual map, UN Millennium Development Goals: 2007 Progress Chart,[23] is also available online and provides a quick summary of the regions of the world that have made satisfactory progress on the various MDGs. The map also offers a ready visual appraisal of the speed of progress in several regions of the world.

At first glance, it is apparent that overall for most of the MDGs and the specific targets associated with them, considerable progress has been made in several of the indicators. However, disaggregation of the data for the indicators by region and nation (recommend using online database MDG Info 2007[22]) reveals that the progress is neither uniform nor rapid in many situations.

Challenges to Overcome: What Lies Ahead?

There are several domains where the progress made towards the MDG targets is laudable. For example, according to a report[24] from the World Bank, since the Millennium Declaration over 34 million additional children in developing nations have been given the opportunity to attend and complete primary school. Similarly, the number of persons living with AIDS who were provided access to current antiretroviral treatment increased dramatically from 240,000 in 2001 to over 1.6 million in 2006.[24]

The United Nations Secretary-General Ban Ki-moon,[25] addressing the General Assembly thematic debate on the MDGs in New York, on April 1, 2008, emphasized that "More than halfway to 2015, the MDG track record is mixed." He specified that as compared to the year 2000, 3 million more children now survive each year and an additional 2 million people receive treatment for AIDS, and millions more children attend school.[25]

News of such accomplishments are tempered by the fact that in 2005[26] less than one in four (32 out of 147) developing nations were on track to achieve the MDG 4 to reduce child mortality. Stagnant or worsening child mortality rates were observed in 23 developing nations,[26] a fact that points toward the uphill battle these nations face in overcoming the loss of lives of their children under five years old.

The last quarter of 2007 and the first half of 2008 have posed two additional short-term challenges to meeting the MDGs. The slowing of the global economy and the dramatic rise in fuel and food prices globally have threatened to undo the gains achieved so far in fighting hunger and malnutrition. Countries that were on track to meeting their MDG targets in these areas are unsure whether they would meet their specified targets on time.[27] The World Bank[26] estimates that price increases of staple food items such as rice (74% over the past year) and wheat (130% over the past year) would further push nearly 100 million people or more into deep poverty (in addition to more than 830 million people in the world who face acute shortages of food). The Bank has calculated that this represents seven lost years in the global fight against poverty and hunger, something that the world can ill afford.[26]

Long-term challenges to MDGs come in several forms—environmental threats (such as natural disasters, effects of climate change, and other environmental problems), biological threats (such as organisms that can pose a danger to humans, animals, birds or plants) political instability, human created disasters (such as wars and other conflicts), emerging and reemerging infectious diseases, and movement of labor away from agriculture to other occupations, to name a few.

It is important to recognize that as progress is made with various MDGs over the next seven years (from 2008 to 2015), the cost of initiating and sustaining such positive changes will continue to increase for at least two reasons: (1) the inevitable inflationary cost increases associated with goods, personnel, and services, and (2) the unit cost of taking care of the tougher challenges (once easier ones have been addressed effectively in the earlier years) will continue to rise. Will governments, multilateral organizations, and donors have the compassion, discipline, and sustained commitment to ensure that the resources (human, fiscal, and material) are made available particularly to the most disadvantaged population groups?

The Future: From Rhetoric to Action

What does the future hold, and what can be realistically achieved in terms of the MDGs by 2015? What would women's lives and their health status be in 2015? While no one has a crystal ball to accurately predict how the world will be in the next eight years, it is not difficult to identify what has worked, what continues to work, and what is likely to work in the future and support those practices.

Global challenges call for global partnership, commitment, and action. "The world now has the wealth, the expertise, and the technology to lift millions of people out of poverty and give them the decent life they deserve, free from hunger, ignorance, and poor health."[27]

Is there a will to share wealth, expertise, technology, and power with those who need them most and likely to benefit the most? Is there a societal and national commitment to treat girls and women as equal partners and include them in every aspect of development? Will men work with women to ensure gender equality and facilitate empowerment of women?

If the answers to the questions are a resounding yes, then the future is certainly bright for girls and women in this century, and the MDGs are indeed achievable by 2015. After all, history will judge us not by our thoughts and plans, but by our deeds.

Conclusion

This chapter began with an overview of how health (and education) became framed as human rights. The applicability and need to make such inalienable rights available to all human beings, irrespective of gender, national origin, or any other factor, were addressed next. Why women's health and education need special attention was then raised and answered. An overview of major events in recent history that framed and reaffirmed women's health and education as human rights was discussed next. The long road from the Alma-Ata Declaration in 1978 to the Millennium Declaration in 2000 and how the intervening time period has offered opportunities for enhancing women's health status was explored.

The current status of women's health, as revealed by the Millennium Development Goals Report of 2007, offers a mixed picture. While several of the goals and their related targets have shown remarkable progress, there are several regions and nations that are struggling to make progress on one or more MDGs. These mixed results, almost 30 years after the Alma-Ata Declaration affirming "Health for All by the Year 2000," continue to evince closer scrutiny of policies and programs that are currently in place. They also raise questions about the willingness of nations and their citizens to empower women and accord them equality. The evidence presented throughout the chapter encourages the reader to recognize that women's health is not merely a health issue, but a development issue with far-reaching consequences. When women make progress, the whole nation benefits, and the mark of true progress is when women are able to exercise their fundamental rights in the areas of health, education, and employment.

DISCUSSION QUESTIONS

1. Why should women's health be considered separately from that of men?
2. Why is it necessary to frame women's health as a human rights issue?
3. How would the accomplishment of the MDGs further women's health status?
4. What barriers do you foresee in the accomplishment of the MDGs? Why?
5. Why is it necessary for an intersectoral approach to be adopted and implemented to further women's health status?
6. How can men help women achieve their highest level of health status at different phases of their lives?

REFERENCES

1. United Nations. Universal Declaration of Rights. New York, NY: United Nations; 1998. http://www.un.org/Overview/rights.html. Accessed October 18, 2007.

2. Pan American Health Organization. Primary Health Care: 25 Years of the Alma-Ata Declaration. Washington, DC: Pan American Health Organization. http://www.paho.org/english/dd/pin/almaata25.htm. Accessed October 19, 2007.

3. World Health Organization. Declaration of Alma-Ata. Geneva, Switzerland: World Health Organization; 1978. http://www.who.int/hpr/nph/docs/declaration_almaata.pdf. Accessed October 18, 2007.

4. International Institute for Sustainable Development. Programme of Action of the United Nations International Conference on Population & Development. New York: International Institute for Sustainable Development. http://www.iisd.ca/Cairo/program/p00000.html. Accessed November 2, 2007.

5. United Nations Population Fund. Advancing the Goals of the ICPD and the Millennium Summit. New York: United Nations Population Fund; 1994. http://www.unfpa.org/icpd/. Accessed November 6, 2007.

6. United Nations. Key conference outcomes on women and gender equality. New York: United Nations. http://www.un.org/esa/devagenda/gender.html. Accessed December 14, 2007.

7. United Nations. Report of the World Conference to Review and Appraise the Achievements of the United Nations Decade for Women; Equality, Development and Peace. New York: United Nations; http://www.un.org/esa/gopher-data/conf/fwcw/nfls/nfls.en. Accessed October 19, 2007.

8. United Nations. Report of the Fourth World Congress on Women. Beijing, China; United Nations; 1995. http://www.n.org/esa/gopher-data/conf/fmcw/off/a—20.en. Accessed March 4, 2008.

9. Molyneux M, Razavi S. Beijing Plus 10: An Ambivalent Record on Gender Justice. Geneva, Switzerland: United Nations Research Institute for Social Development; 2006.

10. United Nations Population Fund. Key Actions for the Further Implementation of the Programme of Action of the International Conference on Population and Development. New York: United Nations Populations Fund; 1999. http://www.unfpa.org/upload/lib_pub_file/561_filename_icpd5-key-04reprint_eng.pdf. Accessed January 25, 2008.

11. United Nations. United Nations Millennium Declaration. New York: United Nations; 2000. http://www.unmillenniumproject.org/documents/ares552e.pdf. Accessed November 29, 2007.

12. UN Millennium Project. Goals, targets and indicators. New York: UN Millennium Project; 2002. http://www.unmillenniumproject.org/goals/gti.htm. Accessed November 29, 2007.

13. United Nations. The Millennium Development Goals Report. New York: United Nations; 2007. http://www.un.org/millenniumgoals/pdf/mdg2007.pdf. Accessed November 29, 2007.

14. United Nations. The Millennium Development Goals Report Statistical Annex. New York: United Nations; 2007. http://mdgs.un.org/unsd/mdg/Resources/Static/Data/2007%20Stat%20Annex%20current%20indicators.pdf. Accessed November 29, 2007.

15. Regional Partnership for Maternal Newborn and Child Health. Blantyre Declaration of Commitment to Millennium Development Goals 4 and 5. Blantyre, Malawi: The Health Care Professional Organizations; 2007. http://www.who.int/pmnch/events/2007/20071121_blantyre_declaration.pdf. Accessed April 4, 2008.

16. Grown C, Gupta GR, Pande R. Taking action to improve women's health through gender equality and women's empowerment. *Lancet*. 2005;365:541-543.

17. Skolnik R. *Essentials of Global Health*. Sudbury, MA: Jones and Bartlett; 2008: 147-166.

18. United Nations Population Fund. Investing in People: National Progress in Implementing the ICPD Programme of Action 1994–2004. New York: United Nations Population Fund; 2004.

19. United Nations. Review of the implementation of the Beijing Platform for Action and the Outcome Documents of the Special Session of the General Assembly Entitled Women 2000: Gender Equality, Development and Peace for the Twenty-First Century—Report of the Secretary-General. New York: United Nations; 2005. http://www.un.org/womenwatch/daw/csw/csw49/documents.html Accessed February 6, 2008.

20. United Nations Population Fund. Beijing at Ten: UNFPA's Commitment to the Platform for Action. New York: United Nations Population Fund; 2005.

21. United Nations Population Fund. World Summit Commits to Universal Access to Reproductive Health by 2015. New York: United Nations Population Fund; 2005. http://www.unfpa.org/news/news.cfm?ID=680. Accessed March 6, 2008.

22. United Nations. MDG Info 2007 [database online]. New York: United Nations; 2007. http://www.devinfo.info/mdginfo2007/. Accessed March 28, 2008.

23. United Nations. Millennium Development Goals: 2007 Progress Chart. New York: United Nations; 2007. http://mdgs.un.org/unsd/mdg/Resources/Static/Products/Progress2007/MDG_Report_2007_Progress_Chart_en.pdf. Accessed March 4, 2008.

24. The World Bank. Global Monitoring Report 2007 - Fact Sheet: Progress on the Millennium Development Goals. Washington, DC: World Bank; 2007. http://web.worldbank.org/WBSITE/EXTERNAL/EXTDEC/EXTGLOBALMONITOR/Ex. Accessed March 18, 2008.

25. United Nations. Mixed record on Millennium Development Goals underlines need for sustained push to meet targets, Secretary-General says at General Assembly thematic debate. New York: United Nations; 2008. http://www.un.org/News/Press/docs/2008/sgsm11487.doc.htm. Accessed April 17, 2008.

26. United Nations. Progress towards Millennium Development Goals at risk of being wiped out, warns Deputy Secretary-General in remarks to special meeting on global food crisis. New York: United Nations; 2008. http://www.un.org/News/Press/docs/2008/dsgsm393.doc.htm. Accessed May 28, 2008.

27. United Nations. MDGs by 2015: Recognizing the achievements, addressing the challenges, and getting back on track. New York: United Nations; 2008. http://www.un.org/ga/president/62/ThematicDebates/MDGsStatements/mdgsummary.pdf. Accessed on May 28, 2008.

Conclusion

The fact that women's health and human rights are so interlinked presents us with a double challenge and a double opportunity for success. By reminding us of the interdependence of women's health and human rights, this section attempts to summarize the underlying theme to this book: a stark and concrete reminder that development cannot be enjoyed without respect for human rights.

The education and empowerment of women throughout the world cannot fail to result in a more caring, tolerant, just, and peaceful life for all.

—Aung San Suu Kyi,
Nobel Peace Prize Laureate,
leader of Myanmar's Democracy Movement

The wide range of themes covered in this book highlights the immense challenge of promoting women's health and human rights. Through its various chapters, this publication reminds us of the interlinked nature of women's health and human rights. They constitute mutually reinforcing goals that cannot be achieved in isolation from each other.

As stated from the outset by Dr. Allan Rosenfield, and then confirmed in specific examples throughout this book, the poor status of women's health is a reflection of broader gender inequalities. Just as women are too often denied access to basic education, economic opportunities, and political representation, they are also deprived of their right to health.

A woman's ability to exercise her right to health does not depend solely on the availability and affordability of health facilities and services. Too often, women face an additional barrier to access to health care—discrimination, both within the health system and beyond, in society as a whole. Because women are often faced with gender-insensitive health care, denied the power to make their own decisions, and treated as undervalued members of their communities, they do not receive the health care they need, when they need it. Poverty is an aggravating factor, and women constitute 70% of people living below the poverty line.

Violence against women is the most extreme, yet pervasive, manifestation of unequal power relations between men and women. It is the most common and least punished crime in the world.[1] It ranges from domestic violence to traditional harmful practices, such as female genital mutilation. Women who experience violence suffer from a range of health problems, both physical and psychological, with lasting consequences on their lives, their children, and their families.[2]

Improving women's health requires policy and programmatic interventions that tackle pervasive gender inequalities and affirm women's basic human rights. The failure to realize the rights of women leads not only to high rates of morbidity and mortality but also hinders progress in reducing poverty and advancing social and economic development.

A large part of realizing women's right to health depends on the provision of universal access to reproductive health. Poor reproductive

CHAPTER 42

Conclusion: Promoting a Human Rights-Based Approach to Women's Health

*Purnima Mane, PhD**

Purnima Mane, PhD, Deputy Executive Director (programme) of the United Nations Population Fund, UNFPA, NY is an internationally renowned social scientist whose areas of expertise include gender issues in international health, especially in AIDS. In 2003, she joined the Global Fund to fight AIDS, Tuberculosis, and Malaria as the Chief Fund Portfolio Director, Asia. Purnima has coauthored and edited four books.

* The author is a staff member of the United Nations Population Fund (UNFPA). The views expressed herein are those of the author and do not necessarily reflect the views of UNFPA or the United Nations.

health constitutes the main cause of women's ill health and death worldwide.[3] And beyond its health benefits, reproductive health and rights allow women greater control over their own destinies and gives them opportunities to overcome poverty.

Maternal health is a case in point. As the Special Rapporteur on the Right to Health explains, "There is no single cause of death and disability for men between the ages of 15 and 44 that is close to the magnitude of maternal mortality and morbidity."[4] Every year, half a million women die giving life, and many more suffer irreversible injuries and disabilities. Maternal mortality, an avoidable tragedy, represents the most apparent violation of women's right to life, health, equality, and nondiscrimination.[5]

The international consensus is clear. As several chapters in this book remind us, the right of every person, woman and man, to enjoy the highest attainable standard of health is an inherent human right. The specific rights related to women's health have been articulated in various documents and conferences, including the Convention on the Elimination of All Forms of Discrimination against Women, and the 1994 International Conference on Population and Development (ICPD) in Cairo.

The ICPD Programme of Action marked a major paradigm shift in approaching women's health and human rights as a key aspect of sustainable development. Not only did ICPD form the basis of a more holistic approach to population and development, it also placed human rights, and especially the human rights of women, at the centre of social and economic development.

Cairo represents "the meeting point of demography, development, human rights, and gender equality."[5] The ICPD Programme of Action highlighted the need to overcome "the power relations and gender inequalities at many levels" as they constitute an impediment to women's attainment of "healthy and fulfilling lives."[6]

This acknowledgment was reinforced at the 1995 Fourth World Conference on Women in Beijing and in the Millennium Declaration. The 2005 World Summit confirmed that countries cannot reduce extreme poverty without significant progress toward gender equality and universal access to reproductive health. These various platforms converge in their affirmation of women's human rights and provide an agreed framework for action.

But progress has been slow, in part because of inadequate funding. Recent estimates show that the financial target of US $18.5 billion for the realization of the ICPD Programme of Action will not be sufficient to meet current needs, which have grown dramatically since the target was agreed upon in 1994. The challenge now is to mobilize sufficient resources in all critical components of the population package, especially for family planning.[7]

Renewed attention to global health issues, including women's health, provides a basis for optimism. Governments and international donors are increasing their spending on health. Development assistance for health is estimated to have grown from US $6.8 billion in 2000 to nearly US $17 billion in 2006.[8]

Concurrently, a series of new initiatives have emerged, such as the International Health Partnership, aimed at enhancing coordination and effectiveness of aid in the health sector.[9] The 2007 Women Deliver conference was instrumental in raising awareness for maternal health and so is the 2008 *Countdown to 2015* conference and report, which for the first time featured maternal health issues alongside newborn and child health.[10] These initiatives, their focus on maternal health, and the achievement of the health-related MDGs provide an opportunity to accelerate the improvement of women's health globally.

Beyond a renewed commitment, the additional funding and coordination of efforts that these initiatives provide, as well as the strong emphasis on health systems strengthening and primary health care, hold much potential. To improve women's health and especially maternal health, we need functioning health systems with strong supply chains, well-equipped facilities, staffed with skilled health workers, especially at the primary healthcare level.

Over several decades, we have seen progress in reducing maternal mortality with these proven cost-effective interventions in over 100 countries. Today, only 60 high-maternal mortality countries remain.[11] Successes show that political will and adequate funding, both from domestic and external resources, can have a positive impact on women's health and well-being.

Thirty years have passed since the Declaration of Alma-Ata, which identified primary health care as the key to attaining health for all.[12] The new aid environment, calling for principles of aid harmonization and nationally owned development, provides a strategic opportunity for a more comprehensive sectoral approach that will bring greater progress. To benefit women, it is imperative that efforts to strengthen health systems adopt a gender perspective, including equitable health budgeting with a focus on women. Health systems need not only to be strong, they must be gender sensitive and respond to women's needs.

Much of the work to enable women to claim their right to health must be accomplished through community mobilization and engagement. The international consensus has to be translated into the reality of communities. Concretely, this requires quality community-based outreach programmes that integrate various components, such as nutrition, disease control, emergency preparedness, and sexual and reproductive health, including family planning and HIV prevention, treatment, and care.

But a more complex undertaking is the changing of attitudes and behaviours, especially those dealing with gender relations. Changing mindsets can be more difficult than providing services and requires culturally sensitive approaches, which emphasize partnership with local agents of change.

UNFPA institutionalized such an approach under the leadership of its current executive director, Thoraya Ahmed Obaid. This approach calls for the understanding of cultural dynamics and cultural values, assets, expressions, and power structures. The results have been gratifying, ranging from new laws protecting sexual and reproductive health to increased women's participation and decision making in their communities and greater male engagement.

As Thoraya Obaid explains, "We all know that human rights cannot just be transplanted as external principles into individuals or their communities."[13] Human rights principles must be internalized by each individual, absorbed and expressed in their own ways, and within the positive aspects of their cultural values and beliefs.

Culturally sensitive programming is essential to a human rights-based approach—a necessary paradigm to holistically address both issues of women's health and human rights, especially gender equality. A human rights-based approach requires a shift in thinking away from just satisfying needs to fulfilling human rights.

Improving women's health must be grounded in the principles of human rights and gender equality and equity. Applied in a culturally sensitive manner, human rights principles are more effective in promoting dignity and social justice for clients and providers at the levels of clinical operations, facility management, and national policy.[14]

A human rights-based approach recognizes the role of gender in influencing access to and quality of health care, and promotes the empowerment of women in making their own health-related decisions. In this sense, the improvement of women's knowledge, skills, and attitudes toward their health is key to changing their behaviors and allowing them to make informed choices. This is particularly true for adolescent girls, but also for boys and men who are key partners in improving gender-biased attitudes in their relations, families, and communities. By increasing women's and men's access to information and knowledge, they can better demand and use reproductive health services.

The fact that women's health and human rights are so interlinked reminds us that succeeding in one area is not only likely to bring positive change in the other, it can also influence broader prospects for social and economic development. By reminding us of the interdependence of women's health and human rights, this book contributes to global efforts to promote the empowerment of women and girls, improve public health and reduce poverty. As such, it is a stark and concrete reminder that development cannot be enjoyed without respect for human rights.

REFERENCES

1. Vlachová M, Biason L, eds. *Women in an Insecure World: Violence against Women, Facts, Figures and Analysis.* Geneva, Switzerland: Geneva Center for the Democratic Control of Armed Forces (DCAF); 2005:1-2, 5-6.

2. United Nations. *Ending Violence Against Women—From Words to Action* [study of the Secretary-General]. New York: United Nations; 2006:iii, 58-61.

3. UNFPA. *The Promise of Equality: Gender Equity, Reproductive Health and the MDGs, State of the World Population.* New York: UNFPA; 2005:33-34.

4. United Nations. *Report of the Special Rapporteur on the Right of Everyone to the Enjoyment of the Highest Attainable Standard of Physical and Mental Health.* New York: United Nations; 2007. A/HRC/4/28.

5. Sadik N. To the Summit and Beyond—Gender Equality, Reproductive Health and the MDGs. Presented at: Rafael M. Salas Memorial Lecture, September 29, 2005, United Nations, New York.

6. ICPD Programme of Action, 4. International Conference on Population and Development,(ICPD) Programme of Action, 4.1. http://www.unfpa.org/upload/lib_pub_file/284_filename_globalsurvey.pdf. Accessed December 30, 2008.

7. Report of the Secretary-General. *Flow of financial resources for assisting in the implementation of the Programme of Action of the International Conference on Population and Development, Economic and Social Council, Commission on Population and Development.* Presented at: 41st Session of the United Nations, April 7–11, 2008;14-15.

8. World Bank/International Monetary Fund. *MDGs and the Environment, Agenda for Inclusive and Sustainable Development* [Global Monitoring Report]. Washington, DC: World Bank: 2008:109.

9. International Health Partnership. http://www.who.int/healthsystems/ihp/en/index.html.

10. UNICEF. *Tracking Progress in Maternal, Newborn and Child Survival: The 2008 Report.* UNICEF; 2008.

11. According to *Maternal Mortality in 2005*, estimates developed by WHO, UNICEF, UNFPA, and the World Bank, October 2007. http://www.unfpa.org/upload/lib_pub_file/717_filename_mm2005.pdf. Accessed December 30, 2008.

12. Declaration of Alma-Ata, International Conference on Primary Health Care, Alma-Ata, USSR, September 6–12, 1978.

13. Obaid TA. Opening remarks presented at: Beyond Cairo: Reproductive Rights and Culture; March 8, 2004. Amsterdam, The Netherlands.

14. UNFPA, University of Aberdeen. *Maternal Mortality Update: Delivering into Good Hands.* New York: UNFPA; 2004:10-11.

Index

healthcare providers and, 425–426, 427
HIV/AIDS and, 422, 428, 430, 433
as human right, 422–423, 424–425
bride burning, 14
Brown, Steve, 379

C

calcium intake, 225–226
Cambodia, 42
Cameroon
    emergency contraceptives access in, 240
    immunization in, 315
    sexually transmitted infections in, 503
Canada
    female genital cutting/mutilation in, 464
    legalization of abortion in, 87
    maternal mortality in, 282
    physical activity in, 454
cancers. *See also specific cancers*
    breastfeeding and, 423
    healthcare access to treatment, 260
    incidence, 411
    palliative care for, 411–415
    physical activity and, 451
    tumors, 201–202
Caplan, Arthur, 396
cardiovascular disease (CVD)
    deaths, 161, 179–180
    diabetes and, 177, 179–180, 400
    hormone replacement therapy and, 396
    in older women, 399
    physical activity and, 451
    predictors, 188
    prevention, 164–169, 189
    risk factors, 161–164, 399
    treatment and gender, 162, 180
caregivers, 361, 400, 402, 410
Caribbean nations, 62
cataracts, 384
Catholic Church, 90, 240, 317
Central African Republic, 464
cerebral vein thrombosis (CVT), 200
cervical cancer
    deaths, 267, 271–272, 273, 315, 411
    incidence, 315
    overview of, 268
    prevention and screening, 269–270, 274
    risk factors, 268
Chacon, Carme, 41
child marriages, 14–15, 357, 511–512
childbirth. *See also* maternal mortality
    female genital cutting/mutilation and, 464, 465, 476, 478
    fetal complications, 19, 182–183, 199
    healthcare providers during, 6, 279, 281, 284, 289, 291, 505
    at home, 291
    newborn deaths, 280–281, 423, 430–431

newborns by gender, 13, 99, 108, 111, 509
    postpartum transmission of HIV and, 75–76
    in refugee camps, 40
    terrorism and, 29, 30, 31
    under torture, 78
children. *See also* families; girl children
    abducted into armies, 131
    blind, 390
    brain damaged, 399
    breastfeeding, 422, 423–424, 430–431
    cognitive development of, 32
    culture and desire for, 301
    diabetes prevention in, 183, 187–188
    disabled, 356, 362–363
    effect of toxic agents on, 32–33
    healthcare rights of, 86
    human rights of, 251–252
    human trafficking and, 60, 61, 62, 68
    immunization practices and, 313, 314, 394
    iodine deficiency and, 399
    malaria and, 337
    newborn deaths, 280–281
    older women as caregivers, 402
    overweight and diabetes risk, 182
    palliative care and, 415
    population ratio by gender at birth, 99, 108, 111
    postpartum transmission of HIV and, 75–76
    sanitation and, 443
    sex trafficking and, 62, 67
    street, 17–18
    terrorism and, 31
    torture of families and, 77–78
    Tuskegee Syphilis Study and, 74–75
    in Universal Declaration of Human Rights, 520
    war and, 39, 48, 49, 51–52
    as witnesses of domestic violence, 468
Chile
    abortion in, 242
    maternal mortality in, 282
    women in government, 41
chimutsa mapfiwa, 16
China
    birth rate by gender, 111
    death rate by gender, 102, 104–105
    diabetes in, 178
    diet in, 184
    disabled people in, 379
    employment of women in manufacturing industries, 485
    HIV/AIDS in, 133
    maternal mortality in, 284
    population ratio by gender, 99
    responsibility system of healthcare, 105
    sex selective abortion in, 13, 395
    sex trafficking and, 67
    sexually transmitted infections in, 244
    tuberculosis in, 334
    water availability in, 444
chlamydia, 503
chronic kidney disease, 252–256
civil unrest. *See* war

gender-based violence (GBV) (*Continued*)
  against older women, 402
  prevalence, 3, 6
  sex trafficking and, 63
  as structural violence, 130–131
  Third International Conference on Women (Nairobi) and, 87
  types of, 12
  types of cultural, 16–18
  types of physical, 13–16
  Vienna Declaration and, 88
  WHO definition, 15–16
  against women soldiers, 40
  women's rights as human rights and, 55
  in workplace, 131, 487
gender-based war offenses
  examples of, 37, 38
  international response, 51–52
  rape, 12, 38, 39, 40, 49–50
genetics
  bone health and, 225, 228
  human papillomavirus and, 270
  identification of kidnapped children and, 78
  osteoarthritis and, 229
  tumors and, 201
  Type II diabetes and, 178
Geneva Convention(s), 47–48, 51
genocide
  ethnic cleansing as, 50–51
  rape and, 29
  women's role and recovery from, 41–42
  word coined, 48
gestational diabetes, 179, 183
Ghana
  abortion deaths in, 502
  blindness in, 384–388
  cervical cancer in, 272
  domestic violence in, 502
  female genital cutting/mutilation in, 473–481
  HIV/AIDS in, 504
  malaria in, 338
  sexually transmitted infections in, 503
Gilber, Kathy, 40
girl children
  birth rate compared to boys', 111
  chronic kidney disease and, 252–256
  deaths, 394
  disabled, 357, 358, 362–363, 388–389
  economics and, 103, 510
  education of, 437, 443
  gender-based violence and, 12, 467, 504
  genital cutting/mutilation of, 463, 474, 475
  health status of mother and mental health of, 33
  healthcare of, 13, 109
  HIV exposure, 49
  immunization of, 314, 316–317, 320, 394
  infanticide in China, 105
  malnutrition, 13, 109, 395
  marriage of, 14–15, 357, 511–512
  maternal mortality and treatment of, 501

physical activity and, 456–457
  pregnancy of, 424
  rape of, 78
  restriction of social interactions, 15
  sexually transmitted infections and, 503
  terrorism and, 31–33
  as tobacco marketing targets, 76–77
  as war victims, 48, 495–496
gliomas, 201, 202
Global Alliance for Vaccines and Immunizations (GAVI), 313
global gag rule, 73–74
Global Plan of Action of Workers' Health 2008-2017 (2007), 488
Global Platform for Action (1995), 52
globalization
  development of global conscience, 54–55
  effect on national health systems, 84
  as governance, 117–119, 123–124
  health and, 120–123
  of human trafficking, 61
  moral universalism and, 53
  war and, 496
Goldman, Emma, 97
gonorrhea, 503
government
  budgeting and goals, 439
  democracy as ideal model, 55
  food policies, 184–185
  gender-based violence in penal codes, 55
  health policies of, 13
  response to sexually transmitted infections, 243–244
  women in, 41, 101, 437
Grant, James, 4
Guatemala, 255

H
Haiti
  filariasis in, 341
  HIV/AIDS in, 131, 134, 135–136
Hakena, Helen, 38–39
health
  as human right, 91, 92, 422
  human trafficking and, 63–64
  literacy skills and, 143–144
  local agriculture and, 122–123
  migration and, 183, 341, 386–388, 397–398
  WHO definition of, 9, 422
healthcare
  access in U.S., 145–147, 253, 401
  development assistance for, 536
  gender equity in, defined, 329
  global governance and, 118–119, 124
  informed choice and quality of, 239
  infrastructure destruction during war and, 39
  older women, 403
  postabortion, 505
  during pregnancy, 505–506
  primary, 520–521
  at refugee camps, 386–388
  reproductive, defined, 500

nationalism and ethnic identity, 50–51
nation-states sovereignty, 54, 55
Native Americans
    diabetes and, 179–180
    forced sterilization of, 78, 79
    physical activity and, 454, 455
negative rights, 84–85
neoliberalism (economic), 117
Nepal, 238, 295
neurological disorders
    cysticerosis, 204
    dementia, 208–209
    eclampsia, 200–201
    idiopathic intracranial hypertension, 202
    leishmaniasis, 205
    meningitis, 203–204
    menopause-related memory disorders, 208
    migraine, 197–198
    multiple sclerosis, 206–207
    myasthenia gravis, 207–208
    pregnancy and, 203
    schistosomiasis, 204–205
    seizures and epilepsy, 198–199
    stroke, 199–200
    superior sagittal sinus thrombosis, 200
    systemic lupus erythematosis, 205–206
    tumors, 201–202
ngozi, 16
Nicaragua, 16, 242, 444
Niger, 14, 15
Nigeria
    abortion in, 502
    assault by partners, 16
    cervical cancer in, 273
    chronic kidney disease in, 254
    female genital cutting/mutilation in, 465–466
    leprosy in, 339–340
9/11 attacks
    adolescents and, 33
    pregnancy and birth outcomes and, 29–30, 31
nongovernmental organizations (NGOs)
    first international, 47
    human rights issues and, 54
    program implementation, 53
    sex trafficking and, 67–68
    Western standards imposed by, 53
norm entrepreneurs, 89, 92
norm evolution, 89
North America. *See also specific nations*
    chronic kidney disease in, 252–254, 255
    death rate by gender in, 100
    diabetes demographics, 177–178
    maternity leave in, 428
    population ratio by gender, 99
Nurses' Healthy Study, 166

O

Obaid, Thoraya Ahmed, 537
obesity/overweight
    diabetes and, 182–185

diet and, 184
idiopathic intracranial hypertension and, 202
in India, 453
overview of, 181–182
as positive cultural value, 453
occupational health
    domestic labor as second job, 486–487
    domestic violence and, 487–488
    in large manufacturing industries, 484–485
    musculoskeletal problems, 484–485
    organizational structures for, 483–484
    of professionals, 486
    safety and health regulations, 488–489
    workplace violence, 487
ocytocin, 290–291
older women. *See also* menopause
    abuse of, 402
    common medical conditions in, 398–400
    health challenges faced by, 395–397
    health earlier in life and, 394–395
    malnutrition in, 397–398
    marginalization of, 396
    physical activity and, 456
    social challenges faced by, 400–402
    UN action plan, 403–404
opioids, 413–414
osteoarthritis, 399. *See also* arthritis
osteoporosis, 224–229, 398–399
overweight. *See* obesity/overweight

P

Pakistan, 178, 335
Palermo protocol. *See* Protocol to Prevent, Suppress, and
    Punish Trafficking in Persons, Especially Women and
    Children (United Nations)
palliative care
    components, 411
    curative care relationship to, 411–413
    as human right, 414
    pain relief, 413–414
    for vulnerable populations, 415
Panama, 68, 240
Papanicolaou Test (PAP Test), 269, 275, 315
parasitic diseases, 204, 341–342
Partners in Health, 135
peace building
    action by women's groups, 38–39, 42
    culture of, 496–497
    empowerment of women and, 37
    women ignored in, 495
pelvic inflammatory disease, 20
Penchaszadeh, Victor, 78
People's Health Movement (PHM), 124, 437–440
personal autonomy, 83, 84, 87
Peru, 16, 239
pesticides, 254–255
Philippines, 335, 442
physical activity
    barriers to, 452–455
    benefits of, 451

war. (*Continued*)
   gender-specific signs of impending, 39
   human rights' risks and, 56
   for humanitarian purposes, 54
   infrastructure destruction during, 39
   legal instruments protecting women and children, 39, 51–52
   population displacement, 40, 48–49
   post conflict violence, 40–41
   poverty and, 495, 496
   prevalence, 37
   rape, 12, 38, 39, 40, 49–50, 52, 131
   spoils of war justification, 50
   women as combatants, 40
   women as victims, 48, 495–496
Ward, Jeanne, 53
Warrior's Honor, The (Ignatieff), 53
waste water, 446
water
   availability, 441–442, 444–445
   conservation, 446
   costs, 442, 443
   needs, 441
   sanitation and, 442–443
   shortages, 446
   treatment, 445–446
weapons of mass destruction (WMDs), 32–33
weight. *See also* obesity/overweight
   adolescent girls and, 226
   body mass index, 182, 184
   bone health and, 225
   culture and, 453
   diabetes and, 181–185
   diet and, 184
   idiopathic intracranial hypertension and, 202
   perceptions of health and, 456
widows, 15, 16, 402
wife battering. *See* domestic violence
Wolf, Margery, 105

Wolferson, James, 355
Women's Health Initiative (WHI), 165–166, 168, 169
Working Group on Women, Peace, and Security, 38
World Bank
   campaign to reduce maternal deaths, 5
   disabled people and, 355, 363
   forced sterilization and, 79
   multitiered health system approach of, 119, 123
World Conference on Education for All (1990), 371
World Health Organization (WHO)
   abortion and, 243
   adolescence, definition of, 241
   cancer research and, 263
   diabetes and, 190
   female genital cutting/mutilation, definition of, 463
   health, definition of, 9, 422
   immunization and, 313
   malaria and, 337
   maternal and child health programs, 4
   maternal mortality and, 5
   obesity, definition of, 182
   palliative care and, 411, 413–414
   primary healthcare approach, 120
   reproductive rights and, 239
   sexual violence, definition of, 15–16
   tuberculosis and, 331, 332, 334, 335
   water needs and, 441, 442
World Summit (2005), 524
World Trade Organization, 122–123

Y
Young People of Paradise, 31
Yugoslavia (former), 50, 52

Z
Zaire, 464, 502
Zambia, 239
Zapatero, Jose Luis Rodriguez, 41
Zimbabwe, 16